BINOCULAR ANOMALIES

Procedures for Vision Therapy

BINOCULAR ANOMALIES

Procedures for Vision Therapy

2nd Edition

John R. Griffin
B.S., M.Opt., O.D., M.S.Ed., F.A.A.O.

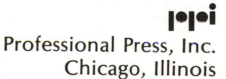

Professional Press, Inc.
Chicago, Illinois

© 1976, 1982 by Professional Press, Inc.

FIRST PRINTING
2nd Edition
ISBN-0-87873-036-2

Library of Congress Catalog Card Number: 82-061252

Published by Professional Press, Inc.
Chicago, Illinois 60603

Printed in the U.S.A.

Dedicated to
ANGELA, LISA, AND SCOTT

Acknowledgments

I wish to thank Richard Hawkins and his word processing staff for their many, many hours spent in typing and preparing the original manuscript of this book. I am grateful to Dr. Phillip Hanson and Richard Morrison for their help with photography; to Robert Tarr, Alan Lee, and the graphic arts staff of the Professional Press for their assistance with illustrations; and to Drs. Jeffrey Jacob, James Bailey, Patrick Stibel, Merrill Allen, James Saladin, James Sheedy, David Kirschen, and Kenneth Brookman for their suggestions, contributions, and assistance. Companies contributing in this regard include Allied Ophthalmic Products Co.; Bernell Corp.; Clement Clarke; Keeler Optical Products, Inc.; Lafayette Instrument Co.; Keystone View, Division of Mast/Keystone; and Wayne Engineering.

· I am also indebted to those members of the faculty of the Southern California College of Optometry who volunteered their time to review material in the manuscript, and to the administration of the Southern California College of Optometry for providing support.

William Topaz and the editorial staff of the Professional Press deserve special acknowledgment for their helpful suggestions. The Professional Press also made available to me editorial help, for which I am grateful. Peter Topaz was inspirational in my beginning this text.

I wish to express my gratitude to members of my family who have shown loving patience during my many months of writing.

Preface

The first edition of this text was written in response to practitioners and students of binocular vision who had expressed their desire for a practical text on the management of binocular anomalies. They asked for a book that outlines the efficient steps toward treatment of these problems. Acceptance has been worldwide.

There have been many developments in vision therapy since the publication of the first edition. Consequently, in this second edition, there are substantial additions to Part Two, which pertains to treatment. The increasing emphasis on therapy for efficient visual skills has necessitated the inclusion of detailed discussions on saccadic and pursuit eye movements, accommodation, and vergence efficiency and strabismus. New considerations are presented, including such topics as learning theories applied to vision therapy and methods in amblyopia.

The Appendix has been expanded to illustrate new clinical forms, consultants' letters, case reports describing therapeutic regimens, and other reference material. The principal addition is a self-assessment test of 100 questions with answers. This test covers the range—in breadth, but not in depth—of this volume. It is intended to serve as an "organizer" for both the student and the practitioner. It may act as a catalyst for students to find out what they do or do not know. Certain perplexing questions may cause students to read the various chapters for related discussion. In doing so, serendipitous knowledge may be gained by "discovery learning." However, the format is intended for reading cover to cover, the usefulness of selective referencing notwithstanding.

Most of the figures and tables of the first edition have been retained, but many new ones have been added. These illustrations and outlines provide a learning opportunity for the student, as well as serving as a reference source for the busy practitioner who may want to look up a particular training sequence, stereoacuity values, and so forth.

Visual scientists and allied professionals may also find this book useful for reference purposes. Nevertheless, I have elected to keep this a clinical textbook relating to evaluation and treatment of abnormal binocular vision rather than a laboratorylike treatise on the physiological optics of normal binocular vision. Other volumes, journals, and college courses serve this need. Likewise, a theoretical discussion on the etiologies of binocular anomalies could comprise an entire book in itself. Many books and journals are available to provide this background information. The references supply a selection of these.

Authorities generally believe that the etiologies of both heterotropia and heterophoria are similar, whether they be innervational, accommodative, sensorial, mechanical, or psychogenic. In most cases, however, the authorities cannot agree on the factors or combination of factors that are responsible. Ultimately, it is the practitioner who must judge the possible etiology of each patient's problem and provide the proper therapy.

Universal agreement does not exist as to whether a motor deviation causes the resultant sensory problems or whether sensory problems are responsible for the motor problems. In order to avoid an endless discussion of which came first, it is probably wise to consider that there may be many possible etiologies, and, therefore, both theories could be correct. Some cases may appear to have been caused by a clearly explainable motor problem, like a paresis of an extraocular muscle. Usually, though, it is difficult to rule in only one cause, or to definitely rule out other possibilities. Although the sensory and motor elements of binocular vision are ordinarily inseparable, I have elected to take the view that when a motor problem arises, it may cause sensory anomalies to follow, such as suppression, amblyopia, anomalous correspondence, and so forth. This approach facilitates instruction.

The second edition is in accord with the first in that the material presented streamlines that vast subject of testing and treating problems of binocular vision. Only necessary theoretical discussions are included. To the extent possible, sequences of testing procedures emphasize the determination of functional problems rather than dwelling upon particular instrumentation; only those procedures requiring standard, currently available instrumentation are discussed. Treatment procedures relate closely to testing procedures in that terminology, symbols, and illustrations are consistently used. In this way, treatment follows testing in a systematic order.

The overall plan of this book is to discuss testing, diagnosis and prognosis, and then treatment, with the emphasis placed on effective procedures to achieve functional cure of amblyopia and strabismus, and efficiency of saccades, pursuits, accommodation, vergences, and sensory fusion. The uses of occlusion, lenses, and prisms in evaluation and therapy are included, but the emphasis is on the utilization of functional training procedures for achieving successful results in vision therapy.

For the sake of brevity throughout this volume, and for this reason alone, the "he/she" designation has been shortened to one gender to promote easier reading. To ensure that frequently used terms and abbreviations are defined, a glossary has been included.

John R. Griffin
Fullerton, California

Table of Contents

Part One - Evaluation

BINOCULAR ANOMALIES

Procedures for Vision Therapy

PART ONE

EVALUATION

1 | Diagnosis of a Deviation of the Visual Axes

When the status of a patient's binocularity is evaluated, the first step is to make a diagnosis of the deviation. Before this can be done, certain diagnostic variables must be determined. There are nine of these, and they are: concomitancy, frequency, direction, magnitude, AC/A ratio, variability, cosmesis, eye laterality, and eye dominancy.

All deviations are classified as being either concomitant or nonconcomitant. Concomitancy means that the angle of deviation of the visual axes remains the same throughout all positions of gaze. This implies there are neither abnormal underactions nor overactions of any of the 12 extraocular muscles controlling eye movements. On the other hand, in nonconcomitancy the deviation changes when the eyes move from one position of gaze to another. Thus, there is either abnormal restriction to movement or overaction of one or more of the extraocular muscles.

Concomitancy of the Deviation

The causes of underaction of extraocular muscles are many. However, in most cases, underactions are the result of one of three basic reasons and may be either congenitally caused or have been acquired. First, the muscles themselves may be paretic as in cases of direct traumatic injury to the lateral rectus muscle. In other instances, mechanical reasons such as faulty muscle insertion and ligament abnormalities may restrict ocular motility. Last and most frequently, the extraocular muscle paresis responsible for underactions is caused by innervational deficiencies due to impairment of the cranial nerves (3rd, 4th, and 6th) which innervate the muscles. Nerve impairment is thought by Hugonnier[1] to be most commonly attributable to vascular problems, such as hemorrhages, aneurysms, and embolisms. Infectious diseases which affect the central nervous system also are frequent causes and should be suspected, particularly in young patients.

Overactions may be due to mechanical reasons; for example, faulty muscle insertion giving mechanical advantage to a particular muscle. More often, however, the overaction can be explained by Hering's law of equal innervation to two yoked muscles. This law states that the contralateral synergists are equally innervated when a movement is executed by both eyes. An example of Hering's law explaining an overaction is given in the following case. Suppose the right lateral rectus is paretic and requires an abnormally high level of innervation to rotate the right eye in a temporal movement. This same high level of innervation will be sent to the left medial rectus, the yoke muscle of the right lateral rectus. This causes an overaction of the left medial rectus, assuming that it normally takes less neural innervation to rotate the left eye. This type of spasticity exacerbates further an eso deviation caused by the paretic lateral rectus. If this continues for many months, a permanent state of contracture may result whereby the tissues of the medial rectus muscle may become fibrotic. The muscle becomes nonelastic, and the prognosis for a cure of the eso deviation becomes poor.

The right medial rectus would also become spastic as a result of the paresis of the homolateral antagonist. This may lead to contracture and may be as serious as that caused by the yoking action involving the contralateral synergist. Precautions and therapy in these situations will be discussed in Chapter Eleven.

Table 1A lists the six pairs of yoke muscles; Table 1B lists the three pairs of homolateral antagonists of an eye.

TABLE 1A. *List of the Six Pairs of Contralateral Synergists*

Right Lateral Rectus	and	Left Medial Rectus
Right Medial Rectus	and	Left Lateral Rectus
Right Superior Rectus	and	Left Inferior Oblique
Right Inferior Oblique	and	Left Superior Rectus
Right Superior Oblique	and	Left Inferior Rectus
Right Inferior Rectus	and	Left Superior Oblique

TABLE 1B. *List of the Homolateral Antagonists of an Eye*

Medial Rectus	and	Lateral Rectus
Superior Rectus	and	Inferior Rectus
Superior Oblique	and	Inferior Oblique

Few individuals have perfect concomitancy in the strictest sense, if the term is used to mean that the angle of deviation remains the same throughout all positions of gaze. The frequent lack of perfect concomitancy results because deviation for most people varies slightly from one direction of gaze to another. Therefore, some allowance should be made so that the term "nonconcomitancy" is not overused leading to misinterpretation of its meaning. For practical purposes, the amount of change of deviation allowable is five prism diopters, thus allowing for the deviation to be classified as concomitant. If the change in deviation in various gazes is greater than five prism diopters, the deviation is considered to be nonconcomitant. I have found it best to identify the severity of non-concomitancy by applying the following qualifications:

Mild	6 to 10 p.d. change in deviation
Moderate	11 to 15 p.d. change in deviation
Marked	16 p.d. or more change in deviation

It is important to remember that not all nonconcomitancies are pareses (paralyses). Paresis is an etiological term whereas nonconcomitancy is a descriptive term. Unless there is absolute sureness of the etiology, it is wise to avoid using the word "paresis" or synonymous terms such as "palsy" or "paralysis." A nonconcomitancy could be due to a mechanical restriction. Therefore, when there is uncertainty as to the etiology, it is best to state the condition as nonconcomitant, or to use synonymous terms such as "incomitant" and "noncomitant."

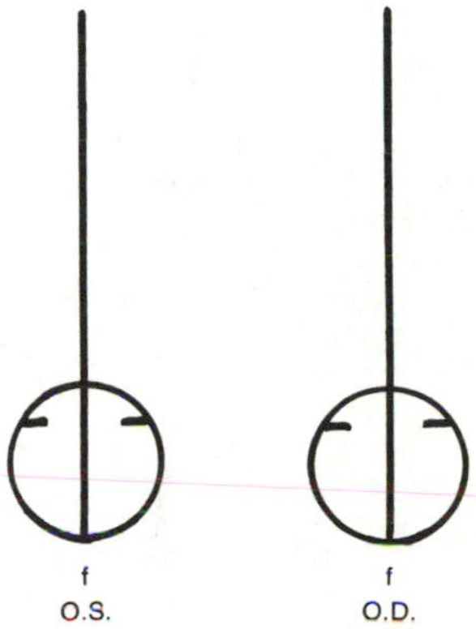

The term "paresis" is used in this text rather than paralysis. Although these are used synonymously in the literature, paralysis seemingly denotes total loss of function to many people. However, the complete loss of function may not always be the case. If there is total loss of muscle function due to a nerve lesion, paralysis is the appropriate term. This may also be called complete paresis. As a rule, when in doubt as to the totality of loss of function, paresis is probably the best term to use.

In testing for nonconcomitancy, it is important to know the relationship of the visual axis of one eye to that of the other. If the axes are parallel, the eyes are postured in the ortho position. Figure 1-1 shows an example of this state of parallelism with the eyes being in the primary position of gaze. Similarly, Figure 1-2 shows the eyes in the ortho posture in the secondary position of gaze of dextroversion. Each eye makes an equal movement so that the ortho posture is maintained.[a]

Another helpful way of illustrating eye posture is by showing a confrontation view. The position of the eyes as represented by Figure 1-2 is the same as that shown by Figure 1-4d. This depicts the patient's eyes as seen by the examiner.

To illustrate a deviation, Figure 1-3a shows the eyes not in the ortho

FIGURE 1-1 — Eyes in the ortho posture. Letter "f" indicates the position of the fovea. The solid line is the visual axis.

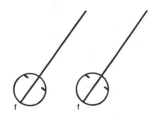

FIGURE 1-2 — Equal movement of each eye from the primary position to the secondary position of dextroversion

[a]Schematic drawings such as in these illustrations depict coronal sections of the eyes as seen from above. Unless nearpoint fixation is involved, the target of regard is assumed to be at optical infinity. Parallel lines meet at infinity; therefore, the visual axes can be drawn parallel to each other without necessitating showing a fixation target. This method of illustration helps in the visualization and explanation of the horizontal posture of the eyes. This is particularly applicable when complicated conditions such as anomalous correspondence are involved.

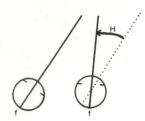

FIGURE 1-3a — Eso deviation of the right eye due to lag of abduction. Letter "H" represents the horizontal objective angle of deviation.

posture. The right eye is lagging. Therefore, the left eye is making a nasal movement (adduction) larger than the temporal movement (abduction) of the right. Assuming the left eye is the fixating eye, this results in an eso deviation of the right eye. This same deviation is also shown in Figure 1-3b.

Observation of such a manifest deviation is easily accomplished by confronting the patient and looking for a tropia of one eye. This method of evaluating a strabismus may be refined considerably by using the Hirschberg test (to be discussed later).

An indication of concomitancy is shown in Figure 1-2. Both eyes rotate an equal amount. The angle of deviation (zero in this example) remains the same as the eyes move from the primary position to a secondary position of gaze. However, concomitancy cannot be definitely established until all nine diagnostic positions of gaze are tested. In this example, only two positions were tested. This is not sufficient for arriving at any conclusion regarding concomitancy versus nonconcomitancy. All nine diagnostic positions of gaze must be evaluated. These are illustrated in Figure 1-4, and are examples of versions (binocular conjugate movements).[b]

OBJECTIVE TESTING PROCEDURES

Objective testing has advantages over subjective procedures because very little cooperation is required on the part of the patient. This is especially important when evaluating infants and toddlers. Findings are made objectively by the examiner, thereby eliminating the necessity of subjective interpretation by him.

THE COVER TEST

O.D.   O.S.

FIGURE 1-3b — Esotropia of the right eye on dextroversion due to a lag of abduction of the eye. Left eye is fixating.

This is probably the most informative single test of all that have been devised for investigation of anomalies of binocular vision. It is especially important for nonconcomitancy testing in cases where only a heterophoric condition exists. Whereas direct observation of the patient is useful if there is a manifest deviation (strabismus), there is no reliability in the investigation of nonconcomitancy for those cases where the deviation remains latent. In the example illustrated in Figure 1-3a, if the patient were esophoric rather than esotropic on dextroversion, the examiner could not observe the change in the angle of deviation. The appearance would be the same as shown in Figure 1-4d, and not like that in Figure 1-3b. To determine if there is a change in the deviation from one gaze to another, the examiner must dissociate the eyes to remove fusion. A strong power of fusion may keep a deviation hidden, as in this example of esophoria. To accomplish this in the most effective way, one eye is completely occluded by means of the cover test.

THE UNILATERAL COVER TEST

This form of the cover test, also referred to as the cover-uncover test, consists merely of holding an opaque occluder before one eye and watching for any movement by either eye. This has been traditionally performed in the patient's primary position of gaze. For nonconcomitancy detection,

[b]Versions should not be confused with "ductions" which are monocular movements.

however, this test should be done in the secondary and tertiary positions as well. Refer to Figure 1-4 showing these positions of gaze.

The recommended procedure for doing the unilateral cover test is best explained by a case example which discusses testing in the secondary position of dextroversion. The case illustrated in Figure 1-3 lends itself to this. The right eye on gaze right is seen to be esotropic. Therefore, if it is occluded, there will be no movement of either eye because the right eye is the deviating and not the fixating eye. After a few seconds the cover is removed, and as before, no movement is observed. This is because in the beginning, the right eye had not been fixating; therefore, a fusional recovery movement is not made.

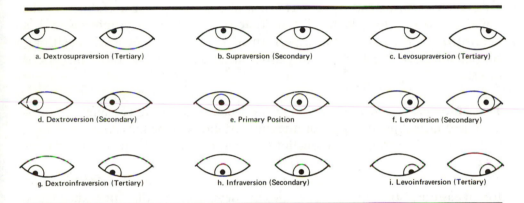

FIGURE 1-4 — The nine diagnostic positions of gaze for conjugate eye movements, with secondary and tertiary positions indicated

The occluder is next placed in front of the fixating left eye. Immediately, the right eye must move temporally to take up fixation. Its fovea is directed to the fixation target, assuming that normal fixation is present in the right eye and abduction is not seriously restricted.

When the right eye moves to fixate, the left eye, under cover, also makes a conjugate movement. This "version" movement confirms the presence of a strabismus in this position of gaze. The other eight positions of gaze should similarly be tested with the unilateral cover test to determine whether or not a strabismus is present in any of these directions.

If in this same example, a heterophoria rather than a strabismus is present, the examiner will observe the following disjunctive movements during the unilateral cover test. Upon occluding the right eye and looking around the occluder at the eye, the examiner will note the eye making a

[c]Occasionally, the uncovered eye may be noted to jump slightly as the other eye is covered. This is thought to be due to the movement of the covered eye which somehow sets off a simultaneous flick in the same direction as the movement of the covered eye. This is common in heterophoria of large magnitude. In such cases the fixating eye flicks back to the original position. If the fixating eye flicks in one direction, but does not fully return in the other direction to put the eye in the fixating position, the presence of a small angle strabismus is indicated.

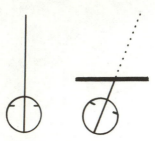

FIGURE 1-5a — Occluder is placed in front of right eye. The deviation is 20 p.d. exo.

movement nasally; however, the left eye remains stationary.[c] When the cover is removed, the right eye makes a movement temporally to retain foveal bifixation (fusion). This refusion process follows the short period of dissociation created by the occluder. Covering the left eye gives the same response as occlusion of the right eye; that is, it moves inward behind the occluder while the right eye remains stationary. When uncovered, it moves outward to regain fusion. This is an example of an esophoric deviation. An exophoric deviation gives similar responses on the unilateral cover test except the movements are in the opposite directions.

The main distinction seen between a tropia and phoria is that the unilateral cover test creates a conjugate movement when a tropia is present and a disjunctive movement in the event of a phoria. The chief usefulness of the unilateral cover test is to differentiate between a heterophoria and a heterotropia. When this test is performed in the nine diagnostic positions, the examiner is able to make this differential diagnosis for those directions of gaze.

THE ALTERNATE
COVER TEST

This procedure is often referred to as the Duane cover test. The angle of deviation and the subjective angle of directionalization can be measured, making it very useful in testing for anomalous correspondence (discussed in Chapter Two).

The concern with the alternate cover test in this chapter is its utilization for measuring the objective angle of deviation in the nine diagnostic positions of gaze. This is useful in concomitancy testing and is not invalidated by the presence of anomalous correspondence, as subjective measurements might be. It also has the advantage over many other extraocular muscle tests in that very little cooperation is required by the patient.

The alternate cover test is performed by alternately occluding one eye and then the other while watching for any conjugate movement. This indicates a deviation; and the greater the conjugate movement, the greater the deviation.

FIGURE 1-5b — Right eye is covered. Deviation is observed behind the occluder.

Since only one eye is fixating at any given moment, the eyes are continuously in a state of dissociation. Fusion is not possible. The examiner has no way of determining whether the movement observed during alternate occlusion is due to a heterophoria or to a heterotropia, because fusion no longer acts to conceal a deviation that may be latent. Consequently, the alternate cover test is not very useful in making a differential diagnosis between a strabismus and a heterophoria. This distinction is best made with the unilateral cover test.

The alternate cover test is far superior to the unilateral cover test for differentiating between concomitancy and nonconcomitancy. This is because the angle can be accurately measured in any of the diagnostic positions of gaze. Any changes in deviation indicate nonconcomitancy.

The procedure for performing the alternate cover test is explained by using a case example (see Figure 1-5a). The patient has 20 p.d. of exo deviation (either exotropia or exophoria) at far. There is a paresis of the right medial rectus which is responsible to some extent for the exo deviation. While the examiner occludes the right eye, the patient is instructed to look at the distant fixation target with the left eye. If an exophoria is present, the right eye is seen abducting soon after the eye is occluded. The eye goes out to the position of deviation (illustrated in Figure 1-5b).

After initial occlusion, the examiner moves the occluder to the left eye (Figure 1-6a). The movement of each eye, particularly the right eye which was just uncovered, is observed (see Figure 1-6b). The magnitude of rotational movement of the right eye as it is uncovered is estimated. This may be noted in degrees or in prism diopters.[d]

The occluder is now returned to the right eye and a loose measuring prism is placed, base-in, between the eye and the occluder (see Figure 1-7). If the prism power is the same as the angle of deviation, no movement is required by the right eye when the cover is moved to the left eye (see Figure 1-8). In this case of nonconcomitancy there is some abduction of the left eye because the right eye has become the fixating eye (secondary angle of deviation). This probably will be small since the right eye is in the resting position and very little contraction is required by the right medial rectus. Hering's law still applies but not to the extent that it does when the right eye is in the primary position. Since the deviation is neutralized with prism, a conjugate movement is not present.

Movement would not be observed in either eye if this were a concomitant deviation without paresis being neutralized by prism.

The same procedure is followed to measure the secondary deviation, except that the occluder and prism are placed in front of the left eye rather than the right. The paretic right eye becomes the fixating eye, making the exo deviation larger because of the secondary deviation. The occluder is then moved quickly to the right eye, and the movement of the left eye is observed. The procedure is followed until subsequent neutralization is achieved by means of an appropriate prism.

For the above testing, several trials using various powers of prisms may be required before complete neutralization of eye movements can be achieved. The technique of bracketing is often helpful in determining the magnitude of a deviation. In the case of an exo deviation not fully compensated by prism, the movements will be in the same direction as the movement of the occluder. If a power of prism greater than that required for neutralization is used, the movements will show an against motion. The examiner looks for the just noticeable with-motion and the just noticeable against-motion. The mean value of prismatic power that induces these two different motions can be considered to be the angle of deviation. The

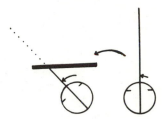

FIGURE 1-6a — Occluder is moved from the right to the left eye. Right eye moves nasally, and left eye moves temporally. Note larger movement of left eye due to paresis of right medial rectus.

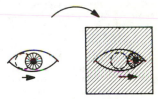

FIGURE 1-6b — Cover is moved from the right to the left eye. The magnitude of movement of the right eye is estimated. This is the primary angle of deviation since the non-paretic eye had been fixating.

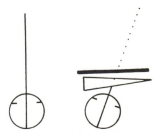

FIGURE 1-7 — Occluder is returned to the right eye. Behind it is placed a base-in prism of 20 p.d.

[d] It is preferable to use prism diopters rather than degrees since measuring prisms (in prism diopters) are used to determine the magnitude of the angle.

technique of bracketing is useful also in measuring eso and hyper deviations.

The alternate cover test has been illustrated when the eyes are in the primary position of gaze. This test should be performed similarly in the other eight diagnostic positions of gaze. To accomplish this, the fixation target must be placed in these various positions. This can be effected by two different methods. One is by keeping the target stationary and moving the patient's head in a doll-like fashion. This simulates the target having been placed in the various directions. A less convenient way is keeping the patient's head stationary and changing the position of the target in space. I generally prefer the latter method for initial concomitancy testing. Vestibular reflexes are not brought into play to the extent they would be if the head were moved. Since these reflexes can affect eye movement and eye posture, in crucial cases, some doubt could possibly arise as to the validity of concomitancy testing.

The illustrations presented have shown the fixation target to be at infinity. This is not meant to imply that concomitancy testing is limited to far vision. Any convenient fixation distance may be used as long as it is kept constant. If the distance changes, there may be accommodative changes which can cause the angle of deviation to vary because of the influence of accommodative convergence.

The possibility of this extraneous factor makes it preferable to perform concomitancy tests at optical infinity. This eliminates the demand on accommodation that would ordinarily be present for nearpoint testing. It should be remembered, however, that if a patient is nonconcomitant at one fixation distance, he is the same at any other distance, as the state of concomitancy does not depend on nearness or farness.

Alternate cover testing in different positions of gaze is often more conveniently done at near than at far. This is acceptable as long as the caveat of accommodation control is heeded.

One other precaution should be taken into account. In cases where anisometropic spectacle lenses of relatively high power are worn, the examiner should allow for any induced prismatic effect. Since concomitancy testing is done in the secondary and tertiary positions, as well as in the primary position, measurements made by the alternate cover test may vary. This is the result of variance of prismatic effect in the different positions. If the patient wears contact lenses, this vagary of testing can be removed.

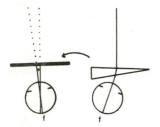

FIGURE 1-8 — Occluder is moved from the right to the left eye. No eye movement is required by the right eye because the fixation target is optically placed on the fovea by the compensating prism. This is the measurement of the primary deviation. The left eye may abduct a small amount behind the cover after the paretic right eye begins fixation.

PRIMARY AND SECONDARY DEVIATIONS

Measurements of the primary and secondary deviations are customarily made in the straight-ahead gaze (primary position), using the alternate cover test with prisms. The magnitude of one angle is compared with the magnitude of the other. If a patient has a paretic muscle in one eye but not the other, the primary angle of deviation is the angle measured when the nonparetic eye fixates. The secondary angle is the angle measured when the paretic eye fixates.

The literature often obfuscates the true meaning of the secondary angle by stating that it is the angle measured when the nondominant eye (or the deviating eye in strabismus) is fixating. This can be misleading, since the nondominant eye may be the nonparetic eye, and the dominant eye the affected one. Under these circumstances, the primary angle is the one measured when the nondominant eye is used for fixation. For this reason, I prefer to reserve the use of the terms primary and secondary to concomitancy rather than commingling these two separate issues. Dominancy is discussed later in this chapter.

As explained by Hering's law of equal innervation to two yoked muscles, the angle of deviation is greater when the paretic eye fixates than when the nonparetic eye is fixating. This is therefore true for either an eso or an exo deviation. To a certain extent, the same rule applies for hyper and cyclo deviations. For clarification, refer to Figures 1-5 and 1-6 illustrating a patient having a paresis of the right medial rectus with an exo deviation. If the deviation is 20 p.d. when the left, nonparetic eye fixates, it will be greater, perhaps 30 or more, when the right, paretic eye fixates. This difference results because, in the secondary deviation, the yoke muscle of the paretic right medial rectus is innervated in excess of normal. This yoke muscle, the left lateral rectus, abducts the left eye and thereby further increases the existing exo deviation.

It should be noted that differences between the primary and secondary deviations may be due to nonconcomitancies caused by other reasons than paresis. A faulty muscle insertion may test positive in this regard. However, this is usually much less remarkable than when a paretic muscle is involved. The disparity is even greater in the case of a newly-acquired paresis than in one of long duration.

If there is a significant difference (of greater than five prism diopters) between the primary and secondary angles, a nonconcomitancy should be suspected. Although a lack of difference would indicate concomitancy, this is not always the case. Some mild nonconcomitancies (usually with other than nerve impairment etiology) may not produce a large enough difference in the deviations to be significant. Even paretic cases with nerve impairment may show a false negative when they are of long duration.

In summary, negative findings may or may not be indications of concomitancy; positive findings tend to be true indications of noncon- comitancy.

It is important that the patient wear his farpoint ophthalmic lenses for any refractive errors; otherwise, a case of uncorrected anisometropia could result in unequal accommodative responses. This could produce a false positive finding of nonconcomitancy.

THE THREE-STEP METHOD

This was introduced by Parks[2] and is useful for identifying an isolated paretic cyclovertical muscle. There are eight of these extraocular muscles. They are ordinarily more difficult to analyze than the four horizontally acting recti. This is especially true if the aid of a systematic approach, such as the three-step method, is not utilized. Refer to Table 1C which shows the three steps required to determine when one of the eight muscles is affected in any particular case.

TABLE 1C. The Three-Step Method			
Hyper eye in primary position	Hyper greater on gaze	Hyper greatest on head tilt	Paretic Muscle
R	R	R	LIO
R	R	L	RIR
R	L	R	RSO
R	L	L	LSR
L	R	R	RSR
L	R	L	LSO
L	L	R	LIR
L	L	L	RIO

This method is best explained by testing a known affected muscle and then proceeding through the diagnostic steps. Suppose the patient has a paresis of the right superior oblique. This muscle normally has an action of infraduction and is an intorter as well. In the primary position the superior oblique has a slight action of abduction, but this can be considered negligible for purposes of the discussion here. Now if the patient fixates in the primary position of gaze, the right eye is likely to have a small degree of hyper deviation. This could be either hypertropia or hyperphoria depending on the results of the unilateral cover test. The magnitude of the hyper deviation of the right eye is measured by employing the alternate cover test together with base-down prism in front of the right eye. The likelihood of a right hyper deviation occurring is because the usual depressing action afforded by the superior oblique is relatively weakened due to the paresis.

The first column of Table 1C lists hyper deviations for either the right or left eye. The fourth column gives the answers by listing the eight muscles. When there is a right hyper deviation, any of three other muscles besides the superior oblique may be involved. They are: the left inferior oblique, the right inferior rectus, and the left superior rectus. A paretic left inferior oblique could cause a hyper deviation because its yoke muscle, the right superior rectus, receives excessive innervation (Hering's law). The same reasoning applies to a paretic left superior rectus with the yoke muscle being the right inferior oblique (an elevator). If there is a paresis of the right inferior rectus, the homolateral antagonist, the superior rectus, overacts to cause a right hyper deviation.

The number of four possibilities can be narrowed to two by having the patient fixate in two lateral positions of gaze approximately 30 degrees each way. On dextroversion, the amount of the hyper deviation is measured with the alternate cover test and base-down prism. The same procedure is performed on levoversion. If the right hyper increases on left gaze, the affected muscle should be either the right superior oblique or the left superior rectus because both muscles have an isolated vertical action on left gaze (refer to Table 1D). The vertical component of the deviation is taken into account in the three-step method.

TABLE 1D. Lateral Eye Positions for Isolated Vertical Action		
Superior Rectus	—	Supraduction only (with abduction of 23 degrees)
Inferior Rectus	—	Infraduction only (with abduction of 23 degrees)
Superior Oblique	—	Infraduction only (with adduction of 51 degrees)
Inferior Oblique	—	Supraduction only (with adduction of 51 degrees)

Theoretically, the right superior oblique becomes a pure depressor only when the right eye is adducted 51 degrees, and the left superior rectus, a pure elevator, only when the left eye is abducted 23 degrees. For clinical purposes, however, 30 degrees for each direction is a satisfactory and workable compromise. To know which of the two muscles is affected, the Bielschowsky head tilt test must be performed. Refer to Figure 1-9. The patient is instructed to tilt his head about 40 degrees toward his right shoulder. The same procedure is followed with a tilt toward the left shoulder. An increase in an existing hyper is watched for. Usually the deviation is manifest upon tilting in the appropriate direction. If the deviation remains latent, the alternate cover test must be used to dissociate the eyes and to measure the hyper deviation. The subjective measurement can be misleading because the tilting itself produces a hyper eye which should not be confused with a true hyper deviation. Because of this artifact, subjective testing to measure the deviation cannot be relied on. The examiner must make this measurement by objective means. This is accomplished by tilting his head the same amount as the patient's. In this orientation, the alternate cover test with prisms can be performed in the same manner as though both the doctor and patient were facing each other in an upright position. A small fixation light may be held by either the patient or an assistant since the doctor may require both hands to hold the occluder and loose prisms. I usually have the patient fixate the tip of my nose.

In case of a right superior oblique paresis, the hyper increases with the head tilt toward the right shoulder due to the postural reflexes causing compensatory torsional eye movements. With a right head tilt, the right eye must make an incycloduction movement; that is, the top of the eyeball must move nasally around its anterior-posterior axis. At the same time, the left eye must make an excycloduction movement. The impulse to keep the visual

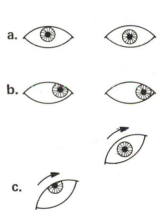

FIGURE 1-9 — The Three-Step Method for diagnosing an isolated paretic cyclovertical muscle. The right superior oblique is affected in this example. (a) Right hypertropia in the primary position; (b) Hyperdeviation increases on levoversion; (c) Further increase of right hyper on right head tilt. Arrows indicate the direction of compensatory torsional movements.

fields upright is very strong which is why the head tilt test is so definitive. In the case of a right superior oblique paresis, the other intorter is called upon to help incycloduct the eye. The other intorter of the right eye is the superior rectus. When brought into action for the purpose of intorting, the eye is elevated. This is the principal reason the right hyper increases on the right head tilt. Another reason is that the left inferior rectus is the yoke muscle of the right superior oblique, and this tends to produce a hypodeviation of the left eye.

The responses of the other affected muscles to the head tilt test can be analyzed similarly if the torsional action of each muscle is known. The rule to remember is that the superior muscles intort, and the inferior ones extort. The mnemonic expression "inferior people extort" may help in remembering the torsional actions of the eight cycloverticals. It should be noted that the four lateral recti (right lateral rectus, right medial rectus, left lateral rectus, and left medial rectus) have no significant torsional action for most diagnostic purposes.

The chief advantage of the three-step method is that it is an objective means of testing requiring little participation by the patient, other than fixating a target. If a hypertropia is present, direct observation of the patient's eyes during the procedure may be all that is required. If the deviation is latent or too small to discern, the alternate cover test is used.

VERSIONS

Versions are conjugate movements of both eyes. Figure 1-4 illustrates all of these except cycloversions.

DIRECT OBSERVATION

These eye movements may be directly observed in two different ways. The first method consists of instructing the patient to voluntarily move his eyes about in space without the aid of a fixation target. Any problem of voluntary movement should be noted. This could be an indication of a lesion above the midbrain. If there is no problem of voluntary movement, but there is one of nonconcomitancy, a suspected lesion would be either in the midbrain or below (i.e., infranuclear rather than supranuclear).

The other way to observe versions is to have the patient pursue a fixation target from the primary position to each of the nine diagnostic positions of gaze. The examiner looks for any signficant change in the patient's angle of deviation that would indicate nonconcomitancy. The presence of strabismus is usually necessary; however, a nonstrabismus may reveal nonconcomitancy if it becomes a strabismus in one or several positions of gaze.

The alternate cover test in various positions of gaze is more sensitive for concomitancy testing than mere direct observation. However, the latter method is a good back-up procedure for infants and toddlers who will not submit to the occluder. The speed of this procedure is sometimes an advantage over the cover test; the addition of the Hirschberg test to direct observation of versions greatly increases the sensitivity of this testing method.

This test was introduced by Julius Hirschberg in the latter part of the nineteenth century. Since then the procedure has remained practically the same, although the interpretation is variable. The test is performed by directing a small light source such as a candle flame, or penlight onto the patient's eyes. From behind the light the examiner sights the eyes while the patient is fixating the light. The doctor's dominant eye can be about ten centimeters away directly behind the light, although this distance is not critical and neither is the distance between the light and the patient. Hirschberg recommended about 30 centimeters. Error of measurement of the deviation is reduced as are other vagaries such as accommodative changes if the fixation distance is increased. A range between one-half to one meter is generally recommended.

Borish[3] summarizes the attempt by Hirschberg to quantify the strabismic angle. This was done by comparing the reflection (commonly referred to as corneal reflex) located in the entrance pupil of the fixating eye with the apparent location of the reflection on the deviating eye. Since the cornea acts as a small convex mirror, a virtual image of the lighted object is formed. The reference point for judging the position of the reflection in the nonfixating eye was either the pupillary margin or the limbus.

Guidelines for quantification were established. For instance, a reflection appearing to be on the temporal limbus of the deviating eye would represent approximately 45 degrees (100 p.d.) of esotropia. This method of estimating the deviation is useful but not reliable. Many other factors such as pupil size, corneal size, sphericalness of the cornea, and angle kappa need to be taken into account.

Various authorities have proposed simple ratios for use in measuring the deviation. The ratio most commonly used has been seven degrees (12 p.d.) to one millimeter. This means that for each millimeter of displacement of the corneal reflection in the deviating eye, relative to its location in the fixating eye, there is a deviation of seven degrees. Thus, a two-millimeter displacement represents a strabismus of 14 degrees.

Recently, a much higher ratio has been proposed by Jones and Eskridge.[4] When testing four subjects, they found, by theoretical calculations and experimental results, the average ratio to be 12 to 1 and concluded that 1-mm displacement equals 12 degrees (or 1 mm equals 22 p.d.).

Griffin and Boyer[5] used photographic means to study 25 subjects with known amounts of strabismus. The positions of corneal reflection were determined by utilizing a traveling microscope. Their results concurred closely with those of Jones and Eskridge.

Figure 1-10 illustrates the Hirschberg test and its interpretation. The 22/1 ratio is assumed; the pupil size is four millimeters. In Figures a and b, angle kappa is zero. In Figures c and d, it is plus one millimeter. In Figure e, the angle kappa is minus one millimeter. Further discussion on angle kappa in regard to eccentric fixation is covered in Chapter Two. The importance of taking angle kappa into account for Hirschberg testing is evident in these

THE HIRSCHBERG TEST

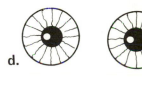

O.D.   O.S.

a.

b.

c.

d.

e.

FIGURE 1-10 — The Hirschberg test. (a) Bifoveal fixation, zero angle kappa; (b) O.S. fixating, zero angle kappa and 22 p.d. ET of O.D.; (c) O.S. fixating, + 1 mm angle kappa, and 22 p.d. ET of O.D.; (d) O.S. fixating, + 1 mm angle kappa, and 44 p.d. ET of O.D.; (e) O.S. fixating, − 1 mm angle kappa, and 22 p.d. ET of O.D.

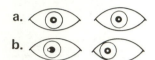

FIGURE 1-11 — Hirschberg test in the primary and a secondary position of gaze. (a) Ortho posture in the primary position; (b) Esotropia of the right eye with dextroversion.

illustrations. This is especially true since a zero angle kappa is the exception not the rule and therefore must be considered when observing the position of the reflection on the deviating eye.

The value of the Hirschberg test for concomitancy testing is not so much the determination of the exact magnitude of the deviation as it is determining a change in magnitude. Even a small shift in the position of the reflection on the deviating eye is easy to observe. A significant change would indicate the presence of nonconcomitancy.

An example of such a change is illustrated in Figure 1-11. Upon dextroversion, the eyes go from an ortho posture in the primary gaze to an esotropia of the right eye. This same example is shown in Figure 1-3b. The facility to observe and evaluate the deviation is greater with the Hirschberg than direct observation without the Hirschberg test.

DUCTIONS

Often there is confusion between the terms "ductions" and "vergences." Academically speaking, ductions are monocular eye movements. Refer to Table 1E for classifications. The common interchanging of the two terms probably arose from the practice of many clinicians who use the term "duction" when they really mean vergence.

TABLE 1E. Classification of Ductions and Vergences

Ductions	Vergences
Horizontal	Horizontal
Adduction (Nasal)	Convergence
Abduction (Temporal)	Divergence
Vertical	Vertical*
Supraduction (Elevation)	Supravergence
Infraduction (Depression)	Infravergence
Torsional	Torsional
Incycloduction (Intorsion)	Incyclovergence
Excycloduction (Extorsion)	Excyclovergence
Tertiary Positions	
Dextrosupraduction	
Levosupraduction	
Dextroinfraduction	
Levoinfraduction	

*This is also referred to as vertical divergence. It is positive if the right eye elevates, and negative if the left eye elevates.

Duction testing is useful when evaluating nonconcomitancy. Generally it is not regarded to be as sensitive as version testing. However, if the muscles are tested in their diagnostic action fields, ductions can be very informative as to the status of concomitancy (see Table 1F).

TABLE 1F. *Diagnostic Action Field of Each Extraocular Muscle*					
Right Eye			**Left Eye**		
Muscle	Gaze		Muscle	Gaze	
RLR	R		LLR	L	
RMR	L		LMR	R	
RSR	R & Up		LSR	L & Up	
RIR	R & Down		LIR	L & Down	
RSO	L & Down		LSO	R & Down	
RIO	L & Up		LIO	R & Up	

Each diagnostic action field (DAF) is evaluated by having the patient look in the appropriate direction. To test the integrity of the right superior oblique, for instance, the left eye is occluded while the patient fixates inward and downward with the right eye. Any underaction would indicate a restriction possibly due to paresis.

The distinction between a true paresis and a mechanical, or anatomical, problem is often difficult to make. In many cases, this can be ascertained by a good case history, combining results obtained from the various methods of testing and by careful observation during duction evaluation. Hugonnier[6] advocates the use of the forced duction test. This, however, usually requires general anesthesia in young patients and is not always a routine out-patient procedure. The patient's eye is moved by the doctor, using forceps, to determine if there are any obstructions to movement. If there are not any, a paresis can be assumed to be the cause of the nonconcomitancy rather than a mechanical anomaly.

Ordinary duction testing lacks some sensitivity compared to other methods. The test may be made more sensitive, however, by looking for nystagmoid movements in each diagnostic action field. These are often present in paretic cases, even in cases of mild paresis.

In many cases, overaction, or spasm, is difficult to spot under monocular testing conditions. The use of a penlight to observe a change in position of the corneal reflection may be helpful. This also increases the sensitivity of duction testing for underactions.

Sherrington's law applies to duction testing. This law states that the contraction of a muscle is accompanied by simultaneous and proportional relaxation of its antagonist. Thus, when the superior oblique contracts, its antagonist, the inferior oblique, relaxes.

Von Noorden and Maumenee[7] point out that some cases of paresis show exception to Sherrington's law. For example, when rhythmic co-contractions of the antagonists are occurring, a retractorious nystagmus results. The eyeball is seen to oscillate backward and forward, in and out of the orbit. Duane's retraction syndrome may be another example of co-contraction; both the medial and lateral recti possibly contract when the patient attempts adduction.

SPATIAL LOCALIZATION TESTING

This is often referred to as testing for past pointing which is usually revealed in patients who have a newly-acquired paresis. For example, assume the right superior oblique is paretic. The muscle is tested in its DAF (levoinfraduction). The left eye should be occluded since this is a monocular testing procedure. The patient is instructed to fixate a penlight located in the DAF position (to the patient's left and down) and to then touch it with the index finger of either hand. Although the distance is not critical, one-half meter is recommended. The patient is told to move his hand quickly from behind his shoulder (out of view) and to touch the light. Otherwise, corrective judgment may be made and localization may falsely appear to be normal. These judgments are learned in time by patients, and this is perhaps the explanation for lack of sensitivity in cases of paresis of long duration for this method of testing.

If testing is done correctly in a newly-acquired case of a paretic, RSO, the patient should miss the target by pointing to the left (patient's left) of and below the target of regard. It must be remembered that the target is not in the primary position but in the diagnostic action field of the particular muscle being tested. Each of the 12 extraocular muscles can be tested for nonconcomitancy in this manner.

SIGNS AND SYMPTOMS

Nonconcomitancy may or may not cause noticeable problems or complaints. In young children, the deviations are usually quite obvious before parents are prompted to have the child examined. Subjective complaints arising from nonconcomitancy are relatively infrequent in children under the age of seven years. The situation is most often that of the parent noticing signs of intermittent deviation rather than the child complaining of diplopia. Likewise, other subjective problems such as nausea and vertigo are thought to be more frequent in adults.

DIPLOPIA

Young children complain infrequently of diplopia because they readily suppress the aggravating image from the deviating eye. This is harder to achieve as the patient matures. Most adults find it difficult to cope with intractable diplopia resulting from strabismus of sudden onset (often caused by newly-acquired paresis) and diplopia becomes the main reason for the office visit.

Diplopia is classified as either physiological or pathological. Physiological diplopia is normal and occasionally perceived by individuals having perfectly good binocularity. Pathological diplopia is abnormal and frequently perceived in cases of strabismus.

Physiological diplopia is illustrated in Figure 1-12. The illustration shows how an object that is not the target of regard can be seen diplopically. It is easily effected by having the patient look out in space while a penlight is interposed in the midline about 40 centimeters away. In the normal type of diplopia, the target of regard is not diplopic; rather, all nonfixated objects in space (those outside of the singleness horoptor) are capable of being seen diplopically. Fortunately, suppression of a normal type is usually active to prevent nonfixated objects from appearing doubled. This type of suppression is physiological.

On the other hand, pathological diplopia is a condition in which the fixated target of regard is diplopic. Figure 1-13 illustrates a case of exotropia of the right eye. Diplopia of this type causes problems for older people who have a sudden onset of strabismus. One of the sensorial adaptations required to eliminate diplopia is suppression. This type of anti-diplopia defense is called pathological suppression (discussed further in Chapter Two).

If a patient has always had poor binocular vision, this type of suppression may be present and may prevent the perception of pathological diplopia that might otherwise result in a person with recent nonconcomitancy. In such instances diplopia is less likely to be a warning of acquired paresis than it would be in cases where binocularity has previously been good.

An affected extraocular muscle can often be determined by merely observing the head posture of the patient. Interpretation of abnormal posture is made easy by realizing that the patient's face points in the same direction as the diagnostic action field of the affected muscle (see Table 1G). For example, a paretic right superior oblique causes a patient to abnormally turn his head to the left and to lower his chin. The RSO muscle is in its DAF when the right eye is turned to the left and down.

Another similar rule explains why there is also an abnormal head tilt to the left. Since the superior oblique is an intorter, the RSO moves the top of the right eye leftward on its anterior-posterior axis. The rule to remember is that the abnormal head tilt is in the same direction as the movement of the eyeball would be if the affected muscle would contract. Therefore, a paretic RSO would cause the head to be tilted toward the left shoulder in habitual natural seeing conditions.

Table 1G lists the directions the face would be pointing for any of the 12 EOM which may be affected.

Diagnosis is complicated when more than one muscle is affected. Nonetheless, observation of abnormal head posture may be effective in detecting a nonconcomitant condition and arriving at a tentative diagnosis. Unlike past pointing, the mere passing of time does not tend to greatly compensate for head posture abnormalities. Consequently, it is likely that

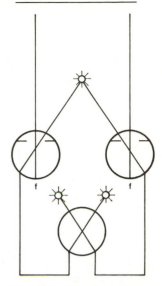

FIGURE 1-12 — Physiological diplopia. Fixation target is at optical infinity with eyes in ortho posture. Test target is a penlight. Cyclopean projection shows the doubled image with the right eye seeing one to the left, and the left eye seeing one to the right.

ABNORMAL HEAD POSTURE

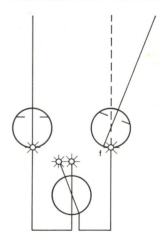

FIGURE 1-13 — Pathological diplopia. Fixation target is a penlight at optical infinity. The right eye is exotropic. Cyclopean projection shows the doubled image with the left eye localizing one in the correct straight-ahead direction, but the right eye sees one to the left.

TABLE 1G. *Abnormal Head Posture Related to Affected Extraocular Muscles*

Muscle	Position of Face		
	Turn	Elevation	Tilt
RLR	R	—	—
RMR	L	—	—
RSR	R	Up	L
RIR	R	Down	R
RSO	L	Down	L
RIO	L	Up	R
LLR	L	—	—
LMR	R	—	—
LSR	L	Up	R
LIR	L	Down	L
LSO	R	Down	R
LIO	R	Up	L

even a nonconcomitancy of long-standing can be detected by means of observing head posture. In cases where more than one muscle is involved, it is usually advisable to perform muscle fields testing by subjective means in order to identify each one that is affected. In this regard the Hess-Lancaster method (discussed later) is the most ideal subjective test.

SUBJECTIVE TESTING PROCEDURES

Concomitancy testing by subjective means is often more precise than by objective testing. The patient may be able to notice a very small displacement of two images resulting from a misalignment of the visual axes. Very small deviations are difficult for the examiner to observe, making objective testing less sensitive. This is particularly true for cyclo deviations where subjective testing must be resorted to for an accurate diagnosis.

However, there are disadvantages to subjective testing. This type of examination is entirely dependent on cooperation by a capable and aware patient. An uncooperative, dull or unperceptive patient gives either invalid or no results. Objective testing has to be relied on in such cases. The presence of anomalous correspondence also may invalidate subjective findings because the objective and subjective angles are different. In addition, the subjective angle itself is sometimes variable when this condition is present (anomalous correspondence is discussed in Chapter Two).

SINGLE-OBJECT METHOD

This is the traditional method of making the patient aware of pathological diplopia when fixating a single target (refer to Figure 1-13). If the patient has an exo deviation, as in the illustrated example, the target (a penlight in a darkened room is ideal for this purpose) is perceived as a double image. The deviating right eye sees the target to the left of the target seen by the fixating left eye. This is an example of heteronymous (crossed) diplopia and is the kind of diplopia normally expected with exo deviations. On the other hand, homonymous (uncrossed) diplopia is normally expected when eso deviations are involved.

In testing for nonconcomitancy using the single-object method, there are two rules to keep in mind. The direction of the target seen by the deviating eye is perceived by the patient in the opposite direction from that in which the eye is deviating. In the example just given, the right exotropic eye sees the image to the left. The other rule is that the distance between the diplopic images becomes greater when there is an increase in either an underaction or an overaction during versions. Measurements are made with loose prisms.

By using a black tangent screen, the subjective angle of directionalization can be measured in all nine positions of gaze. The examiner marks the separation of the diplopic images reported by the patient. If a one-meter test distance is used, each centimeter displacement of the images represents one prism diopter.

Many practitioners find the single-object method confusing because they have to think in reverse as to directions of the deviating eye and the diplopic image. This is eliminated by employment of the two-object method.

TWO-OBJECT METHOD

This method requires two fixation targets, one for each eye. Special filters, usually red and green, are utilized. The right eye sees only one target; the left eye sees the other. Hugonnier[8] recommends combining the method of Hess with that of Lancaster for concomitancy testing. This combination, called the Hess-Lancaster test, is discussed in detail.

Hess developed the kind of screen used for this type of subjective deviation measurement. The screen was originally a black cloth with horizontal and vertical red lines of thread woven in five-degree intervals. The lines were made to be curvilinear in order to demarcate degrees accurately on a flat surface. In addition, red dots on the screen representing the nine diagnostic positions of gaze were advocated by Hess.

The method of performing the Hess test consists of having the patient wear red-green viewers and instructing him to superimpose a green target (a Y-shaped target made of green thread) with a red dot. The physical separation of the two fixated objects (when they appear superimposed to the patient) is the magnitude of the patient's subjective angle. This procedure is followed in all nine positions of gaze. If the deviation varies significantly (more than five prism diopters), nonconcomitancy is indicated.

Lancaster used the Hess method but improved it by developing the technique of projecting red and green slits of light onto a white screen having painted grids of red lines. Lancaster believed straight lines to be sufficiently accurate for clinical testing of deviations. Red dots (or red circles) representing the nine positions of gaze are usually included on these screens. The red lines and dots are invisible to the eye wearing the red filter. Because

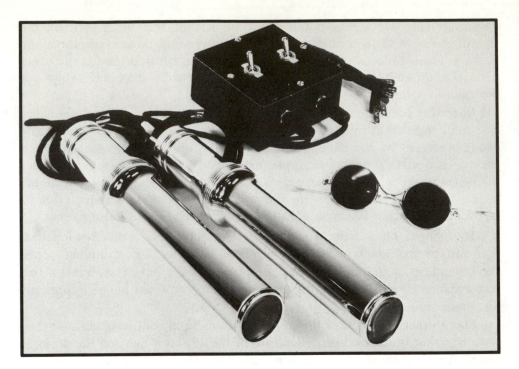

a.

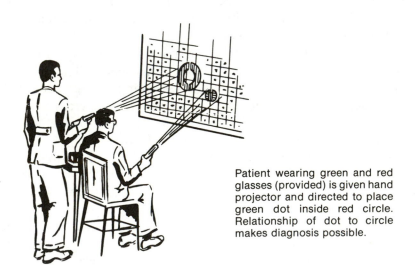

Patient wearing green and red glasses (provided) is given hand projector and directed to place green dot inside red circle. Relationship of dot to circle makes diagnosis possible.

b.

FIGURE 1-14 — The Allied Strabismometer. (a) Photograph of electric flashlights and red-green spectacles (b) Illustration of testing procedure with the Strabismometer. (Photo and drawing courtesy of Allied Ophthalmic Products, Co.)

the white background is more intense than the red lines and dots, they are consequently washed out. However, they are visible to the eye having the green filter. They appear to be dark grey in color, because while the red hue is not transmitted by the green filter, the white background is.

The Hess-Lancaster test may be custom-made or obtained commercially. An available well-designed test is the Strabismometer.[e] The unit comes with a red and green flashlight, red-green spectacles, and a rectangular coordinate tangent screen having red lines and red fixation circles. Figure 1-14a shows a picture of the flashlights and Figure 1-14b an illustration of their application in testing.

Figure 1-15 shows the recording chart for the Hess-Lancaster test used at the Southern California College of Optometry. The separation between the lines represents approximately seven prism diopters. The fixation circles are five squares out from the center; therefore, 35 p.d. (almost 20 degrees) lateral. They are placed 28 p.d. vertically above or below the level of the central fixation circle. Because of changing tangent values, the magnitude represented by each separation of lines is variable. The prism diopter value becomes less as fixation changes from the primary position to the periphery. In spite of this mathematical variable, it is generally not necessary to compensate for these changes. Usually, there are only about one or two prism diopters for most central and paracentral muscle field testing. Fixations would have to be much greater than 35 p.d. away from the primary position before tangent value changes become a significantly invalidating factor.

The chart also lists the names of the 12 extraocular muscles. The location of each represents the diagnostic action field for that particular muscle.

LEFT FIELD   **RIGHT FIELD**

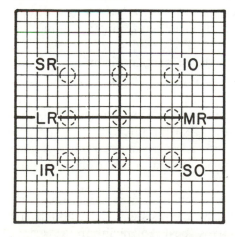 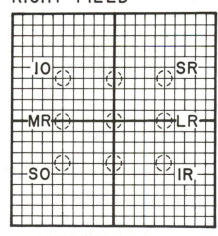

FIGURE 1-15 — Form used for charting results of the Hess-Lancaster test

[e]Allied Ophthalmic Products Co.

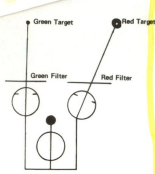

FIGURE 1-16 — Diagram showing patient's perception of superimposition on the Hess-Lancaster test in an example of an exo deviation

The following procedure is recommended for performing this test. To evaluate the right field (meaning the muscles of the right eye are to be tested) the patient puts on red-green spectacles with the red filter over the right eye. This stays in place throughout testing for both the right field and the left field. The room is dimly illuminated. While the examiner holds the green projecting flashlight, the patient holds the red. The test distance from the patient to the center of the screen is one meter. The deviation in the primary position is measured first. The examiner projects the green light onto the central circle. The patient attempts to superimpose the red projected circle of light (being seen by the right eye) with the green spot, fixated by the left eye. If the patient were exotropic (or phoric) in the right eye, the red spot would be projected to the right of the green fixation spot to achieve the percept in his mind that the two targets are superimposed (see Figure 1-16).

If the patient were esotropic (or phoric for that matter, since fusion is broken[f] by the complementary colored filters) the red spot would be projected to the left of the fixated green spot. The rule notes that the patient projects the light in the same direction as the deviation of the eye. This is direct foveal projection; because of this, interpretation is facilitated by not having to think in reverse as in the single-object method.

If the patient does not understand this testing procedure, it is instructive to remove the colored spectacles and let him superimpose the projected spots. Since there is no binocular demand, he should be able to do this satisfactorily. It is sometimes wise to allow the parent of a young child to observe this technique. When the child feels confident that he can superimpose the spots, place the spectacles on his face. Since fusion is broken and the eyes are dissociated, they must be in the ortho position for superimposition to occur. When a deviation is present, the child will have the impression that the spots are superimposed on the screen, but the parent can see they are actually separated. This observation is helpful in explaining the nature of a deviation to the parent.

After measuring the subjective angle in the primary position of gaze, the other eight positions should be tested in a similar manner. For right field testing, the left eye remains the fixating eye.

To test the left field, the examiner simply exchanges flashlights with the patient. He directs the red spot to the central fixation circle, and the patient tries to superimpose the green spot with the red. All nine positions of gaze are measured for the left field following the procedure used in testing the right field.

It is important that the red filter remain over the right eye and the green over the left if this system is to be followed consistently. Although the sequence of procedures is not rigid, it is best to maintain a certain consistency. Otherwise, this type of testing can become confusing and interpretation very difficult.

---

[f]When fusion is broken by means of filters or septums, this process is also referred to as dissociation.

Case examples are given to explain interpretation of the measured deviations. Figure 1-17 shows the charting of a paretic right lateral rectus. This esotropia is similar to the example discussed and illustrated in Figure 1-3. On right gaze the paretic right lateral rectus is in its diagnostic action field and is seen to be underacting. The left medial rectus is also in its diagnostic action field and is shown to have an overaction (because of Hering's law). The x's represent the positions of the spots seen by the deviating eye. The circles represent the positions of the fixating eye. It is helpful to outline the eight outside x's by connecting them with each other to form an enclosure. This aids in visualizing graphs in the more complicated cases of nonconcomitancy. For interpretation, the areas of the enclosures for each field are compared. In this example, the right enclosure is smaller than the left. This means that the paresis (or the cause of the underaction) is in the right eye. The left area is larger, indicating overaction by the left eye; this graphically illustrates the effect of Hering's law.

LEFT FIELD   RIGHT FIELD

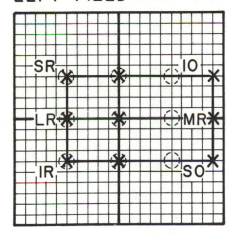 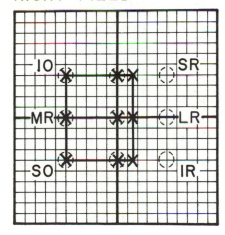

FIGURE 1-17 — Chart of the results of the Hess-Lancaster test in the case of a paretic right lateral rectus muscle

An example of an exotropic deviation with a paresis of the right medial rectus is shown in Figure 1-18. This is similar to the case discussed and illustrated in Figures 1-5 through 1-8. The area of the enclosure for the right field is much smaller than that for the left. The overaction of the left lateral rectus is very large when the paretic right medial rectus is forced into its diagnostic action field, which is gaze left.

This method of charting deviations is very useful when two or more muscles are paretic. Figure 1-19 illustrates an example of paresis of both the right lateral rectus and the right superior oblique. Besides the similar effect of the paretic lateral muscle as in Figure 1-17, there is also an underaction in

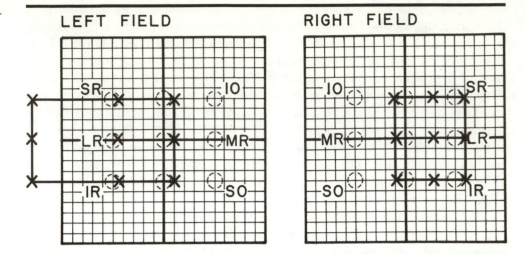

FIGURE 1-18 — Chart of the results of the Hess-Lancaster test in the case of a paretic right medial rectus muscle

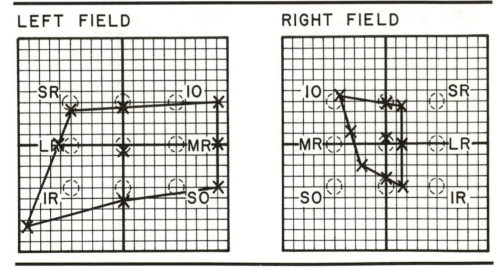

FIGURE 1-19 — Chart of the results of paresis of both the right lateral rectus and the right superior oblique

the diagnostic action field of the right superior oblique. There is an overaction of the yoke muscle, the left inferior rectus. By comparing the size of the two enclosures for the right and left fields, the paretic muscles are detected and a diagnosis is easily made.

Generally speaking, the two-object method, and the Hess-Lancaster test in particular, is the most sensitive of all concomitancy tests. Some pitfalls, however, are occasioned. They include: anomalous correspondence, deep suppression, and poor cooperation by the patient. If any or all of these exist, testing may have to be performed entirely by objective means. In practice, it is wise to perform different types of tests on a patient with a suspected nonconcomitancy. The results of one should confirm the results of another.

A careful case history needs to be taken and accounted for before sound recommendations for case disposition can be given. It is important to know the time of onset of the nonconcomitancy. If it has been recently noted, an immediate neurological consultation is in order. If the onset is sudden, vascular problems such as stroke, or acute diseases may be suspected. If it is gradual, chronic diseases or a neoplasm such as a brain tumor may be the cause. In these events, internists and neurologists should be consulted.

Birth history may indicate the possibility of trauma to the sixth nerve. This is not infrequent. Occasionally the lateral rectus muscle is damaged during delivery. The sixth nerve is affected in many other ways and is the most frequently impaired nerve of the three cranial nerves innervating the extraocular muscles.

The next most frequently affected is the fourth nerve. Occasionally, the pulley mechanism of the superior oblique is damaged by severe sinus complications. Any history of sinus problems should be questioned thoroughly.

Less common are pareses of the muscles innervated by the third nerve. These muscles are the medial rectus, superior rectus, inferior rectus, and the inferior oblique. Careful case history may reveal other associated neurological problems. Frequently, however, there is no other disease but only an isolated extraocular muscle paresis. If there is any suspicion of vascular or viral disease, the patient should receive immediate medical attention.

Since nonconcomitancies may be due to anatomical and mechanical anomalies, an ophthalmological consultation, including the forced duction test, may be recommended.

Management of nonconcomitancy to prevent contractures, and procedures to restore binocularity, are discussed in Chapter Eleven.

Next in importance to concomitancy evaluation is determination of the frequency of a manifest deviation. This knowledge helps the practitioner assess the status of the patient's binocularity. For instance, he can generally assume the patient who is strabismic 95 percent of the time has poorer binocularity than the patient who is strabismic only five percent of the time.

Frequency refers to the amount of time a deviation is manifest. This may range from zero to 100 percent. If a strabismus is not present any of the time under natural habitual seeing conditions, the patient is necessarily classified as being either orthophoric or heterophoric. More patients are heterophoric than orthophoric because normally there is some deviation present even though it may be small. Any latent deviation, one prism diopter or greater, is classified as a heterophoria. As in heterotropias, the deviation may be horizontal, vertical, or torsional.

When the deviation is present from one percent to 99 percent of the time, the strabismus is classified as being intermittent. A synonymous term for intermittent is the word "occasional." This term, I feel, can imply a state of infrequency of strabismus. To some practitioners, an occasional strabismus may mean that the deviation is manifest only once in a while. This possibly may not represent the true condition. It could possibly be misleading to call an intermittent strabismus, which is present 95 percent of the time, an occasional strabismus. It is best to use the term "intermittent" and include the estimated percentage of time strabismus is present at far and at near.

Table 1H lists the classifications of the frequency of strabismus, based on the percentage of time (of normal waking hours) there is a manifest deviation of the visual axes. When it is present 100 percent of the time, the strabismus is constant. Synonymous terms include: continuous strabismus, permanent strabismus, and absolute strabismus.

TABLE 1H. Classification of Frequency of the Deviation

Constant Strabismus   100% *

Intermittent Strabismus   1% to 99% *

  Periodic

    Direct (nearpoint strabismus)
    Indirect (farpoint strabismus)
    Certain cases of nonconcomitancy

  Non-Periodic (unpredictable intermittency)

Non-Strabismus   0% *

  Heterophoria (deviation always latent)

  Orthophoria

* Percentage of the time that deviation is manifest

An intermittent strabismus may be either periodic or nonperiodic. In most cases, it is the latter. If a strabismus is to be called periodic, its occurrence must be predictable and regular. A periodic intermittent strabismus may be either direct or indirect. Direct periodic intermittent strabismus means that the strabismus occurs regularly at near, under specified conditions, but not at far. The typical case is the patient with intermittent esotropia at near caused by the combination of esophoria at far, and uncorrected hyperopic refractive error and a high accommodative-convergence to accommodation relationship (AC/A). Accommodation brought into play for nearpoint demand can precipitate the manifest deviation.

An intermittent strabismus that is periodic and indirect is one that occurs at far but not at near. This is typified by the patient who has intermittent exotropia at far but is exophoric at near. This is usually the case with a high AC/A which allows the deviation to be less at near. At far, however, the patient will lapse into an exotropia unless there is a strong power of fusion.

Another cause for periodicity may be nonconcomitancy. For example, a patient with complete paresis of the right lateral rectus has a marked nonconcomitancy. This would most likely result in the patient having an esotropia every time he looks to the right (as in the example shown in Figure 1-3a).

In the majority of cases, however, the intermittent regularity of the strabismus cannot be absolutely predicted and is the reason most cases are nonperiodic.

EVALUATION

There are two principal ways to evaluate the percentage of time there is a manifest deviation of the visual axes. They are the case history and the results of the testing procedures.

CASE HISTORY

This is a valuable means for evaluating the frequency of strabismus. The best information is knowing how others see the patient. Parents of young children may give such reports as "cross-eyed about half the time, especially when he is tired" or "he's wall-eyed when he looks out the window." Since young patients seldom complain of diplopia, this type of case history is most important.

Older children and adults may give an index to the frequency of strabismus by reporting the amount of time diplopia is noticed. This, however, is not always highly correlated to the frequency of strabismus, and questioning of the patient's appearance as observed by friends and family must be pursued.

TESTING PROCEDURES

The estimation of frequency is not made by a rigid system of testing. It is done by using professional judgment and is the result of various tests and impressions. The case history is critical. There are, however, some guidelines for testing.

It is best to observe the patient before dissociative testing is begun. The next recommended procedure is the Hirschberg test. Since this does not dissociate the eyes, the occurrence or lack of strabismus should be noted. The cover test fully dissociates the eyes. When the cover is removed, refusion movements (if any) should be evaluated. A slow recovery rather than a quick recovery indicates a more frequently occurring strabismus.

Diplopia testing reveals the patient's ability to notice pathological diplopia. If diplopia is easily noticed when the patient becomes strabismic, the frequency of the strabismus is probably lower than if diplopia is not perceived. This is because fusion is better and suppression is less in most cases when diplopia is noticed when the deviation becomes manifest.

Many other routine sensory and motor fusion tests can contribute to the doctor's overall estimation of the frequency of a manifest deviation. This estimation should be determined for both the farpoint and the nearpoint.

Direction of the Deviation

The direction of the deviating eye may be lateral, vertical, or torsional. Table 1I lists the directions in which the eye may deviate.

TABLE 1I. Classification of Direction of Deviation

Deviation	Direction of deviating eye when the fixating eye is in primary position.
Horizontal	
Eso	Inward rotation of eye
Exo	Outward rotation of eye
Vertical	
Hyper	Upward rotation of eye
Hypo	Downward rotation of eye
Torsional	
Incyclo	Top of eye rotated inward
Excyclo	Top of eye rotated outward

It is not uncommon for a vertical deviation to be combined with a horizontal deviation, e.g., an esotropia with a hypertropia. It is less common to find a pure vertical deviation such as a hypertropia without a lateral component. Even rarer is a cyclo deviation without either vertical or horizontal components. The rule follows that if a cyclo deviation is noted, there are likely to be vertical and horizontal deviations. If there is a vertical, the probability of a horizontal deviation is also present. If a lateral deviation is observed, there may or may not be other components.

Some authorities prefer to speak only of hyper deviations, thus avoiding the term "hypo." This is a misleading practice. For instance, it is preferable to call a downward deviation of a nonfixating right eye a right hypotropia rather than a left hypertropia. In this case the left eye is the fixating eye and is not deviating upward.

OBJECTIVE TESTING PROCEDURES

When a manifest deviation is present, the Hirschberg test quickly ascertains the direction in which the eye is deviating. If the deviation is latent, or if the manifest deviation is very small, the cover test should be used for diagnostic purposes.

Unilateral occlusion is good for detecting the direction of deviations, particularly for lateral and vertical components. However, it has limitations for objectively determining cyclo deviations. Other subjective methods are more sensitive in this regard. In the case of a right exotropia combined with right hypertropia and right excyclotropia, covering the left eye would result in the following movements: the right eye would be seen to move inward and downward with the top of the eye (the 12 o'clock position on the limbus) moving inward. This is the required movement the right eye must make to go from the deviated position to the position of fixation. Covering the tropic eye would result in no movement. If, however, there were an exophoria combined with a right hyperphoria and an excyclophoria, occlusion of the right eye would result in the following: the anterior segment of the right eye would drift outward and upward, and the top of the eye would rotate outward.

The alternate cover test is also a good method for determining the direction of the deviation. The use of neutralizing prisms is very effective in this regard. When the lateral component is neutralized either with base-out or base-in prism, the vertical component is much easier to observe. If the vertical component is also neutralized with either base-up or base-down prism, it may be possible to isolate and observe cyclo deviations as small as three degrees. Smaller cyclo deviations need to be detected and measured by subjective means.

The most commonly used clinical method for subjectively determining the direction of deviation is the testing of pathological diplopia. This is explained in the section on the single-object method in regard to concomitancy testing.

SUBJECTIVE TESTING PROCEDURES

A case example is illustrated in Figure 1-13. In reference to that illustration, if a red lens is placed before the right eye which has an exo deviation, suppression is less likely to occur. The filter creates a color difference between the eyes and serves to break down suppression. In some cases where suppression is very deep in the deviating eye, the red filter should be switched to the fixating eye. This reduces the intensity of the light entering the eye and acts as a mild occluder giving an advantage to the deviating eye. In any event, assuming normal correspondence, the deviating eye sees an image opposite in direction to its deviation.

COLORED FILTERS

The same rule involving colored filters applies when using the Maddox rod.[g] Note Figure 1-13. If the Maddox rod is placed with its axis at 180 degrees (rod horizontal) before the right eye which has an exo horizontal deviation in this example, the eye will see a vertical streak to the left of the fixation spot.

MADDOX ROD

If another Maddox rod is also placed before the left eye (axis at 180 degrees) the patient sees two vertical streaks. If a cyclo deviation is not present, the lines appear parallel. However, if the right eye is excyclotropic, the top of the leftward line (seen by the right excyclotropic eye in this example) will appear inclined away from the vertical line seen by the fixating

[g]Although the original rod was a single elongated cylindrical lens, most practitioners now prefer multiple rods for dissociative testing. This, however, is referred to as the Maddox rod rather than rods.

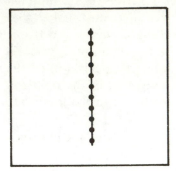

a. O.S. VISUAL PERCEPTION

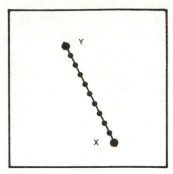

O.D. VISUAL PERCEPTION (POINTS X AND Y ARE NOT SEEN, BUT ARE ONLY FOR EXPLANATION PURPOSES)

b. IMAGE OF MADDOX ROD

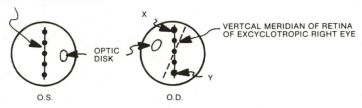

OPTIC DISK

VERTCAL MERIDIAN OF RETINA OF EXCYCLOTROPIC RIGHT EYE

O.S.   O.D.

POSTERIOR VIEW OF RETINAS

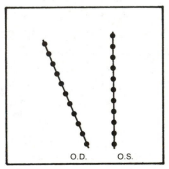

c. PATIENT'S PERCEPTION

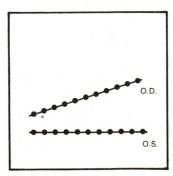

d. PATIENT'S PERCEPTION

FIGURE 1-20 — Illustration of the effect of a cyclo deviation on the results of the Maddox rod test. (a) The patient perceives the imaged line as being vertically oriented for the fixating left eye. However, the line seen by the right eye appears to be slanting, with the top oriented in a leftward position; (b) Posterior view of the eyeballs, illustrating the excyclo deviation of the right eye. The analogy of visual fields and retinal projection is used here for clarification. Point x stimulates the superior nasal retina and is therefore projected into the inferior temporal field. Likewise, point y on the inferior temporal retina is projected into the superior nasal field; (c) The slanted line seen by the right eye is seen to the left of the vertical line because of a horizontal exo deviation of the right eye; (d) Many practitioners prefer to place the axis of the rods at 90 degrees so the patient sees horizontal streaks (in this example, by the left eye). If a vertical prism is placed base down before the right eye, the excyclo deviation causes the perceived streak for the right eye to slant upwards in the temporal field and downward in the nasal visual field. The vertical prism is necessary in order to create the doubling so that one line is above the other. Of course, if the patient has an existing vertical deviation, the use of vertical prism may be unnecessary in this procedure.

left eye. In regard to the direction of the perceived slant, the rule is that the patient perceives the line as slanting in the direction opposite to the cyclo deviation of that eye (see Figure 1-20 for clarification).

If instead of two Maddox rods, a variation of the two-object method such as the Hess-Lancaster test is used, the test streak for the right eye must be oriented in the same direction as the direction of the cyclo deviation. In the above case example, the streak for the excyclo deviated right eye must be oriented with its top in a rightward position (as projected on the screen and as viewed by the examiner). When the slant of the streak is equal to the deviation, the patient will perceive it as being vertical.

An example of the phi phenomenon is seen when the patient perceives movement of a stationary single target during rapid alternate occlusion. The apparent movement is noted when a deviation of the visual axes is present. Refer to Figure 1-13 where the right eye is shown exotropic. Upon rapid alternate occlusion, the right eye is briefly exposed by shifting the occluder to the left eye. The fixation object appears to move to the left (same direction as the movement of the occluder). When the occluder is shifted back to the right eye, the target appears to move to the right (same direction as the occluder). For vertical deviations, the target appears to move up and down. If, instead of a spot, a vertical line is used for fixation, a shift in the inclination during alternate occlusion reveals a cyclo deviation.

In cases of eso deviations, the shift is noticed opposite to the movement of the occluder. In hyper deviations, when the hyper eye is exposed, the movement is downward. If the patient has an excyclotropic right eye (using a vertical line as a fixation target) when the occluder is moved to cover the left eye (exposing the right), the top of the line is perceived making a tilting movement to the left (see Figure 1-20), i.e., the top of the streak moves in the same direction as the movement of the occluder in excyclo deviations and in the opposite direction for incyclo deviations.

If there is no deviation, a movement is not noticed when this method of phi phenomenon testing is employed. The perceived shifting movement of the target is therefore explained by cyclopean projection and is not based on eye movements, because the occluder is moved rapidly and time for fixational eye movement is not given. The alternate occlusion must, however, not be so rapid that dissociation ceases and the patient is allowed to see binocularly (such as looking through the blades of a moving fan).

Unless otherwise specified, the magnitude of the deviation customarily refers to the angle of deviation of the visual axes when fixation is in the primary position. This should be measured for both the farpoint (optical infinity) and the nearpoint. The most frequently used nearpoint fixation distance is 40 centimeters (16 inches). There must be careful control of accommodation if measurement of nearpoint horizontal deviations is to be valid. Figure 1-21 illustrates an esotropic deviation of the right eye at the nearpoint.

PHI PHENOMENON

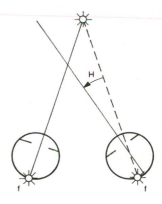

FIGURE 1-21 — Illustration of an esotropia of the right eye at near. The objective angle of deviation is represented by the letter "H."

Magnitude of the Deviation

Alternate Occlusion

For measuring the magnitude of deviations for distance or near, the clinical test, par excellence, is the alternate cover test combined with loose prisms. Loose prisms offer an advantage over prism racks in that both the lateral and vertical components can be conveniently measured simultaneously. In addition, the prism rack is bulky making measurement of more than one component awkward. To use the prisms in measuring an esotropia of the right eye that also has a hypertropia, two loose prisms, one base-out, the other base-down, are simply placed together between the occluder and the right eye.

Another good method utilizing alternate occlusion involves the use of the major amblyoscope. The Synoptophore, manufactured by Clement Clarke, is the most popular commercially available instrument of this type. See Figure 1-22. The procedure for measuring the objective angle with this instrument is similar to the alternate cover test. A clear slide for one eye having a small fixation dot in its center is placed in one carrier. A similar slide to be seen by the opposite eye is put in the other carrier. The instrument is set at the ortho position; i.e., no horizontal, vertical, or torsional demands. If the patient is orthophoric, the two dots should be seen in the same location. No eye movement is required when each eye is occluded (effectively done by switching off the instrument light for each eye). If there is an exotropia, the eyes make a version movement. This is neutralized by moving the arms of the instrument (usually just the one for the deviating eye) toward the patient, thus creating a base-in prism effect. The amount of base-in neutralizing the version movement is the magnitude of the angle of deviation. In this manner, the major amblyoscope also measures the lateral and vertical deviations by objective means. The cyclo deviations are best measured by subjective means conveniently done with the major amblyoscope.

CORNEAL LIGHT REFLECTIONS

When eccentric fixation is present, the cover test may give invalid measurements of the strabismic angle. However, measurements are not invalidated by eccentric fixation when methods utilizing corneal light reflections are used.

HIRSCHBERG INTERPRETATION

This is the most commonly used method employing corneal light reflections for measurement of strabismus. For proper interpretation, a ratio of 22 p.d. to one millimeter is recommended.

THE ARC PERIMETER

The objective angle of strabismus may be measured by using an arc perimeter. Javal's method is as follows: the patient's nonfixating eye is placed in the center of the perimeter. The fixating eye (in the primary position) peers over the arc at a target set at optical infinity. The doctor moves with a penlight along the arc and (with his dominant eye behind the light) observes the changing position of the reflection in the deviating eye. Javal advocated making these movements until the reflection is positioned in

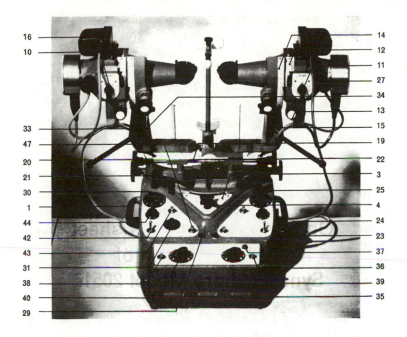

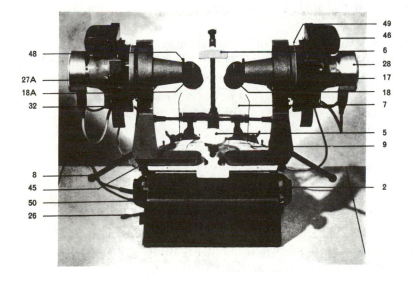

KEY FOR MODEL 2051

MECHANICAL

1. Carrying handles (2).
2. Interpupillary distance selection controls (2).
3. Interpupillary distance scale.
4. Chinrest height control.
5. Chinrest.
6. Forehead rest.
7. Breathshield.
8. Handles for adjustment of horizontal angle between tubes (2).
9. Horizontal deviation scales (2).
10. Vertical deviation scales (2).
11. Vertical deviation controls (2).
12. Torsional deviation scales (2).
13. Torsional deviation controls (2).
14. Elevation and depression scales (2).
15. Elevation and depression controls (2).
16. Slide carriers (2).
17. Slide ejectors (2).
18. Auxiliary lens holders (2).
18A. Eyepiece lens (removable) (2).
19. Horizontal vergence scale.
20. Horizontal vergence controls (2).
21. Tube locking controls (horizontal) (2).
22. Central lock.
32. Lever for swivelling opal screen from optical pathway (2). (Model 2052 only.)

ELECTRICAL

23. On/Off switch.
24. Mains current input plug and socket.
25. Indicator lamp.
26. Voltage selector.
27. 6V. Lampholders (slide illumination) (2).
27A Lamphouse locking lever (2).
28. 12V. Lampholders (after-images and Haidinger's brushes).
29. Hand flashing switches (2).
30. Dimming rheostats (2).
31. Selector switch.
33. Plug and socket connections to 6V. lamps (2).
34. Plug and socket connections to 12V. lamps (2).

Automatic Flashing (Models 2051 and 2052 only).

35. Automatic flashing unit.
36. On/Off switch.
37. Indicator lamp.
38. Rapid/Variable switch.
39. Simultaneous/Alternating switch.
40. Light and dark phases controls (2).
50. Fuse.

Haidinger's brushes (Model 2051 only).

42. On/Off switches.
43. Reversing switches (2).
44. Speed controls (2).
45. Plug and socket connections to motors (2).
46. Motors and rotating polaroid discs (removable from instruments) (2).
47. Haidinger's brush illumination switches (2).
48. Blue filters (removable) (2)
49. Iris diaphragms (2).

Figures in Brackets refer to No. of Controls or Items on Syoptophore.

FIGURE 1-22 — Photograph of the Clement Clarke Synoptophore, model 2051, with key for labeled parts. (Courtesy of Clement Clarke)

the center of the pupil. If angle kappa is zero in the fixating eye, the reading of the perimeter scale gives the angle of strabismus in degrees. However, if angle kappa is other than zero, the strabismic angle cannot be read directly from the scale. In a case of esotropia, angle kappa is added to the reading; with exotropia, angle kappa is subtracted from the reading. The result is the amount of the strabismic angle.

The method I prefer is similar to Javal's with one exception. The light reflection in the deviating eye is positioned to occupy exactly the same relative location as that of the fixating eye. It is a quicker test, and since only one rather than two measurements (finding the magnitude of angle kappa and then adding this to the estimation found by centering the reflection in the pupil) is involved, the chance of error is reduced.

MAJOR AMBLYOSCOPE The same method described above may be employed using the major amblyoscope. The fixating eye views a target in the primary position (carrier set at ortho). The carrier for the deviating eye is moved back and forth (doctor sighting from behind the moving carrier) until the reflection occupies the same relative position as that in the fixating eye. The angle of strabismus can be read directly from the scale on the instrument.

KRIMSKY TEST The technique introduced by Krimsky[9] is similar to the Hirschberg test with one exception. Prisms are used to reposition the corneal light reflection of the deviating eye to the same relative location as the reflection in the fixating eye. The magnitude of the prism necessary to accomplish this is the measurement of the angle of strabismus.

SUBJECTIVE METHODS The magnitude of the angle of deviation may be measured by subjective as well as by objective methods. There are times when measurement by subjective means is preferable, because objective testing may lack necessary precision (e.g., cases having cyclo deviations). However, subjective testing is not always reliable, especially when there is deep suppression or anomalous correspondence.

Practically all subjective methods designed for the determination of the magnitude of deviation are variations of either the single-object method or the two-object method. The measuring tools are either prisms or calibrated scales. The scales may be in free space. For example, in the Hess-Lancaster test, the patient directly views the test targets and their diplopic separation can be converted into prism dioptors by using the measurement lines on the screen. On the other hand, when the major amblyscope is used, the deviation is determined from the scales on the instrument.

Accommodative-Convergence/Accommodation The relationship between accommodative-convergence and accommodation is often referred to as the ACA. More properly, it should be denoted as the AC/A ratio. The ratio means that for every diopter of accommodative response, a certain amount of accommodative-convergence (depending on the value of the AC/A) is brought into play. For instance, if the AC/A is 6 p.d. per 1 diopter of accommodation, a patient who accommodates 2.50 diopters will have an increased convergence of his visual axes of 15 p.d.

GRADIENT METHOD

The magnitude of the AC/A may be arrived at by finding the effect of spherical lenses on convergence. At the farpoint, minus lenses are used for this purpose; at the nearpoint, either plus or minus lenses will give the value.

Regardless of the testing distance, the AC/A should be determined with the patient wearing his full manifest farpoint refractive correction. Unless otherwise specified, this same rule applies to all testing procedures involved in the investigation of binocular anomalies.

The following is an example of how the gradient method may be used. The patient has 15 p.d. of exophoria at far. This is determined either by objective means, such as using the cover test, or subjectively by diplopia testing, such as with the single-object method (e.g., Maddox rod). A spherical lens of -2.50 diopters is placed before each eye. The patient is instructed to focus and clear the fixation target while looking through the lenses. When he reports the target is clear, another measurement of the angle of deviation is made. If the lenses cause the angle to change from 15 exo to ortho, the AC/A is 6/1. This is determined by dividing the change in the deviation by the change of accommodative stimulus[h] (clinically speaking, the power of the added lenses). Thus, 15 divided by 2.50 equals 6 p.d./1 diopter.

CALCULATION FROM FAR AND NEAR DEVIATIONS

There are several ways of calculating the AC/A from farpoint and nearpoint deviations. Flom[10] offers a very useful formula, similar to the following:

$$AC/A = IPD + M (Hn - Hf)$$

Where IPD = Interpupillary distance in centimeters
M = Fixation distance at near in meters
Hn = Objective angle of deviation at near
Hf = Objective angle of deviation at far

Note: ESO deviations have positive (+) values
EXO deviations have negative (-) values

For example, assume the patient with a 60 mm interpupillary distance has 15 p.d. of exophoria at far and is orthophoric at the near fixation distance of 40 cms. The AC/A is 12/1. It is calculated as follows:

$$AC/A = 6 + .4(0 - -15)$$
$$= 6 + .4(+15)$$
$$= 6 + 6$$
$$= 12$$

An AC/A of this magnitude is considered quite high. Normal AC/A

[h]Accommodative response should not be confused with accommodative stimulus. Also, the gradient method is considered to determine a more true AC/A ratio than near-far calculation.

ranges from 4/1 to 7/1. An AC/A greater than 7/1 is high; less than 4/1 is low.

If the patient measured 15 exo at near as well as at far, the AC/A would be 6/1. Table 1J gives the calculated answers for various angles of deviations at far and near. By looking at this table, two useful rules can be visualized. First, the AC/A is equal to the patient's interpupillary distance when the deviations at far and near are the same. For instance, ortho (0) on both scales for angle H intersects at 6/1. The AC/A is 6/1 on the chart whenever the angles of deviation are equal.

Also, a zero AC/A is very improbable, and a negative one is probably impossible. The table indicates those spurious combinations that could produce zero or negative AC/A's. If these result, the examination of the magnitudes of deviation for far and near should be rechecked. For example, if the patient has an interpupillary distance of 60 mm, a measurement of ortho at far and 15 exo at near produces an AC/A of zero and is probably an artifact. However, this deviation of ortho at far and 15 at near is possible if the interpupillary distance were larger. If, for instance, the p.d. is 70 mm, instead of 60 mm, the AC/A would be 1/1, which may occur. Refer to the AC/A formula for explanation of I P D size affecting AC/A.

Regarding the gradient method versus the near-far calculation method, the gradient method will often give a lower AC/A. The depth of focus may cause the accommodative response to be less than the accommodative stimulus. Thus, the denominator of the AC/A is falsely large making the fraction arithmetically smaller. (A gradient value of more than 5/1 is considered high.)

The calculation method may yield a higher value because proximal convergence is often a factor when fixation is shifted from far to near. Both methods are useful; but in general, calculation is more reliable than the gradient method (particularly in cases of strabismus).

Variability of the Deviation and Cosmesis

There are many influences on tonic convergence[i] which, in turn, affect the magnitude of deviation. In cases of heterophoria, these changes are not obvious until dissociative testing is performed, and the findings are compared with each other from day to day. However, significant changes in cases of heterotropias are observable and may have a striking effect on the patient's appearance when the deviation changes from being just noticeable to one that is very noticeable.

In all binocular anomalies, the cosmetic appearance of a strabismus is usually the patient's greatest concern. It is important that the doctor

---

[i]According to Maddox, this is one of the four components of convergence; the other three: accommodative, fusional (reflex), and proximal (psychic). While tonic convergence is evaluated as being either high (eso) or low (exo), measurement of this angle cannot be done by ordinary clinical means. The theoretical angle of tonic convergence according to Hebbard[11] is the magnitude of angular movement of the eyes made by the visual axes when convergence is from the anatomical position of rest (out and upward positions) as in death with no innervation to the eyes to the dissociated position at farpoint (angle of deviation measured by clinical means). For clarification, see Appendix for illustration of the four components of convergence.

TABLE 1J. The AC/A Calculations from Far and Near Deviations for an Interpupillary Distance of 60 Millimeters

			Angle H at Far														
		EXO							ESO							
		35	30	25	20	15	10	5	0	5	10	15	20	25	30	35
ESO	35	34	32	30	28	26	24	22	20	18	16	14	12	10	8	6
	30	32	30	28	26	24	22	20	18	16	14	12	10	8	6	4
	25	30	28	26	24	22	20	18	16	14	12	10	8	6	4	2
	20	28	26	24	22	20	18	16	14	12	10	8	6	4	2	0
	15	26	24	22	20	18	16	14	12	10	8	6	4	2	0	
	10	24	22	20	18	16	14	12	10	8	6	4	2	0		
	5	22	20	18	16	14	12	10	8	6	4	2	0			
	0	20	18	16	14	12	10	8	6	4	2	0				
EXO	5	18	16	14	12	10	8	6	4	2	0					
	10	16	14	12	10	8	6	4	2	0						
	15	14	12	10	8	6	4	2	0							
	20	12	10	8	6	4	2	0								
	25	10	8	6	4	2	0									
	30	8	6	4	2	0										
	35	6	4	2	0											

(left axis label: Angle H at Near)

understand this and have empathy for the patient's feelings in this regard. Attempting to reduce this anxiety is important.

CHANGE IN THE MAGNITUDE OF DEVIATION

Changes in the magnitude of deviation may occur for various reasons. Fatigue, emotional stress, medication, and other possible factors may be involved. A variation in the magnitude of the angle of deviation may cause a latent deviation to become manifest. A case of intermittent strabismus is usually more noticeable than if it were constant. It should be noted, however, that intermittency is not always the result of a change in the magnitude of deviation. Intermittency also involves the power of fusion, whereby a deviation may or may not be held latent.

ANATOMICAL FACTORS IN COSMESIS

In addition to magnitude, its variability, and the intermittency of the deviation there are certain anatomical factors affecting cosmesis. These are listed in Table 1K. The table indicates those which are favorable and those which are unfavorable to the appearance of patients with esotropia or exotropia.

Unfortunately, some practitioners tend to judge cosmesis almost exclusively on the basis of the magnitude of the deviation. Too often, other factors are not considered. For example, the recommendation to undergo surgery for cosmetic reasons may be given a patient having an esotropia of 20 p.d. This procedure, however, would not be efficacious if the patient has a large positive angle kappa, a narrow bridge, no epicanthal folds, a large interpupillary distance, and a narrow face. Under these conditions, the eyes are likely to appear cosmetically straight. It is probable that the eyes would appear exotropic if the eso deviation were significantly reduced by means of surgery.

TABLE 1K. Anatomical Factors in Cosmesis of Strabismus	
Favorable for Esotropia Unfavorable for Exotropia	Favorable for Exotropia Unfavorable for Esotropia
Positive angle kappa	Negative angle kappa
Narrow bridge of nose	Wide bridge of nose
Absence of epicanthus	Presence of epicanthus
Large interpupillary distance	Small interpupillary distance
Narrow face	Wide face

It is always best to observe the patient carefully and weigh the various factors influencing appearance before reaching any conclusions regarding cosmetic surgery.

Facial asymmetries are frequently seen in strabismic cases. It may be important to consider consultation by a plastic surgeon in certain cases.

The effect of eyewear on cosmesis should also be taken into account. A certain spectacle frame may either help or hinder the strabismic's appearance. Trial of different sizes and patterns, and keen observation of the patient's appearance, are the rules to follow.

Eye Laterality   In cases of strabismus, eye laterality shows whether one eye is able to maintain fixation, or if either eye is able to do so. This determination should be made at far and near fixation distances. If only one eye is able to fixate, the strabismus is classified as being unilateral. If either eye can fixate, it is an alternating strabismus.

Alternation should be classified as either habitual or forced. Habitual alternation means the patient switches fixation naturally, without awareness. Forced alternation is when the patient must be aware or coaxed to alternate. The degree of forcing indicates the patient's tendency to alternate and should be included in the evaluation of the eye laterality.

Evaluation is made by means of such tests as the Hirschberg, unilateral cover test, case history, and direct observation of the patient under natural seeing conditions. From these, the doctor judges whether the patient fixates with either eye or only one eye.

One interesting characteristic of many strabismics is their alternations of fixation upon lateral versions. The doctor observes whether or not the patient switches fixation at the midline as pursuits proceed back and forth laterally. In the left field an esotropic patient prefers the right eye for fixation, while on dextroversion, the left eye is preferred. The presence of such a "mid-line switch" should be recorded. This is often associated with congenital esotropia with anomalous correspondence.[j]

Eye dominancy refers to the superiority of one eye over the other. This may be in the motor or in the sensory realm.

Eye Dominancy

Sighting tests which determine the eye preferred for fixation are examples of motor tests for dominancy. In strabismus cases, eye preference and eye dominancy are used synonymously. The unilateral cover test is the most commonly used means of determining the fixating eye in strabismus. If the deviation is large enough to be observed, the Hirschberg test is a practical means for evaluation.

In heterophorias where the deviation is latent and not observable, except upon dissociation, sighting tests such as the hole-in-the-card test should be used. With both hands, the patient holds at arm's length a card having a small hole in the center and sights a distant fixation target. The doctor alternately occludes each eye to determine which eye the patient is using to sight the target.

The convergence nearpoint test is another means of determining which eye is superior in motoric functioning. The eye to first stop pursuing the advancing target is considered to be nondominant.

Testing of fixation disparity and accommodation facility are other indices to motor dominancy (to be discussed in Chapter Two).

Practical dominancy testing in the sensory realm includes testing of retinal rivalry, color fusion, and suppression.

In a strabismus evaluation, eye dominancy is determined by finding which eye is preferred for fixation. This should be determined at far and near, as there may be a difference when the fixation distance is changed. This is an example of mixed dominancy (meaning one eye is preferred for some functions but not for others).

In the evaluation of heterophoria, eye dominancy is determined by testing for sensorial and motoric superiority between the two eyes. In the past, great interest has been shown in crossed dominancy (the dominant eye and the dominant hand being on opposite sides of the body). The relationship between crossed dominancy and learning disabilities was once considered by some authorities to be significant, although the recent trend is away from this thinking.

---

[j]This type of alternation should be referred to as a "cross-fixation pattern" and is not truly alternating as to fixation demands in the primary position of gaze.

2 | Adaptive Conditions Commonly Associated with a Deviation of the Visual Axes

Several possible anomalous conditions often develop when a deviation of the visual axes causes the fovea of one eye to be used for fixation, while at the same time, the fovea of the other eye is not fixating. When bifoveal fixation fails to be achieved, adaptive responses may result. These conditions and the appropriate testing methods for them are discussed in this chapter.

Although it is customary to think in terms of the deviation causing the adaptive anomalous conditions, it is important to remember that the process may work in reverse. In other words, the deviation may be the end result rather than the cause of existing anomalous conditions.

When a manifest deviation of the visual axes occurs to produce a strabismus, the individual may have confusion and/or diplopia (of the pathological type as distinguished from physiological diplopia). Judging from the frequency of complaints in this regard, young children apparently are less likely than adults to be aware of these annoyances. More meticulous case histories may reveal higher incidences of childhood diplopia than have been heretofore presumed. In any event, regardless of age, diplopia rather than confusion is more likely to be noticed and reported.

Suppression is the mechanism first attempted by an individual to eliminate the annoyances of diplopia and/or confusion in his visual space.

Suppression

While it is not precisely known how suppression is brought about, why it is done is easily explained. Figure 2-1a illustrates the concept of confusion and diplopia. The fixation target is represented by a star and is imaged on the fixating left eye. The esotropia of the right eye causes the star to be seen by the nasal portion of the retina of the right eye. Cyclopean projection shows the patient is able to perceive two stars. Since the diplopic image is seen on the same side as the eye that deviates, the diplopia is homonymous (uncrossed).

CHARACTERISTICS OF SUPPRESSION

For the redundant ocular image[a] to be eliminated, the retinal point in the right eye on which the star is placed must be suppressed. Jampolsky[1] refers to such a location as the "zero measure" point where suppression must occur if diplopia is to be avoided.

While the zero point is usually suppressed, the fovea in the deviating eye is suppressed more intensely. If this were not the case, confusion would result for the person with strabismus. As in Figure 2-1a the left eye has a star imaged on its fovea while the deviating right eye has a circle on its fovea. This may result in perception of superimposition of two dissimilar objects. This is the phenomenon of confusion and is more intolerable to normal seeing than diplopia; therefore, a more intense suppression is ordinarily required at the fovea to eliminate confusion (retinal rivalry occurring) than at point zero for the avoidance of diplopia.

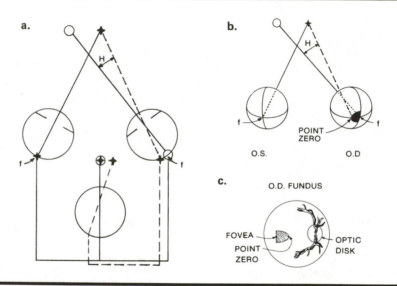

FIGURE 2-1 — Illustrating diplopia and confusion and the accompanying zone of suppression. (a) Esotropic right eye and the patient's perception of confusion and pathological homonymous diplopia. The fixated object is the star which is seen diplopically. The non-fixated circle falling on the fovea of the deviating eye causes confusion. Note: the circle may also by seen diplopically, but is not an aggravation to the patient since attention is not being given to this. (b) Theoretical posterior view of the eyes showing the suppression zone that might result from an esotropia of the right eye. (c) Ophthalmoscopic view of the right fundus illustrating the shape and location of the suppression zone in this example of esotropia.

It is probable that suppression begins first at the fovea when a deviation of the visual axes becomes manifest; then point zero is also suppressed. After this, a pathological zone of suppression encompasses the area between the fovea and point zero of the deviating eye. The vertical dimension of the zone is normally smaller than the horizontal. The shape of the zone resembles the

[a]Ocular image refers to the visual perception of the object. It is distinguished from the term, dioptric image, which solely refers to the focused image on the retina.

letter D, according to Jampolsky[2]; and the vertical demarcation being at the fovea is in the manner of an hemianoptic visual field defect. Figure 2-1b shows a theoretical posterior view of the typical zone in an esotropic eye. A clinical fundus view of the right eye indicating the location of the suppression zone is shown in Figure 2-1c.

It is apparent from clinical findings that suppression is occasionally found to be more extensive than the discussed theoretical D-shaped suppression zone. These cases may respond as though much, and sometimes all, of the retina of the deviating eye is suppressed.

Foveal suppression may occur in nonstrabismic as well as strabismic cases. Typically, these patients have anisometropia. It is thought that the size difference between the dioptric images (causing aniseikonia) may be one reason for foveal suppression of an eye. Another cause may be a great difference in clarity between the two ocular images which leads to suppression of the one most blurred. Suppression is therefore necessary to eliminate the confusion arising from the resulting superimposition of ocular images which are either unequal in size or in clarity.

It should be pointed out that when suppression occurs in cases without strabismus, the condition of an extra foveal point zero does not exist. In such cases point zero is at the fovea and confusion, not diplopia, may be the problem. The suppression zone in these cases may be relatively small and encircle only the fovea.

The mechanism of suppression has been described in terms of portions of the retina being suppressed. This implication notwithstanding, the location of the suppressing mechanism is not known for sure, but probably is in the visual cortex, not the retina.

Suppression may be classified by means of two variables: size, and intensity. In regard to size, suppression is referred to as being either central or peripheral. If it is classified as central, the maximum edge of the suppression zone extends five degrees or less from the center of the fovea. Peripheral suppression refers to a zone extending greater than five degrees from the center of the fovea.[b] If, for instance, the suppression zone represented in Figure 2-1c has a dimension of 6 degrees from the fovea to point zero, the suppression is referred to as peripheral. Suppression testing is necessarily measured under artificial conditions, and information as to the exact zone size during habitual natural seeing is often elusive.

Intensity of suppression is classified as being either deep or shallow. This is a qualitative determination. It is made by finding the ease with which suppression can be broken by utilizing various procedures. Generally speaking, the more unnatural the environment (laboratory type of testing conditions), the less likelihood there is of suppression; conversely, the more

---

[b]This is an arbitrary value but one fairly well in accord with clinical usage as well as with related topics throughout this book. For example, eccentric fixation greater than five degrees is considered to be peripheral.

natural the environment, the more likely is the patient to suppress.

In effect, intensity is described in terms of the testing procedure that is dissociative enough for suppression to be broken and diplopia to be perceived.

Some of the various methods commonly used to test the intensity of suppression are listed in Table 2A. The more natural tests are noted at the top, with the less natural following in descending order. Using this as a guide, it is reasonable to assume, for example, that a strabismic patient who notices pathological diplopia when viewing ordinary objects in free space has very shallow, if any, suppression. On the other hand, when more elaborate means such as colored filters are required to elicit diplopia, suppression is probably quite deep.

TABLE 2A. *Commonly Used Testing Procedures for Determination of Intensity of Suppression. (Assume normal room illumination is used. Tests using lights for fixation targets are made less natural by lowering of room illuminations.)*

Naturalness of Testing	General Method of Testing	Specific Instrumentation	Intensity of Suppression
Natural	1. Diplopia in free space	Ordinary objects in free space	Shallow
—		Penlight fixation	—
—	2. Vectographic methods	Pola-Mirror	—
—		Vis-A-Vis	—
—		Vectograms	—
—		Projected targets	—
—	3. Septums	Turville	—
—		Javal Grid	—
—	4. Septums with optical systems	Brewster Stereoscope	—
—		Wheatstone Stereoscope	—
	5. Colored filters		
—	Pink over one eye	Penlight fixation	—
—	Red over one eye	Penlight fixation	—
—	Red-green filters	Red-green print	—
—		Worth lights	—
Unnatural		Penlight fixation	Deep

The following discussion relates suppression to the diagnostic variables of a deviation of the visual axes (discussed in Chapter One).

The magnitude of the deviation affects the size of the suppression zone. Usually, the larger the deviation, the larger the zone. The intensity of the suppression, on the other hand, does not necessarily correlate highly with the magnitude. It may be that a strabismic with a small angle has as deep a suppression as another with a larger deviation.

If the strabismus is alternating, the suppression is usually alternating; that is, the suppression will shift from eye to eye with fixation in an alternating heterotropia. The intensity, however, is usually deeper in the nondominant eye. Not too infrequently, when the nondominant eye is used for fixation, the alternating strabismic is aware of diplopia.

All other factors being equal, clinical experience indicates that an exotropic eye usually has a more extensive and deeper suppression than an esotropic eye. The reasons are not perfectly clear, but it may be that ipsilateral nerve fibers of the visual pathway are suppressed in the exotropic but not in the esotropic eye (where contralateral fibers are involved). For clarification the zero point is on the temporal retina (stimulating ipsilateral fibers to the visual cortex) of an exotropic eye, but on the nasal retina of an esotropic eye (contralateral decussating fibers stimulated). The homolaterality of the deviation being on the same side as the suppressed visual pathway may account for the difference in the intensity of suppression between eso and exo deviations.

The more frequently the deviation is manifest, the deeper the suppression is likely to be. This conclusion is derived from the reports that diplopia is more readily noticed in cases of intermittent rather than constant strabismus.

Cases of strabismus with nonconcomitancy may have suppression that is less deep than those that are concomitant. The intensity is lessened because the magnitude of the deviation is continuously changing as fixation shifts from one gaze to the other. This means that point zero is moving about the retina and is not in a fixed site as it might be in concomitant strabismus. The mechanism of supression is somewhat interrupted by these changes. Fortunately, the accompanying diplopia with nonconcomitancy often warns unsuspecting individuals of possible neurological problems that require professional attention.

TESTING FOR SUPPRESSION

The number of tests for suppression is legion. Only some of the basic methods are presented.

DIPLOPIA UNDER NATURAL CONDITIONS

One of the basic tests for suppression is to determine if diplopia is noticed under natural conditions in free space. By this is meant whether or not the patient reports ordinary objects appearing doubled during casual seeing. For confirmation, a penlight can be used as a fixation target for it is more likely to elicit diplopia than one that is unilluminated.

Noncorresponding retinal points in each eye must be stimulated before diplopia can occur. Physiological diplopia is the normal type that occurs for a nonfixated object. This was illustrated in Figure 1-12. Suppression of the physiological type is necessary to keep nonfixated objects from being perceived as doubled. The beneficial effect of eliminating doubleness throughout a person's space world by means of physiological suppression is obvious. It happens, although not too commonly, that a patient seeks professional care because of a fleeting awareness of physiological diplopia. Reassurance with an explanation of this normal phenomenon is all that is generally required.

The diplopia reported by patients with strabismus, however, is practically always of the pathological type. Figure 1-13 shows an exotropia of the right eye giving rise to heteronymous (crossed) diplopia. The dioptric image falls on point zero, located on the retina temporal to the fovea. For diplopia to be avoided, point zero must be suppressed. The suppression occurs with varying intensity, depending upon the status of the binocularity. For instance, if an exotropia is concomitant, unilateral and constant, an intense suppression at point zero can be expected.

SENSORY FUSION

There are four levels regarding sensorial fusion of form. This classification is a modification of the categories of fusion recommended by Worth.[3] They are as follows:

> Simultaneous Perception (Diplopia)
> Superimposition (first-degree fusion)
> Flat Fusion (second-degree fusion)
> Stereopsis (third-degree fusion)

These categories of binocular sensorial status can be conveniently tested by using vectrographic, colored filters, and the numerous methods employing septum arrangements. Of these methods, most authorities consider vectrographics as being most similar to natural, ordinary seeing conditions during binocular testing.

SIMULTANEOUS PERCEPTION

Although simultaneous perception is classified as one of the levels of sensory fusion, there is actually no real fusion with this particular binocular demand. Simultaneous perception is determined to be present merely by the patient's awareness of binocular images at the same time. In clinical usage, simultaneous perception refers to the stimulation of noncorresponding retinal points which give rise to diplopia. An example is shown in Figure 2-1a where the fixated star is seen diplopically because the dioptric image is on a noncorresponding point of the deviated right eye.

The usual test applied in determining if the patient can appreciate simultaneous perception is to elicit a diplopic response when one object (e.g., penlight) is fixated. When deep suppression interferes with diplopia testing, it may be desirable to stimulate a noncorresponding point somewhere outside of the suppression zone. This is conveniently done by placing a vertically oriented loose prism before the deviating eye to elicit a diplopic response (Figure 2-1b shows the D-shaped suppression zone). If a sufficiently large base-down prism is placed before the right eye, the dioptric image of the star is located below the suppression zone (inferior retina) and will be perceived (in the visual field) as superior to the fixated star. When suppression is very deep, this technique is useful in determining the horizontal subjective angle of deviation.

Simultaneous perception testing may be carried out by using two objects rather than one. These targets are usually stereograms designed for use in a stereoscope. A familiar example is the Keystone Test 1 (DB-10A). A picture of a pig is seen only by the left eye; a dog, by the right eye. If the suppression zone is very large and encompasses one picture, one of the animals will appear to be missing.

The superimposition of two dissimilar targets is known as first-degree fusion. However, when this occurs, confusion rather than true sensory fusion exists because similar targets are not being integrated; they merely have common oculocentric directions (see Figure 2-1a [the circle and star seen in a common direction]). Since two dissimilar objects stimulate corresponding retinal points and are perceived as superimposed, the definition of superimposition is satisfied.

Superimposition testing usually requires more instrumentation than a penlight in free space. Stereoscopes containing a different target for each eye (e.g., a circle seen only by the left eye and a star seen by the right eye) are usually necessary. As a result of intense foveal suppression in strabismus, the phenomenon of confusion is rarely noticed in free space.

In the case of a nonstrabismic patient having no foveal suppression, confusion may be brought about by the use of prisms. This artificial simulation of heterotropia makes both diplopia and confusion noticeable. However, this means of achieving superimposition (creating confusion) has little, if any, clinical value. As a general rule, it is not necessary to perform first-degree fusion testing in nonstrabismic patients. Superimposition testing is primarily important in cases of strabismus with anomalous correspondence (to be discussed later).

SUPERIMPOSITION

This is true fusion and is the integration of two similar ocular images into a single percept. There may be one target in free space, such as a page of print, or there may be two identical targets in a stereoscope. In any event, this type of target must be two-dimensional and identical in form for each eye to be classified as a flat fusion stimulus.

Such targets are the most frequently employed in testing and evaluating motor fusion (positive and negative fusional vergence). Usually Snellen letters or printed words are used as targets to be fused with the incorporation of unfused suppression clues in the test-design (see Figure

FLAT FUSION

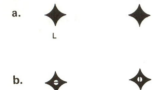

FIGURE 2-2 — Target with flat-fusion demand. (a) Peripheral suppression clues are the R and the L; (b) Foveal suppression clues are the vertical and horizontal lines.

2-2a). In a stereoscope the star with the R is seen only by the right eye, the star with the L only by the left eye.

If the angular separation from the center of the star to the R (or to the L) happens to be greater than five degrees, testing for peripheral suppression is being done. Testing for foveal suppression requires suppression clues to be located in the center of the star such as the small horizontal and vertical lines (see Figure 2-2b). Therefore, the location of the clues that are suppressed determines the size of the suppression. These specifications regarding targets for determination of suppression size are listed in Table 2B.

For flat fusion testing there are numerous varieties of stereograms, as well as special illuminated designs, such as the well-known Worth lights (4-dot test) that are commercially available.

TABLE 2B. Size of Suppression

Classification	Separation from the center of the fused object to the suppression clue
CENTRAL	5 degrees or less
Foveal	1 degree or less
Parafoveal	3 degrees or less (but greater than 1)
Paramacular	5 degrees or less (but greater than 3)
PERIPHERAL	Greater than 5 degrees

STEREOPSIS

Stereopsis is the perception of three-dimensional visual space due to binocular clues. These test targets are similar to those of flat fusion with one exception; there is lateral displacement in certain portions of the target. The displacement of a set of paired points (referred to as homologous points) is relative to the position of other pairs of homologous points on the stereogram. For example, in Figure 2-3, consider the star as the figure that is fixated and fused. The small x's on the top are displaced inwardly (base-out effect when targets are viewed through a Brewster stereoscope), relative to the fused star. Contrarily, the y's are displaced outwardly (creating a base-in or divergence demand).

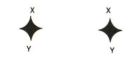

SEEN BY O.S   SEEN BY O.D.

FIGURE 2-3 — Stars for fusion and disparate X's and Y's for binocular depth clues

Assume the patient is concentrating on the fused star. The x's are imaged on each retina temporally in relation to the star. This causes the fused x to appear closer than the star. The opposite is true for each y which is disparately nasalward on the retina. This creates the perception of the composite y appearing to be farther away. The rule to remember is that if the disparity is temporalward from the center of the fovea, the stereoscope image will appear closer; if the disparity is nasalward, it will appear farther. If the disparities become too far apart, the x's and y's can no longer be fused (by remaining within Panum's areas) and are seen diplopically. They fall on points too disparate and cause diplopia in the same manner as in simultaneous perception testing. However, if the disparities are not too great, the targets are fusible even though they do not fall exactly on corresponding retinal points. This is due to the allowance in disparity afforded by Panum's area. It is this small fused disparity that is responsible for stereopsis. As in flat fusion testing, there are suppression clues in stereopsis testing, and these are those portions of the stereogram that are supposed to be seen in depth, relative to a fixated point. In the above example, the clues are the fused x and y. The lack of depth may be an indication of either suppression or anomalous correspondence.

Stereoacuity may also be evaluated by comparing the relative distance of two objects in free space, such as in the traditional Howard-Dolman peg test. This is designed for farpoint measurements. The test consists of two black movable vertical rods viewed through an aperture against a white background. The patient is seated at a distance of six meters from the rods and instructed not to move his head. Otherwise, lateral parallax will be induced, thereby invalidating testing procedures. The rods are moved by the patient, either nearer or farther from each other, by means of strings until they appear to be equally distant; i.e., in the same plane. The distance error is determined from an average of several trials. This is converted from millimeters into seconds of arc and represents the stereoacuity (see Table 2C). For example, if the error (the distance the patient misaligns the two pegs) is 60 mm, the stereoacuity is 20 seconds of arc.

Because there may be a constant error due to a skewed or tilted horopter, testing results may be invalid. The *standard deviation* of the mean would represent a truer measure of stereoacuity. This would take about 15 trials and is seldom done on a routine clinical basis.

An apparatus of the Howard-Dolman type may be custom-made or obtained through commercial sources. One such available instrument is the Lafayette #14012 Depth Perception Apparatus.[c]

For nearpoint testing, the Verhoeff Stereoptor[d] is the most widely used. It has an illuminated white window in which three vertically placed black strips are centered. One of the strips is displaced from the plane of the other two, either forward or backward. The patient is asked to tell which strip is different in distance from the other two. The instrument can be adjusted to form eight different strip arrangements (eight different targets).

A patient with a stereoacuity of 31 seconds of arc or better should be able to report all eight targets correctly at a testing distance of 1 meter. The better the stereoacuity, the farther away the test can be held for the eight

[c]Mfg. by Lafayette Instrument Co.

[d]Mfg. by American Optical Corporation, Scientific Instrument Division, Buffalo, N.Y. 14215.

correct answers. The poorer the stereoacuity, the closer the instrument must be held for all correct responses. Table 2D lists these distances and the corresponding stereoacuities for the Verhoeff Stereoptor.

TABLE 2C. Howard-Dolman Test for Stereopsis. Performed at 6 meters. Assume I.P.D. of 60mm. Stereoacuities were determined by the following formula:

$$Eta = I.P.D. \, (x)/d^2 \times 206,000$$

Eta: symbol for stereoacuity in seconds of arc
I.P.D.: interpupillary distance in mm
x: alignment error in mm
d: testing distance from patient to rods in mm

Alignment error (mm)	Stereoacuity
5	2"
10	3"
20	7"
30	10"
40	13"
50	16"
60	20"
80	26"
100	33"
200	66"
300	99"
400	132"
500	165"

VECTOGRAPHIC METHODS

Applying the principle of polarization to the testing of vision allows the use of suppression clues during fairly natural conditions of binocular seeing. For such testing, the patient wears polarizing filters in the form of spectacles. The polarizing filter for one eye must be rotated to an angle of 90 degrees from the filter for the other eye. This achieves mutual exclusion of light coming to each eye. Thus, when the test targets are also polarized, one eye cannot see certain portions of the test target that are visible to the other eye.

In the U.S.A. the filters in commercially available polarizing spectacles are usually oriented at 45 and 135 degrees; those manufactured in many other countries are set at 90 and 180 degrees.

POLARIZING SPECTACLES AND MIRROR

The use of polarizing spectacles (having crossed axes) with an ordinary mirror to determine the status of binocularity was devised by Griffin. The patient merely looks at himself in the mirror while wearing the spectacles to see if both eyes can be seen.

This test was clinically evaluated by Griffin and Lee.[4] Seventeen orthoptic patients were tested. All of those who had relatively poor stereoacuity (more than 60 seconds of arc) failed, while all with relatively

---

TABLE 2D. Verhoeff Stereoptor Testing Distance and Corresponding Stereoacuities. All eight targets must be responded to correctly. The following stereothreshold values are calculated for an interpupillary distance of 60 mm. The eta value (stereoacuity) are calculated using an x value of 2.5mm. This is the displacement of one strip from the plane of the other two strips. The same formula as applied with the Howard-Dolman test is used to calculate Verhoeff stereoacuities.

Test Distance (cm)	Stereoacuity (seconds of arc)
10	3090"
20	772"
30	343"
50	124"
60	86"
80	48"
100	31"
110	26"
130	18"
150	14"
200	8"
300	3"

---

good stereoacuity (less than 60 seconds of arc) passed this test.

Failing means the patient can see only one eye at any given moment; the other eye appears blackened. The blacking-out occurs in the suppressed eye because it cannot see itself under binocular conditions. The fixating or nonsuppressing eye, cannot see the other eye because of the effect of crossed polarization. Light traveling from the suppressing eye to the mirror and on to the fixating eye is excluded.

The recommended procedure for testing requires the patient to wear polarizing spectacles while holding a mirror approximately 25 cms (10 inches) from his face. The specific instructions are as follows:

1. "Look at yourself in the mirror and tell me which eye you can see." If the response is that both eyes are seen at the same time, suppression is not indicated. If only one eye can be seen at a time while the other looks black, suppression is present.
2. "Close one eye and tell me what you see." This confirms the

response. The closed eye should be reported as appearing black.

3. "Open both eyes and tell me if you see one eye that looks black." If one eye is black, suppression is indicated. Good binocularity is present if both eyes are seen at the same time.

The effectiveness of this procedure in mass screening for suppression and other binocular problems in which suppression may be involved (e.g., amblyopia, anomalous correspondence, and anisometropia) was studied by Griffin[5] using a population of 295 high school students. The procedure was compared to a standard screening procedure, the Modified Clinical Technique[6]. There was a very high correlation between the two methods in detection of binocular anomalies.

A similar study by Heikkla and Dennis[7] indicated that the overall effectiveness of this method is greatly enhanced by the inclusion of visual acuity testing.

This procedure is called the Pola-Mirror test.[e] It is also an effective means to demonstrate to a patient (or parent of a patient) what "suppression" is.

TWO POLARIZING SPECTACLES

The Vis-A-Vis Test, devised by Griffin, is similar to the Pola-Mirror test with the following exception: both the examiner and the examinee wear polarized spectacles (see Figure 2-4). This is also a good test for screening laterality and directionality of perceptual dysfunctions.

The recommended procedure for this test is as follows:

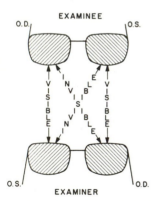

EXAMINEE
O.D.   O.S.

O.S.   O.D.
EXAMINER

FIGURE 2-4 — Illustration of the effect of polarization of light in the Vis-A-Vis method of testing for suppression

1. The patient looks binocularly at the examiner from a distance of 50 cms (20 inches) and is asked which of the examiner's eyes he can see.

2. The patient is instructed to close either his right or left eye and report which of the examiner's eyes he can see. This test may be used for the perceptual testing of "laterality" and "directionality" in conjunction with suppression testing. Laterality refers to one's awareness of left and right body sidedness. When the patient closes his right eye (either a voluntary blink or with finger), determine if he demonstrates good laterality by knowing which eye or hand to use. In testing for directionality (egocentric localization), ask the patient to report which appears black to him with his right eye closed. Determine if he can accurately point to the eye that appears to be black.

3. Have the patient open both eyes and report whether one of the examiner's eyes is blacked-out at any one moment. If both eyes are seen, suppression is assumed to be absent.

If necessary, both the Pola-Mirror and the Vis-A-Vis techniques can be made more sensitive for detecting central suppressions by increasing the test

[e]Crossed polarizing filters and a flat mirror are used in normal room illumination.

distance, although foveal suppressions are usually detectable at the recommended testing distance of 50 cms.

The popularity of vectogram orthoptics is largely attributable to Dr. B.E. Vodnoy,[8] who promotes a popular series of different vectographic targets designed for use in the Polachrome Orthopter[f] for binocular evaluation.

One of the #2 Quoit slides (see Figure 2-5) can be used along with a figure from a different slide, such as Little Bo Peep (See Figure 2-6), that seen only by the right eye is to be superimposed with the quoit that is visible only to the left eye.

If suppression is active, one of the targets may disappear. Peripheral suppression of the left eye is indicated if the quoit is not visible when both eyes are open. If, however, the deviating eye sees the quoit, the targets can be switched so the suspected suppressing eye views the smaller of the two targets, i.e., Bo Peep slide rather than the large circular quoit. This is for more central testing, and central suppression is more likely to be found than peripheral suppression.

As stated earlier, superimposition is actually a simulation of confusion in natural space. This explains why the more central target often disappears as a result of suppression when the targets are superimposed. On the other hand,

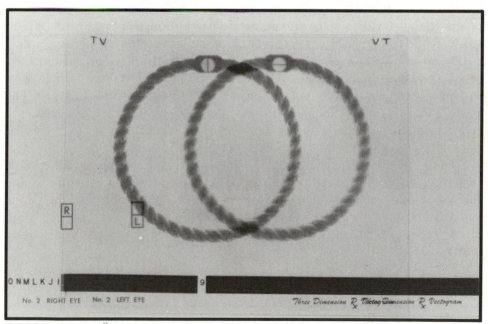

FIGURE 2-5 — The #2 vectographic Quoits Slides

[f]Available through Bernell Corp.

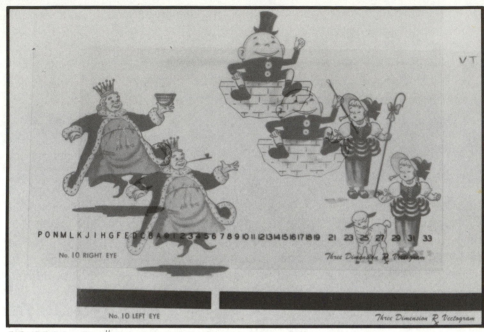

FIGURE 2-6 — The #10 vectographic Mother Goose Slides

when testing involves only simultaneous perception, suppression is not as likely to be found since extra foveal areas are stimulated. Suppression may occur, however, when a relatively small target is placed on point zero.

A popular Flat Fusion vectogram is the #12 target which is a square-x-circle configuration (see Figure 2-7). Vodnoy calls this pair The Basic Fusion slides. The patient fuses the x, common to both eyes, and reports whether either of the suppression clues (the circle or the square) is missing.

The smaller of the rectangular set is designed for nearpoint testing (the larger being for intermediate distances). The central fused target is the x, and the circle and square are parafoveal suppression clues. To test for foveal suppression, the small dots above and below the x's are used as suppression clues. These dots are also useful in fixation disparity testing (to be discussed later).

The #12 target also includes eccentric circles creating a test for qualitatively determining the presence or absence of stereopsis.

The booklet called the Titmus Stereo Tests[g] is perhaps the most popular test for measuring stereo acuity. The patient wears polarizing spectacles during the testing procedures. The booklet contains a picture of a housefly used as a gross stereopsis test (approximately 3000 seconds of arc) and three rows of animal pictures (see Figure 2-8).

---

[g]Mfg. by Titmus Optical Co. and available through many local optical suppliers.

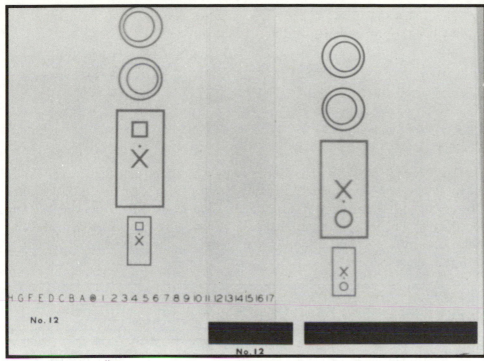

FIGURE 2-7 — The #12 vectographic Basic Fusion Slides

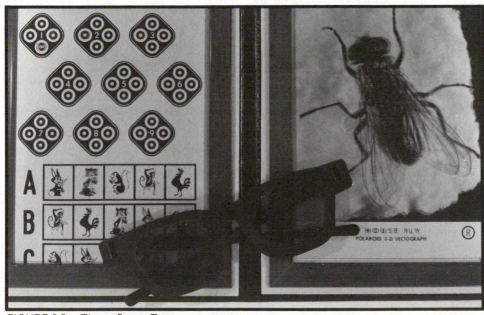

FIGURE 2-8 — Titmus Stereo Tests

The following answers and stereoacuities for the rows of animals are given when the test is performed at 40 cms. (16 inches):

ROW	APPEARING CLOSER	ANGLE OF STEREOPSIS IN SECONDS
A	Cat	400
B	Rabbit	200
C	Monkey	100

The booklet also contains a series of nine diamonds having four circles in each. These are modified Wirt rings (devised by Dr. S. Edgar Wirt). Corresponding stereoacuities for the Wirt rings test at 40 centimeters are listed in Table 2E. The values change if testing distance is changed, and this must be kept consistent for valid comparisons when testing the patient at different times.

TABLE 2E. Key for the Wirt Rings Test for Testing Distance of 40 cm. This is included in the Titmus Stereo Tests booklet.		
SQUARE	ANSWER	ANGLE OF STEREOPSIS IN SECONDS
1	bottom	800
2	left	400
3	bottom	200
4	top	140
5	top	100
6	left	80
7	right	60
8	left	50
9	right	40

When the test booklet is held in the normal upright position, the appropriate circle; e.g., bottom circle in square number 1, should appear to stand out with the patient reporting it as being closer to him. An interesting way to determine if the responses are valid is to turn the booklet upside down. This causes the opposite perception of depth to be apparent to the patient; i.e., the circle that was closest should appear to recede into the booklet and be farther away from the other circles. This trick can also be used with the rows of animals in the booklet. Also, if the booklet is rotated sidewise (only 90 degrees) there should be no stereopsis appreciated.

The best way to evaluate stereopsis when the housefly target is used is to have the patient attempt to pinch the edge of a wing. The normal response is that the pinching fingers should be off the page by several centimeters. This works well with small children as a means of evaluating the quality of sensory fusion. Apell[9] reported that a positive response was found in infants between the ages of 32 and 40 weeks from birth. Usually, though, the patient must be considerably older for reliable testing results to be obtained.

Suppression can be evaluated only indirectly by means of stereopsis testing, but it is axiomatic that the larger and deeper the suppression, the poorer the stereopsis. (Additional vectographic stereopsis tests are discussed in Chapter Fifteen.)

Many projection slides containing crossed polarized targets have been devised in recent years. These afford natural seeing under binocular testing conditions. The popularity of this method has unexplainably remained somewhat limited, possibly because ordinary surfaces (e.g., beaded projection screen) illuminated by projectors break up the uni-directional quality of light that has been polarized by the projecting device. In order to prevent this loss of polarization, special screens must be used. The best screens are those with metallic surfaces, particularly silver or aluminum. If actual metal is not used, a metallic-like surface may be effected by spraying aluminum paint on to a smooth surface. If a pressed wood base is used, the surface must be made perfectly smooth by prior coating with lacquer. Another type of surface that retains polarization quite well is a translucent polyvinyl sheet, often available at yardage stores[h].

With the proper screens suitable for projecting purposes, an overhead projector, such as the popular classroom 3M model[i], can be employed to project vectograms similar to those illustrated in Figures 2-5, 2-6 and 2-7. These vectograms are transformed into farpoint targets, and the same procedures can be applied as with nearpoint testing and therapy.

The above mentioned projecting procedure using large vectograms requires a large wall-mounted screen. When the size of the reflecting screen is a limiting factor, the AO Vectographic Slide[j] may be used for these purposes. The projected size is comparable to that of other visual acuity test slides.

The Vectographic slide has some Snellen letters that are seen by only one eye, some by the other; some unpolarized letters are seen by both eyes. This creates a flat fusion demand with the polarized letters serving as suppression clues. Borish[10] states this can be used for foveal suppression testing.

Another flat fusion demand included in the AO Vectographic slide is a "bull's eye" seen by both eyes, and four lines, two of which are seen only by each eye (see illustration of this in Figure 2-9). Paramacular suppression is

PROJECTED POLARIZED TARGETS

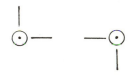

SEEN BY O.D.   SEEN BY O.S.

FIGURE 2-9 — Illustration of portion of the bull's eye target seen by each eye in the A.O. vectographic slide

---

[h]A good commercially available screen is the Mibeck-Stewart Projection System. Mfg. by Stewart Film Screen Corp., 1161 W. Sepulveda Blvd., Torrance, CA 90502.

[i]Mfg. by Minnesota Manufacturing and Mining Co. and available through most suppliers of classroom equipment.

[j]This is the Adult Slide, number 11243. A similar slide for children is number 11246 which has tumbling E's, and pictures for suppression and stereopsis testing. These are manufactured by American Optical Corp., Scientific Instrument Division, Buffalo, N.Y. 14215, and are available through many local optical suppliers.

indicated if two of the lines are not seen. This flat fusion target is excellent for fixation disparity testing (to be discussed later).

Also included in the vectographic slide is a set of third-degree fusion demands. This consists of four rows of circles in which there is a disparate circle in each row to create the perception of stereopsis. Therefore, in each row, one circle should appear to be closer and stand out from the others. The key for this farpoint test giving stereoacuities in seconds of arc is as follows:

First row, 2nd circle forward (240″)
Second row, 4th circle forward (180″)
Third row, 3rd circle forward (120″)
Fourth row, 2nd circle forward (60″)

COLORED FILTERS

The use of colored filters as a dissociation mechanism is popular for both the testing and therapy of binocular anomalies. Most procedures have the advantage of being performed in true space, similar to vectographic techniques.

ONE-COLOR METHODS

A penlight is used as a fixation target while a pink colored lens is placed before the deviating eye. This may cause a strabismic patient, who might otherwise suppress, to become aware of diplopic images of the penlight, one pink and one white. If diplopia does not occur, switching the pink lens to the fixating eye may induce it, because the pink lens attenuates the light going through it and acts as a mild occluder. This inhibits the fixating eye in relation to the deviating eye.

If suppression is too intense for diplopia to be brought out, a dark red filter may be used. This is more dissociative than a light pink filter.

Eliciting diplopia is further aided by reducing the environment (lowering the room illumination) and/or increasing the luminance of the light stimulus of the target. A bright light source in a darkened room tends to break suppression more effectively than a dim light in a well-lit room.

The one-color method lends itself to printed material as well as using light sources as targets. Red reading material (e.g., words typed with red ink) is commonly used for suppression testing and therapy. When the red print is on white paper, the eye with the red filter is unable to see the print since the background appears red, with the figure (print) and ground (paper) being the same. The eye without the red filter is, of course, able to see the red print on the white page. The red filter is placed over the dominant eye so the nondominant eye can be tested for suppression.

TWO-COLOR METHODS

When suppression is too intense for diplopia to be achieved with one-color methods, the patient can wear complementary colored filters. These are usually the color red over one eye and green over the other.

Methods employing colored printed targets rather than lights are termed anaglyphics. Typically the targets consist of red and green (often the green is a blue-green) pictures. When the colored figures are on a white background, the red filtered eye sees the green, not the red figures; conversely, the green filtered eye sees only the red figures. The patient's inability to see both indicates suppression.

A popular commercially available anaglyphic device is the Keystone Basic Binocular Test Set.[k] There are 12 charts that allow for first, second, or third degree fusion testing.

Other anaglyphs are printed on a black background. The most popular example would be the Root Rings[l] (see Figure 2-10). In this procedure, the red filtered eye sees only the red figures, and the green filtered eye sees the green (opposite to a white background).

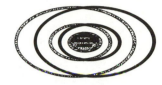

RED
WHITE
GREEN
THE ABOVE FIGURE IS PRINTED ON A BLACK BACKGROUND

FIGURE 2-10 — Drawing of the Root Rings

The patient fixates the center configuration while wearing red-green spectacles. The outer complementary colored rings are laterally disparate creating a stereoscopic effect. This is designed to test peripheral stereo fusion. The outer rings should appear to float forward in relation to the central fixation area if the red filter is before the right eye and the green before the left eye.

In small angle strabismic deviations (less than 10 prism diopters) Panum's areas in the extreme periphery of the retina may allow peripheral third-degree fusion to be appreciated. If, however, suppression is extensive enough to encompass these peripheral areas, then peripheral stereopsis will be adversely affected even though corresponding retinal areas are stimulated.

If the angle of deviation is large, noncorresponding points exceeding the limits of Panum's areas are stimulated, and peripheral stereopsis based upon true fusion in the peripheral visual field does not occur.

Of the different types of instruments used for testing suppression, those having a septum of some sort are very common. They range from the very simple bar readers to the more complex stereoscopes which combine septums with various optical systems of prisms, mirrors, and lenses.

SEPTUMS

This consists of merely interposing a septum somewhere between the patient and the test target in order to dissociate one eye from the other.

BAR READING

If an object such as a pencil, or a finger, is placed in the midline approximately halfway between the patient and a page of printed reading material, the object will obstruct the view of some of the words seen by each eye. Unless both eyes are bifixating and there is no suppression, some of the words are not seen. When a portion of the words in a line of print is not visible, suppression should be suspected.

There are some strabismics who can rapidly alternate (typically a case of congenital alternating esotropia with no amblyopia) and will appear not to

---

[k]Mfg. by Keystone View Division of Mast/Keystone.
[l]Mfg. by Allbee and Son Company.

be suppressing on this particular test. This is because fixation can be switched fast enough for the sentence to be read as though there were no suppression. It is wise to have the patient read without the septum (e.g., bar, pencil, finger) and then compare the speed of reading with the septum in place. A slower reading rate during bar reading indicates suppression, and that flat fusion is poor or absent.

Gibson[11] describes the Javal grid as consisting of five vertical bars fitted with a handle that may be mounted to rest on the page of print. He advised that it is easier to start the patient with the grid held away from the print and slowly move it to the page while maintaining fusion. The use of multiple septums creates a more demanding flat fusion test than when only one is used. In this way, bar reading becomes more sensitive in the detection of suppression.

An example of a patient's view when suppressing while reading through a Javal grid is shown in Figure 2-11. Such devices are available through various ophthalmic suppliers, or they may easily be custom-made.

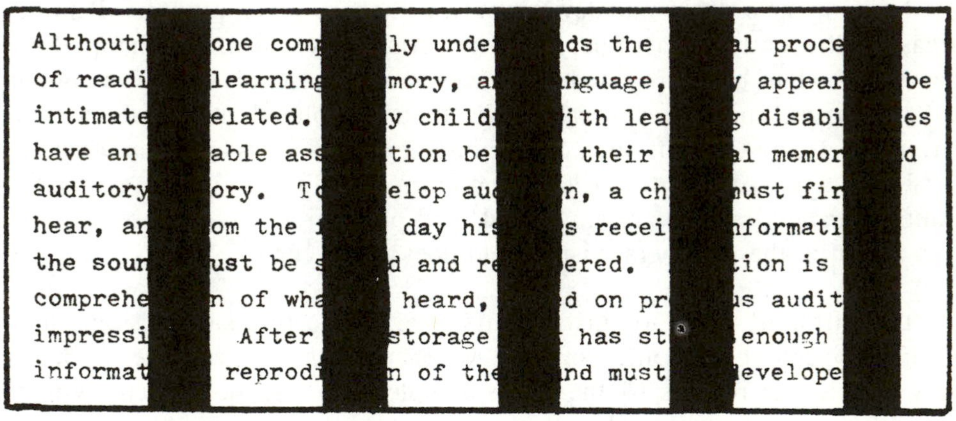

FIGURE 2-11 — Patient's view of printed page through Javal Grid when suppressing one eye

TURVILLE TEST This test was developed by Turville[12] and called the Turville Infinity Balance. The same principle as in bar reading is employed, except that it is designed as a farpoint binocular test rather than one for nearpoint. A vertical septum of approximately 3 cm width is placed midway between the patient and the Snellen chart. This may be positioned in free space at 3 meters in the refracting lane if a 6 meter testing distance is used. If the refracting room is only 3 meters in length and mirrors are used, the septum is placed directly on the mirror in which the patient views the test chart.

Care should be taken by properly placing the septum so that dissociation is achieved. Ideally, the right eye should see only the right half of the Snellen chart, and the left eye only the left half. Under these conditions, the Turville test is not only good for testing suppression, but also for purposes of refracting each eye under binocular conditions. It also provides an excellent means for the evaluation of vertical fixation disparities (to be discussed later).

Instruments of this type are referred to as reflecting stereoscopes. Mirrors are incorporated so that each eye can see independently of the other. This was devised by Charles Wheatstone in 1838. Figure 2-12a shows a sketch of Wheatstone's original optical design.

WHEATSTONE STEREOSCOPES

There have been numerous modifications of this stereoscope resulting in many devices patterned after the same principle. Examples of these are: Synoptophore (Figure 2-12b); Pigeon-Cantonnet Stereoscope (Figure 2-12c); and Bernell Mirror Stereoscope (Figure 2-12d). Keeping in mind the principle of a mirror acting as a septum, it is easily realized that all of these are basically the same.

The Synoptophore[m] is one of the most elaborate of all Wheatstone stereoscopes (see Figure 1-22). This and other similar instruments are classified as major amblyoscopes. Each tube of the Synoptophore has a mirror placed at 45 degrees and a plus 7 diopter eyepiece lens. Test targets are placed at optical infinity. Sketches showing the direction of movement of the carriage arm to create horizontal prismatic demands are presented in Figures 2-13a and b.

The procedure for measuring the objective angle of deviation using this instrument is as follows:

1. Turn on the main switch located on the right hand side (from examiner's view) and have patient look into the instrument.
2. Adjust the chin rest, forehead rest, and the interpupillary distance setting properly for the patient.
3. Adjust the illumination for each tube by setting each rheostat on #8.
4. Place one of superimposition target slides, such as the G47 (fish) and G48 (tank), in each tube. Alternately douse each tube light by means of the two small button switches near the front of the control panel.
5. Have the patient look at the center of each target each time it is illuminated (the other target being dark). It is helpful to take a felt-tip pen and dot the exact center of each slide so that the patient can look there during each fixation, making the position of each fixation more exact. The alternate dousing of each target makes this an alternate cover test, except that it is done in a reduced environment rather than in true space.
6. Neutralize the lateral movement of the eyes by adjusting the position of the tube in front of the nondominant eye. Keep the tube for the dominant eye placed on zero.

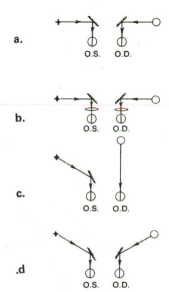

FIGURE 2-12 — Schematic illustrations of optics of various Wheatstone Stereoscopes. (a) Original optical design of Wheatstone (top view shown); (b) Synoptophore by Clement Clarke; (c) Pigeon-Cantonnet Stereoscope (single mirror); (d) Bernell Mirror Stereoscope (double mirror).

---

[m]Mfg. by Clement Clarke, Instrument Division.

7. When the version movement is neutralized, the objective angle of the horizontal deviation (angle H) is determined. The magnitude is read directly either from a red scale in prism diopters or from a black scale in degrees.

A Hirschberg type of testing can also be performed, with a major amblyoscope such as the Synoptophore, by observing the positions of the corneal reflections of the light from the two tubes. For this procedure as in the alternate occlusion technique, the patient must be positioned properly so that the doctor has a good view of the patient's eyes and thus is able to judge the positions of the light reflections.

The procedure for finding angle H by means of corneal reflections with the Synoptophore is as follows:

1. Remove the target from the carriage tube for the nondominant eye.
2. Estimate angle kappa (angle K) of the dominant, fixating eye (eye looking at the dot in the center of the target, e.g., fish).
3. Adjust the tube of the nondominant eye so the corneal reflection is positioned in the same relative position in each eye. The doctor should sight from behind the tube and move with the tube for valid results.
4. When the appropriate position of the light reflection is determined, angle H is read directly from the instrument scale, either in prism diopters (red) or in degrees (black scale).

The procedure for finding the subjective horizontal angle (angle S) with the Synoptophore is as follows:

1. Reinsert the target for the nondominant eye, e.g., the tank.
2. Have the dominant eye continuously fixate the center of the target, e.g., the dot in the center of the fish. The tube for this eye remains at zero on the instrument scale.
3. The target for the nondominant eye (tank) is moved by adjusting the tube so that the two targets appear superimposed, i.e., fish inside the tank. The magnitude of the deviation is read directly from the scale.
4. If the tube is moved toward the doctor (see Figure 2-13a), base-out compensation is introduced and the deviation therefore is eso in direction. If the tube is moved toward the patient in order for superimposition to be achieved, a base-in compensation is given for an exo deviation (see Figure 2-13b).

The objective vertical angle of deviation is better determined by the alternate occlusion method than by reliance on the corneal reflections. The latter method may be too gross for many of the smaller vertical deviations. Vertical deviation adjustments and appropriate scales are located near each tube on the examiner's side of the instrument. The objective angle is measured by how much base-up or base-down must be introduced to neutralize alternate fixating movements taking place for a vertical deviation.

a.

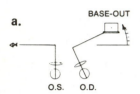

BASE-OUT

O.S.   O.D.

b.

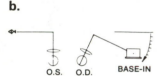

O.S.   O.D.   BASE-IN

FIGURE 2-13 — Illustration of base-in and base-out positions for the Synoptophore. (a) Carriage arm moved toward the examiner is base-out; (b) Carriage arm moved away from the examiner is base-in.

If the tube is raised, a base-down prismatic effect is given that compensates for a hyper deviation. If the tube is lowered, a base-up effect is introduced for compensation of a hypo deviation.

A vertical deviation is subjectively determined in a similar manner as in finding the horizontal subjective angle. If, for instance, the left eye has 4 degrees of hyper deviation, the left tube is elevated 4 degrees by turning the appropriate knob for the compensating base-down effect so that super-imposition can be attained. The corresponding scale for this adjustment reads in degrees rather than prism diopters.

Vertical adjustment may also be effected by adjusting the slide upwards (for base-down) or downwards (for base-up). The scale for this particular vertical adjustment is calibrated in prism diopters.

Cyclo deviations usually have to be determined subjectively. The Synoptophore, as with most major amblyoscopes, can be adjusted so that compensating adjustments for these deviations can be made. It must be remembered that a mirror is used before each eye and that reversal of images occurs. Hugonnier[13] emphasizes this and puts forth the following rule: when the top of the slide is rotated toward the examiner, the compensation is for an excyclo deviation, and when the top of the slide is rotated toward the patient, the compensation is for an incyclo deviation.

The magnitude of a cyclo deviation is read directly from a scale calibrated in degrees. This is found by first achieving superimposition (the fish in the tank, for example) and then rotating the fish until it appears to be swimming horizontally in the tank. The reading for cyclo deviation is then made. Other targets such as the soldier and the sentry box may be more suitable for precise measurements; but, as a rule, most first-degree fusion targets that have linear features are suitable for this purpose.

If one of the targets is not seen, suppression is indicated. Regarding suppression size, slide #G47 subtends angular dimensions of 1½° vertical and 2° horizontal and is useful for foveal and parafoveal suppression testing. Slides such as G1, the soldier, and G2, the sentry box, subtend angles of 12° V, 2½° H and 15° V, 9½° H respectively. These, therefore, are useful in the testing of peripheral suppression. Other dissimilar targets may be an x and a square, or any pair of figures such as these. The above mentioned slides are shown in Figure 2-14.

As with first-degree fusion testing, the Synoptophore is excellent for testing suppression with second degree fusion demands. The initial point of testing under these conditions should be at the patient's subjective angle of deviation. Flat fusion targets in a major amblyoscope are also used in vergence testing. This is the range of motor fusion, i.e., fusional vergences without suppression.

When third degree fusion slides are employed, the targets should be positioned at the ortho position or at the patient's subjective angle if necessary. If depth is not perceived, suppression should be suspected.

The Pigeon Cantonnet stereoscope is a modified Wheatstone stereoscope

EXAMPLES OF SUPERIMPOSITION SLIDES FOR THE SYNOPTOPHORE.

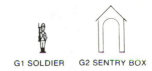

G1 SOLDIER   G2 SENTRY BOX

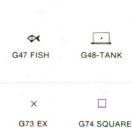

G47 FISH   G48-TANK

×   □

G73 EX   G74 SQUARE

FIGURE 2-14 — Superimposition, or first-degree fusion, slides used in the Synoptophore. G1 and G2 test for peripheral suppression, G47 and G48 test for parafoveal suppression, and G73 and G74 test for foveal suppression.

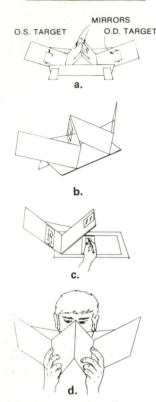

MIRRORS

O.S. TARGET   O.D. TARGET

a.

b.

c.

d.

FIGURE 2-15 — Four views of the Bernell Mirror Stereoscope. (a) Front view; (b) Back view; (c) Used as a Cheiroscope for suppression testing and therapy; (d) Used as a stereoscope for prismatic variation for first-, second-, and third-degree fusion demands.

BREWSTER STEREOSCOPE

that consists of two targets holding baseboards inclined at approximately 135° to each other. A septum holding a mirror bisects the baseboards. First, second and third degree targets may be used in this instrument. Prismatic effects are made by repositioning the targets attached to the baseboards.

A commercially available variation of the Pigeon Cantonnet stereoscope is the Tibbs Trainer[n].

The mirror stereoscope of Bernell is another Wheatstone stereoscope similar to the Pigeon Cantonnet stereoscope. The chief difference is that two mirrors are used for dissociation (see Figure 2-15). The instrument is shaped in the form of the letter W. Prismatic changes are made by varying the angle between the mirrors. This instrument is designed after the stereoscope devised by Javal in the late 1800's (Stéréoscope à Charnière). A range of 40 p.d. base-in to 50 p.d. base-out can be made by simply adjusting the angle of the instrument. For measurement purposes, a scale calibrated in prism diopters is placed at the bottom angles of this stereoscope. The distance from each eye via the mirror to the target is approximately 1/3 meter. Therefore, this, like the Pigeon Cantonnet, is not at optical infinity, but has a definite nearpoint accommodative demand. Unless plus lenses (approximately 3.25 D.Sph.) are worn, all measurements should be considered as being nearpoint findings.

Examples of targets used in the Mirror Stereoscope are shown in Figure 2-16. In Figure 2-16a the fish in the bowl forms a superimposition demand. The square-x-circle pattern is a flat fusion target as well as the chick and egg shown in Figure 2-16b. The doubled circles shown in Figure 2-16c are third-degree fusion stimuli.

Although the mirror stereoscope is intended for home exercises, suppression testing in the office using first, second and third degree sensory fusion targets can be done over a wide vergence demand range requiring motor fusion.

BREWSTER STEREOSCOPE

The refracting type of stereoscope was invented by Brewster a decade after the first Wheatstone stereoscope was devised. Unlike the Wheatstone stereoscope, a true septum is used rather than mirrors for dissociation. Base-out prisms were incorporated for purposes of increasing the lateral field of view and allowing more play in lateral vergences. It can be speculated that because of the compactness of this stereoscope compared to the Wheatstone, the popularity of the refracting stereoscope increased for clinical usage. There are many commercial varieties of the Brewster stereoscope presently available, but all have similar optics.

The schematic top view of such an instrument is shown in Figure 2-17. The eye pieces are +5.00 diopter spherical lenses (can be made from a single spherical lens which is cut in half with each half placed on opposite sides).

[n] Available from several ophthalmic suppliers.

Base-out prismatic effect is created by the optical centers being so far apart relative to the patient's interpupillary distance. This separation, referred to as S, is usually 95 mm. The fixation distance, μ, is 0.2 meters (20 cm) for farpoint testing since this is optical infinity for +5.00 diopter lenses. The letter, h, stands for the distance representing an ortho demand between two homologous points. In Figure 2-17, such points are a star seen by the left eye and a circle seen by the right eye.

The formula to calculate h in millimeters is as follows:

h = S x μ x D (S in mm, μ in meters and D in diopters)

Therefore, from the above, h = 95 x 0.2 x 5

$$h = 95$$

This means that when the homologous points are 95 mm apart, the demand on vergence is zero. In other words, the points are in the ortho position.

For any h value other than 95 mm, a vergence demand is created. A rule to remember is that at 0.20 meters fixation distance, it takes 2 mm to equal 1 p.d. As an example, suppose the star and circle were separated by only 87 mm instead of 95. There is now a difference of 8 mm which represents 4 p.d. (dividing 8 by 2) base-out demand. Conversely, if the h value is 103 mm, 4 p.d. of divergence are required in order to superimpose the star and circle.

While it is true that 95 mm is the theoretical separation for homologous points on a stereogram that represents an ortho demand at optical infinity, the practical h value, and the one almost always used, is 87 mm. This is because most people converge approximately 4 p.d. when looking into the stereoscope, due to the reduced environment of the instrument which tends to cause proximal or psychic convergence. The separation of 87 (representing 4 base-out) is the practical distance that compensates an eso postural shift caused by the instrument.

When nearpoint testing (closer than optical infinity) is performed in a Brewster stereoscope, a new h value must be calculated for the new fixation distance. This is typically 0.133 meters (13.3 cm) which now represents a 2.50 D accommodative stimulus[o] rather than a zero accommodative stimulus when the target is at optical infinity. The h value is calculated for nearpoint as follows:

$$h = 95 \times 0.133 \times 5$$
$$h = 63 \text{ mm}$$

This means that if the homologous points are separated by a distance of 63 mm, the vergence demand at this nearpoint distance of 0.133 meters is ortho.

At this particular distance, it takes 1.33 mm lateral displacement on a stereogram to equal 1 p.d. For example, if the circle and star are 59 mm

---

[o]The 0.133 meter distance has a dioptric value of 7.50; and since the 0.20 meter distance has a diopter value of 5.00 and has five diopter lenses in the instrument, the total demand on accommodation is 7.50 - 5.00 = 2.50 diopters.

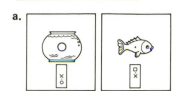
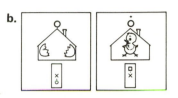
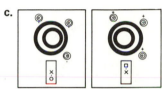

FIGURE 2-16 — Targets used in the Bernell Mirror Stereoscope. (Courtesy of Bernell Corp.) (a) Fish and bowl (FU1 a and b). This pair is a first-degree fusion demand; (b) Chick and egg in house (FU2 L and R). This pair is a second-degree fusion demand; (c) Doubled circles (FU3 L and R). This pair is a third-degree fusion demand.

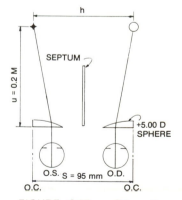

FIGURE 2-17 — Schematic top view of the optics of the Brewster stereoscope

apart, the base-out demand is 3 p.d. (4 divided by 1.33).

Practically all testing using the Brewster stereoscope is performed either at optical infinity (0.20 meters) or at the nearpoint setting (0.133 meters); therefore, for most clinical testing the homologous points are respectively separated 95 mm and 63 mm.

Remembering that at the farpoint, every 2 mm on the stereogram equals 1 p.d., and every 1.33 mm equals 1 p.d. at the nearpoint, any prismatic demand can be determined for any stereogram used in a Brewster stereoscope at these testing distances.

One of the most widely used Brewster stereoscopes is the Keystone Telebinocular[p]. This is shown in Figure 2-18. The visual skills test set is a very popular set of vision screening stereograms that is used with this instrument. The chief purpose and description of each of the 15 stereograms is listed in Table 2F. Although these targets are primarily designed for testing, there are many excellent anti-suppression therapy techniques applicable to these stereograms as well as to the hundreds of other stereograms available from Keystone and from other sources.

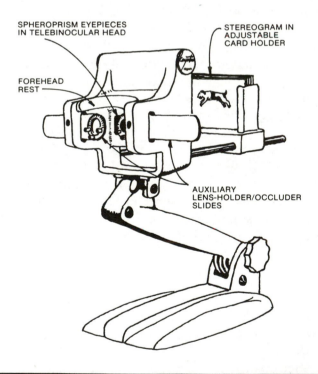

FIGURE 2-18 — Drawing of the Keystone Telebinocular

[p]Mfg. by Keystone View Division of Mast/Keystone.

TABLE 2F. *The Keystone Visual Skills Test Set Related to the Level of Sensory Fusion Demand. Stereograms 1-9 are farpoint tests. Stereograms 10-14 are nearpoint tests.*

Manufacturer's Designations	Sensory Fusion Level	Description
Test 1 (DB-10A) Simultaneous Vision	Simultaneous perception	Dog and pig
Test 2 (DB-8C) Vertical Posture	Simultaneous perception	Numbered figures and horizontal line
Test 3 (DB-9) Lateral Posture	Simultaneous perception	Numbered line and vertical arrow
Test 4 (DB-4K) Fusion	Flat fusion	Red, white, and blue disks
Test 4½ (DB-1D) Usable Vision, O.U.	Stereopsis	Scene of railroad bridge
Test 5 (DB-3D) Usable Vision, O.D.	Stereopsis with flat fusion	Flat-fusion squares, dots acting as suppression clues
Test 6 (DB-2D) Usable Vision, O.S.	Same as Test 5	Same as Test 5
Test 7 (DB-6D) Stereopsis	Third-degree fusion	Rows of figures
Test 8 (DB-13A) Color Perception	No requirement for binocular vision	Colored numbers
Test 9 (DB-14A) Color Perception	Same as Test 8	Same as Test 8
Test 10 (DB-9B) Lateral Posture	Simultaneous perception	Numbered line and vertical arrow
Test 11 (DB-5K) Fusion	Flat fusion	Red, white, and blue disks
Test 12 (DB-15) Usable Vision, O.U.	Fusion not required	Series of circles containing lines or dots
Test 13 (DB-16) Usable Vision, O.D.	Flat fusion	Visual acuity tested under binocular conditions by recognition of dots or lines
Test 14 (DB-17) Usable Vision, O.S.	Same as Test 13	Same as Test 13

The relatively recent introduction of small modified Brewster stereo-scopes that hold color transparencies are useful testing devices for the presence of suppression and have promise as out-of-office vision training devices. Notable among these are the Viewmaster[q] and the Stori-View Stereoscope[r] (see Figure 2-19). Their application for therapy is discussed in Chapters Twelve and Thirteen.

OTHER TECHNIQUES
EMPLOYING SEPTUMS

There have been many other devices with various septum arrangements designed for detection of suppression. The popularity of most of them has waned over the past century. Among those still in common usage are the Remy separator, the diploscope of Remy, and the Maddox Wing test. Discussion of these and many other similar devices would be too lengthy for inclusion in this book. However, the principle of the Remy separator has wide application to therapy, particularly in cases of convergence excess.

The diploscope is principally a diagnostic test, but it is used extensively by some for sensory and motor fusion training in cases of convergence insufficiency and convergence excess.

The Maddox Wing is strictly a diagnostic device designed for the detection and measurement of subjective angles of deviation (lateral, vertical and torsional) at the nearpoint.

SPECIAL LENSES FOR
SUPPRESSION TESTING

Practically all filters and lenses falling in this category involve dissociation to some extent. Three special lenses need mentioning. They are the Maddox rod, the Maddox bi-prism, and Bagolini striated lenses. The first two, at best, allow only for first-degree sensory fusion testing while the striated lenses create a flat fusion demand.

MADDOX ROD

The Maddox rod (or the multiple rod which is more frequently used), is very dissociative, and is made even more so when it is red rather than white. The red multiple Maddox rod is the most dissociative test commonly used, without actually covering an eye with a nontransparent occluder. Because of this, only simultaneous perception (when streak and spot are not aligned) and superimposition (when streak and spot are aligned) may be tested, but not true fusion of form (i.e., second-degree fusion). The absence of either the streak (or part of it) or the spot is indicative of a deep suppression.

BI-PRISM

Maddox designed a bi-prism lens that is less dissociative than the rod test. The lens, in effect, is one prism base-to-base with another. Monocular diplopia can be elicited so that the eye viewing a penlight through this lens will see two lights. The base-to-base axis should be placed horizontally and before the center of the pupil. Monocular diplopia is achieved with one image above the other. The subjective angle of deviation can be determined

---

[q]Mfg. by G.A.F. Co. and available at most camera and department stores.
[r]Mfg. by Visual Data Corp.

by the relative positions of the diplopic lights seen through the bi-prism by one eye and the single light seen by the other eye without the bi-prism. If the diplopic images are properly superimposed and there is no suppression, the patient should perceive three lights in vertical alignment.

BAGOLINI STRIATED LENSES

The Bagolini striated lens[s] is a modern innovation employing the principle of producing a streak similar to that of the Maddox rod. Testing conditions are quite natural, and there is practically no dissociative effect when the striated lenses are used. This is because the etched striations are fine enough to cause no significant interference with vision as is the case with a Maddox rod.

A recommended procedure for using these lenses is described by Winter[14]. A lens is placed in a diagonal orientation before each eye with axes being crossed to produce the ocular image of an x when a small spot of light is fixated. A penlight is an ideal target for these purposes. The orientation marks of the lens are placed at 135 degrees for the right eye and 45 degrees for the left eye. This produces an ocular image for the right eye of a streak oriented from upper right to the lower left. The left eye sees a streak from upper left to lower right. The patient's view by each eye is shown in Figures 2-20a and 2-20b. For purposes of consistency in the interpretation of this test, it is always wise to use the above recommended orientations.

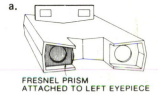

a.

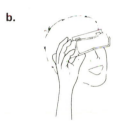

FRESNEL PRISM
ATTACHED TO LEFT EYEPIECE

b.

When the patient fuses the light so that there is no manifest deviation, the perception is an x with the penlight at its intersection (see Figure 2-20c). This percept is also reported by a strabismic patient when his subjective angle (but not the objective angle) of deviation is zero. This indicates harmonious anomalous correspondence.

FIGURE 2-19 — Drawings of the Stori-View Stereoscope. (a) Fresnel prism attached to the left eyepiece; (b) Stereoscope being used by a patient.

Because these lenses are normally less dissociative than either the Maddox rod or bi-prism, suppression is more likely to be detected. An example of central suppression of the left eye is illustrated in Figure 2-20d. Peripheral suppression of the left eye is shown in Figure 2-20e. Sometimes the entire streak will not be seen if peripheral suppression is very extensive.

When the patient is not fusing and the subjective angle of deviation is other than zero, the x will not intersect at the light. Using the above recommended orientations of the Bagolini striated lenses, an esotrope would see the intersection of the lens below the penlights (shown in Figure 2-20f). An exotrope, on the other hand, would see the intersection above (shown in Figure 2-20g). Both lights are shown in these illustrations, but frequently, only one light is noticed by the patient with strabismus. This is because the nonfixated light falls on point zero of the deviating eye and is likely to be suppressed.

MEASUREMENT OF THE
SIZE OF SUPPRESSION

The zone of suppression can be plotted when visual field testing is conducted under binocular conditions. Under monocular conditions, suppression ceases once an eye is occluded. The rationale holds that the greater the dissociation,

---

[s]Available through major ophthalmic suppliers.

the less the suppression (occlusion being the most dissociative of all tests). Depression or contraction in the visual field found during monocular testing is, therefore, due to pathological or other causes and not to suppression.

The three basic ways to measure the size of the suppression zone are by the use of stereocampimetry, the major amblyoscope, and prisms.

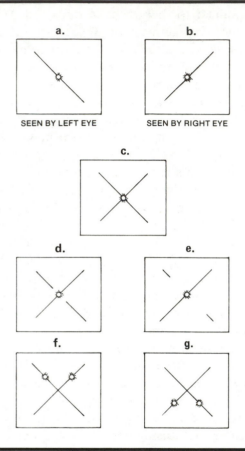

FIGURE 2-20 — Patient's view when looking through striated lenses and fixating a penlight. (a) Orientation of streak seen by left eye; (b) Orientation of streak seen by right eye; (c) Perception when the patient is bifoveally fixating, indicating fusion. This same perception indicates harmonious anomalous correspondence if there is a manifest deviation without the presence of fusion; (d) Central suppression of the left eye; (e) Peripheral suppression of the left eye; (f) This indicates esotropia with normal correspondence, but it may also mean there is a manifest subjective eso deviation in a case of unharmonious anomalous correspondence; (g) This means there is an exotropia with normal correspondence. As in eso deviations, this type of response could also occur in an exotropia with unharmonious correspondence.

STEREOCAMPIMETRY   Stereocampimetry is the testing of the field of vision on a flat surface under binocular conditions.

If polarizing or complementary colored filters are used, binocular testing can be performed using the ordinary tangent screen. The method I prefer is to use red and green fluorescent targets under black-light illumination while the patient wears red-green filters.

In a similar way, the Hess-Lancaster test lends itself to the measurement of suppression zone size. The patient maintains fixation in the primary position on one of the colored spots (e.g., the green) while the doctor moves the other spot (e.g., the red) throughout the field for detection of a suppression scotoma.

Another variation of stereocampimetry using colored filters is the Brock Posture Board. The patient wears red-green filters while viewing a printed or drawn red fixation spot in the center of a white page of paper. The red fixation spot is invisible to the red filtered eye because it blends in with the red background (white page appears red through the red filter). The fixation spot is seen by the green filtered eye as a dark figure on a light green background. While this eye fixates, a red light source is used as a test target to explore the visual field. The light may be white if a red plastic panel is placed under the white page of paper. The light used as the visual field test target is placed behind the red panel. The light shining through the red plastic becomes red, and thus, is seen by the eye with the red filter. When a red plastic panel is not available, any clear panel of plastic or glass works fine as long as the test light is red.

Stereocampimetry is occasionally done in stereoscopes, usually of the Wheatstone variety. The most well-known instrument for this purpose is the once popular Lloyd Stereocampimeter. Dissociation is achieved by an angled mirror permitting one eye to fixate while the visual field of the other eye is tested by small white test targets.

Suppression zones can be measured on a major amblyoscope such as the Synoptophore. Superimposition slides are used. Fixation is maintained in the primary position on one target (e.g., the fish tank) while the other (e.g., fish) is moved base-in, out, up and down. The limits of suppression in all directions are read directly from the dials on the instrument.

MAJOR AMBLYOSCOPE

Jampolsky[15] advocates a practical method for determining the size of the suppression zone with prisms that are introduced before the deviating strabismic eye in various powers and directions until diplopia is just perceived. The extent of the suppression is determined by the power of the prism needed to first induce diplopia in that particular direction. He prefers the Risley prisms rather than loose prisms in this procedure. The advantage of this method of testing is that conditions somewhat approximate those of normal habitual seeing. The size of suppression determined by this method is probably more like the patient's habitual suppression than when found under less natural testing conditions in which stereoscopes or other devices are used.

PRISMS AND SUPPRESSION

This method is just a more detailed form of the commonly used *four base-out prism test* in which the prism is placed before the deviating eye, and the doctor looks for any eye movements. Suppression is indicated if there is no movement. This is confirmed if the base-out prism is placed before the other eye and there is a *version* movement. However, fusion is indicated if there is a *convergence* response (with the base-out prism). Expertise is necessary for interpretation of test results.

COMMENTS Occasionally practitioners are asked to report percentage values of stereopsis for patients rather than values recorded in seconds of arc (see Table 2G). Percentage scales were empirically determined by Dr. Carl F. Shepard for such purposes. Calculations and information pertaining to this method are presented by Fry[25]. The formula for converting seconds of arc stereoacuity (eta) into percentage of stereopsis is as follows:

$$\% \text{ stereopsis} = \frac{10100}{\text{eta} + 81} - 5$$

TABLE 2G. *Approximate Corresponding Values for Stereoacuity in Seconds of Arc and Shepard Percentages*

Seconds of arc	Shepard percentage
1000	4
400	16
200	31
100	51
50	72
40	78
20	95
15	100
10	106

Note: Shepard percentages were calculated using the following formula of Fry:

$$\% \text{ stereopsis} = \frac{10100}{\text{eta} + 81} - 5$$

In summary, both the size and extent of suppression are probably greater when tested under natural conditions and less when testing is done in a reduced environment. Carrying this reasoning to its logical conclusion, there is no suppression if one eye is completely occluded, and there is probably active suppression (at least of the physiological type) taking place under normal casual seeing conditions.

Amblyopia Amblyopia is defined by Cline et al.[16] as the condition of reduced visual acuity not correctable by refractive means and not attributable to obvious structural or pathological ocular anomalies. It is presumed that the best possible farpoint corrective lenses are worn during the testing of visual acuity. In general, vision worse than 20/30 (6/9) is considered to meet the criterion for amblyopia. This is also true when there is a significant difference in the best correctable acuity of each eye. For practical purposes, if the acuity difference is two lines of letters on the Snellen chart, amblyopia of the poorer eye may be present. For example, if the better eye is 20/15 and the poorer eye is 20/25, the definition of amblyopia may be met.

Amblyopia is classified as being either organic or functional. Those patients in whom visual acuity is reduced significantly are classified as being low vision cases (not amblyopic) if there is either obvious ocular pathology, or if there is proven pathology in the visual pathways. Corresponding defects in the visual fields usually accompany such lesions.

CLASSIFICATION OF AMBLYOPIA

Organic amblyopia, however, is the term customarily used, rather than low vision, in certain cases of reduced vision where ocular pathology is not obvious (even though there may be a small central scotoma in some cases).

The term, functional amblyopia, should be reserved for those cases in which the cause of reduced visual acuity is deemed to be purely functional.

There are three broad categories of organic amblyopia, according to Schapero.[17] They are nutritional, toxic, and congenital. A common type of nutritional amblyopia is due to poor diet in cases of alcoholism. The typical visual field defect is either a central or paracentral scotoma.

ORGANIC AMBLYOPIA

In cases of toxic amblyopia, the visual field loss may be either central (as in methyl alcohol poisoning) or peripheral (as in salicylate poisoning).

Congenital amblyopia is regarded by Schapero[18] as existing in a particular case in which therapy is completely unproductive, even when given extensively for a long duration. This condition may be bilateral or unilateral. There is an implication of hereditary problems (not necessarily obvious) somewhere in the visual pathways. A central scotoma may be elicited in such an eye by careful visual field plotting. Finding an absolute scotoma tends to indicate that amblyopia is congenital (therefore, organic, such as pathologies causing field defects); whereas, in functional amblyopia, a scotoma would probably be relative rather than absolute.

The three types of functional amblyopia are hysterical, refractive, and strabismic.

FUNCTIONAL AMBLYOPIA

This form of functional loss of central visual acuity is due to psychogenic causes. It is fairly common in children and adolescents, as well as in adults who are in stressful situations. Perimetric studies usually reveal tubular fields. The Streff "non-malingering" syndrome may be a variation of this problem (discussed in Chapter Fifteen).

HYSTERICAL AMBLYOPIA

Isometropia and anisometropia are two basic types of refractive conditions that cause functional loss of vision.

REFRACTIVE AMBLYOPIA

Isometropia means there is a refractive error of approximately the same magnitude in each eye (not exceeding one diopter difference). If the ametropia is relatively high, and has never been previously corrected, visual acuity may not have had the chance to develop normally due to the continuously blurred dioptric image on each retina. This is particularly true in high refractive errors of hyperopic astigmatism. The immediate best correctable visual acuity may be poor (e.g., 20/60 in each eye). With the passing of time and full-time wearing of ophthalmic lenses, vision usually improves at a rapid rate. If refractive errors are corrected within the developmental years (before age six) there may eventually be 20/20 acuity in each eye. Fortunately, isometropic amblyopia is becoming less prevalent in the United States and other affluent countries where the need for early vision care is being emphasized.

A significant difference in the refractive status of the two eyes may cause anisometropic amblyopia. This is thought to be a functional loss of central vision resulting from long-standing suppression. Humphriss[19] found that a relatively small difference in refraction (e.g., one diopter and sometimes less) between each eye may result in a central suppression. This is because the blurred image of one eye needs to be eliminated in order to prevent confusion that would ordinarily result from two dissimilar (one clear and one blurred) images. Unlike isometropic amblyopia, where the reduced vision is bilateral, the condition is practically always unilateral in cases of anisometropic amblyopia.

The frequent occurrence of anisometropia probably accounts for the high prevalence of this type of refractive amblyopia. Schapero[20] summarized various studies and concluded that anisometropic amblyopia occurs more frequently than does strabismic amblyopia.

STRABISMIC AMBLYOPIA   Amblyopia may occur as a result of long-standing suppression in cases of strabismus. The foveal area is suppressed in order to prevent confusion (refer to Figure 2-1). This is probably the same mechanism that occurs at the fovea in a case of anisometropia, except that in strabismus, there is a difference in form of the ocular images rather than merely a difference in clearness (or possibly aniseikonic size differences). Because of this, suppression must ordinarily be more intense in cases of strabismus than in those with anisometropia. This may explain why amblyopia is usually deeper in strabismic ambloypia than in cases of mere anisometropia. When both conditions coexist (i.e., strabismus and anisometropia), amblyopia is usually found to be deeper than when only one condition is present.

OTHER TERMINOLOGY OF AMBLYOPIA   The type of functional amblyopia frequently referred to as amblyopia ex anopsia is a classification that is meant by most authorities to include only strabismic amblyopia and anisometropic amblyopia. Von Noorden[21] takes exception to the common usage of amblyopia ex anopsia for strabismic amblyopia and anisometropic amblyopia. He believes that ex anopsia implies disuse and understimulation of the retina, such as in deprivation of light from a ptosis, or from deprivation of form such as from a cataract, or from corneal scarring.

Since retinal receptors are, in fact, stimulated in cases of strabismus and anisometropia, I believe amblyopia resulting from these conditions should be referred to, respectively, as strabismic amblyopia and anisometropic amblyopia without the use of the term ex anopsia.

Chavasse[22] referred to cases of functional amblyopia as being due either to extinction or arrest. Amblyopia of extinction is generally considered to be correctable while amblyopia of arrest is not. These concepts will be discussed more fully in regard to prognosis in Chapter Five.

Departure from customary visual acuity measuring is often required when an amblyopic eye is being tested, because of the wide variation of responses when an ordinary chart of Snellen optotype is employed.

Visual Acuity Testing

These tests have remained essentially the same since Herman Snellen devised the first one in 1862. Such a chart may be fine for the testing of nonamblyopic eyes but is not well-suited for reliable interpretation of visual acuity in functional amblyopia.

SNELLEN CHARTS

A standard clinical criterion for assessing the acuity threshold is that more than half of the letters in a particular line must be identified correctly. There is usually no problem in determining this level in the normal seeing eye. In this instance, the patient will consistently identify smaller and smaller letters up to a certain point. Beyond that, letters are consistently missed if an attempt is made to guess the appropriate letters.

In contrast to this response, the patient reading with an amblyopic eye will show wide variance in correctly identifying different-sized letters. The typical response is his reading one or two letters correctly in each of several lines of an ordinary Snellen chart, with no clear-cut stopping point as to correct or incorrect line acuity. For any particular line, the first and last letters are often recognized properly, while the ones in between are not.

A reason often given for such differences between amblyopic and nonamblyopic test responses is the effect of contour interaction, sometimes referred to as the crowding phenomenon. Flom et al.[23] studied this effect and described such differences between responses of amblyopic versus nonamblyopic eyes. They found that while the visual acuity response of the normal eye may be slightly affected by contour interaction, the amblyopic eye is significantly affected and shows a drop of acuity under such conditions.

In order to eliminate the effect of the crowding phenomenon, isolated letters should be presented to the patient. Letter acuities are usually better than line acuities in functional amblyopia when testing visual acuity of an amblyopic eye. When there is a difference of one or more levels of acuity between letter and line on the Snellen Chart, functional amblyopia should be suspected.

This chart (see Figure 2-21) designed by Flom[24] takes the crowding phenomenon into account, and also works around the problem of indefinite

PSYCHOMETRIC CHART OF FLOM

cut-offs in deciding visual acuity thresholds. He recommends using a proportion of correct responses (usually 50 percent) of a series of eight Landolt C's. Because there is a factor of guessing one of four possible orientations of a particular C, the patient is expected to identify five out of eight correctly for 50 percent accuracy. A number of charts are used for differing acuity levels, and each contains the exact configuration of C's and E's. Interspacing is kept to a constant relationship for all charts thus cancelling out the variability of the crowding effect as different acuity thresholds are introduced to the patient.

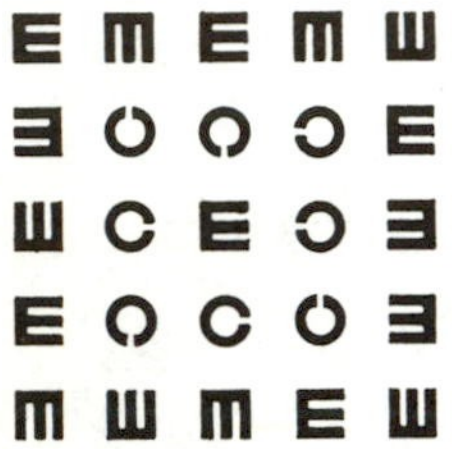

Testing the visual acuity by means of the Flom chart proceeds as follows:

1. Begin with a large lettered chart so that seven or eight of the C's are properly identified (either up, down, right, or left).
2. Use smaller and smaller charts until less than five of the C's are correctly identified.
3. The chart just before this one (where five or more correct answers were reported) represents the level of acuity that should be recorded.
4. The same procedure is used for the nonamblyopic as well as the amblyopic eye. This provides a more meaningful comparison of visual acuities of the two eyes than using the conventional Snellen charts, with variable interspacings and inadequate number of letters for each acuity level. (A refinement using graphical plotting of data is discussed in Chapter Sixteen.)

FIGURE 2-21 — Psychometric chart of Flom for measuring visual acuity in cases of amblyopia

TUMBLING E CHARTS

The rotatable Snellen E is a popular chart for use with young children or older patients who are illiterate. It is preferable to refer to this as a tumbling or rotatable E or other similar terms rather than as an illiterate E. The latter may conjure up derogatory connotations for some patients.

FIGURE 2-22 — S.C.C.O. Tumbling E Test Card for evaluating visual acuity of young children

Since E charts are more simply designed than the complex configuration of the Flom chart, performance on these tests may be easier at younger ages for most preschool children. One such E card is the S.C.C.O. Tumbling E Test Card[t], designed by Griffin. It contains four E's in different orientations, all on one line. The interspacing is equal to the width of each E. This is shown in Figure 2-22. Passing requires four of four correct responses.

The effect of the crowding phenomenon in an amblyopic eye can be evaluated by comparing the responses to the inside E's with those on the ends of the line. If single-letter acuity is desired, three of the E's may be covered by the examiner's fingers, leaving only one E exposed.

To prevent the possibility of memorization, the card can be rotated in four directions when testing either line or letter acuity. Oblique orientations are too difficult for most patients, particularly children, and therefore not recommended. Often a young child responds well to vertical orientations (E pointing up or down) but has trouble with right-left positions. This is because the perception for directionality is usually not fully developed in the

[t]May be custom made by a local printer.

preschooler. As a result, many tests depending on orientation identification are not appropriate for the very young. The child may see clearly, but his poor perceptual-motor responses invalidate this type of visual acuity testing. Each target on the S.C.C.O. card is a 20/15 demand. Since children prefer a nonprojected target at near distances, the card is held at 3 meters (10 feet) making this a 20/30 visual acuity test. The test distance may be varied for determination of other acuities (e.g., 5 feet corresponds to 20/60).

A row of tumbling E's is printed on the back of the S.C.C.O. card in 5-point type (approximately equivalent to 20/30 at a distance of 40 cm) for near point visual acuity testing. Comparing distance and near acuities may help reveal myopic refractive errors if near vision is better than far. Similarly, some cases of malingering and hysterical amblyopia may show this. On the other hand, some children who have visual perceptual learning disabilities often do better on far visual acuity testing than at near. Why this is so is not fully known, but it has been speculated that poor accommodative facility may be a possible reason.

PICTURE CHARTS

Various charts employing two-dimensional picture drawings are frequently used for testing the visual acuity of young children. Preschool children (ages 2-5) usually respond better to nonprojected charts at closer distances than to projected ones viewed farther away. The E test is often unreliable in this age group because of the normal lag in the development of perception of directionality.

A set of pictures designed by Allen[26] is ideal for testing the visual acuity of preschool children. The eight different pictures are: birthday cake, telephone, car, house, flower, teddy bear, Christmas tree, and horse.[u] Instructions for performing the test are as follows:

1. Present the pictures to the child binocularly at a close distance and have him name each picture.
2. Cover the child's left eye and present the pictures to the child in sequence while backing away from the child. The greatest distance at which three of the pictures are consistently identified is then recorded as the numerator of a 30-foot denominator. For example, if the right eye maximum distance is 15 feet, the visual acuity would be recorded as 15/30.
3. Cover the child's right eye and present the same pictures to the left eye in a different sequence.

It is important to remember that a comparison of the visual acuities of the child's two eyes is more valuable than absolute values obtained for each eye. Children between 2 and 3 can usually identify the pictures from 12 to 15 feet. Adults with excellent visual acuity can recognize the pictures at distances greater than 30 feet in good illumination. A difference of 5 feet in visual acuity between a child's two eyes is probable cause for suspecting amblyopia or other causes for reduced vision in an eye.

[u]Published by Ophthalmix. A simplified, but effective, picture test is the apple-house-umbrella series of the Lighthouse Flash Cards (New York Association of the Blind).

Many other methods are available for assessing the central vision of children. A few of the more practical as well as some of those with future promise are discussed below.

PURSUITS

The level of visual acuity may be grossly evaluated by judging the motor control in pursuit fixational movements. Testing is performed in the same manner as in duction testing (discussed in Chapter One). The examiner moves a penlight (or any interesting fixation target, such as a bright shiny toy) in a continuous smooth circle while the patient is encouraged to fixate the target. This is particularly useful in visual acuity evaluation of infants (birth to two years of age) as they are probably unable to respond to traditional Snellen, E's or picture charts.

Although visual acuity cannot be quantified by this means, smooth and steady pursuits indicate that the quality of central vision is probably good; whereas jerky and unsteady fixation during pursuits are frequently associated with poor acuity. Extraocular muscle paresis must first be ruled out, however, before coming to such conclusions.

Schapero[27] points out that an amblyopic eye demonstrates inaccuracies and irregularities in pursuits that are not demonstrated by a normal eye.

Another clue to how well an infant can see in each eye is to observe the child's reaction to being occluded. When amblyopia is present, the patient usually shows signs of discontent when the sound eye is covered.

OPTOKINETIC NYSTAGMUS

Visual acuity can sometimes be estimated in very young infants by means of optokinetic nystagmus (OKN). This is the responsive nystagmoid-like movement of the eye viewing a series of rapidly moving, similar targets, all traveling in the same direction. This phenomenon has also been referred to as railroad nystagmus, since the characteristic flicks of the eyes while viewing a fast-moving train are an example of OKN movements. They are reflexive and involuntary, and the viewer is unaware of them.

OKN testing is one of the few ways to evaluate visual acuity by objective means. This is especially important when testing babies. All that is needed is that the patient be aware and looking in the direction of the OKN stimulus. When there is a positive response, this level of acuity is at least as good as the stimulus level being presented. A negative response to the OKN stimulus, however, is inconclusive.

Dayton et al.[28] were able to make some fairly reliable measurements of acuity in newborns and estimated that, in some instances, vision was astonishingly good. An acuity of 20/150 was found in nine out of 39 infants studied. The ages range from eight hours to eight days old. This exceeds all prior estimations of visual acuity for infants of this age. Black-and-white vertical stripes moving laterally on the surface of a canopy over the baby's crib were employed. Eye movements were monitored by means of electro-oculography. By knowing the stripe size and its distance from the eye, the approximate visual acuity (minimum resolvable) was calculated.

The assumption is that if the black line is too narrow to be seen, optokinetic nystagmus does not occur; only when it is made large enough to be seen does OKN occur.

Although factors such as target speed, contrast, color, and intensity need to be investigated further, the use of OKN as a common clinical procedure appears to be feasible in the very near future. Hand-held rotating drums and other mechanical devices are in use now, but they do not determine other than very gross acuities. Further electronic developments in OKN testing will probably incorporate the necessary refinements and should have great promise for detection of amblyopia and other sensory obstacles to vision in the infant.

The early works by White and Eason[29] on evoked cortical potentials in the occipital lobe have lead to great interest in evaluation of vision by electroencephalographic means. By analyzing the visual evoked response (VER), displayed graphically as a plot of amplitude against time, visual acuity can be determined. Refractive error can also be assessed by the analysis of VER responses to ophthalmic lenses of varying powers.

VISUAL EVOKED RESPONSE

One of the most important uses of VER is determining whether or not a patient has organic or functional amblyopia. Harding[30] believes organic amblyopia can be ruled in or out by use of formless flash stimuli. A computerized write-out showing a reduced amplitude indicates there is a lesion somewhere in the visual pathways.

Patterned stimuli (rather than diffused light) must be flashed and the write-out analyzed in order to evaluate the depth of an amblyopic condition. Harter and White[31] found that factors, such as accommodation and fixation changes, may affect the evoked response and that at least some cooperation is required by the patient in paying attention to a patterned target. I believe that it is not unusual in clinical VER testing to take an hour to test an infant, particularly when patterned stimuli are used. Sometimes only one eye can be evaluated on the first visit, particularly if there is amblyopia. The young patient is not any more likely to submit to the occluder with this testing than under ordinary clinical examination procedures. Although the VER is an objective test par excellence, the doctor-patient relationship is very important for this method to be reliable.

Some degree of measurement of fusion can be attained by use of VER. It is generally thought that when patterned stimuli are presented to both eyes, the amplitudes of the response waves are almost twice as large as those found under similar monocular stimuli.

If suppression is present, the amplitude is considerably less than the typical binocular write-out but greater than that found in monocular testing. This variation depends, of course, on the size and intensity of the suppression. It is thought that when anomalous correspondence is present there is no fusion and, therefore, the VER responses should be the same as though monocular testing were being given.

It should be pointed out that VER mainly encompasses only that portion of the visual pathway represented by the central area of the retina. It is mainly the macular area that is tested by means of the visual evoked response. In order to test the integrity of the retinal periphery, the electroretinogram (ERG) should be performed rather than VER. By using both the VER and ERG, however, the entire visual field can be evaluated by objective means.

The VER, also called the VEP (visually evoked potential), is clinically used as follows: first, detection of demyelinating diseases, as in multiple sclerosis (with latency differences); second, differentiation between organic and functional amblyopia; third, estimation of visual acuity in certain patients, e.g., infants; and fourth, investigation of binocular status.

NEUTRAL DENSITY FILTERS Testing of amblyopia in reduced illumination, requiring the patient to be in the dark adapted state, has been advocated by Von Noorden and Burian[32]. They claim differential diagnosis between organic and functional amblyopia is possible by comparing the visual acuity measured in normal versus reduced illumination. The reduced illumination of the target can be conveniently effected by using a neutral density filter such as the 3.0, #96 Kodak Wratten, recommended by Von Noorden and Burian.

Burian[33] believes the amblyopic eye is functionally at its worst in high luminance and at its best in low luminance. In contrast, an eye with organic lesions has a great decrease in vision in mesopic luminances. In accord with this concept, Verin[34] preadapted amblyopic eyes for three minutes in darkness at each luminance level for visual acuity testing, and reported mesopic visual acuity was above that measured in normal light conditions. He further stated that this indicates the diagnosis of functional amblyopia regardless of the patient's age.

Presenting some difference of opinion on this matter, Caloroso and Flom[35] reported the visual acuity of an amblyopic eye did not improve with decreased luminance; rather, it became worse. The decrease in acuity, however, was not as dramatic as in the normal eye, except at the very lowest luminance level where the acuities became approximately the same.

In summary, most authorities believe that reduced illuminance adversely affects visual acuity the greatest for organic lesions; next for the normal eye; and least affected is the vision of the functional amblyopic eye. Ball[36] points out the importance of checking for media irregularities, uncorrected refractive errors, and neuroses, as well as organic lesions when vision becomes poorer under mesopic testing conditions. I believe that, at present, there are too many variables involved for reliable differential diagnoses to be determined by means of illumination reduction. With further research, however, this could become a routine test in the diagnosis of amblyopia.

Testing of the visual fields is imperative in all cases of amblyopia. Even in young children, a gross evaluation of the peripheral field can be made by use of confrontation testing according to Harrington.[37] This is necessary in order to rule out any pathological causes for reduced vision. In older children, central fields can also be plotted to further differentiate between functional and organic amblyopia. Schapero[38] expressed the opinion that detection of a central absolute scotoma (no light perception within the scotomatous area) indicates amblyopia that is organic or has an organic component, and the prognosis for attaining better acuity is limited by the potential acuity of the retinal area surrounding the absolute scotoma. A relative central scotoma (depressed sensitivity), however, is an indication of a functional rather than an organic amblyopia. Irvine[39] reported a more cautious view in this regard, based on his findings that some functional cases of deep amblyopia apparently exhibit an absolute central scotoma.

Field testing must be done under monocular conditions when testing the integrity of the central field. Otherwise, a zone of suppression may be plotted instead of a true scotoma, if testing is done binocularly (see previous discussion relating to measurement of the size of suppression). Monocular visual field testing may be performed using an ordinary black-felt tangent screen. Unlike paracentral testing where a central fixation spot is routinely employed, testing within the central ten degrees of the tangent screen requires the absence of a central fixation spot. The object to be fixated must be placed paracentrally in order to leave the center of the screen clear for field testing. The most effective fixation lock is a cross with the center missing (see Figure 2-23). This is done by pinning four 1 x 5 cm white strips of paper to the target screen at the 12, 3, 6 and 9 o'clock positions, approximately ten degrees away from the center of the screen. Testing with a 1 mm white target at 1 and 2 meters is generally sufficient to determine whether or not an absolute scotoma is present.

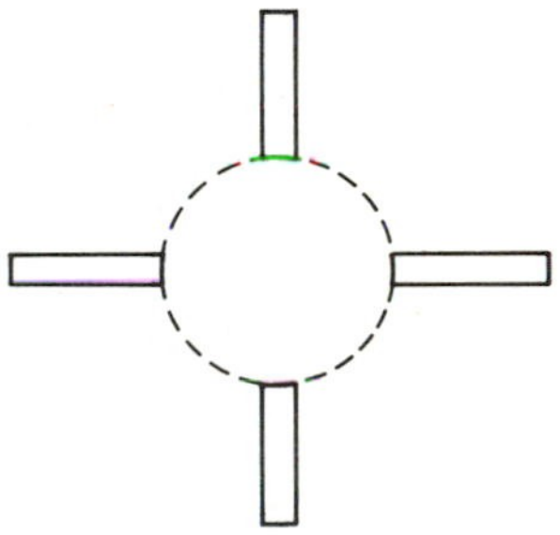

The use of ophthalmoscopy for detection of central visual field defects is a promising innovation.[40,41,42] This may ultimately help in diagnosing functional and organic amblyopias. In this method, the doctor projects a target on to the patient's retina by means of a special modified ophthalmoscope.[v] Both the patient and the doctor should see the same target simultaneously. The target is usually in the form of a small star, or spot, and can be placed on any particular portion of the central fundus that requires testing. The familiar problem with conventional field plotting, of not knowing precisely where the patient is fixating, is eliminated via this method. When the patient reports the target disappearing, a scotoma is indicated. Further studies and standards need to be carried out before

VISUAL FIELDS

FIGURE 2-23 — Paracentral fixation lock for testing integrity of the central visual field on the tangent screen

---

[v]Referring to one modified for visuoscopy or euthyoscopy. Three such ophthalmoscopes commercially available are: (1) Visuskop by Oculus Products, Dutenhofen, Federal Republic of Germany. (2) Projectoscope by Keeler, Mfg. by Keeler in England and distributed in the USA by Keeler Optical Products. (3) Euthyscope by Neitz Instruments, Tokyo, Japan.

definitive conclusions can consistently be reached regarding absolute versus relative scotomas detected by this method.

Central visual fields representing the macular area can be assessed indirectly through the use of entoptic phenomena. If the eye can perceive Haidinger's brushes or Maxwell's spot, the macular area is presumed to be normal and nonpathological.

No presumption can be made, however, if the patient fails to see either of these. Many normally-sighted individuals may be able to see the brushes, but not the spot. Some can see the Maxwell spot but not the brushes, and there is the occasional patient who is unable to see either.

CASE HISTORY   An in-depth case history should be conducted on every amblyopic patient. Diagnostic conclusions often depend upon this evidence alone. Questioning should relate to strabismic history, refractive history, health history, and social history.

STRABISMIC HISTORY   The time of onset of amblyopia often coincides with that of strabismus; therefore, it is vitally important to know the age of onset of strabismus. It generally follows that the earlier the onset, the deeper the amblyopia. Winter[43] believes the younger the age of onset of amblyopia, the more it is embedded and the more difficult it is to successfully treat. He also states that eccentric fixation is not likely to occur if the onset is after the child is three years old.

The mode of onset of strabismus should be questioned. A constantly occurring strabismus is more likely to produce deeper amblyopia than one that is intermittent. Although there is no universal agreement as to the etiology of amblyopia, the popular theory is that suppression leads to the establishment of amblyopia. In the case of intermittent strabismus, the occurrence of fusion results in the occasional elimination of suppression. The depth of amblyopia is probably related to both the duration and intensity of suppression. Another important question regarding mode of onset is concerned with eye laterality, i.e., was the strabismus unilateral or alternating. As a rule, if the child alternates, the likelihood of amblyopia diminishes.

Previous treatment should be questioned very carefully. If occlusion was prescribed, try to establish if the wearing schedule was adhered to faithfully. It so often happens that careful questioning reveals that patching was done only as a token gesture.

If extraocular muscle surgery was performed, complete information about the deviation (diagnostic variables discussed in Chapter One) should be obtained before and after the operation, if possible.

The duration of amblyopia can be assumed to be about the same as the length of time the patient has had a constant unilateral strabismus. For intermittent and/or alternating strabismus, duration of amblyopia is uncertain, and history is not too conclusive in this regard.

Finally, the duration of amblyopia must also include the patient's present age. Immediate therapy is more crucial to an infant than to an adult.

Schapero[44] strongly pointed out that incidence of anisometropic amblyopia is higher than that of strabismic amblyopia. Unfortunately, the age of onset of refractive amblyopia is nearly impossible to determine from verbal history of the patient or his parents. The only reliable means in this regard is to obtain previous optometric or ophthalmological records to ascertain the refractive status and visual acuities (if determined) at certain ages. Records of uncorrected high differences in refraction between the two eyes are suggestive of anisometropic amblyopia, particularly for hyperopic anisometropia. Many young children presently with amblyopia have not had routine preschool professional vision examinations, and undocumented history contributes very little in these cases.

Because lay people are very unlikely to be aware that an infant or toddler has anisometropic amblyopia, the age of onset may be very early, resulting in a period of long duration before it is detected and treatment is given. Since long duration lessens the chance for successful therapy, I believe all infants and preschoolers should have routine refractive examinations by optometrists or ophthalmologists.

This line of questioning should relate to birth history, congenital anomalies, and acquired diseases. Anything out of the ordinary should be noted. The patient's pediatrician can be consulted for further information.

Birth history may reveal information about many pathologies, such as oxygen imbalances resulting in retrolental fibroplasia (low vision), or forceps trauma during delivery, causing extraocular muscle paresis (resulting in strabismic amblyopia).

Schapero[45] states that congenital amblyopia may or may not be related to other co-existing congenital defects, such as nystagmus, albinism, motor defects, etc., but the presence of these tends to implicate the amblyopia as being congenital. No improvement in vision can be expected in this type of amblyopia.

There are a number of acquired types of organic amblyopia and certain questions may give cause-and-effect answers. One example is nutritional amblyopia due to lack of B vitamins, particularly in alcoholism. Vision may be restored with the proper diet. Another example is toxic amblyopia where endogenous or exogenous poisoning is suspected. Winter[46] believes toxic amblyopia is usually irreversible.

The patient may have emotional problems causing either hysterical amblyopia or malingering. A social history of how the patient relates to family and peer group is important when either condition is suspected.

In the case of hysterical amblyopia, the patient wants to avoid a stressful environment by having poor vision, but he is presumably unaware of the mechanism causing loss of sight. On the other hand, the patient who is malingering by feigning poor vision is probably doing so for similar reasons, but is aware of what he is doing.

Psychotherapy is recommended in these cases where history reveals emotional problems, and the prognosis for recovery of vision is good.

OTHER CONSIDERATIONS The incidence of amblyopia has been summarized by Schapero[47] as ranging from 1.0 to 5.64 percent, depending on the investigator and criteria used. Generally speaking, 3 percent is a fairly acceptable normal figure to use for estimating the chance of finding some type of amblyopia in a random population in the United States.

Of all cases of amblyopia, I believe the frequency of finding each type is probably in the following order: refractive, strabismic, congenital, hysterical, nutritional, toxic, tobacco, and light deprivation.

Excessive smoking, particularly cigars, may result in decreased central visual acuity. Many authorities call this organic condition, "tobacco amblyopia." Light-deprivation amblyopia refers to the functional arrest of development of vision of an eye that is deprived of light stimulation. This could be in the form of a ptosis, dense cataract, or any form of total occlusion over a long period of time during infancy or very early childhood.

A list of the prognosis and type of treatment for each category of amblyopia is presented in Table 2H.

Abnormal Fixation Fixation is normal when the center of the fovea is used for fixation and when fixation is steady. If any other area of the retina is used, or if there is an unsteadiness, fixation is considered to be abnormal. Unsteadiness refers to the presence of nystagmoid oscillations (usually irregular flicks and drifts) of the eye. They are noticeable upon careful direct observation, but more easily observed during visuoscopy. An eye with good visual acuity necessarily has central fixation that is relatively steady, while an eye with poor visual acuity may have eccentric and/or unsteady fixation.

CLASSIFICATION OF FIXATION Whether fixation is normal or abnormal is routinely determined when the eye is in the primary position, although other positions of gaze may be used for special investigation of abnormal fixation.

Unless the center of the fovea is used, fixation is classified as being eccentric. Table 2I lists ten categories of fixation. The first is steady, central fixation which is considered to be normal. This means that the center of the fovea is steadily used while fixating a stationary target. This does not mean the eye is perfectly motionless, since even the normally fixating eye has physiological micromovements. The other nine categories include fixation considered to be abnormal.

Occasionally, the site used for fixation in cases of eccentric fixation may vary from time to time. Some authorities prefer to speak of the eccentric retinal area rather than eccentric point. In order to determine the site most often used (designated as point "e" on the retina), several findings should be made by means of visuoscopy and their locations averaged.

I generally recommend averaging three locations timed at one-minute intervals. The position of point e is qualitatively described as being in one of the five locations:

Foveal Center
Foveal Off-Center
Parafoveal
Paramacular
Peripheral

TABLE 2H. Classification and Prognosis of the Types of Amblyopia

TYPE	PROGNOSIS	TREATMENT
Organic		
Nutritional	good	Diet
Tobacco	good	Abstinence
Toxic	poor-to-fair	Medical attention
Congenital	poor	Attempt functional vision therapy to rule this in or out
Functional		
Hysterical	good	Psychotherapy
Light deprivation	poor	Remove obstacle as early as possible
Refractive	*good	Ophthalmic lenses and functional vision therapy
Strabismic	*good	Functional vision therapy

*If onset is very early with duration of amblyopia continuing past the developmental years without therapy being given, the prognosis becomes less favorable.

Refer to Table 2I for magnitude limits for each location. Most ophthalmoscopes modified for visuoscopy have graticules calibrated in degrees rather than in prism diopters. This is why eccentric fixation is customarily referred to in terms of degrees. Otherwise, it is all right to use prism diopters for angle E.

The description of eccentric fixation should also include the direction from the fovea in which point e is located on the retina. This will be one of the following:

> Nasal
> Temporal
> Superior
> Inferior
> Nasal inferior
> Nasal superior
> Temporal superior
> Temporal inferior

Nasal eccentric fixation is common in amblyopia with esotropia and may or may not have a vertical component. Exotropic amblyopes tend to have temporal eccentric fixation and may or may not have a vertical component.

After the site used for fixation is determined, the question of how steady the fixation is at that particular site must be answered. The quality of steadiness, as well as the determination of location of site used, can be best determined by the ophthalmoscopic technique of visuoscopy.

TABLE 2I. Classification of Fixation in Terms of Retinal Site Used and Steadiness of Fixation

Type of Fixation	Magnitude from the Center-of-fovea
Central Fixation	
Foveal Center	0 degree
1. Steady (normal central fixation)	
2. Unsteady (abnormal central fixation)	
Eccentric Fixation	
Foveal Off-center	1 degree or less (but greater than 0)
3. Steady	
4. Unsteady*	
Parafoveal	3 degrees or less (but greater than 1)
5. Steady	
6. Unsteady*	
Paramacular	5 degrees or less (but greater than 3)
7. Steady	
8. Unsteady*	
Peripheral	Greater than 5 degrees
9. Steady	
10. Unsteady*	

*Fixation is usually unsteady in eccentric fixation.

TESTING ABNORMAL FIXATION

There are five general principles used in the testing of abnormal fixation. These include: angle kappa measurements, visuoscopy, uses of entoptic phenomena, after images, and evaluation of spatial localization.

WORTH TEST FOR ECCENTRIC FIXATION

This testing procedure employs the angle kappa test, whereby the angle of one eye is compared to the other eye. When there is a difference in the angles, eccentric fixation is suspected.

Angle kappa is defined as the angle between the visual axis and the pupillary axis. This angle can be determined by clinical testing. It is practically the same as angle alpha, which is defined as the angle formed at the first nodal point by the intersection of the optic axis and the visual axis. Since angle alpha cannot be measured by clinical means, angle kappa is the clinical test used when it is important to estimate the relationship between the visual and optic axes. (Technically, this is angle lambda.)

Most individuals have a small positive angle kappa, meaning that the light reflection formed by the convex surface of the cornea is displaced slightly nasalward in respect to the center of the entrance pupil. Figure 1-10 c or d illustrates an example of a moderately large positive angle kappa of the left eye. A negative angle kappa has the light reflection positioned temporalward to the center of the pupil, as in Figure 1-10e. A zero angle K is one in which the reflection is positioned exactly in the center of the entrance pupil (Figure 1-10 a or b).

The magnitude of angle kappa is customarily referred to in terms of millimeters rather than prism diopters or degrees. Although the normally expected magnitude is from 1/4 mm positive to 1/2 mm positive, there is nothing abnormal about a larger or smaller angle K (even a negative angle) provided fixation is normal.

Positive or negative values determine the direction of angle K. The distance in millimeters between the reflection and the center of the pupil determines the magnitude.

The procedure for testing can be done under monocular conditions. This is unlike the Hirschberg test which is done under binocular conditions. Room lights are dimmed, and the patient fixates a penlight at a distance of approximately 50 cm. The examiner's sighting eye must be directly behind the light source. The position of the light reflection in relation to the center of the pupil is observed and noted (in millimeters, either temporal or nasal). If it is 1mm nasal in the right eye, it is written as: + 1mm positive angle kappa of the right eye (see Figure 2-24). The same procedure is repeated by switching the occluder to the other eye.

For example, assume a patient's visual acuity of the left eye is 20/20, implying central fixation in that eye. Assume angle kappa is + 1/2 mm. Further assume the right eye had amblyopia of 20/200 with an angle kappa of zero. In this case, the right eye can be assumed to be fixating eccentrically by the amount represented by 1/2 mm (the total difference between the two angles kappa). This represents an angle 6 degrees of eccentric fixation (angle E), since 1 mm displacement of the corneal light reflection represents 12 degrees (or 22 p.d.).

The direction of eccentric fixation of the right eye is nasal. The light reflection was displaced from a positive position to a central one by means of the right eye abnormally fixating with a nasal portion of its retina, rather than with the center of its fovea (see Figure 2-25).

a.

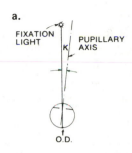

b.

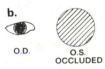

Figure 2-24 — Illustrations of angle kappa. The letter "K" stands for angle kappa. (a) Top view of right eye, illustrating an example of a positive angle kappa; (b) Front view of right eye, illustrating a positive angle kappa, as in Fig. a. The light reflection is displaced nasally by approximately 1 mm, assuming a pupil size of 4 mm and a corneal diameter of 11 mm.

VISUOSCOPY

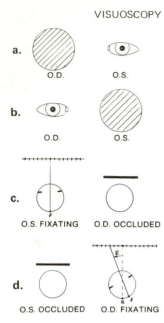

FIGURE 2-25 – Illustrating the determination of eccentric fixation of the right eye by means of angle kappa testing. (a) Positive angle K of ½ mm in the non-amblyopic centrally fixating left eye; (b) Zero angle K in the amblyopic eccentrically fixating right eye; (c) Top view illustration of central fixation of the left eye; (d) Top view illustration of nasal eccentric fixation of six degrees (magnitude of angle E). The letter "e" represents the eccentric point used for fixation.

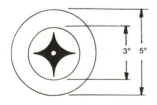

LINKSZ STAR GRATICULE

FIGURE 2-26 – Drawing of the Linksz star used in the Keeler Projectoscope

Visuoscopy for evaluating fixation is done by using an ophthalmoscope in a special way. The doctor observes a projected image (of an object inside the ophthalmoscope) on the patient's fundus while the patient is asked to look directly at the object inside the ophthalmoscope. When the patient has steady central fixation, the doctor sees the projected image, such as a projected star, as staying right in the center of the fovea during the test.

The customary target for these purposes is the Linksz star (see Figure 2-26 which shows the Linksz star used with the Projectoscope). The star may vary in size for different instruments, but the particular one used with the Projectoscope subtends 3 degrees on the retina. Most test stars have a small hole in the center allowing the foveal reflex to be seen (bright pinpoint light) when fixation is central.

When the star is not located in the center of the fovea, the patient is using an eccentric point to fixate. Figure 2-27 shows a schematic drawing of the retina and the dimensions used for classifying the anatomic locations for fixation sites. The standard naming consists of:

1. Describing the horizontal orientation of the site used. This is either nasal or temporal.
2. Describing the vertical orientation, either superior or inferior.
3. The steadiness of fixation, either steady or unsteady.
4. The anatomical location: foveal, foveal off-center, parafoveal, paramacular, or peripheral.
5. If the vertical and horizontal magnitudes of angle E can be measured by visuoscopy, these should be included.

An example of a diagnosis of abnormal fixation might read: nasal, inferior, steady, paramacular eccentric fixation of the right eye (3½° nasal and 3° inferior). This is illustrated in Figure 2-27 which shows the position designated by the letter D.

These anatomical descriptive boundaries for foveal and macular limits have been chosen somewhat arbitrarily, but they are in general accord with common clinical practice. The following discussion relates to this issue.

Davson[48] refers to the fovea as "subtends about 5° at the nodal point of the eye," and the macula as "the region extends over the whole of the central area" (referring to the retina). On the other hand, Wolff[49] describes the fovea as a small concave mirror that produces the bright reflex as seen ophthalmoscopically, and the macula as being about the same size as the optic disc. Likewise, Cogan[50] describes the fovea as "the central declivity of the macula . . . identifiable by a central bright highlight . . ." and "covering approximately 2° of the central visual field . . ." Harrington[51] states that the normal blind spot is 5.5° wide and 7.5° high. If the width of the optic disc can be averaged to 6°, and if this can be assumed to be the same as that of the macula, the subtending angle of the macula can be assumed to be 6° for clinical purposes. Furthermore, it is convenient to assume the fovea subtends 2°.

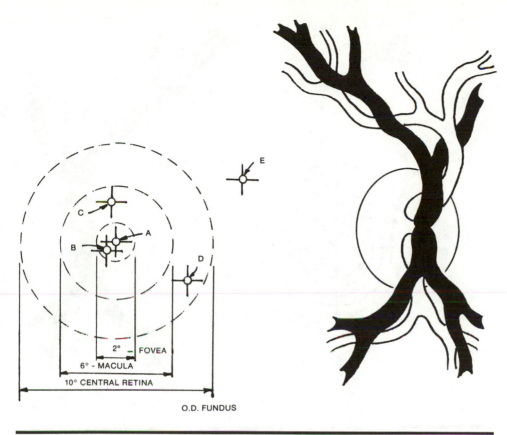

O.D. FUNDUS

FIGURE 2-27 — Diagram of fundus of the right eye as seen in visuoscopy. The star in position A represents central fixation. Position B represents eccentric fixation that is foveal off-center. Position C represents parafoveal eccentric fixation. Position D represents paramacular eccentric fixation. Position E represents peripheral eccentric fixation.

Because eccentric fixation must be tested under monocular conditions, the patient must have one eye occluded when visuoscopic findings are being determined. One practical way of doing this is letting the patient occlude his nontested eye himself, either with his hand or with an occluder. It is frequently helpful for the patient to have both eyes open while the doctor is searching for retinal landmarks in the eye being tested. The young restless patient is usually more cooperative if both eyes are open during most of the testing procedure. Once the fovea is located and the star projected near it, ask the patient to quickly cover up the other eye and look directly at the star, seen inside the instrument. The magnitude of angle E, both the vertical and horizontal dimensions, can either be estimated or measured exactly by means of the projected concentric circles which are calibrated in degrees. For example, the Linksz star for the Keeler Projectoscope has two circles, 3 and 5 degrees. The Neitz Euthyscope has nine circles at ½-degree intervals. Figure 2-28 shows an example of a right eye with nasal eccentric fixation of 3 degrees as seen with the circular projected pattern of the Neitz Euthy-

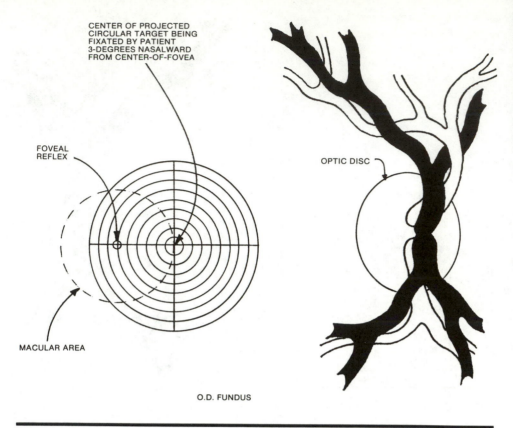

CENTER OF PROJECTED
CIRCULAR TARGET BEING
FIXATED BY PATIENT
3-DEGREES NASALWARD
FROM CENTER-OF-FOVEA

FOVEAL
REFLEX

OPTIC DISC

MACULAR AREA

O.D. FUNDUS

FIGURE 2-28 — Diagram of the fundus of the right eye as seen during visuoscopy when using the Neitz Euthyscope instrument. The magnitude of angle E is measured by means of the projected circles, in ½-degree intervals, on the patient's retina.

scope.[w] Specific detailed instructions for two visuoscopic instruments are presented in the following sets of instructions.

Instructions on usage of the Neitz Euthyscope (see Figure 2-29) for detecting and measuring eccentric fixation:

1. *Viewing lens control:* Rotate clockwise for minus (in green) and counter-clockwise for plus (in red). Range in instrument: +18.00 diopters to -35.00 diopters (using ±10.00 diopter in auxiliary dial). The plus to +5.00 is in one-diopter steps and then +8.00. The minus is in one-diopter steps to -8.00, then -10.00, -15.00, -20.00, and -25.00.

2. *Auxiliary dial* (top dial) contains a +10.00 and a -10.00, a red-free filter, and a plano opening.

3. *Graticule dial* contains a cross target with an open center, nine

---

[w]The trade name for this particular instrument is the Euthyscope, however the procedure employed is visuoscopy.

concentric rings in 1/2° intervals, a 2° black dot, a 4° black dot, and a clear opening.

4. Turn transformer switch on.
5. Occlude the normal eye of the patient and have him look straight ahead.
6. Focus the fundus with the viewing lens control so the cross is seen.
7. Then have the patient look directly at the center of the cross and note whether or not the foveal reflex moves into the center opening of the cross.
8. If the foveal reflex is not centered, put the graticule with the concentric circles into place and measure the angle of eccentricity.

Instructions on usage of the Keeler Projectoscope (see Figure 2-30):

1. *Viewing lens control:* Rotate clockwise for plus, counter-clockwise for minus. Range of instrument is ± 30 diopters (using ± 20 prism diopter auxiliary lens dial). The range of 1-diopter steps is to +10.00 and − 10.00. Note: The black discs of the face serve as a pupillometer. The numbers indicate diameter in millimeters.
2. *Auxiliary dial* (top dial) contains a +20.00 and a − 20.00 diopter lens and polarizing analyzer.
3. *Focusing button* (on handle) is used to focus the graticule patterns on the patient's fundus by moving it up and down. Range from ±20 diopters in 0.25 diopter steps. The scale is read through window directly above focusing button.
4. *Focusing tube* is located on opposite side of instrument. Apertures or graticules are slipped over the end of the focusing tube.
5. *Slide aperture* is located on the handle of the instrument. One of two slides (red-free or polarizing) is inserted with the reference letters uppermost and with the white spot on the side adjacent to the corresponding black spot on the instrument. The letters visible indicate whether or not a filter is in the instrument.
6. Place Linksz Star graticule on the focusing tube. Be sure the focusing button is down.
7. Place red-free slide in instrument with the "O" visible.
8. Set brightness control to 5 and the selector switch to normal.
9. Occlude nonamblyopic eye and instruct patient to fixate straight ahead.
10. Turn on control unit and focus the star on the patient's fundus by slowly pushing up and down on the focusing button.
11. Have the patient fixate the center of the star.
12. Determine if the star is centered over the foveal reflex (central fixation). If not, approximate location and magnitude of eccentric fixation. Determine if fixation is steady or unsteady.

Two important entoptic phenomena are used for investigation of fixation in cases of amblyopia. They are Haidinger's brushes (H.B) and Maxwell's spot

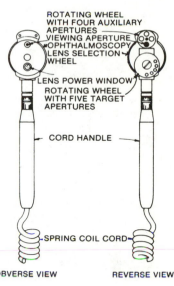

OBVERSE VIEW   REVERSE VIEW

FIGURE 2-29 — Drawing of the Neitz Euthyscope

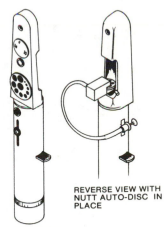

REVERSE VIEW WITH NUTT AUTO-DISC IN PLACE

OBVERSE VIEW

FIGURE 2-30 — Drawing of the Keeler Projectoscope. (This instrument is currently out of production.)

ENTOPTIC PHENOMENA

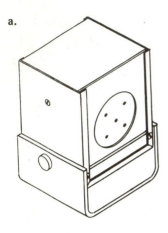

a.

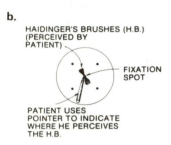

b.

HAIDINGER'S BRUSHES (H.B.)
(PERCEIVED BY
PATIENT)

FIXATION
SPOT

PATIENT USES
POINTER TO INDICATE
WHERE HE PERCEIVES
THE H.B.

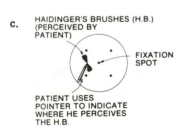

c.

HAIDINGER'S BRUSHES (H.B.)
(PERCEIVED BY
PATIENT)

FIXATION
SPOT

PATIENT USES
POINTER TO INDICATE
WHERE HE PERCEIVES
THE H.B.

FIGURE 2-31 — The Bernell Macular Integrity Tester-Trainer. (a) Drawing of the instrument, clear slide with fixation spots placed before the illuminated circular window; (b) Example of central fixation in which case the patient sees Haidinger's brushes and the fixation spot superimposed; (c) Example of eccentric fixation whereby Haidinger's brushes and the fixation spot are not superimposed. This response would indicate nasal eccentric fixation of the right eye. If this response were found when testing the left eye, temporal eccentric fixation would be indicated.

(M.S.). The elicitation of Haidinger's brushes requires the patient to look through a deep blue filter at a rotatory Polaroid filter. There are several commercially available instruments with this sort of apparatus that may be used for testing and therapy. A set-up for Maxwell's spot testing and therapy may be custom-made by an apparatus that slowly alternates a purple filter with a light grey one before the eye being tested. The eye is viewing a fixation spot on an illuminated white surface. Schapero[52] recommends Roscoe purple No. 28 or Kodak Wratten experimental filter No. 2389 along with the gray, Kodak Wratten neutral filter No. 96, density 1.5 for eliciting Maxwell's spot.

Generally, whatever principle of testing is used for one can be applied to the other. Both are used as tests for macular integrity, because the patient's perception of them is an indication that his macula is fairly well intact. The lack of perception, however, does not necessarily mean the macula is either dysfunctioning or is pathological. Some individuals with normal retinas have difficulty in seeing Haidinger's brushes and/or Maxwell's spot.

Since the centers of either of these entoptic phenomena are tags for the center of the macula, their usefulness in determining the location in which an amblyopic eye fixates is apparent. The testing procedure is simply to have the patient fixate a small target, such as a black spot, while he reports the location of the perceived Haidinger's brushes (or M.S.) in relation to the position of the black fixation spot. If the right eye has nasal eccentric fixation, the Haidinger's brushes will be seen to the left of the fixation spot. If the right eye has temporal eccentric fixation, it will appear to the right of the black spot.

With a known fixation distance and a known measurement of the separation distance between the spot and the Haidinger's brushes, the angular magnitude of eccentric fixation (angle E) can be calculated. For example, if testing at 40 cm and the separation is 20 mm, the angular value is 5 p.d. or approximately 3 degrees of eccentric fixation.

The sensitivity of these procedures is high and is helpful in confirming visuoscopic findings. This is particularly so when there is an indistinct foveal reflex, or when it is difficult to observe the fundus. It should be noted that mydriatics are helpful in cases of small pupils. Clinical experience, however, permits the doctor to become proficient in visuoscopy without the use of mydriatics for pupillary dilation.

There are several instruments available for producing entoptic phenomena, either Haidinger's brushes or M.S., but the most practical, in my opinion, is the Bernell Macular Integrity Tester-Trainer (the MITT). (Figure 2-31a illustrates this.) Figure 2-31b shows the results expected in a case of central fixation and Figure 2-31c for eccentric fixation. It is important to remember that testing is done monocularly when determining whether fixation is central or eccentric. It is best to do this in free space where the patient can point to the exact location of the Haidinger's brushes. The MITT is ideal for this purpose. In addition to this advantage, the brushes are usually vivid (in relation to those seen in reduced environments, such as the Synoptophore, or to those seen at a distance through rotating filters). The Clement Clarke Space Coordinator is an example. One of the Haidinger's brushes' attachments of the Synoptophore also may be held close to the eye while the patient views an illuminated wall in an attempt to perceive the brushes as though the entoptic phenomenon is on the wall.

The patient views an illuminated rotating polarized surface of the MITT and reports the direction of movement of the Haidinger's brushes either clockwise or counter-clockwise. Patients often say the brushes look like an airplane propeller, or a stack of wheat. If a clear piece of cellophane is placed before the eye (i.e., in front of the blue filter), the direction of rotation of the Haidinger's brushes should be reported as going in the opposite direction. This is a useful check on the patient's responses to see if the testing results are reliable.

Afterimages may be used in the therapy of amblyopia as well as in the measurement of magnitude of the angle of eccentric fixation. Brock[53] first suggested the use of the transferred afterimage, and Brock and Givner[54] evaluated this procedure. In performing this test, the patient is instructed to cover the amblyopic eye while the nonamblyopic eye is exposed to a vertical band of light for 15 to 30 seconds. Time should be allowed to create an afterimage. Since the eye fixating the light source is not amblyopic, it can be assumed that the light is imaged on the fovea. If a strobe flash is used, the exposure time is very brief. The speed of flashing may have certain advantages, but the possibility of the eye wandering slightly at the moment of flash should always be considered, as a false positive finding of eccentric fixation can result. A light steadily fixated for a duration of about a half minute would tend to eliminate such spurious results.

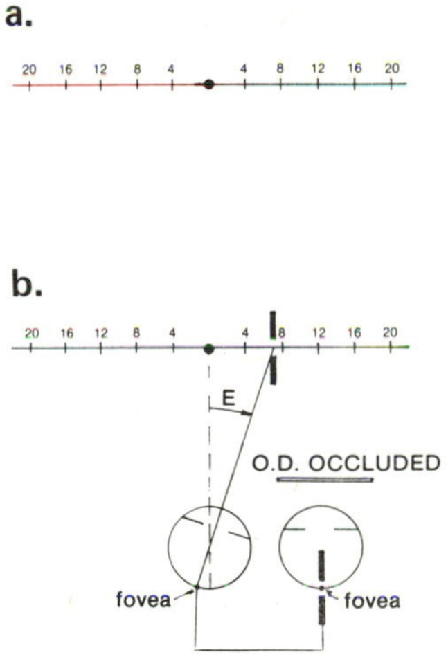

Once the sound eye is exposed to the flash, the occluder is switched, leaving the unstimulated amblyopic eye exposed. The patient is told to look at a black fixation spot on a white chart and try to see the afterimage (transferred from the other eye) of the vertical line. Altering illumination on and off in the room may help the patient to see and maintain the afterimage. If the vertical afterimage is seen passing through the fixation spot, central fixation is indicated. If, however, the afterimage is somewhere on the scale, as in Figure 2-32, eccentric fixation is indicated. The distance between the fixation spot and the afterimage is the magnitude of the angle of eccentric fixation (angle E).

This test becomes invalid for testing and measuring angle E when there is anomalous correspondence. This must be ruled out before afterimage transfer testing for eccentric fixation can be properly interpreted.

Eccentric fixation may produce pastpointing similar to that in extraocular muscle paresis. The amblyopic eye with suspected eccentric fixation is tested with the nonamblyopic eye occluded. The doctor holds a penlight in an

AFTERIMAGE TRANSFER

FIGURE 2-32 — Brock-Givner afterimage transfer test for eccentric fixation. (a) Scale with fixation spot used. Numbers represent distance from the spot in centimeters. P.d. values may be converted into degrees by multiplying by the fraction 4/7; (b) Example of nasal eccentric fixation of the left eye of 7 p.d. (4 degrees).

FAULTY SPATIAL LOCALIZATION

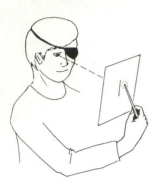

FIGURE 2-33 — Faulty spatial localization in a case of eccentric fixation. Patient views line in same position as the unseen one on the back side of the card. Several trials are necessary to determine if error is repeatable.

upright position at a distance of approximately 40 cm in front of the patient. The patient is told to place his dominant hand behind his head and quickly reach out to touch the tip of the penlight with his pointing finger. An eccentrically fixating eye will usually cause the patient to point to one side or the other, thereby missing the object to be touched. I have seen the direction vary with different patients having similar angle E's of the same direction. For example, a patient with a nasal eccentric fixation of the right eye often past points to his left; while another with the same diagnosis may pastpoint to the right. In any event, the evidence of faulty eye-hand localization is an indication that there is eccentric fixation (assuming EOM paresis is ruled out).

A patient can learn to adjust for the pointing errors after a few trials because his hand is visible, and he can learn to compensate for his errors. When the patient becomes sophisticated in taking this test, an opaque card may be held before the patient in such a way that his arm and hand are not visible to him. A small target, such as a short vertical line, is drawn in the same location on both sides of the card. The procedure is to have the patient attempt to touch the line on the backside of the card with a pointer (e.g., pick-up stick). Figure 2-33 shows a typical localization error in nasal eccentric fixation.

OTHER CONSIDERATIONS

The prediction of the magnitude of angle E cannot be made by knowing the visual acuity, because a functional amblyope may have poor vision even though fixation is central. It is thought that this loss of acuity results from suppression of long duration. Likewise, the prediction of the visual acuity based on the magnitude of angle E is not reliable, because the effects of suppression may not be the same for different cases, even though the magnitude of angle E is the same. It can be safely said, however, that if angle E is large, visual acuity must necessarily be poor. For instance, if visuoscopy indicates a large angle E of 5° and the patient reports good visual acuity by reading 20/25 whole line acuity, there must be an error, either in acuity testing or in angle E testing.

Flom and Weymouth[55] studied the relationship between visual acuity and angle E, as determined by Maxwell's spot. They reported that peripheral acuity for the amblyopic eye was the same as that expected for normal eyes when similar magnitudes of eccentric positions were used for fixation. Flom[56] later used a formula to predict visual acuity from known magnitudes of eccentric fixation. The formula is:

MAR = E + 1

MAR stands for minimum angle of resolution (in minutes of arc).

E is the magnitude of the eccentric fixation (in prism diopters).

An example of calculating the expected visual acuity for 1° eccentric fixation (1.75 p.d.) with this formula is as follows:

MAR = 1.75 + 1
      = 2.75 minutes of arc

and 2.75 minutes of arc represents 20/55 acuity.

Solution: Use ratio, 20/x = 1/2.75 and solve for x.

On the other hand, Schapero[57] would say that the normal eye fixating eccentrically 1° would have 20/30 acuity rather than 20/55 as predicted by Flom. Table 2J compares the peripheral visual acuity averages of Schapero (from the data of Wertheim, Feinberg, and Weymouth) for the normal eye with those calculated from the formula of Flom for amblyopic eyes with eccentric fixation. According to the table, peripheral acuities appear to be much worse in the amblyopic eye than in the normal eye. The finding of poorer peripheral acuity in the amblyopic eye was also reported by Alpern et al.[58] This appears to be consistent with the comparison shown in Table 2J.

My impression is that while the Flom formula may be helpful as a general guide, it is preferable to use the data collected by Schapero in deciding exactly how well an eye might possibly be expected to see for any given amount of eccentric fixation. For example, if 2° of eccentric fixation are found by visuoscopy, the best possible acuity that can be expected is 20/40 (refer to Table 2J). Acuity may vary widely and be only slightly worse or greatly worse than 20/40. In other words, the acuity might possibly be 20/40 for an angle E of 2°, or it might be 20/80, or 20/200, or worse. I believe suppression effects and/or unsteadiness of fixation cause the difference between the data in Table 2J. As stated earlier, the angle of eccentric fixation can be zero, and the amblyopia may be shallow, moderate or deep.

TABLE 2J. Peripheral Visual Acuity Averages

Angle of Eccentricity (degrees from center of fovea)	Normal Eye (from Schapero) Visual Acuity	Amblyopic Eye (from Flom) Visual Acuity
0	20/20	20/20
1	20/30	20/55
2	20/40 - 20/50	20/90
3	20/50 - 20/60	20/125
4	20/60 - 20/70	20/160
5	20/70 - 20/100	20/195
10	20/100 - 20/160	20/370
20	20/180 - 20/300	20/720

This particular abnormal adaptation is very frequently present in strabismus. Its presence indicates a significant difference between the horizontal objective and subjective angles of deviation. From 1 to 3 p.d. difference is allowed for measurement error; otherwise, the angles should be the same in

Anomalous Correspondence

order for normal correspondence to be assumed. When strabismus is small (under 10 p.d.), 1 p.d. measurement error is allowed. In cases of large angle strabismus (over 20 p.d.), a measurement error of 3 is allowed.

DEFINITIONS   Anomalous correspondence is generally defined as the condition in which the two foveas do not correspond to each other in regard to directional values.

There are three different angles to be concerned with when dealing with anomalous correspondence. They are angle H, angle S, and angle A. The letter A stands for the angle of anomaly, defined as the difference between the objective and the subjective angles. The formula is A=H-S.

Another way of looking at this definition: A is the angle subtended at the center of rotation of the eye by the fovea (f) and the anomalous associated point (a). Refer to Figure 2-34 for clarification. In cases of anomalous retinal correspondence, the fovea of the fixating eye corresponds to point "a" in the deviating eye. This point is strictly hypothetical with no anatomical basis implied here as there is for (f), the fovea. It should be noted that the word retinal is redundant in this term, because it is generally agreed that correspondency takes place in the visual cortex, rather than in the retina. Because of the ease in explaining the three angles involved, drawings of the appropriate points on the retina (o, a, f) are usually made. These drawings should not imply, however, that the retina, solely, is involved. Most clinicians refer to this anomaly as anomalous retinal correspondence. Therefore, the abbreviation A R C, although theoretically improper, will be used throughout the book because of its common understanding among clinicians.

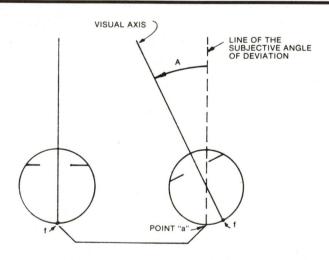

FIGURE 2-34 — Illustration of angle of anomaly in which the fovea of the left eye corresponds to point "a" of the right eye. Angle A is subtended at the center of rotation of the eye by the visual axis and the line of the subjective angle of deviation.

The example illustrated in Figure 2-35 is a case of an esotropia (assume H = 35 p.d.) of the right eye. Further assume that during subjective deviation measuring, such as with loose prisms and red-green spectacles, the subjective angle S is an eso deviation of 15 p.d. The mere fact that H and S are different means that A R C exists. This example represents the typical model of unharmonious A R C having an objective angle larger than the subjective angle.

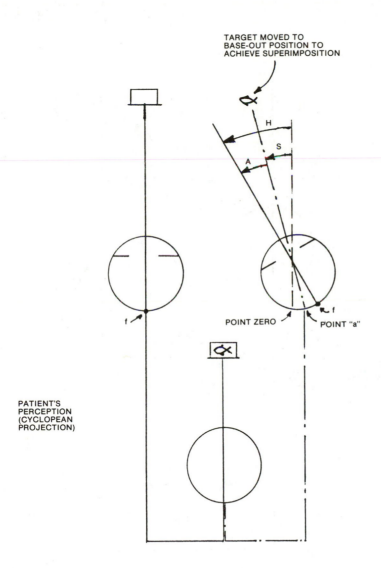

TARGET MOVED TO
BASE-OUT POSITION TO
ACHIEVE SUPERIMPOSITION

H

S

A

f

POINT ZERO

POINT "a"

f

PATIENT'S
PERCEPTION
(CYCLOPEAN
PROJECTION)

FIGURE 2-35 — Illustration of typical unharmonious anomalous correspondence, testing with major amblyoscope

The type of anomalous correspondence probably occurring most frequently is harmonious A R C. This is illustrated in Figure 2-36. Since the subjective angle is 0, the angle of anomaly happens to be equal to the objective angle. Patients with this type of A R C may respond as though they are orthophoric during routine phorometry measurements because the

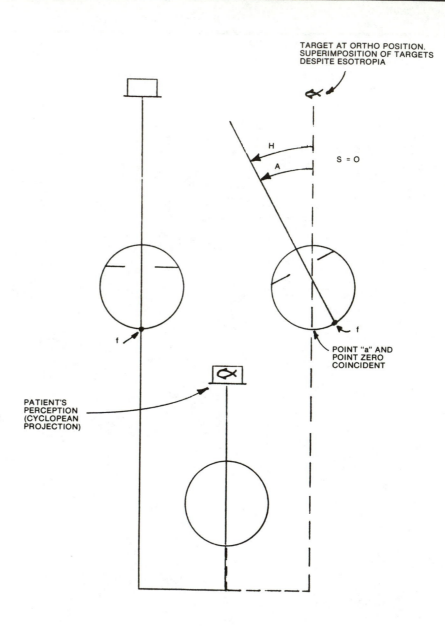

FIGURE 2-36 — Illustration of harmonious anomalous correspondence

anomalous associated point (a) is in the same place as point zero. In other words, the fovea of the fixating left eye corresponds to point (a), which is on point zero of the right eye.

There are two general methods for the testing of anomalous correspondence. Either angles H and S can be measured and compared, or just a measure of angle A can be made. Of the two, those methods that compare the objective and subjective angles are the most frequently used.

The most practical method to measure angle H is by the alternate cover test with loose prisms. The measurement of angle S may also be accomplished by the use of loose prisms. If further dissociation is necessary because of suppression, the patient may wear colored filters. If suppression continues to hamper measurement of the subjective angle, a sufficiently large vertical prism base-down may be placed before the deviating eye. This puts the stimulus below the suppression zone, allowing diplopia to be perceived. While the stimulated point on the retina is different from the original point zero before the base-down prism was added, the new point zero is in the same vertical meridian as the old one. Hugonnier[59] believes A R C occurs in the whole retina rather than in one point, such as that represented by point (a). The point should be thought of as a vertical band in the deviating eye corresponding to a vertical band passing through the fovea of the fixating eye. In accepting this presumption, it should be immaterial whether the subjective angle is measured with point zero being displaced (e.g., by base-down prism) vertically or not.

On the other hand, Parks[60] believes that a fairly small retinal displacement of the image from the macular area may cause an N R C (normal retinal correspondence) response to be revealed in the periphery, even though a central A R C is found. The implication here is that there may be central A R C and peripheral N R C. The opposite of this (i.e., central N R C with fusion, and peripheral A R C without fusion) is highly unlikely.

Parks believes, for instance, that a small angle esotrope, up to 8 p.d., may have good peripheral fusion in spite of there being no fusion centrally. The motor fusional vergences may be normal, and gross stereopsis may be present. He calls this the monofixation syndrome. Cases I have personally seen that fit this description may or may not have A R C. When A R C is present, it is usually of the harmonious type. One case was a 12 p.d. concomitant constant esotrope, of early onset, who alternated, had central suppression, and A R C on most conventional tests. This diagnosis notwithstanding, fusional vergences were fair, and peripheral sensory fusion was good with normal correspondence in the periphery by clinical testing.

In short, I feel these cases are merely examples of small angle strabismus (under 10 p.d.) in which abnormal sensorial adaptation may take place centrally, but because of sufficiently large Panum's areas in the periphery, fusion may be maintained. Often there is a latent deviation ("phoria") in conjunction with the tropia. The alternate cover test reveals a larger angle H than found by unilateral cover in such cases.

Ludlam[61] concurred with the concept of central A R C and peripheral N R C by stating that comparison of results of central versus peripheral afterimage testing may show central A R C with peripheral N R C. A noncross afterimage is seen for central stimulation, but a cross is seen for peripheral stimulation.

CLASSIFICATION   Correspondence is classified as being either normal or anomalous. If it is anomalous, the classification is either harmonious or unharmonious. Unharmonious correspondence may be typical or atypical. Paradoxical type one and type two are the atypical unharmonious models of anomalous correspondence. Refer to Table 2K for classification and formulas pertaining to angular magnitudes for each category.

TABLE 2K. *Classification of Correspondency (for Esotropia)*

Type of Correspondence			Relationship of angles
A.	Normal (N.R.C.)		H = S and A = zero
B.	Anomalous (A.R.C.)		H ≠ S A ≠ Zero
	1.	Harmonious	H = A and S = O
	2.	Unharmonious	
		a. typical	H > A and S < H
		b. atypical	
		(1) paradoxical type one	A > H and S < zero
		(2) paradoxical type two	S > H and A < zero

An example of paradoxical type one A R C is illustrated in Figure 2-37. In such a case the patient subjectively directionalizes under binocular viewing conditions as though he is exotropic, even though the objective angle clearly indicates the presence of esotropia. This may occur when the original angle of esotropia was greater before extraocular muscle surgery than afterwards. The deviation may have been reduced by surgery, but not enough to make the visual axes parallel so the fovea can be at point zero. For example, in a case of harmonious A R C where point (a) was at point zero, the outward rotational movement of the eye from surgery caused point (a) to be moved from the zero point to another point further in the nasal retina. The stimulation of point zero (post-surgical), which is temporal in respect to point (a), causes binocular directionalization to be subjectively like an exo deviation.

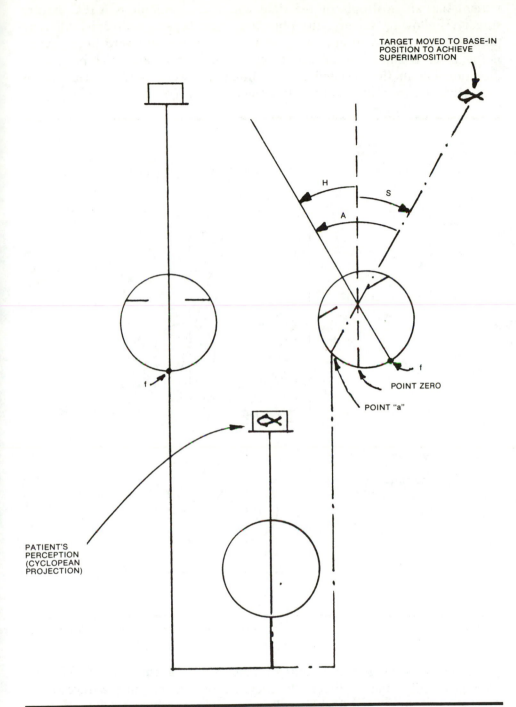

FIGURE 2-37 — Illustration of paradoxical type one unharmonious anomalous correspondence

Unharmonious paradoxical A R C type two may occur following an overcorrection of an exotropia with A R C. For example, suppose the patient had an exotropia of the right eye with harmonious A R C before surgery. Following surgery, the objective angle became esotropic, whereby point (a) was moved from point zero to a place temporalward in respect to point zero. Stimulation of point zero would now cause the patient to directionalize in the deviated eye as though he were highly esotropic. His subjective angle is more eso than his objective angle (see Figure 2-38).

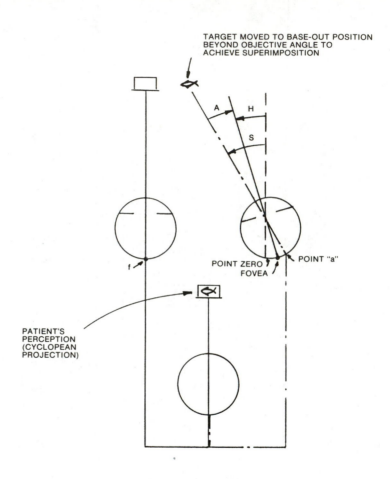

FIGURE 2-38 — Illustration of paradoxical type two unharmonious anomalous correspondence

It should be pointed out that other causes may change angle H other than extraocular muscle surgery. Plus lenses, for example, may reduce an eso deviation, minus an exo deviation. Prisms may optically affect these angular relationships as well as the possibility of orthoptics having similar effects.

An example of normal correspondence is illustrated in Figure 2-39. The objective and subjective angles are the same in this case of esotropia with N R C.

Several testing methods allow the magnitude of angle A to be measured. These rely on the special use of afterimages, entoptic phenomena, or on visuoscopic procedures performed under binocular conditions. All other procedures find angle A by indirectly calculating the difference between the objective and subjective angles of deviation.

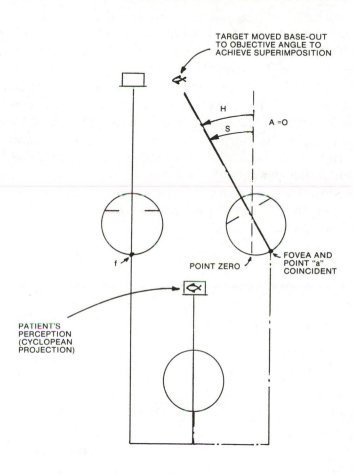

FIGURE 2-39 — Illustration of normal correspondence

The Hering-Bielschowsky test is the most frequently used method of testing retinal correspondence with afterimages. The procedure is as follows:

1. Occlude the nondominant eye while the patient fixates a central dark spot on a brightly illuminated horizontal streak or line (either a continuous light or a strobe flasher). The exact center should be opaque to produce a small gap in the A.I. (afterimage) for reference purposes.

2. After sufficient time of exposure for creation of an afterimage has elapsed, switch occlusion to the dominant eye and expose the nondominant eye to the streak of light oriented in a vertical position.
3. Uncover the eye and instruct the patient to fixate a small spot on the wall that has a neutral color (e.g., grey).
4. Lowering and raising the room illumination usually helps the patient perceive both the horizontal and vertical afterimages.

Interpretation of results is made by measuring the displacement of the vertical A.I. from the central gap of the horizontal A.I. If the patient reports seeing a perfect cross (as illustrated in Figure 2-40), there is a presumption of N R C since the angle of anomaly is zero. It is irrelevant whether the eyes are straight (i.e., in the ortho posture) or not, in order to appreciate a perfect cross. Each fovea is stimulated, and if there is normal correspondence between the two foveas, a cross will be perceived regardless of which way the eyes are pointed. An example of a noncross perception is shown in Figure 2-41. The right eye is esotropic with anomalous correspondence. Point (a) is the representational point that corresponds to the fovea of the left eye. Cyclopean projection shows the vertical afterimage being seen to the left since point (a) has the directional value of zero, and the fovea acts as a temporal retinal point.

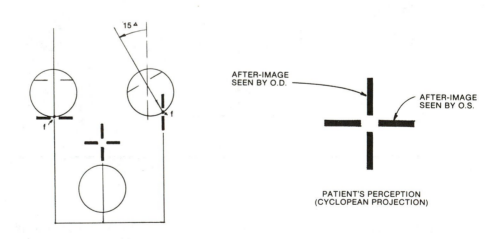

FIGURE 2-40 — Hering-Bielschowsky afterimage test in case of esotropia with normal correspondence

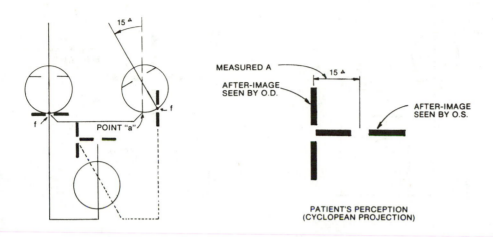

FIGURE 2-41 — Hering-Bielschowsky afterimage test in case of esotropia with harmonious anomalous correspondence

The Hering-Bielschowsky afterimage test is not valid unless the effect of a co-existing eccentric fixation is taken into account. Figure 2-42 illustrates this by taking the same case as in the above examples, but adding to it the condition of nasal eccentric fixation of the right eye. A perfect cross is formed if angle E and angle A are the same. In other words, point (a) and point (e) are in the same location on the retina. In such a case, the patient has point (e) stimulated during monocular fixation with the right eye. Because this is the same as the point that corresponds to the fovea of the other eye, the patient will project the vertical afterimage in the same direction as the horizontal. It is the exception and not the rule that angles E and A are exactly the same. They are usually of different magnitudes, but frequently in the same direction, e.g., points (a) and (e) at different locations on the nasal retina. Unless they are in the identical location, a noncross will be perceived.

The doctor can make no conclusion about the status of the A R C unless there is an accounting for angle E. To do this, the first step is to measure angle E by visuoscopic means. Angle A may then be determined by measuring the separation between the vertical A.I. and the center of the horizontal A.I. and adding the magnitude of angle E to this.

As an example, assume an angle E of 5 p.d. as found by visuoscopy. If the afterimage light is held at one meter and likewise the patient looks for

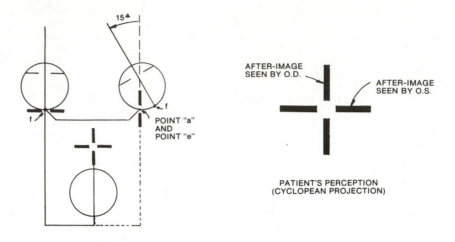

FIGURE 2-42 — Hering-Bielschowsky afterimage test in case of esotropia with harmonious A R C and nasal eccentric fixation. In this particular example the angle of eccentric fixation is the same as the angle of anomaly.

the afterimages on a wall one meter away, each centimeter represents one prism diopter. The patient then reports seeing the vertical afterimage off to the left by 10 p.d. This is the measured angle A, but not the true angle A. The magnitude of angle E (5 p.d., in this example) must be added to this measured angle A to arrive at the true angle of anomaly. It is easily seen that the angle between the fovea and point (a) is equal to 15 p.d. (not the 10 p.d. as measured, leaving angle E unaccounted for). See Figure 2-43.

It is not particularly necessary to use an afterimage for each eye as in the Hering-Bielschowsky test. The Brock-Givner afterimage transfer test is an excellent means of measuring the angle of anomaly. The distance from the fixated spot to the afterimage is subtended by angle A.

The warning of accounting for eccentric fixation must be heeded when attempting to use this test for anomalous correspondence. It is only when there is no eccentric fixation that the separation between the fixated spot and the perceived afterimage represents the angle of anomaly. If eccentric fixation is present, the value of angle E must be added to the value of the measured angle H. Because many patients have some difficulty in appreciating transferred afterimages, A R C testing is usually first attempted by stimulating each eye with a flash. This is the principal reason the Hering-Bielschowsky afterimage test is more popular than the Brock-Givner test for testing of anomalous correspondence. Otherwise, one is just as good as the other for measuring the angle of anomaly. Similarly, the drawback of eccentric fixation invalidating the reported results applies to each test.

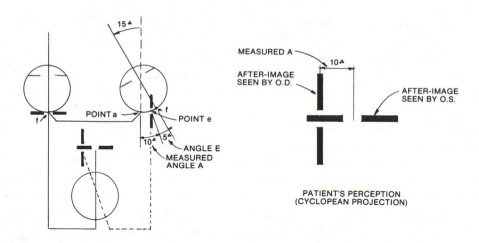

FIGURE 2-43 — Hering-Bielschowsky afterimage test in case of esotropia with harmonious A R C and nasal eccentric fixation in which the angle of eccentric fixation and the angle of anomaly are unequal. Angles A and E must be summed to determine the true angle of anomaly.

The major amblyoscope, such as the Synoptophore, may be used to detect and measure the angle of anomaly. This is done by first measuring the objective angle, then the subjective angle, and comparing the two. Angle H is found by alternately switching off each target light while moving the carriage arm in front of the nondominant eye until neutralization of eye movement is achieved. The subjective angle is measured by using superimposition targets, such as the fish and the tank. The target before the nondominant eye (e.g., fish) is moved from the base-in direction until superimposition is reported by the patient. Beginning from base-in rather than base-out is advised. This is for the purpose of inhibiting convergence that could possibly arise by moving the target from a base-out direction (base-out being a stimulus to convergence).

MAJOR AMBLYOSCOPE

If suppression is too extensive or intense, the target before the nondominant eye may need to be elevated in order for both targets to be seen simultaneously. The carriage arm of the major amblyoscope, or the target slide itself, may be elevated until the fish is seen above the tank. This is as though a base-down prism were introduced before the eye. Assuming enough vertical displacement is given to afford simultaneous perception, the carriage is moved in the appropriate horizontal direction, until the fish and tank are seen in vertical alignment. If there is a difference in central and peripheral correspondency, the subjective angle of deviation found by this procedure may be in question.

Once superimposition of the targets (or vertical alignment, in case of suppression) is achieved, the examiner can quickly check for the presence of A R C. This is done by shutting off the illumination to the target of the dominant eye (e.g., the eye fixating the tank) and watching for movement of the other eye. If the nondominant eye (seeing the fish) has to make a movement in the horizontal direction in order to monocularly fixate the center of the target, A R C is presumed to be present. Because the subjective angle had been fully compensated during superimposition (or alignment), the objective angle is different if an eye movement is necessary upon occlusion of the dominant eye. This, in effect, is the same procedure as the unilateral cover test, but done in the major amblyoscope rather than in free space. This procedure is sometimes referred to as the douse target test.

For example, a patient with an esotropia of the left eye, and with harmonious anomalous correspondence, might report the fish and the tank being superimposed when the instrument is set in the ortho demand position. When the light is doused for the tank target seen by the right eye, the left eye has to make an abduction movement if the patient is to look directly at the fish.

As with other A R C testing, eccentric fixation must be accounted for. In the above case, if A R C is present, nasal eccentric fixation could cause the left eye to abduct, but not as much as the magnitude of angle H. The magnitude of the movement would be equal to angle H minus angle E.

Afterimages may be generated in most major amblyoscopes. Since this is a reduced environment, and testing is less natural than in free space, the use of afterimages with these instruments is usually reserved for treatment of A R C rather than for testing.

DIPLOPIA TESTING   Various diplopia tests can be used in the evaluation of anomalous correspondence. All of them rely on the principle that the subjective angle can be measured by these means. Occasionally, spontaneous diplopia may be noticed in free space without the help of special filters and lenses. This is the most ideal diplopia test for A R C because a truer picture of the status of correspondence may be possible than when testing is done under less natural conditions.

Dissociation by means of colored filters to measure the subjective angle can be considered only slightly more natural than the use of afterimages. Instruments such as the major amblyoscope with septums are probably less laboratory-like than colored filters, but not as natural as vectographic methods which produce conditions fairly close to normal seeing. With the exception of spontaneous diplopia, however, the most natural test of all is the one using the Bagolini striated lenses.[62]

FILTERS AND   Various filters and special lenses may be used in order to measure the
SPECIAL LENSES   subjective angle of deviation which, in turn, can be compared to the objective angle of deviation. This comparison determines whether anomalous correspondence is present or not. Testing procedures are like those for

suppression testing. Measurement of the diplopic separation by means of prisms or linear rules (as in Hess-Lancaster) determines the subjective angle. Some of the more commonly used devices for this purpose include red lens, red-green filters, Maddox bi-prism, and vectographic methods.

The use of these lenses affords almost natural seeing conditions for the patient. The striations are so fine that the patient is unaware of them. If fixation is on a bright spot of light, the striations cause a streak to be visible.

Testing for A R C proceeds in the same manner as in suppression testing. A patient bifoveally fixating a penlight will see the penlight at the intersection of the streaks (see Figure 2-20c). If the patient has a manifest deviation whereby bifoveal fixation is not taking place, diplopic images of the light will be seen, unless suppression is too great. Usually suppression of one of the lights occurs because the image of one falls on point zero of the deviating eye. An example of esotropia is shown in Figure 2-20f. In this illustration, diplopic images of the light are shown to indicate that the intersection of the streaks is below the lights. In the case of an esotropia, one of the lights might be missing. If the right eye is esotropic, the right (homonymous) image would be suppressed.

An exotrope should report the streaks crossing above the light(s) (see Figure 2-20g).

In both of these explanations, there is the presumption of normal correspondence (N R C). If, however, there is A R C of the harmonious type, the patient reports seeing one light centered in the intersection of the streaks, because the subjective angle is zero in this type of A R C.

It should be pointed out here that these lenses are not significantly dissociative, so that a high amount of heterophoria can be present. As long as the deviation is held latent and is not manifest, the patient will report seeing light centered in the X. Now in the case of the frank esotropia with harmonious A R C, the subjective angle may be zero, but the objective angle is certainly not zero. The Bagolini striated lenses measure the subjective angle. All the doctor needs to do in such a case of esotropia is to observe the manifest eso deviation while at the same time listening to the patient report that he sees the light centered in the X (angle S being zero). This is obviously A R C, since the objective deviation can be observed if it is moderately large (10-20 p.d.). If the deviation is less than 10 p.d. and difficult to observe directly, the Hirschberg test can be incorporated. The patient looks at the penlight, and the doctor merely studies the relative position of each corneal reflection. If more sensitivity is needed to determine whether or not there is a manifest deviation, the unilateral cover test may be employed. This is just like the douse target test in the major amblyoscope. The dominant eye is occluded and movement of the nondominant eye is watched for. If movement occurs, the objective angle is greater than zero. This establishes the presence of A R C if the patient reports seeing the light centered in the X, since the angle H and angle S are not the same in this instance.

Von Noorden and Maumenee[63] state that the Bagolini test is not useful in diagnosing cases of unharmonious A R C, where the subjective angle is other than zero. However, I find the following technique useful in dealing with unharmonious cases. First, find out from the patient where the streaks cross. If they cross below, as in an eso deviation, I introduce just enough base-out prism until the patient reports that the light is centered in the X. At this point, I do the unilateral cover test to see if there is a movement of the uncovered eye. If there is, the patient has A R C of the unharmonious type. The subjective angle in such a case would be equal to the amount of base-out prism it took to get the centered X pattern. Since angle S is not zero, the A R C is not harmonious. The angle of anomaly is the magnitude of the movement of the uncovered eye on the unilateral cover test.

I might add here that the majority of A R C patients show the harmonious pattern on the Bagolini test; but not infrequently, A R C cases with the unharmonious type are found by this test.

Cautious interpretation of the response reported on the Bagolini striated lens test cannot be stressed too strongly. Many patients, particularly young children, tend to give unreliable answers unless they are questioned very carefully. My impression is that patients find it easier to say they see the X with the light in the center than to attempt to describe anything otherwise. The doctor must be extra careful not to erroneously lead the patient to this response.

OTHER EVALUATION PROCEDURES

Three other useful procedures for A R C testing are discussed. They are color fusion testing, the Giessen test, and the bifoveal test of Cüppers.

COLOR FUSION TESTING

This is often referred to as testing for luster. The level of binocularity required for the appreciation of color fusion (rather than form fusion) is probably somewhere on the hierarchical ladder between simultaneous perception and superimposition.

The most efficacious way to evaluate whether or not color fusion is present is by having the patient wear red-green filters while looking at a brightly illuminated translucent grey screen (see Figure 2-44a). Usually the red filter is worn on the right eye, but it may also be helpful to have the patient switch filters. Sometimes it is appreciated one way and not the other. What the patient should report is that a mixture of the red and green is seen on the illuminated screen. This is usually reported as being a muddy yellow. Moving the patient so that his visual axes cross at the plane of the screen may help elicit luster (using plus lenses for an esotrope and base-in prism for an exotrope). The key to deciding whether or not there is color fusion in case of indefinite responses is to occlude one eye and ask the patient if anything looks different. If there is a difference between the monocular and binocular percepts, luster is probably indicated, assuming that the entire field is uniformly color mixed, and the patient is not reporting the perception of a bipartite field.

Borish[64] states that if a split field is reported, it is not true color fusion, but indicative of A R C. Figure 2-44b shows the perception of a patient with a split field. I have found that patients who give this response tend to have harmonious A R C, whereas those giving partially split field responses, as in Figure 2-44c, tend to have unharmonious A R C. More reporting in this regard is necessary before these observations can be conclusive.

The Giessen test of Cüppers for A R C testing is reported by Hugonnier.[65] The only equipment necessary is a penlight, or similar white luminous spot, a deep red filter, an afterimage generator, and a calibrated tangent scale, such as a Maddox cross.

Taking, for example, a right esotropia, the examination procedure is as follows:

1. Generate a vertical afterimage on the deviating eye (right eye in this case).
2. Place the deep red filter[x] before the fixating eye (left eye in this case).
3. The patient reports the respective locations (his perception) of the afterimage, the red spot, and the white spot in regard to each other, and their locations on the calibrated numbered tangent scale. Often the white spot is suppressed (being on point zero), but if the scale is marked, the patient merely states what number the A.I. is on and what number the red spot is on.

This procedure is illustrated in Figure 2-45 (a-e). If the left eye is occluded, an afterimage is produced on the fovea of the deviating right eye. Figure 2-45a shows the left eye fixating the target light through the deep red filter. The percept for the left eye is a red spot with everything in the background being almost invisible due to the density of the filter. The right eye has the perception of an afterimage located somewhere on the tangent scale.

Figure 2-45b shows the patient has harmonious A R C (sometimes abbreviated as H A R C). In this particular condition, point zero and point (a) are one and the same. The perception of the ocular images is also illustrated in Figure 2-45b. Cyclopean projection shows that the left eye sees the red spot as being straight ahead. Superimposed on the red spot, however, is the white spot, causing the spot to possibly appear pink rather than either just red or white. This is because point (a) of the right eye corresponds with the fovea of the left eye. The afterimage, however, is seen off to the left, because it is on the temporal retina relative to the zero directional value of point (a).

Calibrated markings on the tangent scale enable the doctor to measure

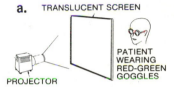

a.   TRANSLUCENT SCREEN

PROJECTOR

PATIENT WEARING RED-GREEN GOGGLES

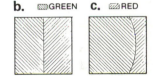

b.   ░GREEN   c.   ▨RED

FIGURE 2-44 — Color fusion testing. (a) Patient views an illuminated grey screen while wearing a red filter over the right eye and a green filter over the left eye; (b) Split field response that may be found in cases of esotropia with harmonious A R C; (c) Partially split field occasionally seen in cases of esotropia with typical unharmonious A R C.

---

[x]The red filter must be very dense so that only the fixation light is visible when viewing through it. I construct such a filter by combining an ordinary red lens with a neutral density filter to create the desired degree of darkening.

angles H, S, and A. Let us suppose that the afterimage was reported by the patient as being on number 14. The objective angle is, therefore, 14 p.d. (assuming testing is done at one meter, and the distance is 14 cms from the white spot). The angle of anomaly is represented by the distance between the afterimage and the red spot (pink spot, in this case, since superimposition with the white spot). This is because both foveas are tagged, the fixating eye has the red spot on its fovea, and the deviating eye has had the afterimage placed on its fovea. In other words, the A.I. and red spot should be superimposed if correspondence is normal, no matter what the objective angle might be under these testing conditions. If the A.I. and the red spot are not superimposed, A R C is present. In this illustrated example, the angle of anomaly is also 14 (since the definition of H A R C is that angle H and A are equal).

Figure 2-45c shows how a patient with typical unharmonious A R C, with the same angle H, might perceive the positioning of the A.I., the red spot, and the white spot. Point (a) is between the fovea and point zero in the typical case of unharmonious A R C. Therefore, the white spot, which is on point zero, is relatively nasalward from point (a), and is perceived as though to the right of the red spot. The afterimage, however, is temporalward and projected to the left of the red spot. The calibrated scale gives the magnitude of the angles. The distance between the red and white spots (as in ordinary pathological diplopia testing) represents the subjective angle. The distance between the afterimage and the red spot represents the angle of anomaly. From the formula A=H-S, the objective angle can be calculated from H=A+S.

The objective angle is determined by the patient who reports on what number the afterimage is seen. This measures angle H because the fixating eye is looking straight ahead, and the direction of the visual axis of the deviating eye is indicated by the afterimage. Thus, the position of the fovea is tagged by the A.I. Examples of paradoxical types of A R C are illustrated in Figures 2-45 d and e.

An example of normal correspondence is illustrated for this same case of esotropia in Figure 2-45a. There is no point (a) in such a case, since the fovea of one eye corresponds to the fovea of the other eye. The A.I. and the red spot, therefore, are seen as being superimposed (no angle of anomaly). The white light falling on point zero is homonymously projected off to the right. Also (as in Figure 2-45a), the patient perceives the superimposition of the afterimage and the red spot, which appears to fall on the same number on the tangent scale. The number on which the A.I. is seen represents the objective angle. The number on which the red spot is seen represents the subjective angle. The angles are equal, as they should be, since this is a case of normal correspondence.

This novel testing method of Cüppers is somewhat unnatural because of the afterimage and dense filter. Furthermore, it is not always practical in certain cases, (e.g., deep amblyopia), or with an uncooperative patient. It does, however, produce definitive results in the majority of cases, and is a

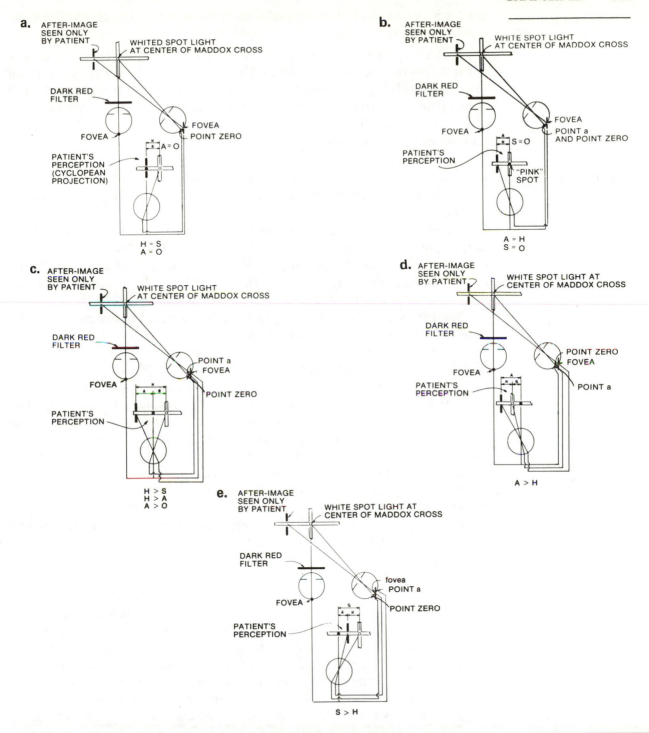

FIGURE 2-45 — Illustrations of the Giessen test. (a) Esotropia of the right eye with normal correspondence; (b) Esotropia of the right eye with harmonious anomalous correspondence; (c) Esotropia of the right eye with typical unharmonious anomalous correspondence; (d) Estropia of the right eye with paradoxical type one unharmonious anomalous correspondence; (e) Esotropia of the right eye with paradoxical type two unharmonious anomalous correspondence.

good way to measure all three angles involved in A R C (A, H, and S) in one quick procedure.

Halldén[66] earlier devised an excellent test for A R C. In many ways it is similar to the method of Cüppers. However, it requires twin projectors, an afterimage, filters, and projection screen. The set-up is too elaborate and cumbersome for most practitioners to have in their offices. Since identical information regarding A R C can be obtained in other ways, this particular method of testing will not be discussed.

BIFOVEAL TEST OF CÜPPERS   Most of the tests for A R C mentioned previously have one or more shortcomings, the most common being the unaccountability for eccentric fixation.

The one test that can eliminate this invalidating factor is the bifoveal test, originated by Cüppers[67]. This is also referred to as the maculo-macular test. Testing is done by performing visuoscopy under binocular conditions for the measurement of angle A. This should not be confused with the measurement of angle E under monocular conditions.

The procedure for performing this test is illustrated in Figure 2-46 (a-d). Suppose the patient has an esotropia of the right eye. An angled mirror (or a large base-out prism of 30-40 p.d.) is placed before the dominant left eye, so that it can fixate a penlight off to the side (see Figure 2-46a). This is necessary for the patient to maintain seeing under binocular conditions without one eye being occluded by the doctor's head during visuoscopy. The next step is for the doctor to look into the nondominant right eye observing the projected image of the star on the patient's retina. At the same time, the patient looks into the instrument to see the star. The patient should be aware of both the penlight and the star, unless suppression is very deep and extensive. The doctor then projects the star directly on to the fovea and asks the patient what he sees. If correspondence is normal (N R C), the patient should report the light and the star being superimposed (see Figure 2-46b) because both foveas correspond with each other. If, however, the foveas don't correspond, as in Figure 2-46c, the patient will not report super-imposition even though both foveas are stimulated.

In this case, the star would have to be moved nasalward to point (a) before the patient would see the light and the star superimposed (see Figure 2-46d). This is because point (a) corresponds to the fovea of the other eye. The distance from point (a) to the fovea represents the magnitude of angle A. This can be measured by the projected concentric circles, or more conveniently be estimated by using retinal landmarks, such as the optic disc. Knowing that the center of the disc is approximately 15½ degrees from the center of the fovea helps in the estimation of the distance from the star to the fovea. Likewise, if the width of the disc is 5½ degrees, the first margin of the disc would be 12¾ (23 p.d.) and the outer margin 18¼ degrees (33 p.d.) from the center of the fovea (see Figure 2-47).

Utilizing this procedure if the angle of anomaly is estimated to be

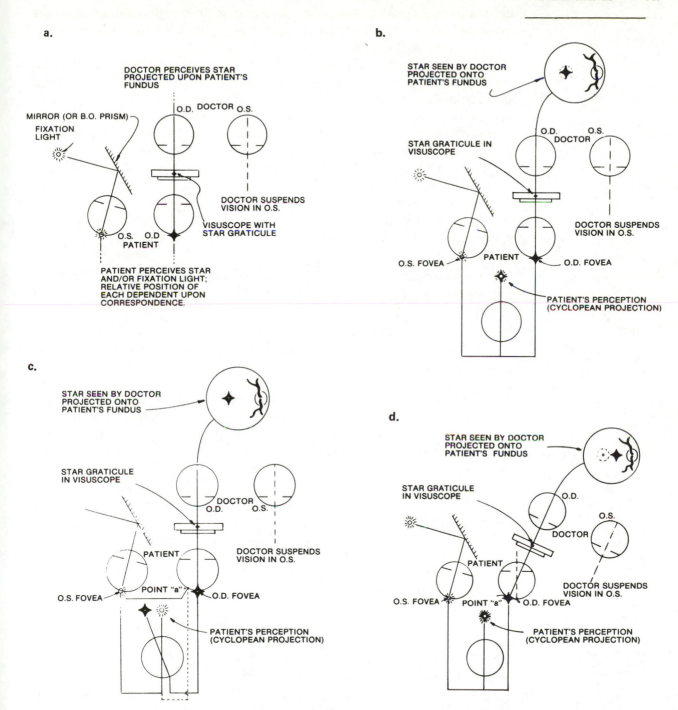

FIGURE 2-46 — Illustrations of the bifoveal test of Cüppers. (a) Doctor's right eye views the patient's right eye by means of visuoscopy. The star is seen by the doctor and the patient. An angled mirror (or a large base-out prism) before the patient's left eye avoids obstruction to seeing by left eye; (b) Example of normal correspondence; (c) Example of anomalous correspondence; (d) Star must be projected onto point "a" in order for a patient with A R C to achieve superimposition of the penlight and the star.

approximately equal in magnitude to the objective angle of the strabismus (as found beforehand by alternate cover test), the A R C is harmonious. If otherwise, the A R C is unharmonious.

The bifoveal test takes much of the guesswork out of measuring the angle of anomaly as compared to other more subjective methods of testing. In addition to this advantage, the presence of eccentric fixation is not an invalidating factor. It is because testing is done under binocular conditions, thereby vitiating any effect of eccentric fixation that would otherwise come into play if testing were done under monocular conditions. The patient's fixating eye which sees the penlight, must, however, have central fixation in order for this test to be valid.

The disadvantage of this test is that a high level of patient control and cooperation must be maintained; otherwise, testing is either impossible or results are unreliable.

Other Considerations

Several miscellaneous topics pertaining to anomalous correspondence are discussed in this section.

DEPTH OF ANOMALOUS
CORRESPONDENCE

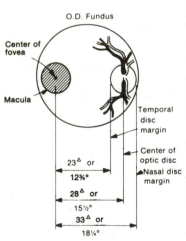

O.D. Fundus

Center of fovea

Macula

Temporal disc margin

Center of optic disc

Nasal disc margin

23$^\Delta$ or
12¾°
28$^\Delta$ or
15½°
33$^\Delta$ or
18¼°

FIGURE 2-47 — Illustration showing useful dimensions in the fundus for estimating the magnitude of the angle of anomaly when using the bifoveal test

Testing of the depth of A R C appears to be analogous to testing the intensity of suppression. If the testing conditions are unnatural, suppression is less likely to be found. This is often apparent in A R C testing. Burian[6 8] is the principal advocate for the concept of depth of anomalous correspondence. He believed A R C is an acquired sensorial adaptation to a motor deviation, and this adaptation may be either deep or shallow. This may be one possible explanation for the frequent occurrence of an A R C response on the Bagolini striated lens test and an N R C response on other less natural tests, such as afterimages.

The rule is that the more natural the testing environment, the more likely it is that A R C will be found; contrarily, the more unnatural the environment, the more likely N R C will be found. Several commonly used A R C tests are listed in Table 2L giving the order of their degree of naturalness.

Most clinicians seem to have accepted the concept of deep-seatedness of anomalous correspondence. Flom and Kerr[6 9], however, reject this concept. They contend that disagreement between various tests can be attributed to measurement error, unsteady eccentric fixation, or changes in the relative position of the eyes from one test to another. They employed five different tests in their study which included the following: Maddox rod-cover test, major amblyoscope, Hallden test using red-green filters and afterimage to measure objective and subjective angles, Hallden test to measure the angle of anomaly (also using red-green filters and afterimage), and the Hering-Bielschowsky afterimage test. Most of the testing methods were less than natural in many respects. Unfortunately, the Bagolini striated lens test was not included in the study.

My impression from clinical experience is that there are some patients who show A R C on some of the more natural tests, while showing N R C on the less natural ones. Prognosis for elimination of A R C appears to be slightly more favorable for those patients giving a positive response on only one test than when A R C is found on all tests.

TABLE 2L. Commonly Used A R C Tests Listed in Rank Order as to Degree of Naturalness

1. Spontaneous diplopia in free space (the subjective angle is found and compared to the objective angle as measured by the cover test)

2. Bagolini striated lens test (this is subjective angle which is compared with the objective angle as measured with the cover test)

3. Vectographic methods (to determine the subjective angle of deviation, and compare it with the objective angle as measured by the cover test)

4. Major amblyoscope (to compare the objective and subjective angles of deviation)

5. Colored filters (to determine the subjective angle, and compare it with the objective angle found with the cover test)

6. Negative afterimages (A.I. seen as dark lines on light background)

7. Positive afterimages (A.I. seen as light lines on dark background)

INTERMITTENCY OF ANOMALOUS CORRESPONDENCE

Most authorities believe a patient can possibly have A R C when an angle of deviation is manifest; yet, this same patient can have N R C when the deviation is kept latent by the power of fusion. In other words, an intermittent strabismic may have A R C if he is intermittently heterotropic, but have N R C when the eyes are in the ortho position. Flom and Kerr[70] concur with this concept of "co-variation" of anomalous correspondence.

This is often found in cases of intermittent exotropia. An angle of anomaly is found when the deviation is manifest, but the angle of anomaly becomes zero (therefore N R C) when fusion is resumed. Intermittency of this nature unexplainably occurs less frequently in cases of eso deviations.

It is possible that an intermittent A R C is less deeply seated than a constant one, but there is no universal agreement on this issue. What is important, however, is that the prognosis is usually good in cases of this type, not necessarily because of the intermittency of the A R C, but because of the intermittency of the strabismus per se. The prognosis for functional cure of an intermittent strabismus is generally much more favorable than for a constant strabismus, the presence of A R C notwithstanding.

ETIOLOGY OF ANOMALOUS CORRESPONDENCE

The traditional view is that A R C is an acquired sensorial anomaly. Burian[71] states the "A R C is acquired by usage . . . the acquisition of an anomalous correspondence represents an adaptation of the sensory apparatus of the eyes to the abnormal position of the eyes."

On the other hand, Morgan[72] believes that A R C is a motor phenomenon and states, "Thus anomalous correspondence might depend not on a sensory adaptation to a squint but rather on whether the basic underlying innervational pattern to the extraocular muscles was one which registered itself in consciousness as altering egocentric direction, or whether the pattern was one which was 'nonregistered' in consciousness as altering egocentric direction." A nonregistered innervation would imply normal correspondence, while a registered pattern would mean anomalous correspondence.

Whether A R C has a sensorial or a motoric cause in strabismus remains an academic question at the present time. Furthermore, there is probably an equal amount of uncertainty as to the time required for A R C to develop. Most authorities believe suppression is involved in the first stages, and A R C follows as an additional antidiplopia mechanism when necessary. Although this process is generally regarded as requiring a considerable length of time, I have personally seen a deep-seated case of A R C develop within a two-week period. A case in particular was a teenage girl with intermittent exotropia who had excellent sensory fusion with normal correspondence. A surgical overcorrection resulted in a small angle constant esotropia with harmonious A R C. The presence of an angle of anomaly was determined by all tests, including afterimages.

Anomalous correspondence is almost always thought of as being a horizontal phenomenon and not vertical. Fitton[73] reported two cases of vertical tropia with vertical A R C in a study of 48 patients examined after a period of six years since extraocular muscle surgery for congenital esotropia. Griffin and Scheffel[74] observed an adult with vertical strabismus and vertical A R C. Case history revealed the patient had esotropia since 18 months of age. Extraocular muscle surgery was performed at five years of age. During an examination the patient took at 21 years of age, there was a constant manifest deviation of approximately 5 p.d. exotropia and 8 p.d. left hypotropia. Correctable visual acuity was approximately 20/20 in each eye, fixation being steady and central. A vertical angle of anomaly of approximately 2½ to 3 p.d. was consistently found on the following tests: Bagolini, major amblyoscope, Giessen test, and Hering-Bielschowsky afterimages.

INCIDENCE OF ANOMALOUS CORRESPONDENCE

This statistic can be quite variable, and is undoubtedly due to the type of cases being considered, the type of testing being used, and who does the testing. A survey of 15 authorities was reported by Enos[75] who found a range from 14 to 71 percent with an average of 47.5 percent. A study done at the Vanderbilt Eye Clinic in which 295 strabismics were followed was included in the same report. A R C was found in 45 percent of the cases. Of the esotropes, 53 showed A R C and only 16 percent of the exotropes showed A R C. These statistics were based on major amblyoscope findings. Perhaps the incidence would be lower if less natural tests were used and higher if more natural tests were used.

In this regard, Hugonnier[76] cites Bagolini's findings. Of 98 cases of strabismus, the striated lens test revealed 84 cases of harmonious A R C; the Synoptophore yielded 64 cases of A R C (12 harmonious and 52 unharmonious) and with afterimages there were only 35 cases of A R C.

My impression is that the Bagolini striated lens test must be interpreted with caution because of the highly subjective nature of the test, and the naive patient's tendency to report an ortho response. In spite of the possible pitfall of the patient reporting erroneously, this can be an excellent test if used judiciously. It seems to indicate the majority of cases of A R C are harmonious; also, that the incidence of A R C may be quite high for strabismics under normal viewing conditions in everyday casual seeing.

Not much is known about these conditions, and the literature is relatively scant on these subjects. Some authorities believe horror fusionis is the same as a lack of correspondence. There is general agreement, however, that either condition represents a very low form (if any) of binocular vision.

Horror Fusionis and Lack Of Correspondence

In horror fusionis, superimposition is not possible, and simultaneous perception is the best form of binocularity that can be attained. Patients who clearly demonstrate a complete lack of correspondence are unable to appreciate simultaneous perception. Parks[77] refers to examples of congenital esotropes who apparently have a lack of correspondence by being unable to perceive diplopia. Consequently, he believes there should be no fear of post-surgical diplopia in cases of this type.

Horror fusionis is defined by Schapero et al.[78] as "the inability to obtain binocular fusion or superimposition of haploscopically presented targets, or the condition or phenomenon itself, occurring frequently as a characteristic in strabismus, in which case the targets approaching superimposition may seem to slide or jump past each other without apparent fusion or suppression."

DEFINITIONS AND CHARACTERISTICS

Lyle and Wybar[79] define horror fusionis as being a macular evasion, and state, ". . . on attempting bi-macular stimulation a constant change occurs in the deviation which may be horizontal, vertical or oblique, thus preventing simultaneous macular perception or fusion."

Kramer[80] believes patients with horror fusionis are of a neuropathic type in which, psychologically, they do not desire fusion, and make no effort to fuse. It is as though there may be a defective development of the sensory areas of the occipital lobes. She believes there is neither normal nor anomalous correspondence in cases of horror fusionis; and therefore, there is no sensorial correspondence at all. She further recommends psychotherapy as playing a role in the treatment of horror fusionis.

On the other hand, Burian[81] believes there is always some type of correspondence, either normal or anomalous. He states, "if an investigator relies exclusively on the Synoptophore test, he may be led to the erroneous conclusion that there is no functional correspondence between the two eyes. But if other tests are also employed, normal correspondence or some type of anomalous correspondence is always evident."

Some authorities equate horror fusionis with intractable diplopia. Krimsky[82] associates horror fusionis with post-operative diplopia and states, "this type of diplopia often disappears spontaneously with a reasonable variable period, and psychotherapy and assurance often prove good treatment."

Borish[83] likewise implies horror fusionis and intractable diplopia are one and the same. He states, "very infrequently a strabismic cannot make a successful adaptation for single vision so that a persistent diplopia is experienced with an inability to fuse, termed horror fusionis."

Not much more is really known about horror fusionis than when Bielschowsky[84] studied it and thought it was not necessarily congenital, but possibly due to aniseikonia, neurotic tendencies or some other unaccounted-for cause. Horopters may be considered (see Chapters Eight and Thirteen).

TESTING PROCEDURES

Most procedures for the evaluation of such poor levels of binocularity require stereoscopic instrumentation, such as the Synoptophore. In the case of horror fusionis, the patient may be able to see both targets simultaneously (e.g., fish and fishtank) but is unable to superimpose them. As the carriage arm of the Synoptophore is moved from a base-in to a base-out direction (or vice versa), the fish is reported as approaching the tank. When it almost touches the edge of the tank, the patient reports the fish jumping to the other side of the tank. No matter how slowly and carefully the carriage arm is moved, the patient cannot see the fish as being inside the tank.

The subjective angle of deviation may be measured in many of these cases, however, by creating a vertical displacement between the fish and the tank. The horizontal alignment is easily attained if the vertical separation is adequate. By knowing angle S from this procedure, the angle of anomaly may be determined by comparing angles S and H. Some cases of horror fusionis have A R C, as determined by this procedure, while others show N R C.

Vodnoy[85] states that a retinal rivalry card containing oblique lines running in opposite directions for each eye can be used in a Brewster stereoscope. A color fusion slide may also be used for detection of horror fusionis. He states, "if neither technique can be achieved, horror fusionis may exist and the patient is untrainable."

OTHER CONSIDERATIONS

It is my personal opinion that a patient with horror fusionis may or may not have intractable diplopia. I have seen both situations, and more frequently, horror fusionis can be demonstated in the major amblyoscope, but intractable diplopia is not present under normal seeing conditions in free space.

I have seen documented cases of congenital esotropias that demonstrate a sensorial ability ranging from peripheral fusion (but not central fusion), with peripheral stereopsis, to those having A R C with no stereopsis. Also seen are those having an apparent lack of correspondence. In the latter type of case, diplopia is usually not present for habitual seeing, and there is no problem of intractable diplopia. In a few instances, however, patients have unexplainably complained of occasional diplopia even though they are unable to appreciate simultaneous perception in the major amblyoscope. As in cases of horror fusionis having intractable diplopia, psychotherapy may be necessary to give relief, not for the binocular problem per se, but for help in coping with diplopia. Patients with emotional problems are generally less tolerant of diplopia than are those without emotional problems.

Accommodation Infacility

Inflexibility of accommodation is frequently found in cases of amblyopia with eccentric fixation. This is probably because nonfoveal areas of the retina do not control accommodative changes. Crane[86] reported that the focus control for any eye is confined to the center of the fovea.

Accommodation infacility is also commonly found in young patients without eccentric fixation. In many of these cases, there is a history of academic underachievement. Although accommodative amplitude is usually normal, the changing of focus from one accommodative demand to another may be sluggish.

MONOCULAR TESTING

A system for monocular accommodation facility testing is presented by Pierce and Greenspan.[87] Three recommended procedures are illustrated in Figure 2-48.

The procedure for the alternate occlusion methods using a hand-held occluder (see Figure 2-48a) is as follows:

1. Have the patient look at the smallest print he can see. This may be at his normal working distance, however, it is usually done at 40 cms unless otherwise specified. Pierce and Greénspan recommend the Harmon distance (from elbow to first knuckle of the middle finger when the hand is stretched out).
2. Have the patient clear the print through a plus lens over the right eye while the left eye is occluded.
3. Switch the occluder to the left eye and have the patient clear the print through a minus lens.
4. Two fixations constitute one cycle. Continue switching the occluder for 20 cycles.
5. Record the time it takes for the total procedure and divide by 20 to find the average time for each cycle.
6. The ideal is to have each cycle within three to four seconds with lenses of +2.50 and −2.50 diopters. In other words, the patient should be able to go through the entire series of 20 cycles in approximately one minute. Lesser powers may be required initially for orientation purposes.
7. The same 20 cycle procedure should be repeated with the lens powers reversed, i.e., minus over O.D. and plus over O.S.

It should be noted that this procedure requires 40 fixations. The total time should be divided by 40 if the average time per fixation is to be determined. Therefore, each fixation should ideally take approximately 1½ seconds. Some patients have trouble going from plus to minus, but not in going from minus to plus. Others find it difficult to go the other way. This difference in response should be looked for during the 20 cycles.

The advantage of putting the patient through many cycles rather than just one or two is that the effect of fatigue can be evaluated. This is thought to play a role in underachievement in reading when nearpoint accommodative demands are not met with ease and accuracy.

Monocular accommodation facility testing using partial occluders (Figure 2-48b) and far-near apertures (Figure 2-48c) are given in manner similar to the procedure using the hand-held occluder. Another way of monocular rock testing is to use a laterally swinging Marsden ball (or any similar target which is suspended by a string from the ceiling) and a septum (see Figure 2-49).

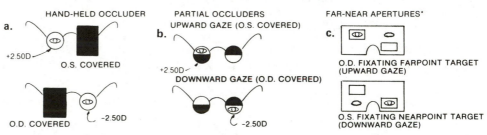

FIGURE 2-48 — Methods for testing monocular accommodation facility. (a) Alternate covering of each eye with a hand-held occluder (Note that two fixations constitute one cycle); (b) Alternate up-and-down fixation by partial occluders applied to spectacle lenses; (c) Alternate up-and-down fixation by vertically displaced apertures (Manas mask).

BINOCULAR TESTING

Binocular testing is divided into bi-ocular and binocular procedures by Pierce and Greenspan.[88]

Bi-ocular rock is accomplished by use of vertical dissociating prisms so that one target is perceived diplopically. The patient is instructed to alternately fixate and clear each of the targets for 20 cycles.

Binocular rock procedures require fusion whereby the patient must achieve bifoveal fixation during every cycle. Patients with vergence problems may be unable to respond well to binocular testing, even though their monocular accommodative flexibility is adequate.

For example, an esophoric patient may have trouble clearing the minus lenses because he has to let go of accommodation in order to see singly. The release of accommodation blurs the target but allows single vision by reducing accommodative convergence enough for the patient to be able to meet the divergence demand required for fusion. If the negative fusional vergence is adequate, however, the reduction of accommodative convergence is not necessary; therefore, the target remains clear during fusion.

An exophoric patient with poor positive fusional vergence may find it difficult going from minus to plus during binocular accommodative rock testing. This is because he may have to over-accommodate in order to increase accommodative convergence so that the convergence demand is met making fusion possible. This over-accommodation blurs the target. The amount of time required for clearing the target is an index to the status of motor fusion.

Figure 2-50 illustrates two set-ups for performing binocular accommodative rock using plus and minus lenses. Twenty cycles are given and timed as in monocular and bi-ocular procedures. The plus lenses are placed before both eyes. After clear vision is reported, they are quickly flipped away so that both minus lenses are introduced.

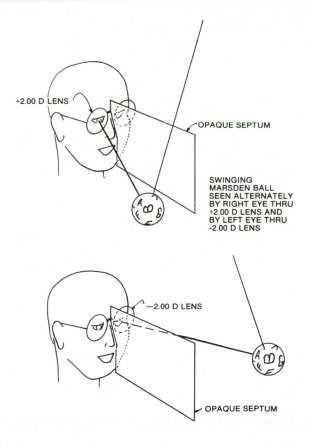

+2.00 D LENS

OPAQUE SEPTUM

SWINGING
MARSDEN BALL
SEEN ALTERNATELY
BY RIGHT EYE THRU
+2.00 D LENS AND
BY LEFT EYE THRU
-2.00 D LENS

—2.00 D LENS

OPAQUE SEPTUM

FIGURE 2-49 — Accommodation facility testing using a septum and laterally swinging ball as a fixation target.

Pierce and Greenspan advocate the ideal goal as having the patient fuse with clear vision for 20 cycles at a rate of 3 to 4 seconds per cycle through lenses of plus 2.50 and minus 4.00 diopters. That is to say, the patient should fuse and see clearly for each of the 40 accommodative demand changes. (Other criteria are given in Chapter Fifteen.)

Fixation Disparity and Fusional Vergence

The condition of fixation disparity is associated with heterophorias and not strabismic conditions.

DEFINITIONS

Fixation disparity is thought of as being a slight error of vergence. It has been emphasized by Ogle et al.[8 9] that in some cases of latent deviations, exact alignment of the visual axes is not present, but fusion is present nevertheless. This is possible when misalignment is small enough to allow the resulting disparate images to fall within Panum's areas of fusion. When this occurs, the condition is referred to as fixation disparity. Its magnitude is expressed in minutes of arc.

The angle of fixation disparity is illustrated in Figure 2-51. It is the angle subtended at the center of rotation of the eyeball by the visual axis and the ortho demand line (going to point zero).

An example of an exo fixation disparity is illustrated in Figure 2-51b. This is a theoretical posterior view of the eyeballs. If there is a very small error of vergence for the fixated x target, and fusion of the x is possible because of Panum's areas, the target will appear to be single and not diplopic. Since there is a fixation disparity, however, the vertical lines which are seen independently by each eye (refer to Figure 2-51a) will not be perceived by the patient as being in vernier alignment.

The direction in which this case of exo fixation disparity is localized is illustrated in Figure 2-51c. There is a heteronymous displacement of the line seen by the right eye. In this case, the top line is seen as being shifted toward the left in relation to the x and the bottom line. In this particular example, the left eye is strongly dominant because the right eye deviates from the true position required for exact on-center bifoveal fixation.

There seems to be semantic confusion in the literature as to whether to call a very small deviation (one that is measured in minutes of arc) a fixation disparity, or a small angle strabismus. In a technical sense, a strabismus is present if a manifest deviation is present. In a practical sense, Ogle did not mean for a condition where fusion is present in the fovea to imply a strabismic condition. Also, for clinical considerations, such small deviations as measured in fixation disparities are too difficult to be detected by objective means such as the cover test. Jampolsky[9 0] claims the cover test can be sensitive to a deviation as small as one prism diopter by objective testing methods. Most fixation disparities are less than 1 p.d.

Morgan[9 1] sums up quantification of fixation disparity by stating, "Normally, fixation disparity rarely exceeds 10 minutes of arc, although it may be somewhat greater when a substantial degree of heterophoria exists,

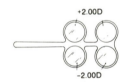

+2.00D

−2.00D

a. BAUSCH AND LOMB
RAY-BAN DEMONSTRATOR

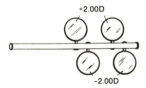

+2.00D

−2.00D

b. BERNELL
BLACK NYLON BAR HOLDER

FIGURE 2-50 — Binocular accommodation facility testing devices. (a) Bausch and Lomb Ray-Ban Demonstrator holding plus and minus lenses; (b) Bernell Black Nylon Bar Holder for use with lenses for an ordinary trial set.

and probably any deviation approaching 30 minutes should be considered abnormal." I would add that any deviation approaching 30 minutes of arc is approaching the condition of strabismus.

I refer to a fixation disparity (angle F) as being a manifest deviation since the patient is not dissociated but, instead, is fusing a central target under relatively natural binocular conditions. Exo fixation disparity, as illustrated in Figures 2-51b and c, is usually found in conjunction with an exo dissociated phoria[y]. Cases of eso fixation disparity are usually found when there is a dissociated esophoria. This is not an absolute rule but is generally true, particularly for eso deviations.

Since 30 minutes of arc is regarded as being a limiting number, and it is approximately nine-tenths of a p.d., it is practical to consider any manifest deviation of 1 p.d. or greater as being strabismic. If the deviation is less than 1 p.d. and there is foveal fusion, the condition is considered a fixation disparity.

Flom[92] made several speculations about flick movements that ranged from 1 to 6 prism diopters on the unilateral cover test. For instance, a case of an intermittent esotropia was reported. When the nonsuppressing eye was covered, the suppressing eye (suppression was central, with probable fusion in periphery, in this case) made a temporalward movement of about 5 prism diopters. One of the speculations made was that this type of movement could be explained as "an unusually large fixation disparity associated with a large heterophoria and otherwise normal binocular vision." My opinion of such eye movements on the unilateral cover test is that they represent a manifest deviation that should be properly classified as strabismic.

Equally nebulous in the classification of deviations, Parks[93] tends to lump similar small angles of deviation (up to 8 p.d.) with peripheral fusion into one category he calls the monofixation syndrome. It is my impression that these are patients with small angle strabismus who have normal peripheral fusion but do not have central fusion. Some may prefer the term heterotropia rather than strabismus when such small angles are involved. Nonetheless, the terms are synonymous, but many practitioners are conditioned to think of strabismus involving larger angles of deviation.

Table 2M gives the classification of deviations to clarify the difference between strabismus and heterophoria. Note that orthotropia may occur when the deviation is less than one prism diopter, but in such cases, foveal fusion is absent. Other associated conditions, such as amblyopia and A.R.C., may be present in cases of orthotropia. In contradistinction to orthotropia, there is foveal fusion in cases of fixation disparity; binocularity is otherwise fairly normal.

Flat fusion is normal in fixation disparity cases, because this is the level of sensory fusion being tested. As in Figure 2-51a, the X is the two

---

[y]Dissociated phoria refers to the angle of deviation found when the eyes are dissociated, as in the Maddox rod test.

dimensional object viewed by both eyes, and the vertical lines are the suppression clues.

Stereopsis is the level of sensory fusion that may possibly suffer in cases of fixation disparity. It is stated by Ogle et al.[94], however, that "fixation disparity has no effect on stereoscopic depth perception." Most clinicians tend to disagree with this contention, because patients who have fixation disparity tend to have poorer stereoacuity than those without it.

Cole and Boisvert[95] conducted a study to determine the effect of fixation disparity on stereoacuity. They reported that the induction of fixation disparity on otherwise normal binocular subjects caused an increase in stereothreshold (decrease in stereoacuity).

In another study pertaining to this issue, Levin and Sultan[96] neutralized existing fixation disparities in 12 subjects by means of prisms to determine the effect on stereoacuity. They found that ten of the subjects had an improvement in stereoacuity.

TABLE 2M. *Giving Classification of Deviations*

Classification	Manifest Deviation in Prism Diopters	Foveal Fusion
A. Strabismus (Heterotropia)		
1. Orthotropia	< 1	No
2. Small angle	1 to 9	No
3. Moderate angle	10 to 20	No
4. Large angle	> 20	No
B. Heterophoria		
1. With fixation disparity	>0 but < 1	Yes*
2. Without fixation disparity	0	Yes*
C. Orthophoria	0	Yes*

* Precludes foveal suppression due to anisometropia, but fleeting foveal suppression may also occur with vergence stress.

TESTING FOR FIXATION DISPARITY

Fixation disparity testing should be done at both farpoint and nearpoint. Devices and instruments available for such testing all work on the same general principle of having the patient fuse a flat fusion demand under natural conditions. Such tests incorporate a vernier type of arrangement so that the patient can report any noticeable misalignment. These vernier alignment markings are suppression clues, and if one line is not seen, a foveal suppression is indicated. Strabismus is present (by strict definition).

Angle F (the angle of fixation disparity) is not measured routinely, but this may be done by using the Disparometer (see Chapter Fourteen).

The associated phoria is of importance and should be measured routinely. The associated phoria (as opposed to the dissociated phoria) is arrived at by neutralizing an existing fixation disparity (the misalignment of the vernier lines) by means of prismatic compensation. For example, an eso fixation disparity would be neutralized by base-out prisms. The direction, but not the magnitude, of Angle F is determined by this means. Special microscopic calibrated devices are necessary in order to measure the vernier separation of the vertical lines. Knowing the type of fixation disparity, and how much prism is required to reduce it to zero (measurement of the associated phoria), is of clinical significance.

The best procedure to follow in testing of fixation disparity is to use vectographic methods. The A.O. Vectographic slide is good for testing at far. The patient wears crossed polarizing viewers and is instructed to keep fixation on the center of the bull's eye target and to report any noticeable misalignment of the vertical lines. If both lines are seen, and there is no misalignment, the doctor can conclude that there is foveal flat fusion with no fixation disparity. If there is misalignment, compensating prisms are used to create an alignment. The power of the prism that causes alignment is not the magnitude of the fixation disparity but is the measurement of the associated phoria. Illustrations of various results using the A.O. slide are shown in Figure 2-52 (a-h).

A good instrument for nearpoint fixation disparity testing is the Mallett Fixation Disparity Test[z]. In this procedure, the centrally fused target is an X (as in Figure 2-51) rather than the circular bull's-eye used in the A.O. Vectographic slide. As in distance testing, the associated phoria should be determined for nearpoint seeing.

FUSIONAL VERGENCE

The magnitude of fixation disparity is closely related to the patient's fusional vergence ability. For instance, if the patient's motor fusion is good, the eye is more likely to compensate a latent deviation than if the motor fusion is poor.

Figure 2-53 illustrates two cases where the dissociated phoria (e.g., measured via alternate cover test, Maddox rod, vertical prism dissociation) is 8 p.d. in each case. The sigmoid curve represents angle F as a function plotted against horizontal prismatic vergence demand. In the first case (Figure 2-53a), the range of fusional vergence is good, being from 18 base-in p.d. for diplopia to 18 base-out for blurring of the target to occur. Thus, the total range of fusional vergence is 36 p.d. Note that angle F is zero from approximately 8^ΔBI to 8^ΔBO. Curves of this type were reported and analyzed by Ogle et al.[9][7]

In contrast, Figure 2-53b shows an example of an exo fixation disparity because of poor fusional vergence. Here, the range is from 12^Δ base-in to 2^Δ base-out. Note there is a moderately large exo fixation disparity of five

[z]Produced by Archer-Elliott Ltd.

minutes of arc in the ortho demand position. The important measurement, however, is the associated phoria. It is $6^\triangle$ exo: that is to say, angle F is not neutralized until a power of 6 p.d. base-in is placed before the eyes.

To reduce the fixation disparity in this case, prescribe either base-in prisms, or motor fusion therapy. In the latter instance, it would be hoped that vergence therapy would result in a curve similar to the one in Figure 2-53a.

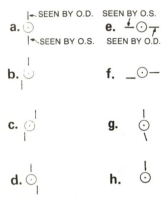

FIGURE 2-52 — Results of fixation disparity testing with the A.O. Vectographic slide. (a) No fixation disparity; (b) Eso fixation disparity (O.D. dominant eye); (c) Eso fixation disparity (mixed dominance); (d) Exo fixation disparity (O.D. dominant); (e) No vertical fixation disparity; (f) Hyper fixation disparity (O.D. dominant); (g) Imcyclo fixation disparity (O.D. dominant); (h) Foveal suppression of O.S.

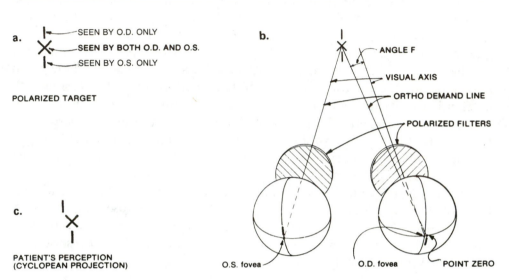

FIGURE 2-51 — Illustrations of fixation disparity. (a) Target viewed by patient; (b) Theoretical posterior view of the eyes illustrating angle F in exo fixation disparity; (c) Patient's perception.

Signs, Symptoms and Other Considerations

Explanations have been offered for the occurrence of suppression, amblyopia, eccentric fixation, anomalous correspondence, horror fusionis, accommodation infacility, and fixation disparity following a motor deviation of the visual axes. Figure 2-54 illustrates the sequence of these adaptive conditions and what level of sensory fusion can be expected in each event.

A motor deviation is not necessarily required for the development of some of these conditions. For example, amblyopia may result from a number of nonstrabismic causes, particularly anisometropia. Likewise, eccentric fixation (although of small magnitude), may be found in cases of nonstrabismic anisometropic amblyopia. Accommodation infacility may occur in almost any type of case, whether it is heterotropic, heterophoric, or orthophoric.

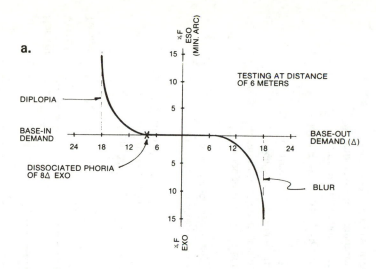

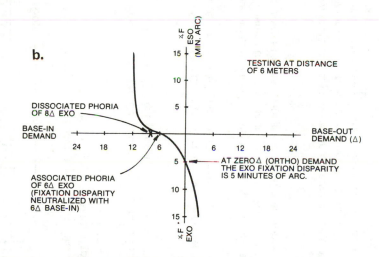

FIGURE 2-53 — Fixation disparity curves plotting angle F as a function plotted against horizontal prismatic demand to vergence, (a) Good vergence ability in case of 8 p.d. of dissociated exophoria; (b) Poor vergence ability in case of 8 p.d. of dissociated exophoria. (Note the fixation disparity at the ortho demand point.)

The doctor should always be on guard for other related signs whenever examining patients with binocular anomalies. Some examples include: indications of multiple sclerosis by central scotoma; ptosis as an early sign of trauma, infection, or vascular problems. Some of the more frequently occurring syndromes involving ocular mobility that should be kept in mind include those of Gradenigo, Millard-Gubler, Moebius, Raymond, and Parinaud.

The doctor should watch for symptoms of diplopia, confusion, faulty spatial localization, poor depth perception, blurring of vision, and asthenopia. Binocular anomalies may be the cause of any of these complaints.

FIGURE 2-54 — Sequence of sensorial status following a motor deviation

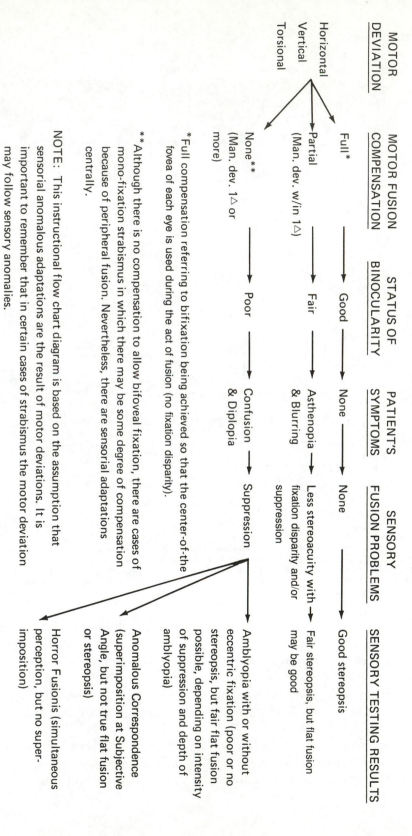

FLOW CHART OF SENSORIAL ADAPTATIONS TO A MOTOR DEVIATION

MOTOR DEVIATION	MOTOR FUSION COMPENSATION	STATUS OF BINOCULARITY	PATIENT'S SYMPTOMS	SENSORY FUSION PROBLEMS	SENSORY TESTING RESULTS
Horizontal	Full*	Good	None	None	Good stereopsis
Vertical	Partial (Man. dev. w/in 1△)	Fair	Asthenopia & Blurring	Less stereoacuity with fixation disparity and/or suppression	Fair stereopsis, but flat fusion may be good
Torsional	None** (Man. dev. 1△ or more)	Poor	Confusion & Diplopia	Suppression	Amblyopia with or without eccentric fixation (poor or no stereopsis, but fair flat fusion possible, depending on intensity of suppression and depth of amblyopia)
					Anomalous Correspondence (superimposition at Subjective Angle, but not true flat fusion or stereopsis)
					Horror Fusionis (simultaneous perception, but no super-imposition)

*Full compensation referring to bifixation being achieved so that the center-of-the fovea of each eye is used during the act of fusion (no fixation disparity).

**Although there is no compensation to allow bifoveal fixation, there are cases of mono-fixation strabismus in which there may be some degree of compensation because of peripheral fusion. Nevertheless, there are sensorial adaptations centrally.

NOTE: This instructional flow chart diagram is based on the assumption that sensorial anomalous adaptations are the result of motor deviations. It is important to remember that in certain cases of strabismus the motor deviation may follow sensory anomalies.

3 | Case History and the Complete Diagnosis

This chapter is concerned with making a complete diagnosis from the results of testing of the diagnostic variables and the associated conditions as discussed in Chapters One and Two. Case history also must be included to determine the time of onset of a manifest deviation, its mode of onset, and its duration. Previous treatment must be assessed as to its effect on existing conditions. Developmental history may reveal other abnormalities in conjunction with binocular anomalies. Additional testing is often required to rule out uncertainties when forming the complete diagnosis.

A vital part of any strabismus diagnosis is to ascertain whether the strabismus is congenital or acquired. There is not complete agreement as to when a manifest deviation is to be classified as congenital. All agree that if a child has strabismus at birth, the diagnosis is congenital; but when it is noticed some time afterwards, opinion begins to differ. While many believe one year is the determinant, Costenbader[1] states that congenital esotropia is present before the age of six months. Jampolsky[2] cautions that a differentiation must be made between truly congenital cases of strabismus and those that are early-acquired. He classified early-acquired as being from age 6 to 12 months. Parks[3] believes that the diagnosis of congenital strabismus may be confirmed if an examination is made by the age of six months.

Six months seems to be a reasonable point in time to classify whether or not a strabismus is congenital. Therefore, if the onset of strabismus is later than the age of 6 months, it should be classified as acquired and not congenital.

To be completely sure of the time of onset, a complete report of previous professional examinations should be obtained. Undocumented information from parents is often erroneous. Pseudostrabismus can be confused with true strabismus. Because the appearance of esotropia may be simulated by such cosmetic factors as narrow interpupillary distance, negative angle kappa, and epicanthal folds, many parents believe their child

Time of Onset of Strabismus

has esotropia, when in fact there is only pseudostrabismus. Further complications are introduced when a pseudostrabismus later becomes a case of acquired strabismus. In such cases, history from parents cannot be relied on for an accurate timing of the onset.

Frequently, a parent believes that the child has strabismus because of the poorly coordinated eye movements usually present at birth. This can cause a parent to erroneously assume congenital strabismus when, in fact, the infant's binocular status was normal in respect to age. A true condition of strabismus must have been established by the age of six months if the strabismus is to be classified as congenital (ideally with reports made by an ophthalmologist or optometrist). I believe the frequency of congenital esotropia is at least one in every four children who have constant esotropia.

An onset any time after the age of six months means the strabismus is acquired. This type of onset is usually between the ages of one and 6 years in cases of esotropia, although onset may be much later in a few instances.

It is generally thought that most cases of exotropia are acquired with the onset being later than in esotropia, and that the incidence of congenital exotropia is relatively rare compared to that of esotropia. A recent survey, however, taken by Forrest and Fitzgerald[4] at the Optometric Center of New York, indicated that 52.0 percent of the sample of exotropic cases had onset within the first six months of life. The percentage of the esotropic sample was 64.71, originating within the first six months of life. These figures do not represent random sampling of the general population and, in my opinion, are not truly representative in this regard. The statistics do point out that exotropias of early onset may be more prevalent than have heretofore been presumed. Costenbader[5] also believes the onset of exotropia may be early, and states that he usually finds it by age two years or before.

When history fails to pinpoint the time of onset of strabismus, certain testing may indicate whether the strabismus is congenital or acquired. Parks[6] believes there are characteristic signs found in cases of congenital esotropia. A modification of these, with a comparison of characteristics typical of acquired esotropia, is listed in Table 3A. These tests are useful when case history is less than adequate.

Results commonly found on the examination of a child with congenital esotropia are alternate fixation, the lack of diplopia awareness, lack of any correspondence (normal or abnormal), double hyper deviation upon unilateral cover test, and insignificant refractive errors. Dr. Parks reported that the dissociated hyper eye may be seen to extort, while at the same time, the uncovered eye intorts. The AC/A is usually normal and not particularly high. Amblyopia of the functional type may not be present because fixation is alternating. Furthermore, a careful case history often reveals the co-existence of developmental neurological defects in congenital esotropic patients.[a]

---

[a]Congenital amblyopia may be among these defects. In such cases, the reduced vision is usually bilateral, in contradistinction to cases of functional amblyopia due to strabismus or anisometropia, in which the poor vision is usually unilateral.

These findings are not infallible indicators of congenital esotropia, but merely tend to be supporting evidence in favor of a congenital rather than an acquired diagnosis. It should be noted that it is certainly possible for any or all of these features to be present in cases of acquired esotropia.

TABLE 3A. Possible Differentiating Characteristics between Congenital Esotropia and Acquired Esotropia

Congenital ET	Acquired ET
1. Alternating deviation (often a midline switch)	1. Unilateral deviation
2. Lack of correspondence (neither N R C nor A R C)	2. Presence of correspondence (either N R C or A R C)
3. No awareness of diplopia (only alternate perceptions)	3. Diplopia awareness possible (true simultaneous perception)
4. Double hyper deviations (may also have excyclo rotation of covered eye)	4. No double hyper deviation
5. Insignificant refractive errors	5. Significant refractive errors (either hyperopia or anisometropia)
6. Normal or low AC/A	6. High AC/A
7. Little or no functional amblyopia	7. Unilateral amblyopia (non-organic)
8. History of neurological defects (including organic amblyopia)	8. Absence of associated neurological signs or symptoms

My experience has been that the onset of exotropia is later than that of esotropia, and the frequency of congenital cases of exotropia is less. Many exotropic children seem to have characteristics similar to those of acquired esotropia, e.g., unilateral deviation, presence of correspondence, etc. Anisometropic myopia is not uncommon. The AC/A, however, is usually lower than in cases of esotropia. Because some fusion has been present at some early period of life in more exotropic patients than in those with esotropia, the opportunity for re-education of fusion is usually better in patients with exotropic deviations.

It is important to know whether the strabismus was intermittent or constant at the time of onset. An intermittent strabismus, although usually quite noticeable, may have less deleterious effect than one that is smaller, but constant. Even if treatment was delayed, it can be assumed that the child with an intermittent deviation may not have completely given up central binocular fusion as did the child with a constant strabismus. This is more true for exo deviations than for those with esotropia. The reason for this is

Mode of Onset

that some of the so-called intermittent esotropias maintain a small residual manifest deviation (monofixation pattern) even though the eyes are apparently "straight." These cases are, therefore, not truly intermittent, since there is a small constant esotropia present. The intermittent exotropia, on the other hand, is more likely to be either all the way out or all the way in for perfect bifoveal fixation.

Regardless of the direction of the deviation, treatment for full recovery of binocular vision is more successful in true intermittent cases than when the strabismus is constant.

As a rule, early-acquired exo deviations tend to be intermittent as compared to eso deviations. It is not unusual for an intermittent exo deviation, with an onset at the age of two or three years, to continue being intermittent for many months. Some cases stay the same permanently, but many young children with intermittent exotropias gradually become constant exotropes with time. This is so unless therapy is instituted. A comparable eso deviation, however, often begins as a constant strabismus. If, however, the esotropia is intermittent at the time of onset and the deviation is moderately large, it is likely to become constant within a short period of time. An eso deviation that is small in magnitude may continue to remain intermittent for a longer period of time before becoming a constant esotropia, while a few remain intermittent indefinitely.[b]

The question of whether the deviation was alternating or unilateral at the time of onset is important in regard to evaluation of amblyopia. A condition of alternating strabismus is not the probable cause of amblyopia, as one of unilateral strabismus might be. The onset of amblyopia, therefore, cannot be equated to the onset of strabismus if the mode of onset was one in which there was an alternating strabismus. A case history of unilateral strabismus is more definitive in regard to onset of amblyopia.

Reports of noticeable variations of the deviation may be useful. Magnitude changes in different positions of gaze point to an acquired paresis as the probable cause of strabismus. If, however, the angle in the primary position was reported to vary from time to time, the deviation may have been concomitant, and due to physical illness, emotional disturbances, or other causes affecting the tonic angle of convergence. For instance, psychogenic strabismus, either eso or exo, is a possibility. Although psychogenic esotropias are more common than those of exotropia, some young children with large exophoria voluntarily let go of fusion to allow the latent deviation to lapse into an exotropia. This is usually for the purpose of getting their way or to receive sympathy.

In the event the patient has not been examined previously by an ophthalmologist or an optometrist, and reports of the patient's refractive, visual acuity, and binocular status are unavailable, the practitioner must

---

[b]Distinction must be made between cases of true intermittency, in which there is bifoveal fusion, and those with the monofixation pattern.

depend largely on statements made by the patient or his parents in order to have any case history at all.

A good line of questioning directed to parents of young patients is the following: "When the turning of the eye was first noticed, did the eye turn out toward the ear or in toward the nose? Was it always the same eye that turned, or did the other eye turn some of the time? Was there a turning of an eye all of the time, or just part of the time? Was the turning more noticeable at different times of the day? Was it more noticeable when the child looked up, down, to the left or right?" Answers to these questions may indicate the mode of onset of strabismus.

The duration of time elapsing between the onset of a manifest deviation and therapy is a crucial factor in the re-education and recovery of normal binocular vision. This is particularly so in the developmental years below the age of six years. Clinical experience indicates that several months without bifoveal fusion can cause irreparable loss of central fusion in the infant or young child. If the duration is inordinately long, peripheral fusion may be the best that can be hoped for. Occasionally, peripheral fusion may be irrecoverable if the onset is too early and the duration too long.

Duration of Strabismus

The duration time factor is not as critical in the ages above the developmental years as it is in the plastic years below the age of six. Nevertheless, loss of the faculty of bifoveal fusion is not too uncommon in adults who have had to give up bifoveal fixation over a long period of time for one reason or another, e.g., unilateral cataract, acquired strabismus due to paresis of the extraocular muscles, etc. Even though the obstacles may cease to exist, it is not always possible to regain bifoveal fusion.

Duration must be differentiated between the total duration (from time of onset to patient's present age) and the time elapsing from onset to treatment. While both time periods are important determinants in prognosis for functional cure, the period between the time of onset and the beginning of treatment is normally more important.

If effective therapy is wisely and immediately instituted, the chance for recovery of binocularity is greater than if treatment is delayed. This is not meant to imply that treatment (e.g., surgery) should be performed instantly with reckless abandon; but rather, caution and discretion should be observed in all cases. It is very unwise to just let things ride, losing valuable time. For instance, in a case where the onset is early and there is a constant unilateral esotropia, alternate occlusion might be prescribed as a measure to prevent amblyopia. Also, base-out prisms (e.g., Fresnels) should be considered as a holding action, particularly if the patient is below the orthoptic training age (usually four years or younger). In certain cases this may be done in conjunction with plus lens therapy. If good binocularity cannot be recovered after a reasonable period of time, extraocular muscle surgery may be the recommended treatment.

Previous Treatment

After questioning is completed regarding time, mode, and duration of onset, another important answer to determine from the case history is the extent and type of previous treatment the patient has actually received.

Unfortunately, it happens all too often that treatment is recommended merely as a token gesture resulting in little or no benefit to the patient. The treatment is usually in the form of patching which has been prescribed, but not adequately undertaken. Not only does the lack of proper occlusion therapy impede recovery, but a history of the patient having been patched can lead to erroneous conclusions on the part of another doctor when he sees this patient at a later time. The second doctor may mistakenly conclude that everything possible has been done for the patient, and that any existing amblyopia could not be eliminated by means of patching, since it has been tried without success. Therefore, in order to avoid such wrong assumptions, questions regarding previous treatment must be pursued in depth. This rule applies not only to occlusion therapy, but to any of the other various forms of treatment for binocular anomalies. For example, Table 3B lists desired information when there has been extraocular muscle surgery.

TABLE 3B. History of Extraocular Muscle Surgery

1. Age when surgery performed

2. Eye having operation
     Right
     Left
     Both

3. Muscle(s) having operation

4. Technique (e.g., recession, resection)

5. Cosmetic results
     Before
     Immediately after
     Following

6. Functional results

7. (Repeat above information for additional surgeries)

Developmental History

The purpose of taking a developmental history is to determine the important milestones at different ages in the child's life. This is related to the physical, mental, and emotional development of the individual, mainly in the plastic years below the age of six. A developmental history may explain why a patient has a particular binocular anomaly.

Fisher[7] states that gross neurologic dysfunction has been found in almost 25 percent of patients with infantile esotropia. On the other hand, the incidence of such coexisting anomalies is very low in those cases of noncongenital esotropia. The history of neurological signs would, therefore, implicate congenital rather than acquired factors as the cause of strabismus.

To what extent a mild lag in neurological development is important in the formation of binocular anomalies is not certain; however, I believe this may produce some detrimental factors to good binocularity. A neurological lag in the older child may not always be obvious. In these cases, a complete developmental history may be necessary.

Perceptual learning-disabilities are common in children who have a history of so-called "psychoneurological lags." Children who experience the frustration of underachievement because of developmental dysfunctions of perception (e.g., laterality, directionality, eye-hand coordination, size, and shape constancies, etc.) very often take on a failure pattern. This sort of poor self-image may become set unless proper therapy, remediation, and guidance are immediately and effectively instituted.

When asking about the patient's past, the following general questions should be included in any case history: "Was the pregnancy normal and full-term? Was the birth normal or were there any complications after delivery? When did the child crawl, creep, walk, run, skip? When did he first talk? When did he first hold things, play with blocks, draw?"

Other questions relating to emotional development should be pursued. "What are his reactions to fatigue? Does he withdraw or become irritable? What are the child's reactions to tension? Is there thumb sucking or nail biting?" There should also be an inquiry about illnesses the child may have had. "What were the childhood diseases? When did they occur and how severe was each? Were there any complications?"

The normally expected development of children has been extensively studied in the past by Gesell and other investigators. A recent compendium by Illingworth[8] lists, in detail, the development expected for various age levels. Some of these important milestones are listed in Table 3C.

It should be kept in mind that great variance in behavior from such a list of expecteds can occur in a child, and he may be perfectly normal in develoment in spite of this. The table of developmental norms is not meant to imply absolutes, but merely to serve as a useful check list and guideline when taking case histories.

Additional Evaluative Procedures

Once all the information pertaining to the diagnostic variables and associated conditions is accounted for and evaluated in concert with a thorough case history, the diagnosis is considered complete. This is true in many cases with binocular anomalies. The constellation of clinical findings provides the doctor with a reasonable degree of assuredness for arriving at the appropriate prognosis in a particular case.

In spite of the apparent completeness provided by the above mentioned procedures, there are some cases in which the doctor may be left with uncertainty. This shows up when the prognosis and recommendations are to be made. Additional diagnostic information may be needed before sound advice can be given. The patient (the parents, if testing a young child) will want to know if treatment is necessary or not; if treatment is recommended, what kind and how extensive will it be; and finally, what are the chances for success in relation to the goals to be set for the patient.

The answers may be revealed by other informative testing procedures which are discussed in this section. These may prove to be useful when routine procedures leave the evaluation somewhat in question.

TABLE 3C. Behavior Expected in the Normal Development of a Child According to Age Levels	
Primitive reflexes (suck, grasp, blink, etc.)	Newborn
Eyes may move independently	Newborn
Head momentarily lifted up	4 weeks
Binocular vision may begin	6 weeks
Laughter	16 weeks
Rolls — prone to supine	24 weeks
Holds bottle	24 weeks
Crawls on abdomen	40 weeks
Creeps — hands and knees	44 weeks
Creeps — all fours (bear walk)	52 weeks
Walks — no help	13 months
Goes up and down stairs without help	18 months
Stacks 3 to 4 cubes	18 months
Runs	2 years
Turns door knob	2 years
Rides tricycle	3 years
Draws, copies a circle	3 years
Normal speech	3 years
Skips	4 years
Copies a cross	4 years
Copies a triangle	5 years
Copies a diamond	6 years

PRISM ADAPTATION TEST   This procedure was introduced by Woodward and reported by Jampolsky.[9] The prism adaptation test (P A T) is used to predict success in cases of esotropia. The testing procedure involves the application of base-out compensating prisms for the manifest eso deviation. The patient wears the base-out prisms for a period of time, usually an hour, while the doctor measures the angle of deviation at certain invervals of time. Usually every 10 or 15 minutes is adequate.

Jampolsky recommends giving the patient an over-correction whereby the prism power is slightly stronger than the magnitude of the esotropia. For small deviations, a 5 p.d. over-correction is recommended; for large deviations, 10 p.d. are advocated.

For example, suppose the patient has 25 p.d. of esotropia. The patient is given 35 p.d. base-out to wear for one hour. Fresnels[c] are usually more comfortable for the patient than clip-on glass or plastic prisms. The immediate measurement on the alternate cover test should show a 10 exo movement. In many cases, the exo will become less in a very short time and, after 10 or 15 minutes, the patient shows an eso movement on the cover test. In some cases, the eso deviation becomes very large. Assume that after an hour the alternate cover test shows a 20 p.d. movement of the eyes. The eso deviation is now 35 plus 20, or a total of 55 p.d. of eso deviation. The angle of the deviation has more than doubled in magnitude as a result of the patient's wearing base-out prisms.

Jampolsky feels this indicates a poor prognosis for cure by surgery and probably by other means as well. If the deviation had remained the same or had increased only slightly, the prognosis would be considered much better. After wearing compensating prisms over a period of time the increase in the angle of deviation can probably be expected in over half of the cases of esotropia. In a study of 88 patients with esotropia, Aust and Welge-Lussen[10] found that 71.5 percent of the patients increased the angle of deviation over an average period of between five to nine days. Anomalous correspondence was thought to be more commonly associated with the increase than normal correspondence.

Alpern and Hofstetter[11] reported a well-documented case of esotropia in which the angle of deviation increased by the same amount as the power of the compensatory prisms. The strabismus was constant unilateral of 14 p.d. with the presence of ARC clearly established.

A total of 18 p.d. base-out was worn for five days. The rate of increase was rapid within the first three hours, with only a slight gradual increase for the next few days, until tapering off to the maximum of 32 p.d. (total increase of angle H of 18). After prisms were removed, angle H decreased rapidly within a few hours, but it took approximately one week before the strabismus was finally reduced to its original angle of 14 p.d.

Postar[12] investigated the use of the P A T for esotropic patients. He concluded that changes in the angle of deviation were related to the status of sensory fusion. The overconvergence reaction to the base-out compensating prisms did not tend to occur when sensory fusion was good, but the tendency was there when sensory fusion was poor. He advocated improving stereopsis early in the therapy program in order to keep the deviation from increasing when prisms are applied. He further concluded that the one hour testing time was too short, and a longer period of time should be allotted for evaluating the effects of prism adaptation.

In taking a different approach to prism adaptation testing, Carter found that heterophoric individuals with good binocularity and without symptoms

[c]Fresnel Press-Ons (T.M.) are used. Manufactured by Optical Science Group, 24 Tiburon Street, San Rafael, CA 94901. These products are distributed by Mentor, Division of Codman and Shurtleff, Inc., Randolph, Mass. 02368. They are also available through many local ophthalmic suppliers.

showed the same magnitude as the original heterophoria before prisms were worn. Thus, a 5 p.d. esophore, corrected with 5 base-out prisms, still showed five esophoria by cover test through the prisms that were worn for 15 to 30 minutes. On the other hand, individuals who had heterophoria and asthenopia (possibly connected with fixation disparity) accepted compensatory prisms. Their symptoms were relieved and there was no adaptation effect with a change in their angle of deviation.

From the above discussions, it appears that prism compensation should be considered in cases of heterophoria with symptoms. In contradistinction, heterophoric patients without symptoms will likely increase the angle of deviation as a result of wearing compensatory prisms. In the case of the heterotropes (strabismics), the eso deviation is likely to increase when the sensory fusion is poor, e.g., from A R C, or suppression. If, on the other hand, the sensory fusion is good, the deviation is likely to stay the same or increase only slightly. On occasion, the basic deviation appears to be reduced in magnitude as a result of wearing prisms.

There is general agreement that when there is little or no increase (or occasionally a decrease) in the angle of strabismus, this type of result on the P A T is an indication of a good prognosis. However, there is not complete agreement as to the interpretations from the results of prism adaptation testing when the angle increases significantly. The majority opinion holds that the prognosis is unfavorable in these instances, but some authorities believe there may be exceptions to the rule. There are some cases that result in a functional cure in spite of dismal expectations that were derived from the results of the prism adaptation test. This points out the need to be cautious when making a prognosis and not to place too much reliance on any one test.

KINETIC COVER TEST Griffin[14] improvised this method of cover testing. The kinetic cover test (K C T) is similar to the objective alternate cover test, except that a moving target is employed rather than a static one.

A fixation target is moved toward the patient along the midline at eye level. This begins at a distance of 50 cm from the patient and proceeds until it is 10 cm from the bridge of the nose. The speed of the moving target is about 5 to 10 cm per second. The timing for each eye being alternately occluded is about every second. This same procedure is continued while the target is moved away and back to 50 cm from the patient. Estimates of the angle of deviation should be made at the distances of 50 cm, 40 cm, 30 cm, 20 cm and 10 cm.

Any fixation target is suitable, e.g., a small toy or pencil tip. A penlight is particularly useful since good observations can be made simultaneously with the cover test. Accommodation responses are more dependable under kinetic testing conditions than when doing static testing. This is particularly true when examining young children. The moving target holds their attention better than a stationary one.

The assurance of eliciting consistent accommodative responses is the important feature of the K C T method of cover testing. Cases of esophoria or esotropia at near may not always be revealed during static testing because of lagging accommodation responses.

Brignull and Mueller[15] compared the angles of deviation measured at various testing distances by means of static versus kinetic cover testing. They found a close relationship between the two. The subjects were all experienced observers as they were senior students in optometry college. The main advantage of the K C T over static testing was that time was much shorter for obtaining the information desired. The magnitude of deviation can, therefore, be estimated quickly and fairly accurately by means of the K C T. If the same consistency holds for young children as with the adult group studied, the K C T could be considered a valid way to detect vergence anomalies in this age group.

Normally, an orthophoric (ortho at far and near) patient will show an exo deviation as the target is moved closer. By the time the target is at 20 cm, an exo of 10 p.d. or greater is common. As the target is moved away, however, the exo diminishes until ortho, or even a slight eso, is observed. If the eso does not exceed 5 p.d. as the target recedes, there is no indication of a vergence anomaly. However, when the eso becomes greater than 5, an eso problem should be suspected (i.e., convergence excess, or divergence insufficiency). If, instead, the patient is highly exo as the target is moved closer and remains exo as it recedes, an exo type of vergence anomaly should be suspected (i.e., convergence insufficiency or divergence excess).

Vergence anomalies may be associated with either heterophoria or heterotropia. They are commonly classified into six categories.

The exo conditions are basic exo, divergence excess, and convergence insufficiency. The basic exo is considered to have approximately the same magnitude of deviation at far and near, while the divergence excess case would have the exo at far being greater than at near. A case of convergence insufficiency would have the exo at near greater than at far.

The eso vergence anomalies consist of basic eso, divergence insufficiency, and convergence excess. The basic eso condition has approximately the same magnitude at far and near. A case of divergence insufficiency would have the eso at far greater than at near, while in convergence excess, the eso at near would be greater than at far. Graphical representations of examples of each vergence anomaly are shown in Figure 3-1. The ordinate represents accommodative stimulus (e.g., far to near fixation distance), and the abscissa the base-in to base-out vergence stimulus. Typical results of the K C T in relation to these different types of vergence anomalies are presented in Table 3D.

I believe the kinetic cover test is a useful method for the detection of vergence anomalies. Without it some of these may be overlooked and, therefore, go undetected when there is complete reliance on static cover testing.

TABLE 3D. Typical Expected Results on the Kinetic Cover Test.

		K C T Target	
A.	Vergence Anomalies	Moving Closer	Moving Away
	1. Basic exo	exo increase	exo decrease
	2. Divergence excess	exo approximately the same	exo approximately the same
	3. Convergence insufficiency	exo increase	exo decrease
	4. Basic eso	eso decrease	eso increase
	5. Divergence insufficiency	eso decrease	eso increase
	6. Convergence excess	eso approximately the same	eso approximately the same
B.	Orthophoria	small exo may be induced	ortho or small eso (allowing 5 p.d.) may be induced

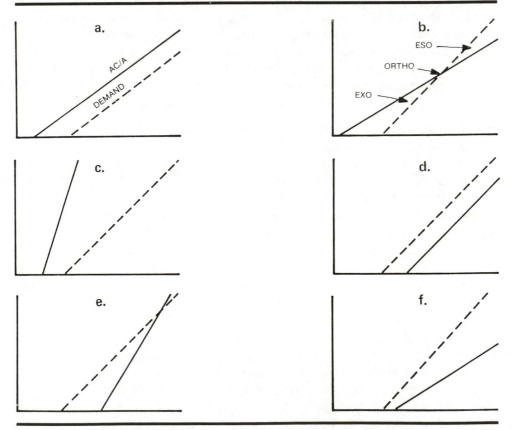

FIGURE 3-1 — Classification of vergence anomalies. (a) basic exo (exo same at far and near); (b) divergence excess (exo greater at far than at near); (c) convergence insufficiency (exo greater at near); (d) basic eso (eso same at far and near); (e) divergence insufficiency (eso greater at far); (f) convergence excess (eso greater at near). The dashed line represents the ortho demand line, and the solid line is the AC/A line (may be referred to as the phoria or tropia line).

The Hirschberg test was discussed at length in Chapter One in regard to estimating the angle of strabismus. Since the patient fixates a nearpoint penlight target, the measured angle of strabismus is at near and not necessarily at far. In order to measure the deviation at far, the patient must look over the examiner's head and fixate a farpoint light source. This introduces an error in the usual interpretation. If, for example, the patient has an interpupillary distance of 60 mm, and the examiner's sighting eye is at one-half meter from the patient, there is an error of 12 p.d.

An orthophore would thus appear by the Hirschberg test to be 12 p.d. exotropic. The convergence demand at this distance is 12 p.d. Therefore, a factor of 12 should be added to the observed value. Similarly, a 12 p.d. esotrope would appear ortho under these conditions. This amount would have to be added to the observed value (ortho plus 12 equals 12 esotropia for proper evaluation).

If the doctor sights from a distance of 1 meter, a factor of 6 must be added to the observed value. At one-third meter, the factor is 18 p.d.

Romano[16] introduced a method for estimating the farpoint angle of strabismus directly by means of Hirschberg or Krimsky testing. This consists of using a telescope and a flashlight at far to observe the patient's eyes in order to study the relative positions of the corneal reflections. If a 7 x 50 monocular prism telescope is used, a 20 diopter plus lens must be placed before the eye piece in order to focus at six meters. The image of the patient's eyes would otherwise be blurred, since such telescopes are normally focused for infinity.

Vertical deviations are measured either by objective or by subjective means, just as horizontal deviations are. The doctor should be aware of and watch for two vertical artifacts which may occur in some cases when the horizontal angle is sufficiently large. For example, an intermittent exotropia may have a vertical component when the deviation is manifest, but there may be none at all when the deviation is latent with the eyes in the ortho posture.

Even in cases of exophoria, testing of the hyper deviation is often carried out under dissociative conditions in which a misleadingly high amount of hyper may be measured. The exo deviation becomes manifest with dissociation, and an exotropic eye may drift upwards in its abducted position. Therefore, it is a good rule to follow that, whether the exo deviation is a phoria or a tropia, the horizontal deviation should be made minimal before measuring the vertical component.

This may be accomplished by the use of minus lenses, providing the AC/A ratio is sufficiently high. Suppose, for instance, there is an exophoria of 15 p.d. and an AC/A of 6/1. The wearing of minus 2.50 spherical lenses should theoretically straighten the eyes into the ortho posture. Under these conditions any hyper component is significant and should be considered in regard to therapeutic steps that may be subsequently undertaken. The hyper found upon dissociation is not particularly significant, unless the exotropia is intermittent and the vertical deviation is more noticeable than the horizontal deviation. This, however, is a rare situation. On the other hand, a manifest exotropia that is being compensated by means of base-in prisms may require vertical prismatic compensation as well, until fusion holds the eyes in the ortho posture. If the vertical deviation is less when the eyes are straight, the excess vertical prisms must be removed immediately. Otherwise, this exacerbates the status of binocularity.

Measurements of vertical deviations tend to be uncomplicated for most eso deviations. However, in some cases of large eso deviation, a misleading hyper deviation may be measured. This is usually the case in which an esotropic eye shows a greater hyper than when it is in the primary position. This is most often due to the overaction of the inferior oblique of the strabismic eye.

CENTRATION POINT For these special cases, plus lenses may be efficacious for getting the eyes to the ortho posture. The proper amount of plus power and the centration point (the point in space where the visual axes cross) must be determined. For example, suppose the esotropia is 15 p.d. and the interpupillary distance is 60 mm. The centration point is 40 cm away from the patient, and is determined by finding the lens power that will place the eyes in the ortho posture. The formula is:

$$\text{Diopters} = \text{Angle H}/\text{I P D}$$

Angle H is the objective angle of deviation expressed in prism diopters and I P D is the interpupillary distance expressed in centimeters. From the above example, if 15 p.d. is divided by 6, the answer is 2.50 diopters. The distance of the centration point is the focal distance of the lenses (100/2.50 = 40 centimeters). If these lenses are worn, the patient is seeing at 40 cm as though at optical infinity. The horizontal deviation should, therefore, become ortho at the 40 cm test distance, wearing the +2.50 lenses.

This is theoretical in the sense that the visual system does not always work in a mechanical, predictable manner. For example, in some cases of esotropia, plus lenses seem to have little or no immediate effect. Only upon the prolonged wearing of the plus lenses will a reduction of the deviation begin to be evident.

Other sensory and motor testing should be carried out when the eyes are in the horizontal ortho posture whenever it is possible to do so.

PROLONGED OCCLUSION The occlusion of one eye is another means of assessing the status of binocularity. This is the most dissociative of all tests, and if prolonged over a period of time, is even more effective in completely dissociating the visual field of one eye from that of the other.

Marlow[17] stated that "... a week's occlusion is sufficient, at any rate in some cases, to render a latent deviation manifest, and that while exercises may improve the muscle tone or stimulate the function of the nerve center they do not cure the deviation." The implication is that the basic deviation is always present, but it is not always discovered by cursory testing; only prolonged occlusion will reveal the true basic deviation.

Bergin et al.[18] reported a case that bears this out. The patient had been seen by several practitioners before prolonged dissociation revealed he had a 52 p.d. hyperphoria of the left eye. Ordinary cover testing, in the immediate fashion, failed to detect the presence of any significant vertical deviation.

Another purpose of prolonged occlusion testing is to ferret out what symptoms are due to binocular dysfunction or disorders as opposed to those that are not binocular in nature.

Marlow[19] thought that photophobia was just one of many binocular symptoms. Regarding increased illumination he stated that ". . . formation of better defined images on the retina necessitates more exact binocular fusion and so a greater demand is made on the extrinsic muscles." He claimed that occlusion could sometimes eliminate photophobia. I believe the clinical experience of many practitioners would show that it is not uncommon for intermittent exotropes to close one eye in bright light. Whether or not Marlow's rationale is valid is not known, but it may have some merit.

An important rule to follow is that equal occlusion time should be allotted to each eye to see if any induced hyper is equal to that of the other eye. Another reason for alternate occlusion is to determine if symptoms are worse when seeing with one eye than with the other. The mere patching of the dominant eye may cause symptoms in itself. Also, a case of uncorrected unilateral astigmatism can give rise to asthenopia when the nonastigmatic eye is patched. These, and other motility and refractive problems, must be taken into account when the occlusion test is given.

When it is not feasible to occlude for a week at a time, a shorter period may suffice. It is important to do at least a delayed (several minutes) cover test. Although the immediate cover test is useful in evaluating fusion under habitual everyday seeing conditions, it does not necessarily bring out the true basic deviation of the visual axes.

Poor perceptual awareness on the part of the patient is a deterrent to good testing and evaluation of binocular anomalies.

PERCEPTUAL AWARENESS OF PATIENT

Notable problems encountered by the doctor in such cases are the testing of visual acuities, checking for suppression, and determining the level of stereopsis. The examiner frequently has to retreat to more objective procedures and temporarily forego many subjective tests.

The cause may be a normal developmental lag in the young child. For example, there may be poor directionality making visual acuity testing difficult with the use of tumbling E targets. While there are many possible reasons for perceptual-motor dysfunction, it is not infrequent that otherwise normal children and adults are slow in their perceptiveness. They are unable to respond quickly and accurately to some of the more complex subjective tests.

Often a short period of perceptual training is helpful. For instance, it is not too uncommon that a normal adult has to be coaxed into seeing Haidinger's brushes, or seeing the float effect on the Root rings. In most cases, patients do learn to respond properly. This is necessary when making a complete evaluation of binocular anomalies.

SEEKING LOGICAL TEST RESULTS

Several findings of the objective angle of deviation should be obtained to determine their reliability. The angle of deviation should be measured at various distances. An AC/A ratio is determined from these results. It may also be done by the gradient method of accommodative stimulus changes (discussed in Chapter One).

An example of inconsistent findings would be measurement of ortho at 6 meters, 5 eso at 1 meter, and ortho at 40 centimeters fixation distances (see Figure 3-2). Theoretically, all three coordinate points should fall in a straight line. Graphing the horizontal deviation at various accommodation-demands is helpful in picking out such discrepancies, as in this example. Unless a fourth measurement of the angle is made, the correct position of the AC/A line is not known.

Suppose that the alternate cover test at 20 cm (0.2 meters) indicates 25 p.d. of eso deviation. This is plotted (see Figure 3-2) and falls in line with

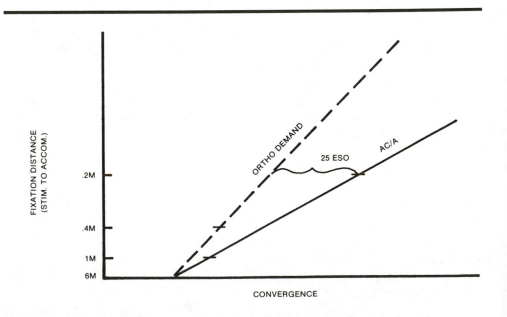

FIGURE 3-2 — Graphing the angle of deviation as a function of accommodation against convergence. The ordinate represents stimulus to accommodation — either by proximity of fixation target or by spherical lens power. The abscissa represents the base-in and base-out p.d. scale at 6 meters. The AC/A line is determined by connecting three aligned data points.

the other plots to make an AC/A line of 11/1. An AC/A may also be arrived at by calculation from the formula[d] presented in Chapter One. In this case it is 11/1 rather than 6/1. This lower value could have erroneously been decided upon, unless additional tesing had been done and the misalignment noticed on the plotted graphical results.[e]

Occasionally, there is another type of illogical test result that goes unnoticed unless scrutinized thoughtfully. This is the matter of negative AC/A's. For example, a measurement of 5 eso at far and a 15 exo at near would have a negative AC/A value. Combinations such as these are shown in Table 1J. Another discrepancy to watch for is an illogical visual acuity finding that is not in accord with the angle of eccentric fixation, e.g., very good acuity associated with large angle E.

Instances such as those discussed are just some of the many examples that may occur in which the doctor should make sure test results are logical.

The question of strabismus in the family should be raised whenever a patient is suspected of having some sort of binocular anomaly. Clinical experience points to the fact that strabismus tends to be familial. Knowledge of this often helps in finding similar problems of the patient.

OTHER HELPFUL INFORMATION

Another important consideration is whether a family history of strabismus is an unfavorable factor toward functional cure. Flom[20] found that, statistically, a family history of strabismus is not unfavorable in either esotropia or exotropia. He found that in cases of esotropia, the chance for functional cure is actually better when there is a strabismic history in the family. Just why this is so is not yet clear, but it is good to know that traditional thinking in this regard can be reversed, and that a family history of strabismus does not necessarily mean the prognosis is poor.

Another important aspect of history-taking is to ask questions that could be related to heterophoria. Although this is not noticeable per se, it may result in various signs and symptoms. Flax[21] believes that the student with poor bifixation is likely to have more trouble with demands of higher level reading than the monofixating student, assuming other things being equal.

Table 3E lists some of the signs and symptoms that should be looked for, both in the office and out of the office by nurses, teachers, and parents.

It is always important to know as much as possible about the refractive history of the patient. This is especially true in cases of strabismus and/or amblyopia. Esotropia is often associated with hyperopia, while exotropia is not uncommon in cases of myopic anisometropia.

REFRACTIVE INFORMATION

In the developmental years, there are more hyperopic children than

[d]Although the formula is AC/A = I P D +M(Hn − Hf), angle S at far and near may be substituted. It is recommended, however, that either H or S be used together and not separately in the same formula; i.e., not (Hn − Sf) or (Sn − Hf).

[e]Printed forms for graphical plotting are available through various optometry colleges, or ordinary graph paper will suffice.

myopic. Hirsch[22] found that the mean refractive error of the newborn is 2.07 diopters hyperopic, and that the mean for the young school child is plus 1.06 diopters. He believes that children entering school with hyperopia of 2.50 diopters or greater rarely outgrow the refractive error. Ludlam[23] believes that a child with plus 2.50 or greater either has or is likely to have binocular problems, usually esophoria or esotropia. He recommends that patients with this magnitude of hyperopia should be followed very carefully and be given prescriptive lenses when necessary.

Unfortunately, a complete refractive record is often unattainable.

TABLE 3E. Signs and Symptoms Frequently Occurring as a Result of Heterophoria or Other Binocular Anomalies Which are Not Obvious

1. Blurring of vision at farpoint
2. Blurring of vision at nearpoint
3. Frowning, or squinting of eyelids
4. Excessive blinking when reading
5. Covering or closing one eye during reading
6. Confusion, omission, or repetition of words when reading
7. Sustaining nearpoint work with difficulty
8. Reading at a very slow rate
9. Losing place when reading a book
10. Eyes burning, aching, itching, tearing, or photophobic

Hopefully, there will be earlier and more frequent vision examinations available to all children in the future. In any event, all refractive information, either past or present, is important when making a complete diagnosis of the patient's binocular status.

Sample Diagnoses   Twelve diagnostic summaries are presented in this section. These sample cases are only representative of the almost infinite permutations that are possible. There are literally no two cases alike. Prognoses and recommendations pertaining to each of these cases are discussed in Chapter Five.

CASE NUMBER ONE   The deviation is a concomitant, constant, alternating (O.D. dominant), esotropia of 15 p.d. at far and 13 at near. There is also a double dissociated hyper deviation. The AC/A is normal and cosmesis is good because angle kappa is positive. There is complete lack of correspondence, and the patient has no demonstrable fusion range.

Case history reveals that onset of esotropia for this seven-year-old patient was at about three months. Examination at age four years found refractive error of plus 0.75 sphere in each eye. Lenses of this power were prescribed at that time, but were worn only a few days before being rejected by the patient. Present refraction is plano and 20/20 in each eye. (See Appendix for a sample consulting letter pertaining to this case.)

The deviation is a nonconcomitant, constant, unilateral, esotropia of the right eye of 15 p.d. at far and near, with normal AC/A (6/1) and good cosmesis. The associated conditions include: lack of any fusion; deep amblyopia, nasal, unsteady, parafoveal, eccentric fixation; lack of correspondence; poor accommodative flexibility in the amblyopic eye; no motor fusion; and slightly noticeable facial asymmetries. Muscle testing indicates a complete paresis of the right lateral rectus.

The patient is ten years old with a history of esotropia since birth. The strabismus has been constant since then. No previous treatment has been given. Further history reveals possible traumatic injury during delivery. Developmental history appears to be normal, other than the child always having difficulty in abducting the right eye. The refraction is:

O.D. Plano 20/300
O.S. Plano 20/20

The deviation is a concomitant, constant, alternating, esotropia, with the left eye being preferred. The deviation is 45 p.d. at far and 35 at near with the AC/A being low (2/1). Cosmesis is poor. The associated conditions include: deep, peripheral suppression; probable harmonious, anomalous correspondence; horror fusionis; and no motor fusion.

The patient is nine years old with a history of constant esotropia since the age of one year. No previous treatment has been given. The patient has no complaints of diplopia. Refraction is:

O.D. +2.00 − 0.50 x 180 20/30
O.S. Plano   20/20

The deviation is a concomitant, constant, unilateral exotropia of the right eye of 25 p.d. at far and 15 at near with a high AC/A (10/1). Cosmesis is poor due to the magnitude of the deviation and to a large positive angle kappa (+1½ mm). The associated conditions include: deep peripheral suppression; deep amblyopia; unsteady, temporal, parafoveal, eccentric fixation; typical, unharmonious, anomalous correspondence; and no motor fusion. The patient is ten years old with a history of exotropia of the right eye. The onset was intermittent beginning at seven months through one year of age. The strabismus has been constant since then. Direct patching was attempted for a few weeks at age three, but only token occlusion was accomplished. No other treatment has been given since. Refraction is:

O.D. - 1.00 − 1.00 x 180 20/100
O.S. Plano   20/20

The deviation is a concomitant, constant, unilateral esotropia of the right eye of 10 p.d. at far and 20 at near with high AC/A. Cosmesis is good because of a large positive angle kappa (+1½ mm). The associated conditions include: deep suppression; deep amblyopia; nasal, inferior, unsteady, paramacular, eccentric fixation; and no motor fusion. Correspondency is normal, and there is no evidence of horror fusionis.

The patient is a five-year-old strabismic with a history of constant esotropia beginning at age two. No previous examination or treatment has been given. Present refraction is:

O.D. + 2.00 D. Sph. 20/100
O.S. + 1.00 D. Sph. 20/20

The deviation is a concomitant, intermittent (constant at far and estimated 75 percent of the time at near), unilateral esotropia of the right eye of 15 p.d. at far and 4 at near. Cosmesis is good because of a positive angle kappa and a relatively wide I P D of 65 mm. The AC/A is low (2/1). Associated conditions include intermittent deep, central suppression; shallow amblyopia; a small (foveal off-center) nasal eccentric fixation; intermittent, harmonious, anomalous correspondence and a very limited motor fusion range. (There is possible co-variation of A R C.)

The patient is ten years old and has had a slightly noticeable esotropia of intermittent onset of the right eye since the age of three. The strabismus is occasionally observed by family members when the patient is looking far away. No previous treatment has been given. Refractive history is incomplete, but the patient was taken for an examination at age five. No treatment was given then, and the advice was that the strabismus would eventually go away. The present refraction is:

O.D. + 1.00 D. Sph. 20/30
O.S. + 1.00 D. Sph. 20/20

The deviation is a concomitant, intermittent, unilateral, exotropia of 20 p.d. at far and 5 at near with a high AC/A ratio (12/1) and poor cosmesis. The appearance of the strabismus is noticeable because of the intermittency and a positive angle kappa (+1 mm). The exotropia is estimated to be present 75 percent of the time at far and 10 percent at near. Associated conditions include: deep peripheral suppression when the deviation is manifest, shallow amblyopia with unsteady central fixation; co-varying, harmonious, anomalous correspondence. An exo fixation disparity is measurable when fixation is at the nearpoint with an associated exophoria of 4 p.d. Motor fusion ranges are very limited, being from 22 B.I. to 18 B.I. at far and from 8 B.I. to 1 B.O. at near.

The patient is six years old and has had an exotropic deviation of the left eye since the age of four. Since then, strabismus has been intermittent. No previous treatment has been given. Present refraction is:

O.D. Plano 20/20
O.S. Plano 20/30

The deviation is a concomitant, intermittent (25 percent of the time at far and 95 percent at near), unilateral exotropia of the right eye of 15 p.d. at far and 25 at near. Cosmesis is fair. The associated conditions include: moderately deep, peripheral suppression, when the deviation is manifest; co-varying, harmonious A R C; a limited motor fusion range; and poor stereopsis.

The patient is eight years old with a history of exotropia since the age of three. The onset was intermittent and has been so ever since. An examination was given at age four. No significant refractive error was found, and glasses were not prescribed. There has been no other examination since that time. The present refractive error is:

O.D. Plano 20/20
O.S. Plano 20/20

The deviation is a nonconcomitant, intermittent, unilateral hypertropia of the left eye of 6 p.d. at far and near. Also, there are deviations of 1 degree excyclo and 4 p.d. of eso at far and 7 at near. Cosmesis is good in the primary position and on levoversion, but the hyper deviation is quite noticeable on dextroversion. The frequency of the manifest deviation is approximately 50 percent of the time in the primary position and 100 percent on dextroversion. There is an associated condition of vertical fixation disparity (associated phoria of 4 p.d. of left hyper, measureable only when patient is fusing).

The patient is 35 years old with a complaint of intermittent diplopia of sudden onset following trauma to the head in an automobile accident. This resulted in a partial paresis of the left superior oblique. Refractive history is unremarkable with the exception of a small myopic refractive error. Present prescription being worn:

O.D. - 1.00 D. Sph. 20/20
O.S. - 1.00 D. Sph. 20/20

The deviation is a concomitant, intermittent (10 percent of the time at far and 90 percent at near), unilateral, esotropia of the right eye of 6 p.d. at far and 16 at near. Cosmesis is good. Associated conditions include: shallow central suppression when the deviation is manifest; eso fixation disparity (associated esophoria of 5 p.d. at far but nearpoint findings could not be measured); and a fair motor fusion range.

The patient is seven years old with a history of esotropia since the age of four. The onset was intermittent and has been so ever since. The patient was examined at age five with a small amount of hyperopia found in each eye, but no prescription was given. Diplopia is noticed occasionally during nearpoint tasks. Refraction is:

O.D. Plano 20/20
O.S. Plano 20/20

CASE NUMBER ELEVEN

The deviation is a concomitant, intermittent (five percent of the time at far and 40 percent at near), unilateral exotropia of the right eye of 8 p.d. at far and 20 at near. The AC/A is low (1.2/1). Cosmesis is good with far fixation but noticeable with near face-to-face viewing. Associated conditions include: shallow, central suppression when the deviation is manifest; fixation disparity (associated exophoria of 1 at far and 5 at near); and poor motor fusion range.

The patient is eight years old with a history of intermittent exotropia at nearpoint that was first noticed at age six. The frequency of the deviation has increased somewhat since then. No previous treatment has been given. During fusion, the stereoacuity is 60 seconds of arc. Refraction is:

O.D. - 1.00 D. Sph. 20/20
O.S. - 0.25 D. Sph. 20/20

CASE NUMBER TWELVE

The deviation is a concomitant, exophoria of 5 p.d. at far and 10 at near. The AC/A is normal, being 4/1. Motor fusion ranges are fair (vergences at far of 11 B.I. to 4 B.O. and nearpoint relative vergences of 16 B.I. to 3 B.O.). The nearpoint of convergence is 10 cm. Associated conditions include: accommodation infacility (unable to clear 20 cycles of plus and minus 1.00 diopter lenses in one minute); and an exo fixation disparity at near (associated exophoria of 1 p.d.). The only other abnormal analytical findings were low positive and negative relative accommodation.

The patient is a 22-year-old college student who is complaining of blurring of vision and asthenopia during prolonged reading. The refraction is:

O.D. Plano 20/20 (J1 at 40 cms)
O.S. Plano 20/20 (J1 at 40 cms)

Note: Discussions pertaining to the above cases are presented in subsequent chapters.

4 | General Methods for Treatment of Binocular Anomalies

Before a prognosis for either a functional or cosmetic cure can be considered complete, the doctor must take into account the type of therapy that must be administered in order to effect the desired results. There are six basic approaches to vision therapy in cases of binocular anomalies. An overview of each of these is presented in this chapter.

Occlusion is one of the most frequently used procedures, particularly in cases of amblyopia. This may be due partly to the fact that it is often the only efficacious one for certain patients. The patient could be an amblyopic infant who is too young for functional orthoptic training. Also, the wearing of glasses may not be feasible. Other reasons for the common use of occlusion are that it is relatively inexpensive, readily available, and quick and easy to apply.

The main use of occlusion in strabismus therapy is to nullify suppression and anomalous correspondence. It may be combined with the total binocular treatment program and prescribed for intervals when the training of bifoveal fixation is not being done.

Allen[1] summarizes the uses of occlusion by stating that it can be used diagnostically, preventively, and therapeutically. A modification of his recommendations is given in Table 4A.

There are many different occlusion techniques because of the variables giving rise to many possible combinations. An outline of the classification of these variables is presented in Table 4B. An example of how some of these may be combined would be the prescription of full, opaque occlusion for constant, alternate wear in the case of an amblyopic infant.

Full occlusion refers to the entire area of the visual field of an eye, in contradistinction to partial occlusion, in which only a portion of the visual field is occluded. The occluder may be either opaque or nonopaque. If there is full covering by means of an opaque material, it is referred to as total occlusion. This is done when opaque adhesive patches[a] and special cup

Occlusion

---

[a]For example, the Elastoplast Eye Occlusor (Duke Laboratories), available at most pharmacies.

devices[b] are used to cover the eye completely so that no light enters. Probably the most commonplace full occluder is the familiar black tie-on patch. Children and some adults may be more receptive, however, if the patch is custom-made of cloth that is plaid, or has a pretty color. Older girls generally like to coordinate the material of the eye patch with their clothing.

TABLE 4A. Uses of Occlusion, Modified from Allen

A. Diagnostic
 1. Determine if asthenopia is monocular or binocular (e.g., in cases of anisometropia, aniseikonia, heterophoria).
 2. Reveal basic deviation (determine what amount is latent).
   a. Horizontal
   b. Vertical
   c. Torsional

B. Preventive
 1. Amblyopia
 2. Anomalous correspondence
 3. Suppression
 4. Diplopia
 5. Secondary contractures in cases of nonconcomitancy

C. Therapeutic
 1. Indirect occlusion (e.g., in certain cases of eccentric fixation)
 2. Direct occlusion
   a. Develop fixational ability in strabismic or amblyopic eyes.
   b. Develop eye-hand coordination in strabismic or amblyopic eye.
   c. Improve visual acuity of amblyopic eye.
 3. Binasal occlusion (combines merits of indirect and direct occlusion)

Micropore[c] is a material I recommend for full occlusion. It is a porous white adhesive tape that "breathes" while worn and is "ouchless" upon removal. The patch can be custom-made for the patient, with enough vertex distance, so to speak, to allow the occluded eye to blink freely without the eyelashes being restricted. This is one of the frequent problems with conventional patches, whether worn by children or adults. Construction of the patch is done in the following manner:

1. Place the nonadhesive side of one or two small segments of tape near the eye to be patched. Allow clearance for the lashes.
2. Hold them in place and use other segments (with the adhesive side

---

[b] Available through the many ophthalmic suppliers.

[c] Micropore Mfg. by 3M Co., available at most pharmacies. Pre-formed patches using this material are available and known as Opticlude eye patches.

toward the patient) to form a patch that sticks to the facial skin around the eye.

3. Lightly demarcate the desired boundaries of the patch with a felt-tip pen.
4. Remove the patch and cut off unwanted portions.
5. Reapply patch to patient.

TABLE 4B. Classification of the Variables of Occlusion

A.   According to area of visual field occluded:
   1.   Full (one eye completely monocular)
   2.   Partial (only a portion of visual field of either or both eyes occluded)

B.   According to the effect on light transmission and/or form:
   1.   Non-transmitting (opaque)
      a.   Tie-on patch
      b.   Clip-on patch
      c.   Adhesive patch
   2.   Partially transmitting (attenuating)
      a.   Neutral density filters
      b.   Crossed polarizing filters
      c.   Colored filters
      d.   Translucent lenses (frosted or etched)
      e.   Blurring (spectacle lens, contact lens, drugs)

C.   According to wearing time:
   1.   Constant (full time)
   2.   Periodic (part time)

D.   According to which eye is occluded:
   1.   Direct (patching of better eye)
   2.   Inverse (patching of poorer eye)
   3.   Alternating (switching patch from one eye to the other in a prescribed manner)

The use of the Micropore material does not allow total occlusion in the strict sense because some light does enter through the white tape; however, it is rare when absolute nontransmission of light is necessary, and this form of full occlusion is generally preferable to the conventional black patch and to other patches that do not allow freedom of movement of the lids. Furthermore, conventional patches are usually too bulky to be worn underneath spectacles. This problem may be avoided when using Micropore.

Other forms of occlusion are possible when the patient is wearing spectacles. For practical purposes, the occlusion may be considered full if the entire eye size of the spectacle lens is covered. Sometimes, however, young children will peek around the occluder and the doctor must resort either to special cups that fit between the spectacle lens and the eye, or to adhesive patches worn underneath the spectacle frame.

One of the most convenient materials to apply to a spectacle lens is Scotch Brand Magic tape. This may be either in the form of full occlusion or partial occlusion, such as binasal occlusion. Diorio and Friedman[2] reported good acceptance of occlusion by older children who tend to reject traditional forms of patching. They recommend the use of a transparent self-adhering contact paper[d] that is applied to the inside surface of the spectacle lens. They claim the contact paper is easily applied and removed, and that it is cosmetically acceptable. The level of visual acuity through it is decreased to 20/4000. Because the material is convenient, easily removable, readily available and inexpensive, they prefer this method of distorting vision to the use of the American Optical Occluder Lens[e], or to the use of clear nail polish.

Other forms of spectacle patching include the use of neutral density filters, crossed polarizing filters, translucent lenses, and ordinary ophthalmic lenses of such power to cause blurring of vision. A contact lens can be used in the same manner to purposely blur the vision of an eye. Enoch[3] reported successfully fitting hydrophilic (soft) contact lenses to infants and young children. I believe this means of occlusion could be an alternative to other, less tolerated forms of occlusion for this age group. Cycloplegic drugs have been used for similar effect. Gillie[4] recommends atropine in the dominant eye each morning.

Penalization (or graded occlusion) is a term sometimes used when attenuating lenses, filters, or drugs are used for the dominant eye. The concept is that a balance should be created in the visual cortex so that representation of the visual signal from each eye is approximately equal. Some writers call this partial occlusion, but I believe this is a misleading term when reference is being made to attenuation.

All variables of occlusion must be considered before this form of therapy is prescribed. Specific aspects of occlusion therapy are discussed in subsequent chapters.

Lenses   The use of lenses in the care of binocular anomalies has played an important role, especially from the time of Donders to the present. In the 1800's, Donders[5] discovered the relationship between hyperopia and accommodative esotropia. Practitioners since then have found a relationship between myopia with anisometropia and the incidence of exotropia. Whether esotropia or exotropia exists, it is important to investigate the child's refractive status as soon as possible. Children usually accept the wearing of glasses by the age of two. Dowaliby and Griffin[6], however, have pointed out the unfortunate lack of a selection of spectacle frames from which the infant patient's parents can choose. The most available frame for an infant girl or boy is the Nipper by Bausch and Lomb Optical Company.

---

[d]Con-Tact, brand name, available in the household section of many department stores.

[e]Mfg. by American Optical Corp., 14 Mechanic St., Southbridge, Mass 01550.

Whenever the patient has an eso tendency together with a high AC/A ratio, and significant hyperopia (2.00 to 2.50D or greater), the possibility of prescribing plus lenses for the refractive error should be seriously considered. Likewise, if there is anisometropia, prescribing of lenses should be considered to eliminate this sensory obstacle to fusion. If aniseikonia is induced in the process, contact lenses may be necessary in order to avoid the size difference created by spectacle lenses.

Astigmatic corrections are important for visual acuity to develop normally and prevent isoametropic amblyopia. If only one eye is astigmatic, a sensory obstacle is present, and the patient may develop strabismus as well as amblyopia in the ametropic eye.

Over-correction of spherical power is used in certain cases of strabismus, typically, in cases of esotropia where the AC/A ratio is high. The over-correction is usually in the form of bifocals with plus adds ranging from 2.00 to 4.00 diopters. It is generally unwise to give an over-correction of plus for distance seeing. The patient may either reject the glasses completely, or worse, he may accommodate in an attempt to see clearly. This exacerbates the eso condition rather than helping it.

The exotropic patient may wear an over-correction of minus sphere, usually on a temporary basis, for distance-seeing in certain cases of divergence excess. This is feasible when the AC/A is high enough to elicit sufficient accommodative convergence to bring the visual axes to relative alignment.

Proper refractive care at an early age can prevent many binocular anomalies, and the retinoscope is one of the most effective tools in vision therapy. Further advancements, such as with V E R, should facilitate earlier detection, so that effectiveness of lens therapy can be increased. Hard resin lenses rather than glass lenses should be worn by children since they are safer and lighter in weight.

Prisms

This means of compensation for the angle of strabismus has been used, though to a limited extent, for over 100 years. Traditionally, the power of the prism was less than the objective angle of deviation. They were mostly fabricated from crown glass, and prescriptions of high power were split and placed over both eyes for better balancing of weight. Eakin[7] thinks that prismatic powers from 6 to 10 diopters are feasible, but that it is wise to divide the amount of prism equally between the two eyes. He also advises prescribing base-up rather than base-down in cases of vertical deviations to avoid the thickness at the lower portion of the spectacles when looking downward to read.

From clinical experience, I have found it better to use base-down rather than base-up when Fresnel prisms are used. The ledges on the base-up Fresnel prism tend to reflect overhead light into the patient's eyes and may produce an irritating annoyance.

With the advent of Fresnel prisms for ophthalmic use, Jampolsky et al.[8]

state that "the majority of children with strabismus are amenable to therapy with optical (prism) over-correction, which often results in dramatic improvement and changes toward a more normal sensorial relationship." This concept of over-correction has become popular in recent years, probably spurred on in part by the fact that very high powers of prism with very little weight are now available.

An example of one of the methods of prismatic over-correction is that used for young children by Fleming et al.[9] Patients as young as one year of age are prescribed prismatic glasses with all the prism before the dominant eye. If the total prism power exceeds 50 diopters, the power is then split between the two eyes. An overcorrection of about 15 p.d. is advocated. If, for instance, the esotropia is 30 p.d., then the patient is given 45 p.d. before the dominant eye. Presumably, this tends to penalize that eye and help foster alternation of fixation. If the angle of deviation increases (as may occur with the prism adaptation test), more prism is prescribed to keep the patient approximately 15 p.d. ahead of the deviation, so that he remains a "sensorial exotrope." After two months, if A R C is eliminated, the exact prism correction (the same as the objective angle of deviation) is given. The patient, then, should have "sensorial orthophoria" while wearing prisms. Depending on the case, other therapy (e.g., surgery) may later be required to effect a functional cure.

Inverse prismatic prescriptions are sometimes recommended in cases of strabismus or amblyopia. This was proposed by Dobson[10] in the 1930's. According to this method of prism therapy, an esotropic patient would wear base-in prisms to create diplopia in order to stimulate divergence. This means that point zero is prismatically displaced nasally from the habitual suppression zone, and the patient is likely to notice simultaneous perception. A divergence would place the diplopic image back on the suppression zone.

The chief benefit of the inverse prism technique in strabismic patients is that a cosmetic improvement may be attained. If the eyes actually diverge, in the case of the esotrope wearing base-in prisms, cosmesis will be improved. Another factor working toward improved cosmesis is the optical effect of the prism itself. The image of the patient's deviated eye (seen by someone looking at the patient's eye behind the prism) will be displaced toward the apex of the prism. This causes the eye to appear more temporal than it actually is, and the esotropic eye looks cosmetically straighter because of the optical effect of the inverse prism being worn. In applying this principle to a case of exotropia where cosmesis is the primary concern, inverse prism, base-out, would be considered.

Prescribing of prismatic corrections in cases of heterophoria, often due to symptoms related to fixation disparity, takes the more conservative traditional turn. The power of the prescribed prism is rarely greater than the deviation of the visual axes, and it is usually much less in strength. There is great diversity of opinion among the authorities on this subject. After neutralizing a fixation disparity by means of prisms, Mallett[11] recommended placing the correcting prism over the nondominant eye (the one with the fixation disparity). If Rx requires greater than 3 p.d., the power should be divided between the two eyes, leaving the stronger prism before the nondominant eye. In case of mixed dominance, the power should be divided equally.

When more than occlusion, lenses and prisms are necessary to achieve the desired results, functional training procedures may be the choice of therapy. Sometimes this is done without other forms of therapy, but often, at least one or more are included with the training program. Vision training relative to binocular problems includes orthoptics and pleoptics.[f] Other types of functional sensory-motor therapy may also be important to orthoptic or pleoptic cases.

TABLE 4C. *Classification of Vision Training*

A. Binocular

    1.   Pleoptics (for certain cases of functional amblyopia)
        a.   Abnormal fixation
        b.   Effects of suppression on visual acuity

    2.   Orthoptics
        a.   Heterotropia
        b.   Heterophoria

    3.   Visual skills efficiency training
        a.   Poor pursuit or saccadic eye movements
        b.   Accommodation infacility
        c.   Vergence inefficiencies
        d.   Other, e.g., poor stereopsis

B. Non-binocular

    1.   Visual perceptual training
        a.   Poor laterality and directionality
        b.   Poor figure-ground perception
        c.   Other, e.g., poor visual closure

    2.   Visual perceptual integrative training
        a.   Visual-auditory mismatching
        b.   Visual-tactile/kinesthetic mismatching

Nonbinocular forms of vision training (e.g., visual perception in certain cases of learning disabilities) are not covered in this text. They may be mentioned, but only when being applied to motivate the patient who needs this sort of stimulus as part of his therapy for binocular anomalies. Refer to Table 4C, outlining the categories of vision training.

---

[f]Authorities consider most cases of functional amblyopia to be the result of some sort of binocular problem. There is little doubt about this when anisometropia or strabismus is involved.

The term pleoptics means "full sight." This was originated in the 1950's by Bangerter[12] whose aim was to eliminate eccentric fixation in order to cure amblyopia. "Pleoptics" now implies all therapy necessary for elimination of amblyopia, the goal being improvement of visual acuity.

The Greek translation of "orthoptics" is "straight sight." It is believed that this term was introduced by Landolt[13] in 1886. It is Javal, however, who is generally credited as being the originator of the discipline of orthoptics. This is undoubtedly due to his pioneering work in the investigation of suppression and the functional approach to treatment of strabismus. Many authorities now consider orthoptics to include problems of heterophoria as well as those of heterotropia.

Since Javal's time, there have been numerous ophthalmologists, optometrists, and orthoptists who have contributed greatly to the understanding and practice of this form of therapy for binocular anomalies. A discussion of the basic philosophies of orthoptics is presented in Chapter Six.

Extraocular Muscle Surgery

This form of binocular therapy may be necessary in certain cases when the angle of deviation is too large to be consistently and easily overcome by fusional effort, or when there is a significantly great nonconcomitant condition. There are many differing procedures used by ophthalmologists in extraocular muscle surgery. Some basic principles, however, are accepted by most surgeons. Only those general approaches to correction of deviations of the visual axes are discussed. There is no intention to cover this subject in depth, but merely to discuss it briefly as one of the several alternates for the treatment of binocular anomalies. There are many fine books for reference purposes covering the details of surgical procedures on extraocular muscles and other anomalies affecting ocular motility. Three particularly good current references in this regard are publications by Dyer[14], Hugonnier et al.[15] and Hurtt et al.[16]

The general approach to muscle surgery is that the action of an extraocular muscle should either be made weaker or stronger. Commonly accepted weakening procedures include recession, tenotomy, tenectomy, myotomy, and myectomy. When the muscle is recessed, the insertion is moved from the original site and transplanted to another location to produce less mechanical advantage. Tenotomy may be either marginal or free, in which case there is a disinsertion at the scleral attachment. There are many varieties of controlled tenectomies where the tendon is appropriately cut for weakening the action of an overacting muscle. Myotomy, or myectomy, is the term used when the muscle, rather than the tendon of the muscle, is altered.

Strengthening procedures may include resection, tucking, and advancement. Resectioning of a muscle changes the angle of deviation by shortening the muscle. The method of tucking may involve the tendon or the muscle, and also serves to effectively shorten the muscle. Advancement of the insertion serves to strengthen the action of the muscle by giving it greater mechanical advantage.

In cases of esotropia with convergence excess, where the deviation is greater at near than far, a standard procedure is the recession of both medial recti. In cases where the deviation is larger at far than near (divergence insufficiency) resection of both lateral recti may be recommended. If the eso deviation is very great, recession of one or both medial recti may be necessary, in addition to the lateral resection of both lateral recti.

Where the deviation is approximately the same at far and near, a recession-resection operation in one eye may be suitable.

It may be recommended that an exotropic deviation with divergence excess (far-exo greater than near) have a recession of both lateral recti. A recession of 6 or 7 mm places the insertion near the equator and is normally the maximal amount of transplantation that is done. Otherwise, the eye loses ability to abduct if recession is carried out to any greater extent. If the exotropia is very large, a resection of one or both medial recti may also be required to straighten the eyes. If only one resection is to be performed, it is usually in the nondominant eye. A 10 mm resection of the medial rectus is not uncommon.

Exotropias with convergence insufficiency (exo more at near than at far) ordinarily do not require surgery unless the far deviation is very large. The recommendation in such a case is usually the resection of both medial recti. As in eso deviations when the exotropia is approximately the same at far and near, a recession-resection in one eye may be recommended.

Since each case with horizontal deviation is different, the ophthalmologist decides the best particular surgical procedure for each patient. Similarly, the number of combinations of vertical problems and appropriate surgeries is legion and cannot be covered in this cursory overview.

In regard to A-V patterns, an esotropia with an A pattern (eso greater on upward gaze) that has no oblique involvement may be treated by recession of the medial recti and inserted upward (approximately the muscle width above the original insertion). If there also happens to be overaction of the superior obliques in an eso A pattern, weakening procedures for these obliques may be necessary. An underaction of the inferior obliques may also aggravate an A pattern and may require strengthening procedures.

Esotropias with V patterns may require recession of both medial recti and downward displacement from the original site of insertion. An underaction of the superior obliques will aggravate the V pattern, and these may require strengthening procedures. Similarly, an overaction of the inferior obliques exaggerates the V pattern and may require weakening procedures.

Exotropias with A pattern may require the recession of both lateral recti with downward displacement of the insertions. If the eyes are exotropic with an A pattern due to overaction of the superior obliques, weakening procedures for these may be required.

Exotropias with V pattern may be treated by recessing both lateral recti with an upward transplantation of the insertions. If the inferior obliques are overacting, the exo deviation tends to increase on upward gaze; these, therefore, may require weakening procedures.

Other forms of transposition are used in cases where one muscle is totally paretic or absent. Other normally acting muscles may possibly be transplanted to substitute for the ineffective one. One such procedure is the Hummelsheim operation in which portions of the superior and inferior recti are sutured to the insertion of a paretic lateral rectus. Another example of substitution of muscles is using the superior oblique in place of the medial rectus in cases of third-nerve damage (causing paresis of the medial rectus).

Drugs   Although there have been numerous drugs used at one time or another for the treatment of binocular anomalies, those in use today are relatively few. Reference was made regarding the use of mydriatics for purposes of occlusion. However, miotics for accommodative esotropia are more frequently used. Two particular anticholinesterase drugs have proven to be effective in this regard. They are diisopropylfluorophosphate (DFP) and echothiophate iodide (PhospholineR), which greatly increase accommodation, but only slightly, if at all, increase the accommodative convergence. This results in a lower AC/A ratio.

Abraham[17] pioneered the use of DFP to reduce esotropia. A report by Gellman[18] summarizes the effectiveness of DFP by citing case reports in which the nearpoint eso deviation was reduced by the use of the drug.

In recent years, echothiophate iodide has become the more popular of the two. It apparently causes less side effects (formation of brown iris cysts, for example) than DFP. One effect that should always be avoided is the cardiovascular or respiratory failure that may happen when a drug of this type is combined with those used for general anesthesia. Smith[19] states that PhospholineR and DFP are very stable complexes, and produce action of long duration. Manley[20] warns of the danger of giving general anesthesia in case of surgery for esotropia, when the patient has previously been taking one of these anticholinesterase drugs. If succinylcholine chloride is used prior to endotracheal intubation, there will be an overeffect if the patient has been taking anticholinesterase drugs. Cessation of respiration may result. A careful history should be taken to determine if any such drug was used several months prior to the scheduled time of extraocular muscle surgery.

The use of drugs in the treatment of binocular anomalies appears to be somewhat limited and may be on the decline. There are times, however, when their use may be advantageous in the treatment of accommodative esotropia. They may be effective when the AC/A is high, in cases of significant hyperopia, and when wearing of lenses is not tolerable. Under most of these circumstances, it is feasible to prescribe bifocals, but in the case of infants and some children, drugs may be a means to reduce an eso deviation.

When one method of treatment is not adequate, others may be used. It is possible that any combination of the six basic methods may be employed, and there are cases in which all are required. There is further discussion on their uses and various combinations in subsequent chapters.

5 | Prognosis and Recommendations

Prognosis is the prediction for success by a specified means of treatment. As to binocular anomalies, prognosis pertains to the chance for a favorable outcome by the use of occlusion, lenses, prisms, training, surgery, drugs, or any combination of these methods of treatment. After all necessary testing has been completed and a complete diagnosis made, the doctor arrives at an appropriate prognosis for the case. From this, appropriate recommendations can be made.

There are two types of prognoses depending on the goals of treatment. The doctor can hope for either a functional cure or a cosmetic cure.

Goals

The criteria for functional cure, according to Flom[1], are that there must be clear, comfortable, single, binocular vision present at all distances, from the farpoint to a normal nearpoint of convergence.[a] There should be stereopsis[b] and normal ranges of motor fusion. The deviation may be manifest up to one percent of the time, providing diplopia is experienced whenever this happens. Corrective lenses and small amounts of prism may be worn; however, prismatic power is limited to 5 p.d.

FUNCTIONAL CURE

Flom listed another category of cure which is called "almost cured." The criteria are that there may be stereopsis lacking, the deviation may be manifest up to five percent of the time, providing diplopia is noticed. Larger amounts of prism may be used as long as there is comfortable binocular vision. Otherwise, the other criteria for functional cure must be met.

The third category is called "moderate improvement." The stipulation here is that there must be improvement in more than one defect.

The fourth category of cure, according to Flom, is "slight improvement." This means there is improvement in only one defect.

Finally, there is a category of no improvement, meaning that there was

---

[a]Not specified, but 2 to 3 cm from the bridge of the nose may be considered normal.

[b]Flom does not specify the stereoacuity.

no improvement in any defect as a result of therapy.

I concur with the criteria set forth by Flom, but I do think it is important to specify the level of stereoacuity. Manley[2] indicates that a stereothreshold of 67 seconds of arc is the differentiating value between monofixation pattern and bifoveal fusion, and that on the Titmus Stereo Test "central fusion (bifixation) must be present for circles 7 to 9 to be answered correctly."

This compares closely with findings on the Pola-Mirror (refer to discussion in Chapter Two) in which there was central suppression found on all patients who had worse than 60 seconds of arc stereoacuity, while all those with better than 60 seconds passed the Pola-Mirror test. Therefore, I believe the cutoff value of 67 seconds of arc is reasonable, and it should be included in the criteria. This can be one of the means of determining if the strabismus is completely eliminated (i.e., when there is bifoveal fixation without suppression).

It should be pointed out that a patient who has made either "moderate improvement" or "slight improvement" may or may not be any better off from a physiological standpoint. These labels are sometimes nothing more than academic, since they are useful only in statistical analyses of reported studies. For example, suppose ARC is eliminated but the patient still has esotropia, suppression, etc. The important question that should be answered by the doctor is whether or not the patient is actually any better off as a result of having had an "improvement." There are, however, possible psychological benefits for these patients when they feel they have been helped. These results should be evaluated and put in their proper perspective.

It is unfortunate that most reported studies giving rates of cure have not incorporated such complete and definitive criteria as those of Flom. Consequently, there are very few of significant value. One of the exceptions, however, is the survey by Ludlam.[3] In this study of 149 strabismic patients the criteria of Flom were strictly adhered to. Treatment did not include surgery or drugs as methods of therapy. This kept the study "clean" in comparision to most others in which the effects of surgery cannot be delineated from nonsurgical methods. According to Ludlam, the reported functional cure rate was 33 percent. The almost-cured rate was 40 percent with the remaining percentage being distributed among the other categories.

Ludlam's study took place in a large clinical setting with many inherent disadvantages for efficient and effective functional vision training (e.g., frequent change of doctors, poor patient control, group therapy). A higher rate of success was reported by Etting[4] who surveyed a random sampling of 42 case results of an optometrist in a private practice. There were 20 exotropes, six of whom had constant strabismus, and 22 esotropes, 18 of whom had constant strabismus. Using Flom's criteria, the overall functional cure rate was 64 percent. It was 85 percent for the exotropias and 45.4 percent for the esotropias. Seven patients were known to have had surgery prior to training, but there was no subsequent surgery for any of the cases in this study.

One of the few well-documented strabismus reports in which surgery was the dominant method of therapy is the study by Taylor.[5] He found that in cases of congenital esotropia there was not one instance of functional improvement when surgery was accomplished after the second birthday. However, he is of the opinion that it is possible to achieve functional cure in such cases if there is early surgery (meaning before two years of age), particularly if diligent (minimum of five years) follow-up care is given. Surgery must result in a deviation 10 p.d. or less horizontally, and 5 p.d. or less vertically in order for there to be any hope for functional results. In a selected sample of 50 such patients having early surgery, there were 30 who were later found to have stereopsis ranging from 40 to 400 seconds. Of these 30 patients, there were four with 40 seconds of arc on the Titmus Stereo Tests. Taylor, therefore, advocates early surgery in case of congenital esotropes and believes late surgery is hopeless in respect to achieving a functional cure.

My opinion is that early surgery is currently the most efficacious means in cases of congenital esotropia. I suspect this applies, as well, to congenital exotropia.

Cases of acquired strabismus are usually helped by some or all of the other methods of therapy. The possible use of surgery for achieving functional cure in cases of acquired strabismus should be considered in those cases that fail to respond to nonsurgical means of therapy. This may be necessary in certain nonaccommodative cases of strabismus. See Table 5A for a classification of these types of strabismus according to time of onset. A general, expected prognosis is listed for each category, but it is in no way meant to apply to all cases within each category.

TABLE 5A. Classification of Strabismus According to Time of Onset and Prognosis

Type		Prognosis
A.	Congenital (onset 6 months of age or earlier)	Poor (unless early surgery)
B.	Acquired (onset after 6 months of age)	
	1. Non-accommodative	Fair (depending on circumstances and therapy used)
	2. Accommodative	Good (unless long duration)

The nonaccommodative acquired type may be eso, exo, hyper, or torsional in direction. In the young child, a sensory obstacle to fusion—such as a unilateral cataract, or a condition of anisometropia—usually results in an esotropia, while in the older patient, exotropia is often the result. Extraocular muscle paresis may cause exo or eso as well as hyper or cyclo deviations. Psychogenic strabismus may be exo or eso with the latter occurring more frequently. Although there may be other possible explanations as to etiology, many cases of nonaccommodative strabismus are idiopathic.

Accommodative strabismus is usually thought of as being esotropic. This is usually the case, but there may be an exceptional case of exotropia of the divergence excess type. This is the condition in which the exo at far is much greater than the exo at near, indicating a high AC/A ratio. A patient with moderate hyperopia may be ortho at near, but exotropic at far. This can be thought of as an indirect type of accommodative strabismus.

The prognosis in most cases of accommodative strabismus is usually quite good, providing effective treatment is administered without delay. A long duration of constant strabismus makes the prognosis considerably worse. If the sensorial adaptive anomalies become deeply embedded, the condition is referred to as deteriorating. In these cases the prognosis may be only fair or even poor. An example of a deteriorated accommodative esotropia is the case in which the onset was at age one. Many years of constant esotropia have gone by without treatment, making it almost impossible to effect a functional cure by means of therapy. When surgery is resorted to, the result may be one of cosmetic improvement. However, the monofixation pattern will be hoped for. Bifoveal fixation achieved in cases of long duration such as this one would be the exception.

COSMETIC CURE The biggest fault of most reports in the literature is that there is no distinction made between functional and cosmetic cure. Many surgeons label the patient as "cured" just because the eyes "look straight." Studies purporting to give cosmetic cure rates are unreliable because this is a subjective value judgment with each reporter using his own criteria.

As discussed in Chapter One, certain cosmetic factors have a great effect on the appearance of the strabismic. The principal factor is angle kappa; e.g., a negative angle kappa may make an orthophore appear to have esotropia. Similarly, cosmesis may be good in moderately large angles of strabismus. For instance, a 15 p.d. esotrope with a positive angle kappa may look as though he has no strabismus. Because of the various combinations of cosmetic factors affecting the appearance of the individual, there are no hard-and-fast rules relating the magnitude of strabismus to cosmesis.

In the majority of cases, however, I find that if the strabismic angle is reduced to 10 p.d. or less, the cosmesis is generally good. The esotrope may get by with a larger angle, such as 15 or 20 p.d., before the deviation is too noticeable. This is because most people have positive angles kappa which favor the appearance of esotropia. Conversely, an exotropia of the same magnitude will probably be quite noticeable.

Hyperdeviations of 5 p.d. or less are not noticeable. Deviations beyond

10 p.d. are usually unsightly and present a cosmetic problem for most patients.

Cyclodeviations are ordinarily not a cosmetic problem unless they are extremely large. In such cases, there is usually a vertical deviation present as well as one that is horizontal. These are usually the cause of the poor cosmesis and not the cyclotropia, per se.

When the goal is just cosmetic and not functional, the most frequently used form of therapy is surgery. Lenses are occasionally used for this purpose in the form of plus single vision lenses for the correction of hyperopia. Plus adds (bifocals) generally serve no purpose in cases in which cosmesis is the sole concern. Minus adds for farpoint exotropia have been employed. This procedure is not highly recommended, because the cosmetic gain is only temporary. Nothing is achieved in the long run, since the cosmetic problem returns as soon as the over-correction is removed. Minus lenses do play an important role, however, in certain cases of exotropia in which there is hope for a functional cure.

Inverse prisms have been used for cosmetic improvement with limited success. The main problem is the thickness and weight factor of glass or plastic prisms. Fresnel prisms eliminate these drawbacks, but they introduce the problem of degraded visual acuity, and the occasional complaint of noticeable lines for the patient looking through the prisms. This becomes a significant problem in powers greater than 10 p.d. If all the prism is confined to the deviating eye, the complaint is removed. The patient wearing a Fresnel prism does object to the appearance of the lines visible to someone looking at him. Thus, the use of inverse prism may become impractical because of the appearance of the Fresnel lines.

Patients may be taught the tactic of controlling head movements or using specified positions of gaze to minimize a cosmetically noticeable strabismus. This is applicable in cases of concomitant as well as nonconcomitant strabismus. For instance, suppose a patient with 20 p.d. of concomitant, constant, esotropia of the right eye wishes to appear to be orthophoric during a job interview. The effect of "straight eyes" may be accomplished by the individual making a small dextroversion. He could fixate on the interviewer's left ear, for example, rather than look directly face-to-face. This type of advice can be helpful to patients in their personal life.

The report on prognosis in strabismus by Flom[1] included certain factors which he found to be favorable and those which he found to be unfavorable for functional cure. A modification of this list is given in Table 5B. In his report Flom presented a quantitative system for determining the prognosis for a given case.

While such schemes may have a certain amount of instructional value, I believe it is unwise to depend on a mathematical model to make a prognosis for a patient with strabismus. Instead, the doctor must take into account all the variables, associated conditions, and other factors and then use

Favorable and Unfavorable Factors in Strabismus

professional judgment to arrive at the most correct prognosis for a particular patient. This requires an item analysis of each factor in the prognosis and evaluation of their total combined effect.

TABLE 5B. Prognosis for Functional Cure of Strabismus by Means of Orthoptics (modified after Flom)

Favorable factors

1. Good cooperation
2. Intermittent strabismus
3. Exotropia better than esotropia
4. Small angles of deviation rather than large angles
5. Concomitancy better than nonconcomitancy
6. Family history of strabismus
7. Patient's age between 7 and 11 years

Unfavorable factors

1. Eccentric fixation
2. Amblyopia in esotropia, but not as bad in exotropia
3. Cyclotropia
4. ARC in esotropia but not an unfavorable factor in exotropia
5. No motor fusion range (unfavorable in esotropia but not unfavorable in exotropia)
6. Suppression in esotropia, but not as bad in exotropia
7. Constant strabismus

PROGNOSIS OF THE VARIABLES OF THE DEVIATION

Concomitant strabismus is generally regarded to have a better prognosis than nonconcomitant strabismus, but many exceptions may occur. Nonconcomitancy caused by a recently acquired paresis in which remission is quite likely would not follow the general rule.

In regard to frequency of the deviation, there is general agreement that an intermittent strabismus has a more favorable prognosis than one that is constant. However, there are differences in favorability from one intermittent case to another. A deviation that is manifest 99 percent of the time is more difficult to treat than one present just one percent of the time.

The direction of deviation may determine the prognosis. Exo deviations are ordinarily easier to treat than are eso deviations. Vertical deviations present more of a challenge and torsional deviations even more so.

Although there is some correlation between the magnitude of the deviation and prognosis, the relationship is not always close. It is generally assumed that the larger the angle, the worse the prognosis. This rule is often refuted in cases of small angle strabismus. Wybar[6] states that "microtropia is unlikely to prove responsive to therapeutic measures." Likewise, Parks[7] concludes that the prognosis for bifoveal fixation in the patient with monofixation pattern is poor.

The effect of an AC/A ratio has to be considered (as with all factors) in regard to the particular case in question. A high ratio can be either a blessing or a curse, depending on the circumstances. It may be the principal cause of esotropia at near, or exotropia at far. However, the mechanical advantage of a high ratio when using lenses may help to drastically reduce deviations of this type, e.g., plus lenses for the nearpoint esotropia, and minus for the farpoint exotropia. It is difficult, therefore, to make prognostic statements about the AC/A, but it may be good to have a high ratio to work with.

In regard to variability of the deviation and cosmesis, it may be favorable if the magnitude of the deviation changes from time to time. This tends to keep suppression and A R C from becoming too deeply embedded, though it cannot be assumed to be so in all cases. If cosmesis is good, there may be no problem as far as the patient is concerned. This is often the reason a patient does not wish to try for a functional cure.

Traditional thinking is that treatment of an alternating strabismus is more difficult than treating one that is unilateral. This conclusion has been prevalent because many congenital esotropes are alternators. This group of patients has led to equating alternation with poor prognosis. Most recent studies show that alternation is not a deterrent and may be slightly favorable when all types of strabismus are considered.

Eye dominancy is probably not a factor in prognosis. However, it can be a consideration regarding the strabismic's perceptual adjustment to everyday seeing and may be related to certain eye-hand or eye-foot coordination tasks.

Associated Conditions

As with diagnostic variables, it is difficult to pin down what influence each of the associated conditions has on the overall prognosis.

Peripheral and deep suppression may cause the prognosis to be worse than if it is central and shallow. Although this is generally true, there are many exceptions. For instance, there could be an esotropia with A R C in which suppression is very slight. The prognosis may be poor because of the A R C, in spite of the apparent favorable factor of the almost negligible suppression. Since there is always an interplay between the many factors that go into making a prognosis, it is hard to speak in terms of absolutes for any one factor. Generally speaking, though, suppression alone is not considered highly unfavorable.

The presence of amblyopia has traditionally been a stumbling block to the successful treatment of strabismus. In recent years, however, the presence of amblyopia has become less of an obstacle, because it has become more treatable than in the past, mainly due to the greater understanding of the relationship between abnormal fixation and visual acuity. Treatment procedures used in pleoptics have evolved to the point that amblyopia can be cured in many cases. Once amblyopia is eliminated, the chance for treating strabismus is better.

Winter[8] believes that practically all cases of strabismic amblyopia or anisometropic amblyopia can be cured by direct occlusion alone, providing the child is less than four years old, and that from four to six the prognosis may be good. However, extensive treatment may be required. Aust[9] similarly feels that occlusion therapy can lead to a cure of amblyopia in more than 90 percent of the cases, whether or not fixation is central; this can be up to the fifth year of life.

Goodier[10] used direct occlusion for 46 amblyopic patients up to the age of nine. An improvement in fixation and visual acuity was reported in 44 cases. It was concluded that the use of inverse occlusion did not appear to be as efficacious as direct occlusion.

There are many who disagree with the contention that direct occlusion is always the best method of occlusion therapy. If a patient over five years of age has eccentric fixation, direct occlusion is thought to cause the abnormal fixation to become even more deeply embedded. If this happens, very specialized pleoptic therapy utilizing afterimages and entoptic foveal "tags" may be called for in order to treat the abnormal fixation. The contention is that inverse occlusion would have prevented the degree of embeddedness that resulted from direct occlusion.

Kavner and Suchoff[11] believe the prognosis is poorer when there is a stable eccentric fixation as opposed to one that is unstable. They recommend inverse occlusion and specialized pleoptic training when dealing with this type of condition.

I believe that direct occlusion is the procedure of choice in amblyopic patients up to six years of age. In patients older than six, direct occlusion should be tried if fixation is central, or if there is unsteady eccentric fixation. The prognosis may be fair or good depending upon the circumstances. However, in cases of steady eccentric fixation above the age of five, the prognosis for eliminating the eccentric fixation and amblyopia by means of direct occlusion is usually poor. What so often happens when direct occlusion is used in this type of condition is that there is an immediate small improvement in visual acuity, but no further gain afterwards. This may be because the eccentric fixation becomes very entrenched, making it difficult to reduce it any further. Therefore, the prognosis may be somewhat better if indirect occlusion is initially tried.

Chavasse[12] introduced the concepts of amblyopia of arrest and amblyopia of extinction. Amblyopia of arrest is a failure in the development of visual acuity due to strabismus, anisometropia, or any number of conditions. In any event, the development of visual acuity is arrested at the time of onset of the causative condition.

The prognosis for improving visual acuity in a documented case of amblyopia of arrest is considered to be very poor. This is probably true if the patient is beyond the developmental age (six years or older). However, if the same type of case is treated at a much earlier age, the prognosis may be better. Amblyopia of arrest, therefore, is not always a deterrent to treatment if the patient is very young; but if treatment is delayed until the child is older, the prognosis becomes worse.

The prognosis for a case of amblyopia of extinction is thought to be good, no matter at what age the treatment is given. The difference is that an older patient may require a more lengthy therapy program than a younger patient. Amblyopia of extinction is a condition in which vision has deteriorated, because of suppression resulting from strabismus, or anisometropia. The vision that was once lost may often be recovered through the re-educative process of pleoptics.

These concepts of Chavasse are not without dispute. The argument against them stems from the fact that many authorities have found that the results of pleoptics do not always correspond to the level of visual acuity that is traditionally expected. It often happens that better acuity is achieved than was thought possible in cases of relatively early onset of amblyopia. This would seem to contradict the concept of amblyopia of arrest.

However, if modern normative visual acuity levels expected for certain ages are properly matched with the time of onset, the concept of amblyopia of arrest is on solid ground. The apparent mismatch comes in because of the old assumption that an infant has poorer vision than he actually has at a very early age. Chavasse thought that the acuity level of a four-month-old child is normally about 20/2500. Dayton (refer to discussion in Chapter Two) has found that this is not true and that newborns may have an acuity of 20/150. This may explain why treatment in cases of very early onset is often successful. Perhaps the condition being treated is not that of amblyopia of arrest, but rather, one of amblyopia of extinction.

Amblyopia tends to be an unfavorable factor in the prognosis of strabismus, but this becomes less of a factor after it is eliminated or significantly reduced by means of pleoptics. The prognosis for cure of amblyopia is good if treatment is begun when the child is young. It is less favorable as the patient becomes older, particularly in cases of amblyopia of arrest, but age is not much of a factor in cases of amblyopia of extinction.

The presence of anomalous correspondence is a very unfavorable factor in the prognosis of esotropia. Flom[1] reported that while A R C is highly unfavorable in cases of esotropia, it is of no significance in cases of exotropia. Flom[1,3] reported that the cure rate for esotropia with A R C was only three percent compared to the rate of 40 percent of the cases with normal correspondence. The cure rate for exotropes with anomalous correspondence was 38 percent compared to 57 percent with N R C.

The cure rates of Ludlam[3] were reported as 23 percent of esotropes with A R C as compared to 86 percent N R C. The exotropes with A R C have a cure rate of 62 percent as opposed to 89 percent for those with normal correspondence.

Etting[4] reported a cure rate of 10 percent of the esotropes with A R C while it was 75 percent of the esotropes with N R C. The cure rate for exotropes with A R C was 50 percent.

It appears that anomalous correspondence is a serious factor in cases of esotropia but not in exotropia.

Horror fusionis and lack of correspondence are considered to be unfavorable factors. Using presently known procedures there is no hope for the older child or adult to have a functional cure when there is a complete lack of correspondence. The best recommendation in such cases is either no treatment, or to make an attempt at a cosmetic cure.

In cases of horror fusionis, the usual recommendation is no treatment since the prognosis is poor. There are some cases, though, that appear to be due to the sensory obstacle of aniseikonia. There may be some chance for functional improvement in these cases. This is discussed further in Chapter Eight.

Accommodation infacility is not an unfavorable factor in strabismus. It is frequently an accompaniment of amblyopia with eccentric fixation and should be treated prior to strabismus therapy. Accommodative flexibility training is often used as part of pleoptics and considerable time may be required before both the fixation and accommodation are improved. In nonamblyopic cases, accommodation flexibility usually improves quickly with training.

Poor fusional vergences are only slightly unfavorable prognostically, because they can be increased by means of orthoptics in the majority of cases.

OTHER FACTORS   The time of onset, mode and duration, previous treatment, developmental history, and additional evaluative procedures all play important roles in determining the prognosis in any case of strabismus.

The prognosis is better when the onset of amblyopia and/or strabismus is late than when it is early. A short duration is better than a long one, since immediate therapy helps the chance for cure. Existing anomalies that were once successfully treated are often easy to eliminate by re-education. A developmental history that is normal can be considered favorable.

Certain supplemental tests indicate the nature of the prognosis. The prism adaptation test is particularly significant in this regard.

Cooperation is a vital factor in treatment when functional training methods are used. The patient must be perceptive and of high intellect in order to go though this form of therapy. This, along with genuine interest on the part of the patient, and parents, in the case of a child patient, is extremely helpful. It explains why a family history is favorable. The parents may feel motivated to do something about their child's condition because of their familiarity with binocular anomalies.

The age of the patient is an important factor in itself, often dictating what form of therapy that patient will receive. The best orthoptics and pleoptics can be done when the child is six or older. Some patients as young as four years of age may cooperate, but it is rare that there will be sufficient cooperation from those much younger than four.

Farpoint strabismus is commonly more difficult to cure than one at near. Convergence excess is typically easier to treat than is divergence insufficiency. Similarly, convergence insufficiency is less difficult to treat than divergence excess.

Proper refractive care may prevent some of the binocular anomalies. In this regard a history of good care can be considered favorable to the prognosis in many cases.

The prognosis for improving existing visual skills in heterophoria is almost always good providing there is adequate cooperation and motivation on the part of the patient. In the sensory realm, stereopsis might be improved by means of orthoptics, lenses, and prisms.

In the motor realm, orthoptics may help increase fusional vergence which may be necessary in cases of fixation disparity. Prism therapy also is applicable to cases of heterophoria with fixation disparity.

Of the four generally recognized types of vergence (tonic, accommodative, fusional, and proximal), most authorities believe tonic convergence is the least significantly changed as a result of training. Although there is some dispute over whether or not the basic deviation can be changed by means of training, I believe it remains approximately the same, before and after orthoptics. On immediate testing, however, there may appear to be a difference following training. However, when it is put to the prolonged occlusion test, tonic convergence is usually found to be the same as it was before training.

As to the trainability of accommodative vergence, Manas[14] reported an increase (by measuring the accommodative-convergence to accommodation ratio) with orthoptic training. Flom[15] also found a similar increase. However, after about one year, the AC/A ratio appeared to have decreased and approximated the original values.

There are numerous references regarding the trainability of fusional vergences. Costenbader[16] stated, "In general, the treatment of strabismus includes . . . improving fusion and the fusional vergences." Jones[17] writes, "In regard to motor fusion, it is the aim of orthoptic treatment . . . to increase them sufficiently." This was in reference to fusional vergence ranges.

Excessive proximal convergence has been found to be reduceable by familiarization with the testing environment which produced the increased vergence.

It might be summarized that the chance of increasing fusional vergence is usually good. The easiest is positive (convergence) fusional vergence followed by negative (divergence) vergence. Positive fusional vergence is the same as what is sometimes referred to as tests number 9 (farpoint) or number 16A (nearpoint). Likewise, number 11 (farpoint) and number 17A are tests for negative fusional vergence.

Vertical fusional vergence is the next in difficulty to improve by means of training, and, in most cases, torsional fusional vergence is even more difficult.

Heterophoria

Heterophoric, and even orthophoric patients may benefit as a result of the amelioration of other sensory-motor dysfunctions such as accommodation infacility and poor saccadic eye movements. This could have a bearing on the patient's achievement and performance in everyday living as well as in school. The prognosis for improvement of these types of visual skills generally is good. (Refer to Chapter Fifteen.)

Case Studies   The previous discussion consisted of generalities regarding favorability of the various factors of concern in making the prognoses. This section will be specific in that the prognosis will be given for each of the 12 sample diagnoses. These are the sample cases that were discussed in Chapter Three. For each diagnosis, one of the five prognoses ranging from poor to good is given. Table 5C lists the five categories of prognosis that are used.

It is hoped that the presentation of the prognoses of the following 12 cases is instructive in the process of evaluation. These cases are theoretical in the sense that they are presented as "cold facts" without the reader actually knowing the person represented by each case example. The reader may disagree with some of conclusions because of differences in clinical experience. If patients were actually examined, the variance would be greater because of the many subtle factors in the doctor-patient relationship. These interpretations also play a role in the doctor's final conclusions.

It becomes evident that all cases are different, therefore, vitiating the usefulness of too many generalizations as well as the adoption of any one specific scheme intended to be applicable for all cases. The doctor must take into account the myriad facts peculiar to each case, analyze them, and then arrive at logical conclusions based on professional judgment.

TABLE 5C. Range of Prognosis
1.   Poor
2.   Poor-to-fair
3.   Fair
4.   Fair-to-good
5.   Good

CASE NUMBER ONE   Refer to the diagnosis of case number one in Chapter Three. The prognosis for a functional cure by means of any or all methods of vision therapy is poor. The reason for a poor prognosis in this case is that the esotropia is congenital and of long duration. If treatment had been given early in life, perhaps there would have been a chance for fusion and possibly bifoveal fusion.

Since there is no cosmetic problem, no treatment should be recommended. Furthermore, the onset of amblyopia of extinction is unlikely to occur considering the age of the patient, and the fact that the strabismus is alternating.

The patient should be advised to have a routine follow-up examination in one year.

Refer to the diagnosis of case number two in Chapter Three. The strabismus of this 10-year-old patient is congenital. The prognosis for a functional cure by any or all means of therapy is poor.

CASE NUMBER TWO

It is also probable that the prognosis is poor for any significant change in the status of the amblyopia because the deviation has probably been unilateral since birth; therefore, it can be speculated that the reduced visual acuity is due to amblyopia of arrest. The ultimate differential diagnosis would be made by treating the condition in order to find out if there is any improvement. If there is enhancement of visual acuity, the amount of improvement represents that portion of visual loss due to amblyopia of extinction. If there is no improvement, the presence of amblyopia of arrest is confirmed, assuming organic amblyopia has been ruled out.

No treatment for the strabismus is recommended in this case since cosmesis seems to be acceptable to the patient. Because the deviation is only moderately large, the appearance of the eyes is fairly good in the primary gaze; however, the esotropia may become noticeable on right gaze because of the right lateral rectus paresis. Cosmesis is good otherwise.

Direct total occlusion should be recommended for constant wear. If the patient cannot see well enough in school with the amblyopic eye, an attempt should be made at periodic occlusion. This should continue for one or two months to find out if there is any improvement. If there is, pleoptics may be advised. If there is no change, further therapy is not indicated, and the patient should be advised to have a routine follow-up examination in one year.

Refer to the diagnosis of case number three in Chapter Three. The prognosis for a functional cure by any or all means of therapy is poor. The prognosis, however, for a partial cure is poor-to-fair. What is meant by partial cure is that the large manifest deviation could be converted into one that is small. This implies that peripheral fusion could possibly be re-educated, thereby holding the eyes relatively straight. The patient would technically be strabismic; but if motor ranges could be developed, the patient could function with at least some degree of binocularity. This would be a case of monofixation pattern. With a history of no previous treatment and a duration of eight years of constant esotropia, there is little hope for anything beyond this expectation.

CASE NUMBER THREE

The shallow amblyopia is probably due to the anisometropia rather than the strabismus since the deviation is alternating and not unilateral. Pleoptics is not absolutely necessary since the vision is not too poor for beginning binocular treatment.

The prognosis for cosmetic cure by means of extraocular muscle surgery is fair-to-good. Prism adaptation testing would be useful in this case to predetermine whether or not the angle would be changing after the operation.

Spectacle lenses should be prescribed to correct the refractive errors if they are axial and not due to corneal refractive differences. A contact lens for the right eye might be considered if the anisometropia is refractive rather than axial. In any event, there should be an examination for aniseikonia to see if this type of sensory obstacle produces the horror fusionis. This type of testing is discussed in Chapter Eight.

The patient should be advised that several appointments are needed for further evaluation and that orthoptics will be tried for a while to find out if there is any positive response. Correcting lenses should be worn during this time and their effect noted.

If training is of no avail, surgery should be recommended for cosmetic reasons.

CASE NUMBER FOUR Refer to the diagnosis of case number four in Chapter Three. The prognosis for a functional cure of the strabismus by means of therapy is poor. The prognosis for achieving monofixation is fair, and the chance of considerably ameliorating the amblyopia is also fair, because of the history of intermittency with onset not being too early in life. Much of the amblyopia may be of extinction rather than arrest. It is unlikely though that 20/20 (or 6/6) vision will be attained.

Assuming the amblyopia can be effectively reduced, minus lens over-correction may be used to align the visual axes. The high AC/A ratio is useful for accomplishing this. The A R C is probably not as unfavorable as is the deep suppression in this case of exotropia. A surgical over-correction (resulting in a small eso deviation) may be called for, both for functional reasons as well as for insuring a good cosmetic result in the event functional training fails. At best, it would be hoped that good fusional vergences could be developed, and the patient would have gross stereopsis.

The patient should be advised that approximately 24 orthoptic appointments and home training are required. Surgery may also be needed and followed up by postsurgical orthoptics.

CASE NUMBER FIVE Refer to the diagnosis of case number five in Chapter Three. The prognosis for functional cure is poor-to-fair. The prognosis for a partial cure whereby a monofixation is to be achieved is fair-to-good. The chief reason a complete cure (where there is exact bifoveal fixation) is difficult to achieve in this case is because there has been a duration of constant strabismus of three years.

There are many cases in which bifoveal fixation is difficult to regain after the patient has lost it for a few months. This is particularly so in very young patients.

The prognosis for cure of amblyopia by means of pleoptics is good because of the patient's young age and relatively late onset.

The patient should be advised that glasses, probably bifocals, are necessary and that approximately 36 orthoptic sessions, along with home training, are needed to develop peripheral fusion and good motor fusion ranges. Since cosmesis is good and functional results can be expected without surgical intervention, there is probably no need for an operation in this case. However, prisms may be required during and after training.

Refer to the diagnosis of case number six in Chapter Three. The prognosis for functional cure by means of therapy is fair. The factor of intermittency helps the prognosis immensely. The primary purpose of orthoptics in this case is to improve the presently existing visual skills which are in play at least some of the time for nearpoint seeing. Binasal occlusion for farpoint seeing should be recommended, as well as the possibility of base-out prisms followed by anti-suppression training and the development of adequate fusional vergence. A certain amount of training to improve monocular fixation and accommodative facility would be helpful prior to the binocular therapy regimen.

CASE NUMBER SIX

The prognosis must remain guarded because of the long duration of strabismus and lack of previous treatment. It is interesting to note that so many allegedly knowledgeable practitioners in the health-care field make statements such as "strabismus will go away by itself with time." This occurrence, unfortunately, is rare.

The patient should be advised of the need for glasses, occlusion, and 36 to 48 orthoptic appointments and home training. Surgery should be recommended only if absolutely required for functional results.

Refer to the diagnosis of case number seven in Chapter Three. The prognosis for a functional cure by means of lenses and orthoptics is fair-to-good. This case is a classic example of divergence excess. The prognosis must be guarded because of the larger deviation at farpoint and the intense and extensive suppression when the deviation is manifest. Anomalous correspondence is not a factor with which to be concerned since normal correspondence predominates while there is fusion.

CASE NUMBER SEVEN

Pleoptics may be done prior to sensory and motor fusion training in order to eliminate the amblyopia.

The patient should be advised that glasses, probably bifocals, are to be recommended, and that 24 to 36 pleoptic and orthoptic visits, as well as continuous home training, should be anticipated.

Refer to the diagnosis of case number eight in Chapter Three. The prognosis for a functional cure by means of orthoptics is fair-to-good. Other

CASE NUMBER EIGHT

supplemental testing such as the prolonged occlusion test, could help make the prognosis more decisive. It would also be helpful to know the patient's stereoacuity.

Although there is normally a direct correlation between a high level of stereoacuity and good binocularity, there may be an occasional exception to this rule. Griffin and Baldwin[18] reported a case of a patient who had relatively good flat fusion but absolutely no stereopsis. There was no way to account for this other than speculating that there must be an innate inability to perceive stereopsis.

Surgery is probably not called for in this case; however, a combination of presurgical orthoptics, surgery, and postsurgical orthoptics would most likely help the prognosis. Practically speaking, probably all that is required to cure this case of convergence insufficiency is orthoptics that emphasize positive fusional vergence training.

The patient should be advised to plan for 24 orthoptic appointments and continuous home training with the remote possibility of extraocular muscle surgery.

CASE NUMBER NINE   Refer to the diagnosis of case number nine in Chapter Three. Additional information would be helpful before the prognosis is made; for example, stereoacuity and motor fusion ranges. Assuming these are relatively normal, the prognosis for this adult patient is fair-to-good for a functional cure by means of therapy. There is a good chance of spontaneous remission of the superior oblique paresis with the passing of time. If this does not occur after six months or more, surgery may be required.

Management of the nonconcomitancy should emphasize the prevention of secondary contractures (discussed in Chapter Eleven).

The patient should be advised to make follow-up appointments as necessary for evaluation and training involving occlusion, prisms, and orthoptics. Communication with other specialists, particularly the neurologist, should be maintained. The patient should be advised of the eventual possibility of extraocular muscle surgery.

CASE NUMBER TEN   Refer to the diagnosis of case number ten in Chapter Three. The prognosis for a functional cure by means of lenses (bifocals) and orthoptics is good. This is a classic case of convergence excess being caused by a high AC/A ratio. The far deviation may be helped by incorporating base-out prisms in the patient's spectacles.

The prognosis must be slightly guarded because of the possible unacceptance of the spectacles by this seven-year-old child. Other than that, the prognosis is theoretically good. As in other cases, the prognosis is dependent upon good motivation and cooperation. These factors must always be taken into account.

The patient should be advised to make six orthoptic appointments at which time bifocals will be dispensed, and he will be taught to accept and properly use them. Some anti-suppression training and a great deal of fusional vergence training is required. Fortunately, much of this can be done in the form of home training, assuming the patient and parents are motivated and cooperative.

Refer to the diagnosis of case number eleven in Chapter Three. The prognosis for a functional cure by means of lenses and orthoptics is good. This case of convergence insufficiency should be aided by the wearing of lenses that correct the myopic anisometropia. Afterwards, fusional vergence ranges should be expanded by means of orthoptics.

The patient should be advised to make 12 orthoptic appointments and plan on an intense home training program.

Refer to the diagnosis of case number twelve in Chapter Three. The prognosis for a functional cure by means of orthoptics is good. Even though this is a case of heterophoria and not strabismus, the patient does not meet the criteria of Flom as being functionally cured because of his blurring of vision, discomfort, and the inadequate nearpoint of convergence.

The patient should be advised to make six therapy appointments and plan on home training for approximately 30 minutes per day during this time. Afterwards, five to ten minutes per day of home training will probably be recommended for six months or more.

PART TWO

TREATMENT

6 | Philosophies of Orthoptics

There is little dispute that Javal is responsible for laying the foundation of modern orthoptics. Since his original work in the late 1800's there have been many advances. He knew a great deal about the treatment of binocular anomalies, and many procedures in use today were advocated by him over 100 years ago. Other clinicians in France were to follow in Javal's footsteps and improvise on his successful treatment methods.

Meanwhile, in England, Worth was responsible for promulgating the philosophy of training the faculty of fusion. The amalgamation of the French and English schools of thought gradually evolved into what might be called a standard philosophy of orthoptics.

Individual approaches have also evolved through the years. Although they may have provided certain embellishments, by and large, the various approaches to treatment have much in common with each other. Differences between them are usually only a matter of relative emphasis of certain portions of the standard philosophy of orthoptics. The fundamentals remain basically the same.

One of the best summaries of the functional training procedures used by Javal appears in the writing of Revell.[1] Without going into great detail, a brief discussion may suffice to illustrate the principal features of Javal's approach to strabismus therapy.

The first step was to equalize the vision in each eye by means of glasses for refractive errors or by occlusion to eliminate amblyopia. Even if the amblyopia had been cured, occlusion was continued in order to prevent suppression.

Javal's recognition of the role of suppression in strabismus is one of the great strides forward in the field of binocular therapy. He employed stereoscopes for anti-suppression training. Brewster stereoscopes were used for small deviations, and Wheatstone stereoscopes were used for the larger ones. Training began with large peripheral targets which were gradually made smaller as progress was made in breaking down suppression.

Javal spoke of free-space training at the crossing point of the visual axes

Javal and the French School

in cases of esotropia. The purpose of this was to create an awareness of diplopia of an object placed either in front of, or in back of, the fixation target. Vergence ranges were developed by movement of the fixation target back-and-forth while the patient learned to avoid suppression by continuing to notice the diplopic images of the nonfixated target. Bar reading was then used for fine control and monitoring of suppression.

Javal believed that treatment time could be expected to take as long as the duration of strabismus. Many of his cases took three to five years to cure.

Notable among those following the teachings of Javal were Remy and Cantonnet. Remy is known for refining Javal's methods of anti-suppression training and for the development of two important instruments used for this purpose: the Remy separator and the diploscope.

Cantonnet[2] introduced the concept of mental effort. Anti-suppression methods contributed by Cantonnet included the hole-in-hand, adaptation of the Pigeon stereoscope to make the Pigeon-Cantonnet Stereoscope, deneutralization (breaking down suppression) by bright light and septum, and the effective use of anaglyphs.

Gibson[3] stated that mental effort is an important factor in the therapy of strabismus for it may aid the esotrope in making divergence movements. A way to instruct the patient to do this is to have him imagine he is looking at a distant object above the horizon. In a similar manner, the exotrope should try to imagine he is fixating an object close to him in a downward position of gaze. Mental effort may be used with or without instrumentation. The purpose of this training is for a voluntary change in vergence to eventually become one that is automatic and reflexive.

Worth and the English School

The concept that strabismus is due to poor sensory fusion is largely attributed to Worth[4] who contended that binocular vision was either developed in the early plastic years or not at all. He thought the fusion faculty, necessary for binocular vision, normally reached full development before the end of the sixth year of life and that any attempt to train the fusion sense after that time was futile. According to his philosophy, it is wise to begin fusion training as soon as possible in cases of strabismus. Worth believed that poor fusion was the cause of strabismus. He wrote, "Thus the essential cause of squint is a defect of the fusion faculty."

Worth thought that the faulty faculty of fusion was sometimes congenital. Today this is recognized as a possibility for some congenital esotropes who show complete lack of correspondence.

In stressing the importance of early detection and treatment of strabismus, Worth stated, "Of the cases of squint in which efficient treatment is carried out from the first appearance of the deviation, only a small proportion will ever need operation." He believed in treating three-to-five-year-old children, and sometimes younger, providing they were cooperative. He trained the fusion sense by using the amblyoscope which he invented for this purpose. The idea behind fusion training was that good sensory fusion creates a "desire for binocular vision." Worth wrote, "The favorable time for fusion training is between the age of three and five years. In children under three years of age this treatment is apt to be rather difficult, though I have succeeded in many cases. After five years of age the fusion training takes longer, and a much less powerful desire for binocular vision is obtained."

Worth conceded that some older patients having had strabismus for a long time could achieve binocularity as a result of the deviation being corrected. He stuck to the contention, however, that the apparently new development of fusion was not really new, but was present before the deviation became manifest and that it was originally too weak to prevent the deviation from becoming manifest. The concept of re-education of fusion is still in general acceptance today.

Worth's philosophy prevailed in England until challenged by Chavasse[5], who stressed that the development of binocular vision was dependent upon reflexes that require both time and usage. He did not accept the concept of a faulty fusion faculty but rather believed that the mechanism for fusion is present at birth. In order for the binocular reflexes to develop normally, it was extremely important for the infant to have the opportunity for early single binocular vision.

Both Worth and Chavasse were in accord to the extent that any hindrance to fusion should be eliminated and treated as quickly (without long duration) and early as possible. Chavasse believed obstacles to fusion could be sensory, motor and central. A modified outline of the obstacles presented by Lyle and Bridgeman[6] are presented in Table 6A.

Chavasse emphasized the need for the elimination of obstacles by means other than orthoptics; as a result, many of his followers become disinterested in the functional training approach to strabismus. This negative influence notwithstanding, the overall influence of Chavasse can be considered positive. His great contributions were in the area of the developmental aspects of binocular vision.

The philosophy of modern orthoptics is in many ways a combination of the early French and English philosophies. The general agreement that training can often help the patient regain lost skills or develop those that are arrested (if treated in the plastic years) is still the prevailing attitude.

Most authorities recommend the patient go through a monocular phase prior to binocular training. This could include working on the improvement of visual acuity, fixations, and accommodation. The degree of the importance placed on the monocular phase of training varies from one practitioner to another. Some practitioners stress this, particularly those who share many of the philosophies of the clinical associates of the Optometric Extension Program.[7] Although other practitioners may not put as much emphasis on monocular training, practically all insist that attempts should be made to significantly reduce amblyopia before the binocular phase is started.

The next phase of training is the bi-ocular phase, in which both eyes are

Standard Orthoptic Philosophy

used at the same time, but noncorresponding points are stimulated. This is an important step for developing binocular awareness and maintaining progress made in the monocular phase. For example, vertical prism dissociation is considered to be a bi-ocular procedure used for improving alternate fixation, as well as breaking down suppression. Getz[8] states that a mistake can be made by moving the patient into the binocular phase too quickly without adequate bi-ocular training.

TABLE 6A. Obstacles in the Reflex Paths for Development of Binocular Vision (from Lyle and Bridgeman)

A. Sensory Obstacles
   1.   Dioptric obstacles
       a.   Uncorrected errors of refraction
       b.   Opacities of the media

   2.   Prolonged Uniocular activity
       a.   Unilateral ptosis
       b.   Occlusion for one reason or another (e.g., injury)

   3.   Retinoneural obstacles (lesions in the visual pathways)

B. Motor Obstacles
   1.   Abnormalities of the orbit and adnexa (e.g., tumor that is space taking)
   2.   Conditions affecting one or more of the extrinsic ocular muscles
       a.   Congenital abnormalities (e.g., faulty insertion of a muscle)
       b.   Injury, particularly to lateral rectus in birth trauma
       c.   Contractures in cases of paresis
       d.   Disease of the muscle itself

   3.   Conditions affecting the central nervous system
       a.   Congenital absence of the oculomotor nerves or their supranuclear pathways
       b.   Head injury
       c.   Inflammation (e.g., encephalitis)
       d.   Supranuclear lesions

   4.   Decompensation of an extrinsic ocular muscle imbalance

C. Central obstacles
   1.   Psychogenic
   2.   Hyper or hypo excitability of the central nervous system
   3.   Central uniocular inhibition
   4.   Inability of the infant to learn

The binocular phase is essentially that of sensory and motor fusion training. Unlike the bi-ocular phase in which noncorresponding points are stimulated, the binocular phase requires the stimulation of corresponding points.

First-degree fusion training is involved with eliminating anomalous correspondence by teaching the patient to appreciate superimposition while corresponding points are being stimulated. Horror fusionis may also require this type of training. Treatment by the use of peripheral superimposition targets is often required in cases of deep suppression.

Development of good sensory fusion, both second degree and third degree, is the next step in the binocular phase. Once this is accomplished, training is concerned with the establishment and improvement of motor fusion. Table 6B lists the sequence of standard orthoptic procedures. Specific procedures used in the standard approach are discussed in detail in subsequent chapters.

TABLE 6B. *Standard Orthoptic Philosophy for Functional Cure*

A. Lenses
  1. Prescribe full corrective lenses (full plus and possibly bifocals in esotropia)
  2. Possible over-correction of minus in exotropia

B. Monocular phase
  1. Ocular calisthenics to increase ductions
  2. Occlusion and/or Pleoptics for amblyopia and abnormal fixation
  3. Pursuit and saccadic eye movement training

C. Bi-ocular phase
  1. Develop simultaneous perception without suppression
  2. Bi-ocular accommodative rock

D. Binocular phase
  1. Elimination of anomalous correspondence and/or horror fusionis and development of good superimposition without suppression
  2. Development of good flat fusion (continuation of anti-suppression training, commencing with peripheral targets and gradually working toward foveal ones)
  3. Encouragement to use mental effort to converge in exotropia and to diverge in esotropia (voluntary vergence)
  4. Development of good stereopsis
  5. Development of motor fusion using flat-fusion targets
  6. Development of motor fusion with stereopsis
  7. Stabilization of sensory and motor fusion by achieving normal fusion ranges and recoveries without suppression and good flexibility of vergences and accommodation (e.g., jump vergence training and binocular rock)
  8. Insurance of good sensory and motor fusion in all positions of gaze

---

Certain additions to the standard orthoptic procedure were advocated by Brock.[9,10,11] His major contribution, perhaps, was the introduction of his normal environment training philosophy. Authorities such as Ludlam, Flax, Vodnoy, and many others are, to some degree, advocates of most of Brock's methods.

Brock believed that a therapy environment should be familiar and meaningful to the patient. Training devices should simulate reality as much as possible and should be within the patient's level of achievement. Brock thought it unwise to train a strabismic patient at his angle of deviation since it would only reinforce strabismic behavior. Instead, he thought training should begin at a point (usually at near) at which the patient shows a desire for binocular vision. Brock believed that stereopsis was more natural than flat fusion and, therefore, recommended using third-degree fusion targets initially. Large targets were employed to stimulate peripheral portions of the visual field. In order to see depth, correct binocular posture must be present. Large targets were used not only because suppression was a factor, but because motor fusion is facilitated by large visual fields and hindered by small ones. He felt that small targets devoid of peripheral fields lost reality as far as the patient was concerned.

In differing with the classical school of thought, Brock did not advocate diplopia awareness training. He considered training that produces diplopia in habitual surroundings unwise because it was contrary to normal vision.

Brock concentrated on using anaglyphic or vectographic devices for free-space orthoptics. These were thought to be more life-like so that transferring binocular posture to normal surroundings could be made easier. He preferred to have patients work in the open and not in instruments. In cases of esotropia binocular posture at infinity was not attempted initially, but only toward the conclusion of training did he expect the patient to achieve parallelism of the visual axes.

Smith[1][2] placed great emphasis on monocular training. To a large extent he concurred with Brock as to binocular training but differed with his belief that peripheral fusion training should be stressed. Smith believed that once foveal fixation is good in each eye, central fixation training should be given under binocular conditions.

In subsequent chapters, other advances and new concepts of orthoptic procedures are presented as they pertain to treatment of specific binocular anomalies.

Some of the basic underlying principles of the doctor-patient relationship in vision training should always be kept in mind. This type of therapy is educative (re-educative to a certain extent) and requires learning on the part of the patient. It should be remembered that learning takes place from within, and the goal is for the patient to know what he is doing with and to himself. He should be aware of errors so that these can be corrected.

The patient should feel comfortable and open with the doctor and have the sense of freedom to make errors and share thoughts and reactions. Patients tend to be afraid to make mistakes and may clam-up if this fear is reinforced by harsh judgment and undue criticism. Ordering a patient to perform a certain task may cause a negative reaction and cut off a communication bond between the doctor and the patient, therefore, it is a good rule for the doctor to ask the patient rather than to tell him.

The term "orthoptics" is the traditional designation for treatment of strabismus, and, to some extent, this applies to heterophoria, according to some practitioners. Other functional vision training procedures may be needed, however, to finish the patient by refining and enhancing visual skills that may have been attained and/or regained via orthoptic efforts. (Refer to Table 4C for a general classification of vision training.)

For want of a suitable term, these refining and enhancing regimens may be called "visual skills efficiency training." Practitioners are preferring to discontinue the "orthoptics" label when treating non-strabismic patients, particularly for visual skills therapy. The limitation that orthoptics ("straight sight") connotes may be a reason for this attitude. It must be realized that the *orthoptic* goal in strabismus is not necessarily the goal for a patient undergoing therapy for inefficient visual skills. For example, the criteria of Flom (Chapter Five) include clearness, singleness, and comfortableness of binocular vision, but *efficiency* of vision is not explicitly stated. The patient will probably want more than just having his strabismus cured. He will want to have inefficient visual skills—those newly attained as well as pre-existing ones—also cured. (A detailed discussion of this aspect of therapy is given in Chapter Fifteen.)

What if a certain patient has problems requiring the full scope of vision therapy? Suppose he is strabismic with amblyopia, and what visual skills he has are insufficient. The phases of therapy would be most efficacious in the following sequence: (1) pleoptics for *amblyopia;* (2) orthoptics for *strabismus* and development of bifixation and normal fusional amplitudes; and (3) training for good *saccades* and *pursuits;* training for *accommodation* sufficiency, good facility, and adequate stamina; training for *vergence* sufficiency, good facility, and adequate stamina; and excellent *sensory fusion* as exemplified by a low stereoacuity threshold (in that order).

If a learning difficulty persisted after all these problems were abated, perceptual and cognitive evaluations and recommendations would have to be made by an interdisciplinary team.

7 | Therapy for Amblyopia

Therapy for amblyopia may include any or all the methods used in the management of binocular anomalies. The most commonly used method is occlusion. Lenses are helpful in many cases of anisometropia, and lens therapy is often used in conjunction with occlusion to effect a cure of functional amblyopia. Many practitioners believe that frequent changes in the lens prescription may be necessary for the amblyopic eye. Winter[1] writes that this may be due to latent hyperopia and changes in angle E. He stresses the importance of exact lens corrections, even in cases with small refractive errors, particularly if there is oblique astigmatism or anisometropia. If lenses and/or occlusion therapy fail, pleoptics may be necessary in order to eliminate amblyopia. Many authorities believe that vision should be reasonably good before binocular treatment can be started. Visual acuity of 20/40 is generally considered acceptable in this regard.

Occlusion and Monocular Training Activities

There is very little argument against prescribing direct occlusion to the infant who has either strabismic or anisometropic amblyopia. Total occlusion (i.e., full, opaque, patching) is almost always recommended in these cases. The wearing time should be constant, and there should be alternate, rather than unilateral, occlusion, to prevent amblyopia from occurring in the sound eye that is covered. This is referred to as occlusion amblyopia. The ratio of wearing time I recommend is 2/1. Thus, this patch should be worn over the sound eye (direct occlusion) for two days, and then switched to the amblyopic eye (inverse occlusion) for one day of wearing. In other words, the patch should be worn during all waking hours on one eye or the other, but predominantly on the nonamblyopic eye. Constant occlusion, however, should last only a few days at a time, because possible stimulation of *binocular* cortical cells in the interim should be encouraged.

Active monocular training in many infants may be possible during direct occlusion. This tends to hasten development of good visual acuity, and time is critical in regard to binocular vision. The child should be taught to associate wearing the patch with love and reward, rather than with the feeling of rejection and punishment. Training begins with simple passive demands, such as looking at television, and then progresses to more active means that require eye-hand coordination. A suggested list of these activities is presented in Table 7A.

It matters little whether there is central or eccentric fixation in amblyopic infants. Some practitioners may consider this a factor in children from three up to age six; however, I generally find that direct occlusion is very effective in eliminating amblyopia regardless of the nature of fixation. The only difference in occluding the three-year-old is that the ratio is changed from 2/1 to 3/1. For a four-year-old, the ratio is four days direct occlusion and one day inverse. Likewise, the ratio for the five-year-old is 5/1. The rule of alternate patching is easy to remember, because the ratio is the same as the patient's age in years.

TABLE 7A. Activities during Direct Occlusion for the Infant with Amblyopia

1. Association of attention, love and kindness with patching
2. Association of eating rewards with patching (e.g., giving favorite foods when patching non-amblyopic eye)
3. Stimuli of sight and sound by watching television
4. Peek-a-boo games
5. Watching suspended toys or mobile
6. Following a rolling ball with amblyopic eye
7. Crawling, creeping, standing, walking
8. Playing with flashlight or bright objects
9. Handling blocks and toys
10. Catching rolling ball

Many authorities feel that the ratio should be greatly increased for the infant, possibly 6/1. It would be wise, however, to stay on the conservative side with lower ratios, since this is done as an out-of-office procedure without the doctor's direct supervision.

Consideration must be given before occlusion procedures are recommended in patients who are age six or older. Certain types of eccentric fixation require inverse patching, and these patients may be able to cooperate in special pleoptic therapy.

Central Fixation   Direct occlusion is normally the best method of therapy to start first in cases of amblyopia with central fixation. This is true for patients of any age. The main drawbacks to occlusion are producing occlusion strabismus, particularly in young children, or possibly causing intractable diplopia in certain cases with older patients.

Therapy time is shortened if occlusion is combined with monocular training activities. Cases of unsteady central fixation are treated in the same manner as those with steady central fixation. There is usually a slightly better prognosis for the latter condition and the treatment time may be less. In either case, the chance of eliminating amblyopia is good in patients above age five, if the reduced vision is due to extinction and not to amblyopia of arrest. In this older age group, direct, constant, unilateral patching is recommended, as there is hardly any chance of occlusion amblyopia occurring.

TABLE 7B. Monocular Training During Direct Occlusion for the Patient over the Age of Two Years

1. Watching television or other passive activity

2. Walking, running, hopping, skipping

3. Balancing exercises (e.g., balance board or walking beam, walking on balance beam)

4. Eye-foot coordination (e.g., playing kick-ball)

5. Laterality and directionality training involving perceptual motor tasks for right-left awareness (e.g., ball and bat)

6. Eye-hand coordination play, including drawing, coloring, dot-to-dot pictures, bead stringing, tiddly-winks, pick-up sticks, toothpick in straw, tic-tac-toe, dominoes, card games, jacks, jig-saw puzzles, cross-word puzzles, cutting with scissors, glue-on collages, tracing, pounding nails, coloring out O's, coloring out all vowels, throwing and catching ball, etc.

7. Accommodative rock

8. Visual tracing exercises (e.g., Groffman)

9. Figure ground discrimination (e.g., Hidden Pictures)

10. Reading, which may include low vision print with low illumination, low vision print with high illumination, low vision print with normal illumination, normal print with normal illumination, and car games such as reading street-signs or license plates

11. Proofreading and special visual discrimination tasks

12. Tachistoscopic training for speed and span of recognition, and also for visual memory

---

The number of different monocular training activities for either in-office or out-of-office is legion. These activities are used to stimulate the fovea and promote correct spatial localization ability. A list of some of the more popular exercises in this regard is presented in Table 7B.

Patching may be traumatic to any patient, whether a child or an adult. It is wise, therefore, to let the first exposure be spent in relatively comfortable surroundings, with as little demand on the patient as possible. Passive activity, such as watching television, is recommended. If the amblyopia is deep, the patient necessarily behaves as though he is a low vision patient who is partially sighted. This is quite disconcerting to most individuals, and the intolerance to this sudden change of circumstances is the main reason for the failure of occlusion therapy. If the patient is properly indoctrinated beforehand, this negative response can be avoided in most cases. The patient should be advised to move as close to the television set as necessary, so that viewing is relatively easy and enjoyable.

Gross motor activity may help patients learn to overcome poor visual spatial localization caused by amblyopic viewing. These activities may involve balance exercises, laterality training, as well as many coordination exercises.

It is a good idea to build the patient's confidence before the patch is worn. The patient should first be able to demonstrate proficiency in gross motor tasks. Otherwise, he will experience frustration, and will most certainly reject being occluded. In addition, there is the reality of danger to the patient if he is placed in certain situations while wearing a patch. For example, if he is expected to maintain his equilibrium while standing on a balance board, and see with an amblyopic eye, the patient is likely to fall unless he has been adequately prepared, and has become sufficiently familiar with the particular set of demands. In all cases, the therapist should be ready to catch the patient should he lose his balance and begin to fall. An illustration of training on the balance board prior to occlusion is shown in Figure 7-1. Curry[2] described the construction of the balance board. A 16-inch square piece of one-inch board may be mounted on a block of wood that is typically a three-inch cube.

Table 7C lists some of the many balance board activities applicable to amblyopia therapy.

Many of the balance board activities can also be used with the walking rail. The chief advantage of the rail over the balance board is that the patient can experience movement by walking forward or backward while maintaining balance. At the same time, monocular stimulatory exercises can be performed. Children enjoy this type of activity, and it is used at times for a "break" in the training routine, regardless of the type of problem being treated. The various procedures are too numerous to mention, as each practitioner invents new procedures for the walking rail. Some of these are listed in Table 7D.

Walking rails may be constructed by ordinary 2 by 4 inch lumber. The recommended length is ten to twelve feet (at least three meters). The beginning exercises should be done with the patient walking on a four-inch wide rail, since this is much easier than walking on the side that is only two inches wide.

Most gross motor training can be done at home as out-of-office procedures. This is true for eye-foot coordination development, as well as many of the eye-hand training procedures. Some activities can incorporate balance training along with eye-hand coordination training; for instance, throwing and catching a ball while balancing.

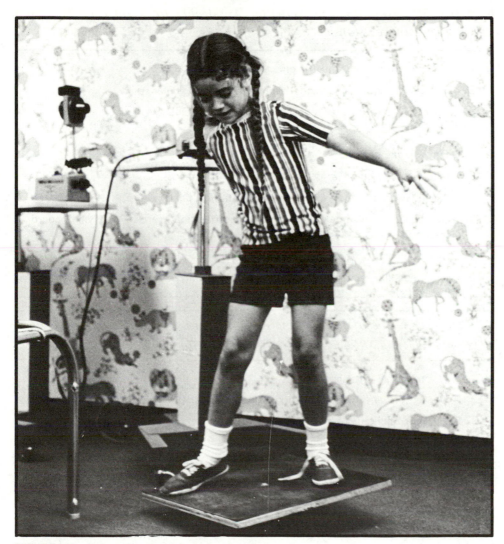

FIGURE 7-1 — Balance board training prior to occlusion

A very effective combination of procedures is the simultaneous use of the rotating pegboard[a] while balancing. This is a rotating, perforated patterned disc into which the patient is instructed to insert colored golf tees. It is designed to develop facility in controlling each hand with either or both eyes. In the case of direct occlusion, the amblyopic eye is trained, and the patient is instructed to place the appropriately colored golf tee into the matching colored hole. At first, the rotator may have to be turned off so

---

[a]Custom-made by placing a circular wooden board on a motorized rotator. Also, there is one manufactured by Manico, P.O. Box 395, Clute, Texas 77531 and called the Manico Home Trainer.

that the patient can learn to achieve proper placing of the golf tees in a quick and accurate manner. This instrument is shown in Figure 7-2.

TABLE 7C. Some Balance Activities Applicable to Amblyopia Therapy during Direct Occlusion

1.   Balance without any specific directions
2.   Swing arms in various directions while maintaining balance
3.   Move feet to various positions while maintaining balance
4.   Hold toy, and change from hand-to-hand
5.   Throw and catch ball
6.   Fixate on swinging Marsden ball while maintaining balance
7.   Bat the swinging Marsden ball while maintaining balance
8.   Maintain balance while doing eye-hand coordination exercises (e.g., chalkboard drawings)
9.   Combine balance board with monocular accommodative rock training
10. Combine balance board with tachistoscopic training

TABLE 7D. Some of the Walking Rail Activities Applicable to Monocular Training for Amblyopia during Direct Occlusion

1. Walk on the rail watching feet
2. Advance to level of walking without watching feet
3. Walk while maintaining fixation on a target
4. Repeat above, while walking backward
5. Walk forward or backward while balancing an eraser on head
6. Walk while throwing and catching a ball (or bean bag)
7. Walk while changing toy from hand to hand
8. Walk while fixating a swinging Marsden ball
9. Pick up small toys placed on the rail without losing balance
10. Monocular accommodative rock with minus lenses while walking on rail
11. Visual memory training when seeing with amblyopic eye while walking on rail and maintaining balance (e.g., with flash cards on one end, patient turns around and walks to other end, then draws on chalkboard from memory)

There is an almost endless variety of eye-hand exercises for home training. I recommend stringing Apple Jacks[b], and letting the child eat the cinnamon flavored rings once he has a string of them.

---

[b]Kellogg's Apple Jacks cereal, available at most food markets.

As with eye-hand coordination exercises, there are many procedures that may be used for laterality or directionality training. It is interesting to note that a person seeing with an amblyopic eye performs in many respects as though he were afflicted with a perceptual learning disability; e.g., reading is poor with many regressions of fixation.

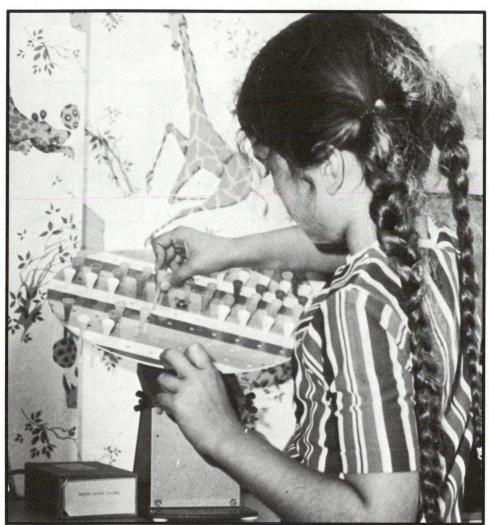

FIGURE 7-2 — Rotating peg board for eye-hand coordination training during direct occlusion

A practical method of home training for improvement of laterality and directionality is the use of a bat and a Marsden ball. Refer to Figure 7-3 for illustration. The bat is colored in various segments. Most practitioners using this device prefer to have four colors on each end of the bat. For instance, green may be the color used on either end of the bat, followed by yellow, red, and white symmetrically placed on each section. The child builds an awareness of right and left by learning to follow the verbal directions given to him by the therapist. This could be in following manner: "Hold the bat on the yellow portion with each hand. Hit the swinging ball with the left red portion, now the right green portion," and so on. This is an enjoyable procedure for most young patients, and they can readily monitor their own progress as they improve. Most of this work can be done at home under a parent's supervision. If the amblyopia is deep, it is usually wise for the patient to master this exercise when using the nonamblyopic eye before patching is begun.

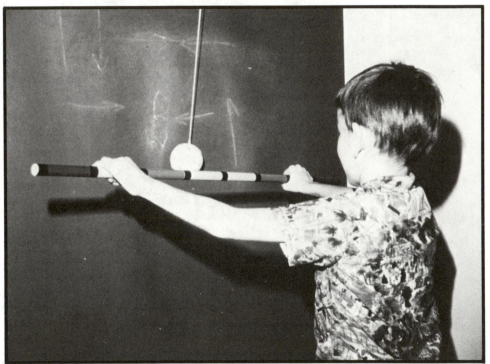

FIGURE 7-3 — Bat and Marsden ball for laterality and directionality training may be combined with balancing as well as occlusion.

The patient may be presented with greater demands by having to balance on a board all the while. Further demands may be created by requiring the patient to fixate arrows on a chalk board after each hit of the ball, and to verbalize the direction in which each successive arrow is pointing. This is excellent both for fixation training and for improvement of directionality.

Monocular accommodative rock may be done with or without lenses. The Marsden ball serves as a useful target in either event. A good way to interest the patient in accommodation facility training is by the use of a minus five diopter lens held before the amblyopic eye. The nonamblyopic eye is occluded as the patient views a swinging Marsden ball, with which there must be accommodation if the numbers on the ball are to be seen clearly. The lens is removed so that the eye is now seeing the ball without the minus five diopter accommodative demand. This is repeated for several minutes at a time, with the eventual goal of clearing the letters on the ball forty times within one minute. Since the focus control for accommodation is thought to be in the fovea, this type of training is good to stimulate the fovea and ensure central fixation. The ball's movement tends to generate more interest for the patient than a stationary target does. Lateral movement of the ball is useful for pursuit training, while at the same time, accommodative rock is being done. Full rotation pursuits can be worked on by having the patient lie in a supine position and look up at the Marsden ball moving in a circular pattern.

If lenses are not used, the patient may do near-far fixations for monocular rock with the amblyopic eye. This could be done with a Marsden ball swinging to and fro while the patient maintains clear vision. Another good procedure is the near-far fixations using the Hart charts.[c] The patient holds a chart of letters resembling a reduced Snellen chart, clears one letter, and then views a similar chart at the farpoint. After the print becomes clear, another letter on the nearpoint chart is fixated and cleared.

Visual Tracing by Groffman[d] is an excellent method for amblyopia therapy. The patient looks at a series of lines, each of which is connected to a letter on one end and a number on the other. The object is to correctly match the number with the appropriate letter, the eye sighting along a line and following it to its end. This represents a very high demand on fixation, as no tactual clues are involved. I have discovered that children enjoy making their own exercises. An example of a seven-year-old's work is shown in Figure 7-4. The child has the additional benefit of working on eye-hand coordination while drawing the lines, plus the satisfaction of doing something original and creative. The amblyopic child feels a sense of pride in the designs he has made. A key is made up, and the patient can administer the test to siblings or friends who do not always fare too well on some of the more elaborate patterns. This is sometimes a much needed boost to the ego of the amblyope who wears a patch.

There are several available sources for good figure-ground discrimination training material. Effective training procedures can be given with Hidden Pictures[e], Seek-A-Word[f], and the Michigan Symbol and Alphabet tracking books[g]. Alphabet exercises can also be done with ordinary newspaper print

---

[c]Hart charts devised by Dr. Walter Hart, Tacoma, Wash., and available from Keystone View, Division Mast/Keystone.

[d]Visual Tracing by Groffman, available from Keystone View, Division of Mast/Keystone.

[e]Available from Highlights for Children, 2300 W. Fifth Ave, Columbus, OH 43216.

[f]Seek-A-Word magazines, available at local bookstores and newsstands.

[g]Ann Arbor Publishers, Inc., P.O. Box 7249, Naples, FL 33940.

for home training. The object is for the patient to encircle every letter in alphabetical order as he comes to each successive letter while reading a passage of print. It is evident that more than just figure-ground discrimination is being trained; e.g., eye-hand coordination. This is fine, if amblyopia is also being treated.

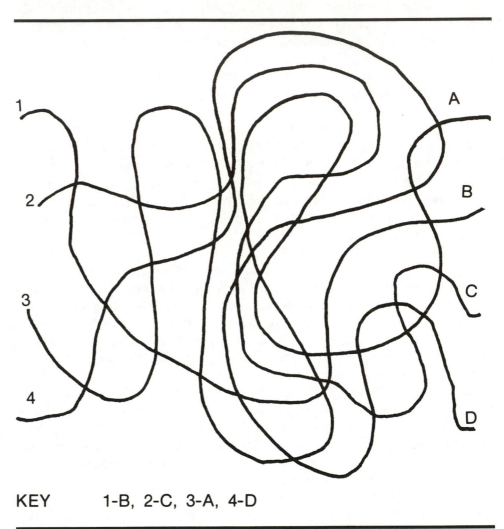

KEY   1-B, 2-C, 3-A, 4-D

FIGURE 7-4 — Sample visual tracing exercise drawn by a patient

The patient should be encouraged to read with the amblyopic eye as much as possible. The reading level should be commensurate with the patient's nearpoint visual acuity. This may require the use of large print, used for patients who have low vision due to pathological causes. As treatment progresses, the print size can gradually be made smaller and the illumination reduced from very high to a normal level.

Sedan[3] warns that if the functional result attained through the training process is not reinforced, the function is apt to become defective again. To prevent this, he recommends the patient undergo proofreading exercises, such as the ones contained in his book. In addition to proofreading, he includes a series of pictures in which the patient is instructed to point out all the possible differences between a set of two pictures. This requires good attention, which is important in the treatment of amblyopia.

Some clinicians feel that one eye should function as well as the other eye if binocular therapy is to be successful. This is why some practitioners emphasize the training of monocular skills prior to starting binocular therapy. Those who follow this line of reasoning employ tachistoscopic procedures to finalize the monocular phase of training. Targets may consist of numbers, letters, words, phrases, or geometric symbols. Flash speeds usually vary from 1/10 to 1/200 of a second. This type of training is done in the attempt to equalize speed and span of recognition for each eye, as well as to improve and show that visual memory is equal when each eye is used.

If all of the above procedures employed with direct occlusion are carefully carried out for two months with very little positive results, the likelihood of further improvement of visual acuity is not great. Additional foveal stimulation techniques (to be discussed in section on treating eccentric fixation) may be tried, but the chances for further significant improvement are slim. It is fortunate, however, that in cases of amblyopia with either steady or unsteady central fixation, the majority of patients can be helped by the relatively simple means of using direct occlusion along with monocular training activities.

If the amblyopic patient is under six years of age and has variable eccentric fixation, the prognosis for cure by means of direct patching and monocular training activities is good. If, however, the patient is over six, the prognosis for cure by this means becomes poorer with increasing age, particularly if point "e" is always in a fixed, non-variable area. However, the prognosis is not necessarily poor if all means of pleoptics are at the doctor's disposal. This may include such elaborate procedures as dazzling and the use of afterimages and entoptic phenomena. ("Non-variable" refers to point "e" being in a fixed site; "variable" means point "e" wanders from moment to moment or day to day.)

VARIABLE ECCENTRIC FIXATION

Even if the patient is over the age of six, I recommend the traditional method of direct occlusion as the initial choice for therapy. This is done (in conjunction with the monocular training activities) in the same manner as though the patient being treated has central fixation. In very many cases, angle E disappears, and good visual acuity is the result of training. This may take several months, however, and is related to the patient's age. Treatment time is longer in the older patient, but there appears to be no upper age limit for treatment as long as the condition is amblyopia of extinction, and not amblyopia of arrest.

There are some patients with variable eccentric fixation who do not respond favorably to direct occlusion and typical monocular training

DIRECT OCCLUSION

activities. Angle E may change slightly, possibly reducing by 20 to 30 percent, but further training seems to enforce the fixation at a new location. Trying to move the point of fixation away from this area is difficult in many cases. The patient somehow becomes tenacious in maintaining that certain point "e" with which to fixate. Some authorities refer to this as being an embedded case. The prognosis is poor unless elaborate pleoptic procedures are used.

To keep a nonembedded case from becoming embedded, the doctor must carefully monitor the eccentric fixation during every office visit. Embeddedness can be seen when point "e" is in a fixed site even though there is unsteady eccentric fixation. Angle E is usually not very large in these cases, but often the visual acuity is fairly poor. Common findings are approximately two degrees of eccentric fixation with visual acuity of 20/80. Sometimes the eccentric fixation may have been large before therapy, i.e., 4 degrees with 20/200, and after direct patching, angle E may be reduced to two degrees and the vision improved to 20/80. Unfortunately, continuing the same treatment is of no avail. The position of point "e" remains fixed, and the visual acuity shows no further improvement. It behooves the doctor to watch for such signs and be ready to change to other therapeutic procedures.

INVERSE OCCLUSION

Switching from direct to inverse occlusion is called for in the previously mentioned example. The patch should now be worn on the amblyopic eye for a month, and then other forms of pleoptics, similar to those of Bangerter and Cüppers, should be started.

COLORED FILTERS

The use of a red filter, such as the Kodak gelatin Wratten filter No. 92, which excludes wavelengths shorter than 640 mμ, has been advocated by Brinker and Katz.[4] This is worn over the amblyopic eye. Burian and Von Noorden[5] recommend using the less expensive and more durable Transilwrap 0.06 Red transparent vinyl.[h] Stray white light should be blocked out by side shields, otherwise the purpose of seeing through the red filter is defeated. The idea is to have the amblyopic eye become dark adapted, because vision supposedly improves in the amblyopic eye upon dark adaptation. Similarly, cone vision is stimulated because of the red hue. This in turn tends to promote foveal fixation, since the highest density of cones is located at the fovea. During the time when the red lens is over the amblyopic eye, there should be total occlusion of the nonamblyopic eye. Because of the general nonacceptance of this type of occlusion, patients will usually accept this arrangement for only a few hours a day. When the red filter is removed, the patient should immediately revert to inverse occlusion.

Although there is theoretical merit to this form of therapy, it has never

---

[h]Mfg. by the Transilwrap Co., 2740 North 4th St., Philadelphia, PA 19133. The recommended thickness is 0.06 inch.

really been used extensively. Nevertheless, the doctor should have this available as a procedure and attempt this type of treatment when the occasion warrants its use. Red filters are also useful in treatment of amblyopia under binocular conditions (to be discussed in a subsequent section).

Cüppers[5] advocates the wearing of monocular prism. He feels this is effective if angle E becomes less, or possibly zero, in one of the nine diagnostic positions of gaze. For instance, if angle E of the left eye becomes zero upon dextrosupraduction, prism over the left eye should be worn while the right eye is totally occluded. The prism should be base-out combined with base-down. The strength of the horizontal and vertical components of the prism would depend on the power required to neutralize angle E. The effect of the prism is that the eye moves toward the apex of the prism; therefore, when the patient is looking at an object directly in front of him, the eye behind the prism will be pointing leftward and upward. This simulates the condition of the eye in the dextrosupraduction position.

If the eccentric fixation is reduced by means of the prism, visual acuity should improve, but other pleoptic methods are usually required in addition, in order to completely eliminate amblyopia.

Pigassou and Toulouse[6] recommend inverse prism over the amblyopic eye, while the nonamblyopic eye is totally occluded. If the left eye has nasal eccentric fixation, a base-in prism equal in magnitude to angle E is worn over the left eye. If the eccentric fixation is temporal, a base-out prism is worn. When the prism is not being worn, the patient goes back to inverse occlusion.

The purpose of this procedure is to shift the principal visual direction from point "e" to the fovea. In the case of nasal eccentric fixation of the left eye, wearing the base-in prism causes the left eye to abduct. This turning outward of the eye puts the fovea in the "straight-ahead" or true primary position. Monocular training activities, such as eye-hand coordination exercises, are carried out for the purpose of associating the straight-ahead position with the true spatial location of the target. The exact true location of the object being fixated can be verified by the tactual kinesthetic sense when the patient touches the object with his finger or a pointer.

Toward the end of training, when eccentric fixation has been changed into central fixation, it is always possible that eccentric fixation will return. This is particularly true when the patient is required to do ordinary reading. Sedan[7] believes that there is almost always a horizontal component to angle E in cases of eccentric fixation, and reading of horizontal lines of print is not recommended. It is thought that ordinary reading can cause the patient to regress to using point "e" rather than the fovea.

In order to determine which orientation is most easily read, Sedan advises using a star-like configuration of four rows of letters (see Figure 7-5). The most favorable orientation is determined by having the patient read aloud, and evaluating his performance for both speed and accuracy. The least favorable direction is usually found to be 90 degrees from the most favorable. For instance, the patient may be able to read well in the vertical meridian, but poorly in the horizontal.

In this event, the patient is given home reading exercises (during direct occlusion) in which vertical lines of letters are to be read. The patient should be discouraged from reading horizontal meridians of print at this time. Such sheets of print can be custom-made or purchased.[i] After sufficiently reading in the most favorable orientation, the patient begins in the less favorable orientations until he has no trouble with them. Once this is accomplished, the patient can proceed to the monocular training activities advised for the amblyope with central fixation, listed in Table 7B.

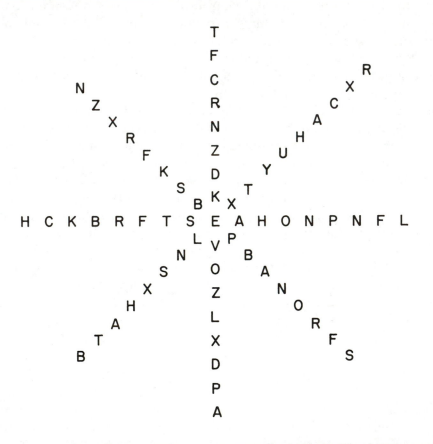

FIGURE 7-5 — Example of star-like configuration of rows of letters for vertical and oblique reading in cases of eccentric fixation

[i]Available from Bernell Corp.

Fixed-site eccentric fixation is the most difficult type to treat successfully, particularly if point "e" is *always* at a fixed, non-variable site. However, patients under six years of age may respond well to therapy recommended for the central fixator or the variable eccentric fixator. But the prognosis is not as good if these means are used in the treatment of patients over the age of six who have this condition.

Although most of the cases with large angles of eccentric fixation have variable sites with unsteady fixation, there are some large angles in which the fixation is relatively steady with the same fixation site always used. "Large" refers to paramacular eccentric fixation with angle E greater than 3 degrees, or peripheral eccentric fixation with angle E greater than 5 degrees. These cases of steady eccentric fixation with fixed sites require special pleoptic therapy for amblyopia to be either cured or almost cured. Attainment of vision better than 20/30 is considered a cure. Even when all forms of pleoptics are used, the prognosis for a cure is poor-to-fair.

In some circumstances, it is not feasible for patients to undergo an extensive pleoptic program that is required for functional results. This could be because of lack of time, funds, interest, or concern on the part of the patient. The doctor may have to choose a simplified therapy program with the hope of attaining some results but not a cure. In these instances, the patient with a large angle of unsteady eccentric fixation with a variable fixation site (not as embedded as one with a fixed site) may be put into a program similar to the one used for normal fixation or unsteady central fixation. In most cases, angle E is reduced somewhat, and there is a corresponding improvement in visual acuity. The progress levels off after a few weeks, and further improvement is virtually impossible if these therapeutic means are continued. This limited improvement may be all the patient wanted; e.g., to pass the visual requirements for a particular occupational requirement. It should be kept in mind, however, that with this approach, the eccentric fixation may become more deeply embedded than before. Further treatment could be adversely affected in such cases.

Cases with angle E of 3 degrees or less usually constitute the most embedded of all types of eccentric fixation. In general, the site of fixation does not vary (i.e., fixed-site) as in many cases with large angle E; and direct occlusion may not reduce the magnitude of angle E. For much hope of cure or almost-cure of amblyopia in those patients over the age of six, special therapy for eccentric fixation involving procedures similar to those of Bangerter and Cüppers must be used.

If the amblyopia is deep, and if the doctor is aiming for only limited results, training appropriate to cases having normal or unsteady central fixation may be tried. The rationale here is that some of the reduced vision is probably due to effects of suppression, and not all of the poor visual acuity can be attributable to eccentric fixation. Refer to Table 2J (Chapter Two) for the relationship between visual acuity and magnitude of eccentric fixation. For example, a case of amblyopia of 20/200 with an angle E of only 2 degrees must have another factor contributing to the poor vision other than the eccentric fixation alone. In a case like this, visual acuity might be improved to some extent by the less elaborate forms of pleoptics, but the likelihood of attaining acuity better than 20/30 is very remote unless special pleoptic procedures are used. The prognosis is generally fair in these cases, provided all methods of therapy can be used.

Special Therapy for Eccentric Fixation

Cases of eccentric fixation often require pleoptics similar to those of Bangerter and Cüppers. These are the embedded cases of eccentric fixation characterized by steady eccentric fixation with a fixed site. Treatment may involve a host of different procedures such as inverse occlusion, euthyoscopy, fixations, entoptic phenomena, photic stimulation, and special filters.

METHOD OF BANGERTER

Therapy advocated by Bangerter[8],[9] is based on his belief that the eccentric fixator uses an extrafoveal point because of a lowered acuity at the fovea in relation to extrafoveal areas. Consequently, the emphasis and theme throughout his approach to treatment is to improve the sensitivity of the fovea. He feels this is accomplished by effective foveal stimulation.

Bangerter thought that specific instrumentation was needed so that foveal stimulation could be brought about. In the late 1940's, he developed the Pleoptophor[j] for this purpose. This instrument enables the doctor to project an opaque spot onto the patient's fovea to shadow it, while at the same time, the perifoveal portion of the retina is dazzled by a bright light. The use of the Pleoptophor normally requires the pupil to be dilated by means of a mydriatic prior to treatment. Correct positioning of the projected spot on the fovea of the amblyopic eye is facilitated by the binocular arrangement of the instrument. The patient's fixating eye views a guiding target which can be moved about so the spot can be placed on the center of the fovea.

The extrafoveal portion of the retina is dazzled to include point "e" within the bleached portion of the retina. Bleaching is done by a strobe that is activated for about one minute. Following this, a stimulatory phase is started. This is achieved by projecting 50 to 100 brief flashes of a very small spot of light onto the fovea. Since the fovea has been protected during the dazzling phase, the patient should be able to see the light impulses with the fovea. He is instructed to see the light and look directly at it. The dazzling and stimulation phases may have to be repeated once or twice before the patient is fully aware of the flashing spot of light. Once this is done, he should then be able to perceive this, as the illumination of the stimulating light spot is reduced.

---

[j]Mfg. in Switzerland and available through Alfred Poll, Inc.

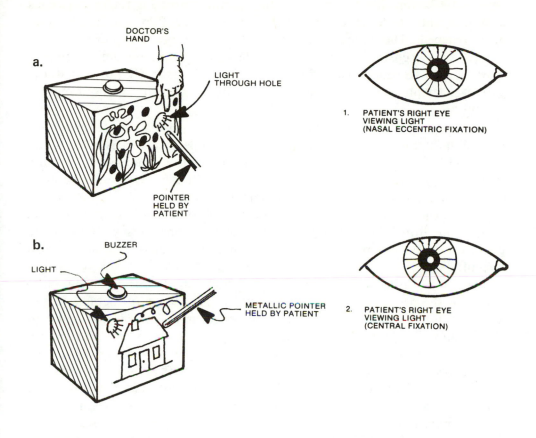

a.

DOCTOR'S
HAND

LIGHT
THROUGH HOLE

POINTER
HELD BY
PATIENT

1. PATIENT'S RIGHT EYE
    VIEWING LIGHT
    (NASAL ECCENTRIC FIXATION)

b.

BUZZER

LIGHT

METALLIC POINTER
HELD BY PATIENT

2. PATIENT'S RIGHT EYE
    VIEWING LIGHT
    (CENTRAL FIXATION)

FIGURE 7-6 — Fixation exercises recommended by Bangerter. (a) Schematic illustration showing principle of the Localizer; (b) Schematic illustration showing principle of the Corrector.

After effective dazzling and stimulation, the nonamblyopic eye is occluded and fixation exercises are performed. Bangerter developed many instruments for this purpose, and some of them include sounding devices for the purpose of developing visual-auditory coordination. The most popular instrument for fixation training is the Localizer-Corrector.[k] See Figure 7-6 showing its use as either a Localizer or a Corrector. This is a box containing electric circuitry. To use it as a Localizer, a perforated board is mounted on the front surface of the instrument. Points of light can be shown randomly through the holes in the board. As each light is seen by the patient's amblyopic eye, the patient attempts to fixate the light. Since the patient may fixate eccentrically, eye-hand coordination training is introduced in the hope of encouraging foveal fixation. The doctor places his finger on the light

[k]Available from Alfred Poll, Inc.

while the patient is told to fixate the doctor's finger tip. The patient continues fixating the finger tip as the doctor moves his finger in various positions until angle kappa (referred to in Chapter Two) appears to have been reached. The corneal reflection should be properly positioned in repsect to the position representing angle kappa in the nonamblyopic eye (with central fixation). When the amblyopic eye is properly positioned, the patient attempts to touch the light source with his finger tip without moving the eye.

As progress is made, the patient uses a pointer instead of his finger (less tactile clues), and the procedure is repeated until performance is consistently good. This is usually done in dim room illumination, supposedly because fixation may be better in low illumination than in high. Also, angle kappa is easier to determine when the room illumination is low.

The major drawback of this procedure is the lack of sensitivity in monitoring foveal fixation by means of angle kappa testing. It lacks the precision normally required when dealing with angles of such small magnitudes.

The same instrument is simply converted into a Corrector by interchanging the perforated board with any one of a series of metallic plates. Some of the plates have pictures, while others have line mazes similar to Groffman's Visual Tracing. The patient is instructed to follow the engraved lines on the plate with a metallic pointer. If the pointer strays off the line, the electric circuitry causes an alarm buzzer to go off and/or a red light to turn on. This provides instant feedback to the patient, and is excellent for eye-hand coordination training. Metallic plates with finer lines are introduced commensurate with the patient's progress.

Besides eye-hand coordination exercises, Bangerter recognizes the need to take into account the crowding phenomenon, visual memory, and the effects of strabismus on amblyopia.

He devised an instrument known as the Separation Trainer which contains 64 E's oriented in different directions. The patient looks at one E from a distance at which it can just be seen. This single letter is brightly illuminated; the other E's are in a dark background. The surrounding E's are gradually made brighter as the patient tries to keep seeing the original one. This type of training helps in reducing the effect of the crowding phenomenon (i.e., contour interaction).

Visual memory is used in the attempt to make very small targets recognizable. Large designs are introduced to the patient for him to copy. They are later presented in smaller sizes for the patient to identify. Any of a number of instruments may be used for visual memory training; for instance, tachistoscopic exercises.

Although Bangerter concentrated on elimination of eccentric fixation and designed many instruments for this purpose, he recognized that the ultimate goal in treatment is attainment of good binocular vision. Otherwise, successfully eliminating amblyopia by means of pleoptics may be of little or no avail if a coexisting strabismus is left untreated, or if care is not taken for a condition of anisometropia.

The Cüppers treatment is based on the theory that eccentric fixation is due to an abnormal shift of the principal visual direction from the foveal to the eccentric fixation point. The emphasis of training is on shifting the directional value from point "e" to the fovea. This form of pleoptics is a re-educating process whereby the patient is taught straight-ahead localization for the fovea. To accomplish this, Cüppers relies on two basic procedures: the use of afterimages and entoptic phenomena. Like Bangerter, Cüppers recommends inverse occlusion.

In order to simplify Bangerter's method of treatment, Cüppers introduced the Euthyscop[l] and the Coordinator[m]. Diagnosis of eccentric fixation is made by means of visuoscopy (see Chapter Two) and treatment is begun with euthyoscopic treatment.

The Euthyscop by Cüppers is similar to the Oculus Visuscope, except that black spots are in the graticules, rather than the star and concentric circles as in the Visuscope. There are two spots of different size, one subtending an angle of three degrees, and the other of five. A green filter is used first for locating the fovea, then a spot is inserted into the middle of the light field to protect the fovea. A transformer is used to set off a strobe flash to dazzle the extrafoveal retina.

The Coordinator by Cüppers uses the phenomenon of Haidinger's brushes and is a small circular device in which a small window shows the view of an airplane. The patient is instructed that the brushes resemble a rotating propeller. Central fixation is indicated when the "propeller" is centered on the nose of the airplane.

Euthyoscopy is done to produce a perifoveal afterimage, and to protect the fovea. The doctor's first step is to locate the fovea. The red-free (green) filter is used to illuminate the fundus. Once the fovea is located, the graticule containing a black spot is introduced and the protective shadow is centered on the fovea. It is helpful to have the patient under binocular conditions during this part of euthyoscopy. This can be done by angling a mirror in front of the nonamblyopic eye so that the eye can fixate a small target, ideally, a small red light. It may be important to have the patient under binocular conditions in cases of latent nystagmus in which the eye movement is often exaggerated when one eye is occluded. Many patients with nystagmus find it difficult to maintain the steadiness required for this

---

[l]Euthyscop by Cüppers (trade name, Euthyscop), mfg. by Oculus Products, Dutenhofen, Kr. Wetzlar, West Germany, and available through various ophthalmic suppliers.

[m]The Coordinator by Cüppers (trade name, Koordinator), mfg. by Oculus and availability same as in footnote l.

procedure when the doctor's head blocks the view of the nonamblyopic fixating eye. A base-out prism may be used instead of the mirror, used in the same way as the bifoveal test of Cüppers for A R C (see Chapter Two).

Once the shadow is centered on the fovea, it is left in the exact location, usually for about one-half minute (assuming a strobe flash is not employed).

The three-degree spot should be used when angle E is small, otherwise point "e" will be shadowed and protected along with the fovea. The five degree spot is used for paramacular and peripheral eccentric fixation (angle E greater than three degrees).

While shadowing the fovea, the illumination of the instrument should be just high enough to clearly see the fundus details, since a slight unsteadiness, either on the part of the doctor in holding the instrument, or by the patient's eye movements, may result in the light hitting the fovea. This should be avoided, because the purpose of this procedure is to protect the fovea and inhibit the retina in which point "e" is located.

It may be helpful, as well as expedient, to use a flash attachment for this procedure. Raising the illumination of the Euthyscop by several volts and momentarily (e.g., one second) flashing the retina protects the fovea while the remaining portion of the retina is dazzled.

The room illumination should be low when attempting to create an afterimage by euthyoscopy. This is the rule except in certain cases when fixation is better in higher illuminations, e.g., in some cases of nystagmus. Unfortunately, it is hard to produce a strong afterimage when the room illumination is high.

The dazzling phase is similar to that advocated by Bangerter with the Pleoptophor, but the stimulation phase is by-passed by Cüppers. Instead, the patient is told to become aware of the euthyoscopic afterimage. Bangerter ignores the part of therapy utilizing afterimages. This is the basic difference between the methods of treatment of these two authorities.

The next step in the method of Cüppers is for the patient to have direct occlusion while he views an illuminated distant white or light neutral grey screen. The amblyopic patient can usually see a positive afterimage at this stage, but may be unable to appreciate a negative afterimage. It may be difficult for the patient to appreciate either afterimage without the aid of intermittent flashing lights in the room. Rapidly blinking his eyelids also helps. Afterimages may be enhanced and prolonged by means of a Light Interval Regulator.[n] This is a transformer with a timing device for controlling the on-and-off periods of an ordinary lamp.

A positive afterimage is perceived when the room is darkened and is seen more readily than the negative afterimage. Consequently, training should begin by having the patient become aware of the positive afterimage. The patient should perceive a "white doughnut" with a dark center. This is noticed when the room light is low or when the eyes are closed. For this to

---

[n]Available through various optical suppliers, but similar devices may be custom made.

become apparent to the patient with very deep amblyopia, the dark phase of room illumination may be required to be much longer than the light phase. A ratio of six seconds of dark phase to one second of light may be necessary for the patient to become aware of the positive afterimage.

a.

b.

c.

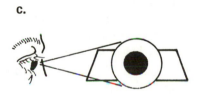

d.

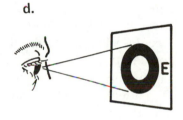

e.

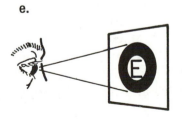

f.

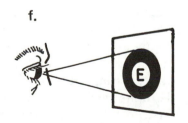

FIGURE 7-7 — Euthyscopic afterimage advocated by Cüppers for eccentric fixation therapy. (a) Negative afterimage (black doughnut); (b) Afterimage with psychological characteristics of a real object; (c) Positive afterimage (white doughnut) which violates the psychological characteristics of a real object; (d) Nasal eccentric fixation of the right eye; (e) Central fixation; (f) Central fixation using small letter as fixation target.

With the room illumination high, the light phase should elicit a negative afterimage, and the patient should become aware of a "dark doughnut" with a light center. This is the important afterimage with which to work in pleoptics. Some patients can see only the positive afterimage, and the prognosis for significant improvement of the amblyopia is poor in such cases.

The doctor hopes the patient can learn to see the black doughnut. Once this is easily seen, the light phase is made much longer, e.g., six seconds of light to every second of darkness.

Priestley et al.[10] discuss the importance of the negative afterimage of pleoptics, saying that it has the visual characteristics of a real object in free space. They feel that the perception of a negative afterimage is associated with functions of the highest cortical centers. Therefore, when the patient learns to control the placement of the negative afterimage around a real target (e.g., a Snellen letter), a shift in the principal visual direction may be made from point "e" to the fovea. Figure 7-7a illustrates the patient's perception of a negative afterimage. Figure 7-7b shows how the negative A.I. appears on a tilted surface. Figure 7-7c shows how the positive A.I. violates the psychological characteristics of a real object seen in free space. Figure 7-7d shows how a patient fixating with the right eye with nasal eccentric fixation would see the negative A.I. in relation to a letter E on a screen. Figure 7-7e is the way the patient sees the E surrounded by the negative afterimage when the fovea is fixating the Snellen letter. This is what the eccentric fixator should attempt to do. He is instructed to make every effort possible to put the doughnut around the letter he wants to see. The patient will usually notice the letter clearly when this is done. Smaller letters within the patient's capability are gradually presented (as in Figure 7-7f). It is vital that the letter remain centered in the negative A.I. This is done until the smallest visible letter is held inside the doughnut. The patient is encouraged to walk nearer to see it more easily, and is then instructed to walk away slowly until the letter cannot be recognized. Walking rail activity can later be incorporated into this procedure as progress is made.

ENTOPTIC PHENOMENA   The next step in the method of Cüppers is working with Haidinger's brushes. Maxwell's spot may be used in a similar manner, but most patients do better with H.B. This is probably because the H.B. can be seen more easily, and there are more variations in treatment than with Maxwell's spot. For instance, the doughnut afterimage and the H.B. make a better combination for superimposition than the Maxwell's spot and the doughnut. However, the H.B. are preferred over Maxwell's spot because of the availability of pleoptic instrumentation in this regard.

Since this phenomenon of H.B. is due to the polarization of light by Henle's fiber layer, the foveal area is assumed to be tagged. If the Coordinator is used, the patient is instructed to put the propeller on the airplane's nose. Central fixation is indicated when this is accomplished.

The patient is then instructed to keep the propeller on the nose of the airplane while placing the tip of a pointer on the propeller. Because of faulty retinomotor values in most cases of eccentric fixation, the patient may past point at first and miss the propeller with the tip of the pointer. With practice, this error in spatial localization is soon overcome, and the patient learns to place the pointer on the H.B. (propeller) while maintaining the propeller on the object of regard (the nose of the airplane). This accomplishment indicates that the fovea has attained the principal visual direction and a normal (zero) retinomotor value.

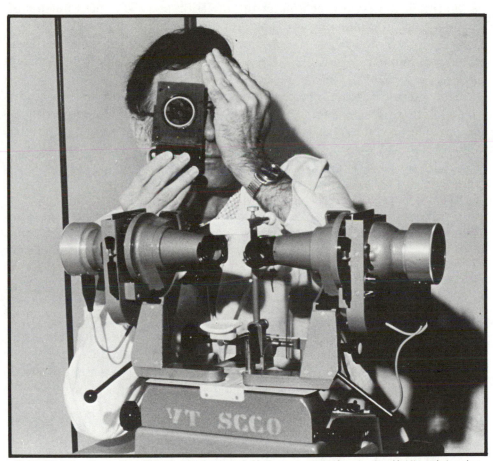

FIGURE 7-8 — Space Coordinator attachment of the Synoptophore for viewing Haidinger's brushes

If there is trouble keeping the brushes centered on the real object, the patient may require dazzling of the eccentric point with the Euthyscop. In this case, the fovea is protected and the patient should be able to see the black doughnut afterimage surrounding the propeller on the nose of the airplane. The pointer should be accurately placed in the center of all of these. Pointing should be quick so that spatial localization errors are not compensated for by the intellectual judgments, but rather by the fact that localization is accurate. When the patient is able to accurately place the H.B. on a real fixation target, such as a Snellen letter, Cüppers recommends using a pointer to trace line drawings of letters, mazes, pictures, etc. The drawings are put on a clear plate of glass or plastic and used as an overlay on the surface of the H.B. generating device, e.g., Coordinator by Cüppers, or the Bernell Macular Integrity Tester-Trainer (MITT). The MITT was discussed in Chapter Two. I prefer this instrument over the Coordinator because of the larger surface area on which the patient can trace while viewing the H.B.

Tracing is done with the pointer tip, the H.B., and the fixated portion of the target, all in conjunction. If they are not lined up, easier demands will have to be presented before proceeding further. The demand may be made easier in a number of different ways, e.g., bolder lines to be traced, or by allowing the patient to trace more slowly.

After pursuit training is perfected, the patient should proceed to saccadic training. He performs these tasks by looking from one discrete target to another while keeping the H.B. centered on each fixated target. A pointer should be placed directly on the H.B. and the fixated target. The overlay slide with dots (see Figure 2-31) is good for this purpose. Another good exercise in this regard is the tic-tac-toe game.

After good spatial localization (without past pointing) is achieved, the use of the pointer may be discontinued. The patient is then instructed to make rapid saccadic eye movements from one dot to another, always keeping the H.B. on each fixated dot. A metronome is recommended so that speed as well as accuracy of fixation can be improved.

Perception of H.B. in space is more difficult than when viewing the entoptic phenomenon on an instrument's surface, such as on the Coordinator or the MITT. The patient is normally not ready for projecting the H.B. into the distance until he can perform well on directly viewed instruments at near. When this is learned, training is done with the Space Coordinator.[o] This is a small table-mounted apparatus through which the patient can look with one eye and view an illuminated screen at the end of the room.

The Space Coordinator can be purchased as a separate unit, or the doctor can use the accessory rotating Polaroid filter attachment of the Synoptophore (refer to the photograph and the key for Figure 1-22). A picture of this attachment being held before the amblyopic eye is shown in Figure 7-8. The purpose is for the patient to be aware of the H.B. on the distant screen, and to see it move with each eye movement. The patient practices putting the H.B. on a Snellen letter that is projected onto a distant screen. It is important for the screen to be highly illuminated so that perception of the H.B. is possible.

In cases where angle E is large, a small field-restricting diaphragm may be

---

[o]Mfg. by Clement Clarke, Ltd., Instrument Division.

placed in front of the sighting hole of the Space Coordinator in an attempt to reduce the magnitude of Angle E. This may happen because the H.B. will not be seen if the patient's visual field is severely contracted by the effect of the diaphragm. In order to see the Snellen letter simultaneously with the H.B., angle E will necessarily have to be small enough to be within the angular subtense of the angle limiting the area of the visual field.

Another helpful procedure is to dazzle the retina by means of euthyoscopy to produce a perifoveal negative afterimage. The patient is told to put the brushes inside the doughnut and center the combination of the brushes and doughnut on a Snellen letter. This is not too difficult with practice, because the fovea has been protected by the preceding euthyoscopic procedure. The eccentric fixation point is "blinded" by its having been dazzled; therefore, if the patient can see the letter, it ought to be seen by the fovea. This can be verified by the use of foveal tags, i.e., the H.B. and the A.I.

A device that may help promote central fixation while using the Space Coordinator is the Plateau spiral[p] (shown in Figure 7-9). The spiral is rotated at such speeds so that the circles appear to be decreasing in size. According to Bangerter, this helps the patient concentrate on the center of the spiral, and thus, promote foveal fixation. The patient looks through the Space Coordinator, and projects H.B. toward the center of the spiral. The rotating effect of the spiral helps the patient hold the H.B. in the center of the spiral target.

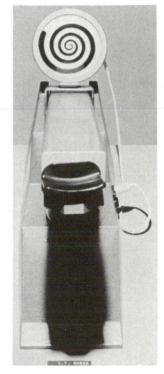

FIGURE 7-9 — Plateau spiral to promote central fixation. Clockwise rotation causes circles to appear to decrease in size.

The Plateau spiral also produces the afterimage effect of objects appearing to increase in size after watching the diminishing circles of the rotating spiral. This is similar to the well-known waterfall afterimage illusion. Patients feel that Snellen letters are "larger" and frequently report better acuity for a short time afterwards.

After the patient can centrally fixate a static target, when looking through the Space Coordinator, visual tracing is begun. Illuminated line drawings on the wall are used for visual tracing while the H.B. is kept on the line at all times during the "pursuits" (actually voluntary saccades).

When tracing is adequate, the patient practices saccadic eye movements by looking from one target to another while keeping the H.B. centered during each fixation. A projected Snellen chart is good for this purpose. The patient should make every attempt to see smaller letters while maintaining the H.B. on each fixated letter.

FORM RECOGNITION

Cüppers emphasized the importance of training the perception of form recognition as part of the treatment of amblyopia. Once central fixation is achieved, any number of form recognition exercises can be carried out as out-of-office training procedures. Direct occlusion is recommended during

[p]The Plateau spiral instrument may be custom-made or purchased as a complete motorized unit, available from Alfred Poll, Inc. This is referred to as the Centrophore.

these exercises. The procedures listed in Table 7B serve as examples used for this purpose.

Cüppers and Bangerter agree that once amblyopia is cured, good binocularity is important if the gains made in the treatment of amblyopia are to be of lasting value. Some form of orthoptic training is necessary in practically all cases of amblyopia.

STANDARD PLEOPTIC PROCEDURES

Standard methods for treating amblyopia have evolved from Bangerter and Cüppers. Contributions by many authorities have helped in forming a logical rationale for therapy. In planning any specific therapy program, the doctor should consider the following: preparing the patient for pleoptics, inverse prism therapy, euthyoscopy, afterimages, Haidinger's brushes, fixation training using combinations of procedures, monocular training activities with direct occlusion, and binocular considerations. Table 7E lists these standard procedures in greater detail.

SEQUENCE OF TREATMENT

A good diagnosis is the most important aspect of any pleoptic program. The prognosis can be determined, and the treatment plan can then be presented to the patient.

PREPARATION OF THE PATIENT FOR PLEOPTICS

Pleoptic therapy may involve tremendous time and effort on the part of both the doctor and the patient. Therefore, a complete consultation is vitally important so that the patient can be admonished. If there is deeply embedded steady eccentric fixation, many months of intensive therapy will probably be required. The patient should clearly understand this before any decision is made. If anything less than enthusiasm is shown, an extensive program of pleoptics should probably not be started. The requirement for enthusiasm also extends to the parents if the patient is a child.

Therapeutic decisions of such a hard-line nature are not quite as necessary in cases of central fixation and other conditions in which most of the training can be done at home. Relatively little expenditure of the doctor's time is necessary in these instances.

It is important for the patient to wear the best possible correcting lenses for any existing ametropia. However, some authorities take issue with this rule and advise prescribing less than full plus correction in cases of hyperopia. It is thought that the refractive error is not validly measured in cases of eccentric fixation. This is possibly because off-axis measurements are made and refractive status may vary with the magnitude of eccentric fixation. Accommodative responses are also thought to be stimulated to a greater extent, and full plus inhibits accommodative responses.

I tend to abide by the rule of prescribing full plus, unless the refraction is suspected of being significantly influenced by eccentric fixation. Furthermore, I believe it is better to improve accommodation facility by means other than the reduction of power of the correcting lens, e.g., accommodative rock exercises.

TABLE 7E. Sequence of Standard Pleoptic Procedures

A.   Preparation of patient for pleoptics
    1. Diagnosis of amblyopia and abnormal fixation (history, visual acuity testing, and visuoscopy)
    2. Consultation
    3. Occlusion considerations
       a. direct (if central fixation, possibly if unsteady eccentric)
       b. red filter (worn over amblyopic eye if eccentric fixation with total occlusion of non-amblyopic eye)
       c. inverse (for eccentric fixation, particularly if steady eccentric)
B.   Inverse prism therapy
       a. Cüppers
       b. Pigassou
C.   Euthyoscopy to protect the fovea and dazzle eccentric fixation point
D.   Intermittent photic stimulation of fovea
       a. Bangerter
       b. Allen
E.   Afterimages
    1. Euthyoscopic afterimage
       a. perception of positive afterimage
       b. perception of negative afterimage
    2. Transferred afterimage (vertical line transferred from fovea of nonamblyopic eye)
    3. Direct afterimage for home training (e.g., Inouye's disc)
F.   Haidinger's brushes
    1. Perception on surface of instrument (e.g., MITT)
    2. Perception in space (e.g., Space Coordinator)
G.   Fixation training using combinations of procedures
    1. Afterimage on real object
       a. doughnut on Snellen letter
       b. transferred vertical line on Snellen letter
    2. Afterimage and letter with pointing
    3. Combination of afterimage and Haidinger's brushes
       a. without pointing
       b. with accurate pointing to letter (overlay on MITT)
       c. quick pointing exercises with letter
       d. pointer with A.I. and H.B. on picture for pursuit tracing
       e. saccadic movements with A.I. and H.B. with Snellen chart
    4. Quick pointing with H.B. and letter
    5. Pointer with H.B. on picture for pursuit tracing
    6. H.B. on picture for eye movements without pointer
    7. Saccadic eye movements with H.B. and Snellen chart
    8. H.B. and Snellen letter in space
    9. H.B. on picture for visual tracing in space
    10. H.B. on Snellen chart for saccades in space
    11. Transferred A.I. in space
    12. Steady fixation, pursuits, and saccades without A.I. or H.B., but occasional monitoring (to ensure central fixation)
H.   Monocular training activities with direct occlusion (refer to Tables 7B, 7C and 7D)
I.   Binocular considerations
       a. Begin binocular training when visual acuity is 20/40.
       b. Continue amblyopia therapy with binocular training and use binocular methods to improve amblyopia.

The type of occlusion to be used should be discussed with the patient, and patching started as soon as possible after the consultation. Direct occlusion should be tried initially in all cases of amblyopia except possibly non-variable, steady eccentric fixation. Red filter occlusion could be considered in cases of variable eccentric fixation, since this can be part of the home training routine. The patient over the age of six who has embedded eccentric fixation should have inverse occlusion for at least one month prior to active training, with occlusion being total during all waking hours.

PRISM THERAPY

Prism therapy should be tried if angle E is reduced in certain postiions of gaze. The most obvious approach to follow is that of Cüppers; but even if there is no noticeable reduction of angle E on certain gazes, the Pigassou method should be tried for a few weeks to determine if fixation can be improved by the use of inverse prisms. The prism is worn at home, and office visits are necessary only to check the progress and to make sure the patient is properly carrying out the prescribed occlusion instructions. If the patient removes the prism, inverse occlusion must be reinstituted immediately.

EUTHYOSCOPY

This was originally done with the Pleoptophore. Euthyoscopy may also be done with the Oculus Euthyscop, the Neitz Euthyscope, or the Keeler Projectoscope. The initial purpose is to protect the fovea and dazzle the eccentric fixation point. Intermittent photic stimulation of the fovea is given after the dazzling procedure.

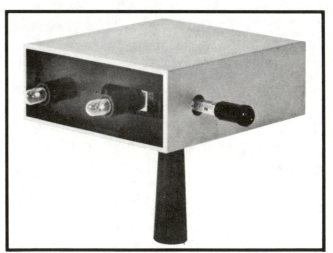

FIGURE 7-10 — Translid Binocular Interaction Trainer. (Courtesy of Keystone View, Division of Mast/Keystone)

INTERMITTENT PHOTIC STIMULATION OF THE FOVEA

The Pleoptophor was specifically designed for stimulation of the fovea with a flashing light. Since this is relatively expensive and is found in few offices, less complex instruments have been designed for this purpose. The Keeler Projectoscope works well in this regard.

A Nutt Auto-Disc is placed on the graticule holder of the Projectoscope (see Figure 2-30). This attachment has three graticules; one has a green filter with a central, lighter green hole for centering the fovea, the second has a three degree black spot for euthyoscopy, and the third graticule has a very dark green filter with a 1.5 degree clear hole. The third graticule is used in the stimulatory phase. A transformer is pre-set as to light intensity, and timing for on-and-off flashes. The first graticule is used to find the fovea; then a trigger control is pushed to change to the second graticule with the three-degree black spot. A flash of bright light is activated for the desired time, usually about one or two seconds, by a pre-set transformer that comes with the Projectoscope. The control trigger is released and the graticule with the 1.5 degree clear hole moves into place. This automatically activates rapid flashing of light. The doctor maintains the small spot of flashing light on the fovea for one or two minutes. As with the Pleoptophor, this procedure is repeated several times before going on to fixation exercises in free space.

The use of intermittent photic stimulation is advocated by Allen[11] who introduced the Translid Binocular Interaction Trainer (T.B.I)[q], shown in Figure 7-10. The instrument holds a pair of small light bulbs that are flashed on and off by a free-running multivibrator at a rate of approximately 7 to 10 cycles per second (approximating the alpha rhythm) for one eye at a time. The bulbs are separated by a distance equal to the patient's I.P.D. and gently placed on the upper eyelids so they barely touch. The room illumination should be low for most effective results. The recommended time of stimulation with the T.B.I. is about two minutes at a time with 15-minute breaks. It should be used about 15 times a day for best results.

A precaution to watch for is any sign of photoconvulsive behavior during or after the periods of flashing. This reaction may occur in a small portion of the population when a strong flashing light source is viewed directly. These individuals may go into a petite or grand mal epileptic seizure. Closing the eyes and having the light go through the lids reduces the likelihood of this type of reaction. Because of this possibility, treatment time should always be short, and made even shorter or discontinued if there is any resultant sign of discomfort or subjective complaints. The doctor should never dispense this form of therapy for home use until there is certainty as to the patient's reactions and complete understanding of the proper use of the T.B.I.

It is unclear why this procedure is effective in cases of amblyopia with eccentric fixation. Unlike Bangerter's method of photic stimulation, there is no selectivity as to which part of the retina is stimulated. The T.B.I. stimulates the entire retina; whereas in Bangerter's method, only the fovea is flashed. Nevertheless, cases of amblyopia may respond favorably to this

---

[q]Available through Keystone/Mast. Further directions on the use of the T.B.I. can be obtained from Dr. Merrill J. Allen, Indiana University, Division of Optometry, 800 East Atwater, Bloomington, Indiana 47401. Another model of the T.B.I. is available from Manico, P.O. Box 395, Clute, Texas 77531.

method of treatment, and it may be tried in the absence of the more elaborate instrumentation recommended by Bangerter.

A variation of the T.B.I. is the Alpha Brightness Enhancement instrument of Dr. Ariyasu[r] which may incorporate colored lights and a rheostat to control light intensities as desired.

Other uses of alpha rhythm light flashes will be presented with the discussions on anomalous correspondence and suppression.

Another type of flashing device used to stimulate the central retinal receptors is the Electronic Orthoptor by Otwell.[s] This instrument has a sodium amber light that is flashed into the amblyopic eye in cycles of 4 seconds on and 1.5 seconds off. Otwell[12] claimed the sodium light is very effective in treating amblyopia. Unlike the T.B.I., the flashes are not at the alpha rhythm to cause brightness enhancement (Bartley phenomenon) that is supposedly effective in the treatment of amblyopia. Also, foveal fixation is not monitored by the Electronic Orthoptor, so it is unclear why this method is reportedly effective.

Foveal monitoring could be done by performing euthyoscopy prior to flashing with the Electronic Orthoptor. Although exact foveal monitoring is not being done according to the method of Bangerter when using either the Pleoptophor or the Nutt Auto-Disc of the Projectoscope, the fact that the fovea has been protected may be encouragement enough for stimulation of the fovea to occur with the flashing amber light.

AFTERIMAGES   The method of Cüppers is followed in the attempt to teach the patient the appreciation of a negative afterimage. Following euthyoscopy, the patient should be able to see a white doughnut when the room is dark and a black doughnut when the room has normal illumination.

Transferred afterimage techniques are occasionally employed. A vertical line is transferred from the nonamblyopic to the amblyopic eye (Brock-Givner afterimage transfer test, discussed in Chapter Two). This may be good for home training, if there is no anomalous correspondence. The primary purpose of the afterimage transfer in amblyopia therapy is to tag the fovea of the amblyopic eye. If A R C is present, the transferred vertical line goes to point "a" rather than to the fovea of the amblyopic eye. Therefore, the presence of A R C defeats the purpose of this procedure. Another objection to the transferred A.I. is that it is weak compared to a direct afterimage. For this reason alone, I prefer to use direct afterimages whenever possible. This is because most young amblyopes are not attentive to a faint ocular image. They are more likely to participate in therapy if the image is intense.

There are many ways to create a direct afterimage. The use of Inouye's disc is one such way. This was described by Priestley et al.[13], and is a four

---

[r]Available from Dr. George Ariyasu, 8783 Parthenia Place, Sepulveda, CA 91343.

[s]Designed by Dr. Harry Otwell, Fayetteville, Arkansas.

cm black disc with a 3 mm red fixation target. It may be constructed by applying black electrical or Mystic Tape to a frosted flood lamp. The patient views it from a distance of approximately 50 cms. It creates an afterimage on the amblyopic eye and the patient is instructed to look about the room at various objects while keeping the afterimage centered around each item fixated. The patient can look into the MITT and center the afterimage around the H.B.

It is advisable to follow through with intermittent photic stimulation. Backman[14] suggests using a home light regulator made from a Christmas tree flasher and a 60 watt bulb that is connected in circuit to an ordinary bulb socket. A pinhole can be punched in a metal sheet that is held close to a bright flashing light. This serves as a home training device for the stimulatory phase of pleoptics.

This type of afterimage training is good, if there is central fixation where the intent of therapy is merely to stimulate the fovea. However, it is not suitable in cases of eccentric fixation, unless certain procedural modifications are made. The best way to go about this is first, to measure angle E on the MITT. Suppose the patient has five degrees of nasal eccentric fixation of the right eye and is fixating the MITT from a distance of 50 cms. The patient would report seeing the H.B. to the left of the fixation dot by five degrees. This is 8.75 p.d. represented by a distance of 4.4 cms from the H.B. to the dot. In order to protect the fovea, the patient would necessarily have to fixate a prescribed amount to the right of the black disc. If the fixation distance to the lamp is also 50 cms, the patient would have to look to the right of the center of the black disc 4.4 cms in order for the center of the black disc to fall on the fovea (see Figure 7-11).

The red fixation dot is therefore moved from the center of the large black disc to an eccentric point on the light bulb. The placement of the red fixation dot is equal in magnitude to angle E found by H.B., but the direction of the dot is 180 degrees away from the location of the H.B. With a minimal amount of calculation of angles, this can be an effective home training procedure to protect the fovea, dazzle the extra-foveal area, and follow up with foveal stimulation by means of a flashing pinpoint light source as discussed previously. Treatment according to Cüppers can be carried out at home, since a black doughnut (negative A.I.) is produced.

The important thing to remember is that this treatment is of no use, and may actually hinder therapy, unless the center of the fovea is protected. In the past, too many practitioners did not take proper precautions to insure that the euthyoscopic shadow is on the fovea of the amblyopic eye.

When eye movements are well controlled while being monitored by the afterimage, pointers are used to establish good spatial localization and to strengthen the central fixation ability that has just been achieved. Real objects, such as children's toys, are used initially. The patient then advances to less tangible targets such as projected letters or symbols.

Further monitoring of foveal fixation is done by using the combination of an afterimage with H.B.

Vodnoy[15] has introduced a novel home training procedure to produce afterimages in the proper position when treating eccentric fixation. The patient's eccentric fixation must first be determined by some means, such as by H.B. When this is done, an afterimage is produced by putting an opaque mask[t] in front of a bright flood lamp (see Figure 7-12). A pair of arcs is cut out of the black mask so that the distance from the center of the arc to the center of the mask is the same as that between point "e" and the fovea. For

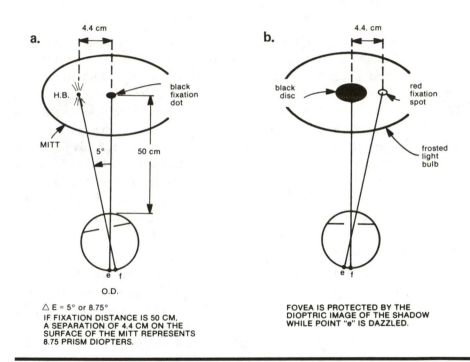

a.

4.4 cm

H.B.

black fixation dot

MITT

5°   50 cm

e f

O.D.

△ E = 5° or 8.75°
IF FIXATION DISTANCE IS 50 CM,
A SEPARATION OF 4.4 CM ON THE
SURFACE OF THE MITT REPRESENTS
8.75 PRISM DIOPTERS.

b.

4.4. cm

black disc

red fixation spot

frosted light bulb

e f

FOVEA IS PROTECTED BY THE
DIOPTRIC IMAGE OF THE SHADOW
WHILE POINT "e" IS DAZZLED.

FIGURE 7-11 — Use of a black disc taped on a frosted flood lamp for home training in cases of eccentric fixation. (a) Angle E is first determined by means of Haidinger's brushes; (b) Disc is used to protect the fovea with extra-foveal area, including point "e" being dazzled. The amblyopic eye must fixate in a direction opposite to the H.B., but by an amount equal to the magnitude of angle E.

example, assume the right eye has nasal eccentric fixation of five degrees. The patient is instructed to look at the illuminated arc to the right side of the black mask. The arc dazzles point "e," and the arc on the left-hand side of the mask dazzles a temporal extra-foveal point an equal distance away from the fovea. This gives the patient the advantage of having a bracket as an afterimage. He will notice two black arcs (negative A.I.) in normal room illumination. The patient is instructed to put these brackets around anything

[t]May be custom made.

a.

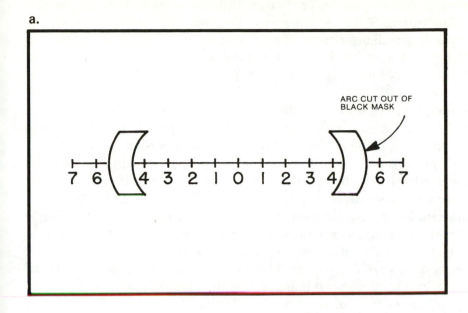

b.

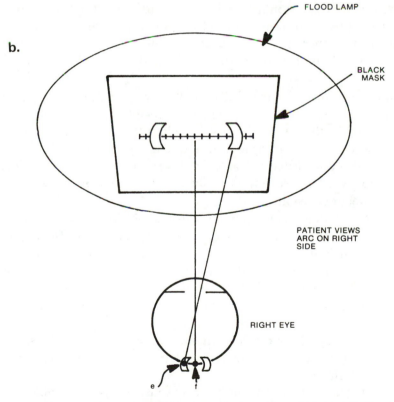

FIGURE 7-12 — Method of Vodnoy for home training in cases of eccentric fixation. (a) The opaque mask held before a flood lamp with arcs cut out for viewing by a right eye with nasal eccentric fixation; (b) Drawing showing the fovea being protected while point "e" is dazzled by the arc on the right side of the mask

he wishes to fixate; e.g., Snellen letter, H.B., Maxwell's spot, or any real object. The patient is then looking with his fovea. Flashing to stimulate the fovea according to Bangerter can then be carried out. The use of this mask is a tremendous aid in controlling the position of fixation for use as an out-of-office procedure.

HAIDINGER'S BRUSHES

This entoptic phenomenon was discussed in Chapter Two for testing, and previously in this chapter for treatment. The important thing to keep in mind is that it may take considerable time for a person to perceive the brushes. This is true for many nonamblyopes and particularly true for the amblyopic patient. Another difficulty may arise if angle E is relatively large and the fixation distance is too great. The H.B. in this instance may be off the entire surface of the instrument and, therefore, cannot be seen. Simple trigonometry is sometimes necessary to make sure the eccentric angle is within the limits of the instrument for a particular fixation distance.

It is best to start the patient with directly viewed brushes. The MITT unit is an excellent home training device for this purpose. Later on in therapy, office training for the perception of the H.B. in space (such as with the Space Coordinator) is recommended. Afterwards, this type of training can be done as an out-of-office procedure. Kavner[16] highly recommends the Rinaldi-Larson Dynascope[u] for this purpose. This instrument is a small battery driven hand-held unit used to produce the H.B.

FIXATION TRAINING USING COMBINATIONS OF PROCEDURES

Fixation training may include the use of real objects, hand-held pointer, direct afterimage, transferred afterimage, and entoptic phenomena, with various combinations that may be useful clinically. Twelve of these combinations are presented as a logical sequence for the treatment of eccentric fixation They are listed in Table 7E. Inverse occlusion is prescribed at all times except when active training is being conducted. At those times there should be direct occlusion.

As soon as the patient can easily perceive a negative afterimage, he should do exercises at home and in the office until he can center the A.I. on a real object. The doughnut A.I. is usually better than the transferred vertical line A.I. because of its greater brightness and its not being invalidated by the presence of anomalous correspondence. This is often the case with the transferred A.I. since A R C is present in many of the cases of eccentric fixation.

The next step is to work on establishing normal retinomotor values. This is best done by having the patient point to a letter while foveal fixation is monitored by an afterimage.

Further monitoring of fixation can be accomplished by the combination of A.I. and H.B. This is done at first without pointing, so that the patient is not distracted and can hold superimposition easily. This indicates that the

[u]Mfg. by Oculus

principal visual direction of the amblyopic eye is at the fovea. This procedure is followed by the patient's slowly pointing to a letter (e.g., using overlay slide on the MITT) that is superimposed with the H.B. and encircled by the A.I. When spatial localization becomes accurate (without past pointing) while, at the same time, fixation is central (as monitored by the H.B. and A.I.), the patient can begin to do a series of quick pointing exercises. These are rapid pointing movements beginning from behind the patient's head to the fixated target. The finger may be used at first because of the advantage of tactile/kinesthetic clues; but later, the patient should be able to do accurate quick pointing with a short thin stick. Overlay slides containing line drawings and dot-to-dot types of targets may be used in the training of pursuits and saccades respectively.

As central fixation becomes more established, there is less dependency on euthyoscopy. The doughnut may not be necessary and the patient can begin doing quick pointing exercises while the H.B. is on the letter. If the patient regresses, it may be necessary to go back to protecting the fovea and producing the doughnut as an aid to maintaining central fixation.

When the patient can hold steady central fixation on a Snellen letter or dot target as monitored by the H.B., a pointer should be used for pursuit tracing exercises. This is followed by visualizing the H.B. on the picture but without the pointer; then, the patient progresses to saccadic movements with the H.B. on a Snellen chart or dot-to-dot targets for saccadic eye movement training.

As the patient's fixational ability improves, he can start working with the H.B. in free space. He can look through the Space Coordinator and fixate a distant Snellen letter. He should advance to visual tracing in space and then to saccadic movements while keeping the H.B. on each fixated object.

At this stage of pleoptics, the patient may use transferred afterimages in space for steady, pursuit, and saccadic training. However, the caveat of the possible presence of anomalous correspondence must be heeded. Anomalous correspondence invalidates this type of procedure for treatment of abnormal fixation. The transferred A.I. is usually in the form of a vertical line, but this may vary according to the doctor's particular choice of instruments. Some use a small cross, marked on a strobe flash unit. This may also be accomplished by masking of a frosted flood lamp to leave the exposed part of the bulb in the form of a plus sign. When the A.I. has been transferred to the amblyopic eye and the nonamblyopic eye is occluded, the patient can use his amblyopic eye to search out objects and place the A.I. on anything or anyone he chooses. This A.I. is facetiously called the "death ray" which apparently delights many young patients, especially when they fixate the doctor, siblings, etc. This ensures foveal fixation, providing there is no A R C.

When foveal tags are no longer necessary to ensure central fixation, the patient can practice pursuit and saccadic movement exercises using real objects in free space; but occasional monitoring is recommended to make sure fixation is central during these exercises.

At this point in the treatment program, the patient should essentially be a central fixator. Occlusion is switched from inverse to direct, and monocular training activities listed in Table 7B are appropriate at this time.

It may be wise to include vertical and oblique reading exercises before too much emphasis is placed on reading horizontal lines of print.

The Plateau spiral may be used for its afterimage enlargement effect as a means to promote good visual acuity.

An additional training procedure that should be incorporated is prism jump exercises. Small prisms are quickly placed before the amblyopic eye with the nonamblyopic eye occluded. The patient is instructed to be aware of a movement of the fixated target as the prism is introduced. The normal eye can perceive prism jumps that are very small; usually one-half prism diopter is easily noticed. Irvine[17] found that the amblyopic eye may require larger amounts of prism before there is perception of a shift in direction of the fixated object. A penlight is a good fixation target for this purpose. Training proceeds by starting with large prism where there is a noticeable jump and going to smaller prisms until the patient can notice jumps equally well with each eye.

BINOCULAR
CONSIDERATIONS

A good starting point for binocular training is when there is attainment of 20/40 vision in the amblyopic eye. In some cases where the vision cannot be improved to this level, binocular training should be started with the realization that perfect bifoveal fusion will not be achieved under this condition. Nevertheless, good peripheral sensory and motor fusion may be developed, and the patient may have fairly good binocularity in many respects.

A convenient test to check for the simultaneous presence of anomalous correspondence and eccentric fixation is the combination of the transferred afterimage with Haidinger's brushes. Assume the patient has esotropia with nasal eccentric fixation of the right eye. (This is illustrated in Figure 7-13). The patient looks at the MITT to perceive the H.B., and the separation between the fixation dot and the H.B. represents angle E. Prior to this, the patient's nonamblyopic left eye has been flashed with a vertical line strobe. The left eye is occluded, and the line is seen by the right eye.

With the patient looking at the MITT through the appropriate blue filter, he can perceive the H.B. as well as the A.I. The distance between the H.B. and the A.I. represents angle A.

If normal correspondence were present, the H.B. and the A.I. would be superimposed. If there were no eccentric fixation, the H.B. and the dot would be superimposed. Likewise, if there were neither A R C nor eccentric fixation, there would be superimposition of the H.B., the dot, and the A.I.

Amblyopic therapy can continue during binocular therapy as long as anomalous correspondence is taken into account (therapy for A R C to be discussed in Chapter Nine). Similarly, suppression will have deleterious effects on gains made in pleoptics, and there must be a reckoning with this

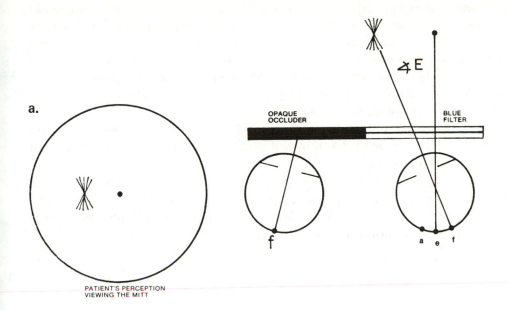

a.

PATIENT'S PERCEPTION
VIEWING THE MITT

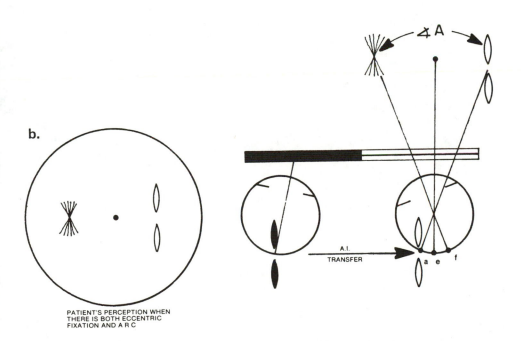

b.

PATIENT'S PERCEPTION WHEN
THERE IS BOTH ECCENTRIC
FIXATION AND A R C

FIGURE 7-13 — Test for simultaneous presence of anomalous correspondence and eccentric fixation. (a) Drawing showing use of Haidinger's brushes to indicate eccentric fixation; (b) Drawing shows how afterimage transfer can be used to indicate anomalous correspondence at the same time that eccentric fixation is also indicated.

problem (therapy for suppression to be discussed in Chapter Ten).

Once the associated anomalous conditions of suppression and anomalous correspondence are eliminated, binocular training is often very effective in eliminating any residual amblyopia. It is important to remember that bifoveal fixation must be achieved in order to prevent the return of amblyopia. In some cases of monofixation strabismus, this possibility will have to be realized in advance since a complete cure is often difficult, and sometimes impossible, to achieve.

Fortunately, there are many cases in which binocular therapy is effective in establishing bifoveal fixation without suppression; and the results of pleoptics can be lasting.

Although treatment may take many months and sometimes one year or longer, many authorities believe the results are justified. Pigassou-Albouy[18] compares the important humanistic values of treatment of amblyopia to the management of poliomyelitis and retinal detachment.

8 | Management of Horror Fusionis

The prognosis is poor in most cases of horror fusionis. Generally, the best recommendation is no treatment at all. If, however, there is a large angle of strabismus causing cosmetic concern, extraocular muscle surgery should be cautiously advised. Caution is in regard to the possibility of intractable diplopia. Some authorities believe horror fusionis may be responsible for the occurrence of postoperative diplopia.

Aside from the slight chance of achieving a fusional improvement, the principal consideration in cases of horror fusionis is the possibility of intractable diplopia. It is fortunate that most patients, in whom horror fusionis can be diagnosed by means of the major amblyoscope, do not suffer from diplopia. At least, relatively few of them complain of this problem. Nevertheless, those having this symptom complain enough to make the doctor wary of ever encountering this problem again.

Whereas diplopia is a distinct possibility in the patient who has horror fusionis, this is seldom true if there is complete lack of correspondence. Diplopia is rarely a symptom in these cases, since the patient is unable to achieve simultaneous perception. This is unlike the patient with horror fusionis who has simultaneous perception (but without superimposition). Cosmetic surgery can, therefore, be performed with almost absolute impunity, as far as the possibility of precipitating intractable diplopia is concerned.

The prognosis for functional cure in these cases is even worse than in cases of horror fusionis. Most authorities believe it is impossible to attain binocularity in patients who have a complete lack of correspondence.

Surgery for cosmetic reasons is probably the most common form of therapy given in cases of horror fusionis. When there is diplopia of the post-surgical type, Folk[1] recommends the following: 1. Hope the patient will learn to suppress. 2. Hope the patient will learn to live with the diplopia. 3. Restore the original deviation by means of surgery. 4. Shift the visual field

Intractable Diplopia

with prisms so that the image falls on the suppression zone.

Some cases of intractable diplopia may require occlusion in order to avoid diplopia. Smith[2] described a young woman with horror fusionis who had constant diplopia. Superimposition of binocular targets was impossible, and anomalous correspondence was revealed on afterimage testing. Therapy was of no avail; and ultimately, occlusion was prescribed to avoid diplopia. A patch was applied to the nasal half of the left spectacle lens. Occlusion effectively eliminated diplopia in the primary position of gaze.

If surgery and prisms fail to eliminate diplopia, and if the patient finds occlusion unacceptable, psychotherapy may be the best recommendation for those who are so upset they are unable to function in everyday life.

Considerations for Therapy

Three methods may be attempted when there is any hope for functional improvement. They involve treatment with iseikonic lenses, use of binasal occlusion, and peripheral fusion training.

ANISEIKONIA

This may be a problem causing binocular symptoms in either orthophoric or heterophoric patients.

Aniseikonia may be produced by anisometropic corrective lenses. Spectacles are particularly culpable in this respect, and this is mainly true in cases of anisometropia caused by different curvatures of the corneas. On the other hand, contact lenses may have a minimal aniseikonic effect on these cases; however, contact lenses may cause significant size differences in cases of axial length anisometropia. Some cases of aniseikonia cannot be explained on the basis of lens corrections or refractive errors, but may be due to other causes in the retinal receptors or in the visual pathways.

When the difference in ocular image size is very small (e.g., less than one percent), symptoms are not usually produced as a result of this slight degree of aniseikonia. As the percentage becomes greater, symptoms may result. If the aniseikonia is greater than five percent, this obstacle to fusion may make it impossible for the individual to have central fusion. Aniseikonia can, therefore, be offered as an explanation for the occurrence of horror fusionis, and also a cause of strabismus.

Precise measurement of anisekikonia requires the use of the Office Model Space Eikonometer.[a] Also the patient must be nonstrabismic and have relatively good stereopsis. The subject of nonstrabismic aniseikonia is quite extensive. A brief summary is given in Chapter Sixteen.

It has not been customary to think in terms of the association of strabismus with aniseikonia. One reason, perhaps, is that methods of testing have not been utilized.

Fisher and Ludlam[3] reported a method to measure aniseikonia in cases of poor binocularity in which testing with the space eikonometer is not feasible. They claim this method is critical to one-half percent size

---

[a]Formerly mfg. by American Optical Corp., but no longer produced.

differences. Their testing procedure involves the use of transferred after-images. Two afterimage lights (10 cm long and 1.5 mm wide) are used to generate afterimage marks with a separation distance of 25 cms from the same fixation distance of one meter. A difference in separation between the afterimage marks and the real marks is an indication of aniseikonia. It is helpful to have the patient dark-adapted for about four minutes prior to flashing, so that a strong A.I. is produced. In the same report, Fisher and Ludlam claimed to have developed stereopsis in a 41-year-old male who had horror fusionis, strabismus and amblyopia. Aniseikonia was measured by the A.I. transfer procedure, and the patient was given a five percent overall clip-on size lens to wear over one eye. Fusion training was also given.

Whether bifoveal fusion was established or not was not reported, nor was the level of stereopsis given for this case.

Walton[4] recommends a more direct method of testing for aniseikonia in the strabismic patient. He uses a Maddox rod and two penlights (see Figure 8-1). The lights are held one above the other (separation of 15-20 cm) and the patient fixates the lights from a distance of approximately two meters. The patient looks through a Maddox rod that is oriented with its axis 90 degrees. The eye should see two horizontal streaks. The other eye does not have a Maddox rod before it, but looks directly at the lights.

If superimposition is possible, the patient should report the streaks going through the lights if there is no aniseikonia. However, if there is a large degree of aniseikonia, the distance between the streaks will be different from the distance between the lights. Iseikonic size lenses are introduced before each eye in the attempt to equalize the size of ocular images in the vertical meridian. To test other meridians, the orientation of lights and the Maddox rod are rotated by the same amount to axes of 180, 45 and 135 degrees.

There are pitfalls to this procedure; principally, that superimposition may be impossible when there is horror fusionis. Sometimes, if the separation of the lights is made large enough so that the peripheral retina is stimulated, superimposition may be possible. Prisms are often necessary for compensation of deviations of the visual axes. Since a change in the ocular image size may be induced by looking through a prism, it is wise to split the prism power equally for each eye to minimize artifacts of size differences resulting from the prisms.

Both the afterimage transfer and the Maddox rod procedures lack the sensitivity of the Eikonometer in the testing of small amounts of aniseikonia. However, a large aniseikonia may be detected by these methods. It is important to check for the possibility of aniseikonia since this could be a reason, or at least a contributing factor, for a patient having horror fusionis.

Borish[5] states there have been "at least five reports in the literature reporting successful elimination of horror fusionis by the application of size lenses."

One of the first practitioners to do this was Bielschowsky[6], who reported a case of horror fusionis that responded to correction with iseikonic

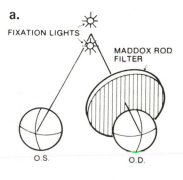

a.

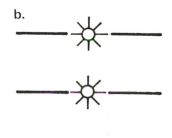

b.

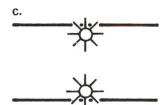

c.

FIGURE 8-1 — Method of Walton to detect aniseikonia in strabismic patients. (a) Diagram showing the right eye looking through a Maddox rod and the left eye seeing the penlights; (b) Patient's perception if there is no aniseikonia; (c) Perception if there is aniseikonia.

lenses. The summary of this case is as follows:

> A 25-year-old patient had a sudden onset of strabismus at the age of seven as a result of trauma to the head. At age 13 surgery was performed on both eyes. There was no complaint of diplopia or other subjective symptoms until the age of 24. Diplopia was suddenly noticed then, as well as the onset of headaches and other symptoms. Three subsequent surgeries were performed to try to eliminate diplopia, and fusion training was tried but with no success.

> For aniseikonic testing, Bielschowsky stated "a considerable difference in the relative size of the ocular images was easily ascertained. After correction of his refractive error, a black square at a distance of 15 feet appeared larger when seen with the right eye than with the left." When this difference was corrected with size lenses, the patient, for the first time, was able to fuse, but without stereopsis. After many examinations, a permanent prescription was given which included in the left lens, an overall magnification of 11 percent and a meridional magnification of 4.5 percent, axis 150°. Some degree of depth perception could be appreciated, "though not of the highest degree when tested with stereoscopic pictures." The patient was happy and had no subjective complaints.

From his experience with this case, Bielschowsky concluded that "we shall have to look, in every case of weak or defective fusion for aniseikonia as a possible origin of the fusion anomaly."

BINASAL OCCLUSION

Some practitioners advocate binasal occlusion for treatment of binocular anomalies. This may be tried in cases of horror fusionis. Jaques[7] writes in regard to functional success in surgery in horror fusionis that "almost never is it achieved where there is horror fusionalis or where deep set, conditioned reactions preclude binocular vision." In the same report he discussed a case of a young patient who had horror fusionis with esotropia. Binasal occluders were made by using masking tape that exactly bisected each monocular field with the eye in the primary position of gaze. The binasals were worn for one year and "removal of the covers reveals a ready fusional response."

The patient was five and a half years old, and I believe the young age of the patient may have been a favorable factor in this case.

While there is no intention to discount the merits of this procedure, cases such as these need to be extremely well-documented before this method can be completely endorsed. The literature is scant in this regard, and the need for extensive, well-documented case reports is obvious. The use of binasal occlusion is presented because this is one of the few methods that has been reported effective in the therapy of horror fusionis.

PERIPHERAL FUSION

If orthoptics is attempted, superimposition training should be given. As discussed in Chapter Two, it is virtually impossible to get the patient to superimpose foveal or macular targets in the major amblyoscope. The eyes move as the targets approach each other. Movement is usually horizontal, but it may be vertical or oblique, or a combination of these directions. If large peripheral targets are used, there may be some chance of obtaining a superimposition response.

Suppression is usually no problem on the major amblyoscope, since the patient is aware of each image at all times. It is best to have a small foveal or parafoveal target, such as a small fish, seen by the dominant eye, and to use a large peripheral target, such as a fishtank for the nondominant eye.[b] The patient moves the arms of the Synoptophore until he can center the fish inside the tank and maintain it there for several seconds. As the patient's confidence is gained, the duration of superimposition is increased until he

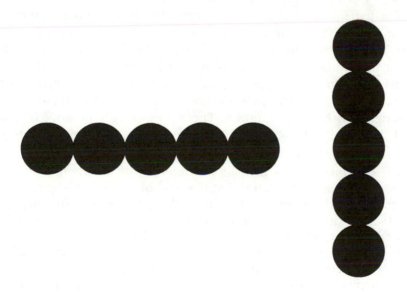

FIGURE 8-2 — Drawing of Javal "N" Card for training in cases of horror fusionis. Vergences, either horizontal, vertical or torsional, will not cause avoidance of a circular target for each eye.

can hold it for approximately one minute. The slides are then switched so the nondominant eye sees the smaller of the two slides, and the procedure of increasing the time of superimposition is repeated.

[b]A small dot and a large circle will work well also. Certain targets, such as a very large fish tank may have to be custom made for the Synoptophore. This can be done easily with felt-tipped pens and clear sheets of acetate.

The patient may be given the Brewster stereoscope for home exercises. Revell[8] describes the Javal N card that is good for this purpose (see Figure 8-2). With this particular target, the patient is prevented from avoiding superin.position because of vergence movements.

The major amblyoscope is further used for office training by having the patient attempt superimposing smaller targets. If the patient cannot achieve first degree fusion with central targets (target subtending 10 degrees or less at the nodal point of the eye), orthoptics should be discontinued, as long as other means, such as size lenses, have also been tried.

Patients with horror fusionis may or may not have anomalous correspondence. This can be a difficult determination to make in many of these cases. If a patient with A R C happens to achieve superimposition at his subjective angle but is unable to do so at his objective angle, it is better to let him remain as is, because true fusion cannot occur under this set of conditions. This could be advantageous because anomalous correspondence can be a very effective antidiplopia mechanism.

If the patient can achieve first-degree fusion of central targets at the objective angle, flat fusion training may be started (to be discussed in Chapter Ten). Some patients may be almost cured, but very few achieve a complete functional cure in cases of horror fusionis. I believe this could be possible for patients of the developmental age when the anomaly is of short duration. Most diagnosed cases of horror fusionis, unfortunately, involve older patients with a long duration. There is practically no hope of achieving bifoveal fusion in these cases. A monofixation syndrome is the most optismistic goal that should realistically be expected.

Flom[9] explained horror fusionis in subjects with esotropia and A R C on the basis of non-uniform relative distributions of corresponding retinal points (irregularly shaped horopters). He found these horopters exhibited a "sharp localized convexity (toward the eyes), whose apex lay on or close to the visual axis of the fixating eye. . . ." This is referred to as the "notch" of the horopter. Flom explained the horror fusionis movement when superimposition is attempted (as in the major amblyoscope). It is reasoned that the sudden movement occurs when the target of the deviating eye is moved across a limb of the notch of the horopter, and is not due to any eye movements. "This jumping phenomenon is commonly observed by squinters with A R C when viewing constantly illuminated first-degree targets, one of which is moved toward the other to obtain superimposition."

A convenient test in free space for detecting this notch of the horopter is a test called the "three-light test." Flom recommends having the patient wear red-green filters and view a meter stick which holds three penlights placed in the horizontal frontal plane. This set of lights is held closer to the esotropic patient than is the fixation target and at a certain distance so that the central light falls within the notch. The patient may be able to report seeing six lights under these conditions, "the central pair being seen in uncrossed diplopia and the outer pairs in crossed diplopia."

If a patient has horror fusionis due to A R C, perhaps it can be eliminated with the A R C therapy. Unfortunately, A R C is often very difficult to eliminate.

9 | Anomalous Correspondence Therapy

Amblyopia should be eliminated or at least reduced significantly before an active therapy program for A R C is begun. When amblyopia is not completely eliminated, the doctor should use 20/40 acuity as a criterion in this regard. Even though treatment is hampered by the patient's not having 20/20 in each eye, it may be necessary to begin binocular treatment in spite of this. However, there are certain patients who show an improvement in the visual acuity of the amblyopic eye as a result of appropriate binocular therapy.

It is also important that good monocular skills be developed in each eye before administering binocular treatment of anomalous correspondence. Therapy for anomalous correspondence may consist of: occlusion, optical procedures, training in a reduced environment, training in free space, and extraocular muscle surgery.

Occlusion

Anomalous correspondence is associated with the presence of strabismus. Whenever there is an onset of strabismus, particularly esotropia, the doctor should consider occlusion for the purpose of preventing the occurrence of anomalous correspondence.

Probably the best form of occlusion is full, constant, alternate patching. It may prevent A R C, and it is effective in preventing suppression, amblyopia and possibly horror fusionis. If the patient has intermittent strabismus rather than a constant manifest deviation, the doctor should be very cautious in prescribing occlusion, for "occlusion strabismus" may result from the wearing of a patch. This may also be true in cases of heterophoria of high magnitude that could become strabismic if dissociation is continued over a long period of time.

When the strabismus is constant, it is all right to give constant occlusion, provided there is proper alternation of occlusion appropriate for the age of the patient (discussed in Chapter Seven regarding occlusion therapy for amblyopia). The chief problem is not the risk of undesirable sequelae but is getting the patient to cooperate in wearing the patch on a full-time basis.

Folk[1] believes occlusion is essential between treatments. Once the patient is started on an active program of orthoptics, it is easier to motivate him to patch during the intervals between training, either in the office or at home. If the patient never looks with both eyes open, except during controlled training exercises, A R C does not exist under the monocular conditions, greatly facilitating the successful elimination of A R C and the ultimate achievement of fusion.

Some authorities believe that binasal occluders are useful in the prevention and treatment of A R C. If the esotropic patient can alternate, Greenwald[2] recommends binasals tilted slightly to allow for the amount of convergence at the nearpoint. His criterion for placement of the tape on the spectacle lens is, ". . . that there be a visible pupillary reflex in both eyes, just beyond the edge of each tape while the patient fixates a near and far muscle light." He believes that if the objective angle of deviation is reduced as a result of wearing the binasals, the prognosis for functional cure is fair to good. However, if angle H increases, ". . . either eye being 'thrust' behind the tape (so as to avoid simultaneous awareness) . . .," the prognosis is poor.

Partially-transmitting, or attenuating, filters may be used in the hope of eliminating A R C. This procedure is sometimes referred to as graded occlusion. A dark filter[a] is placed before the dominant eye so the nondominant eye has a better chance of participating under binocular conditions. This may result in spontaneous normal correspondence. The state of correspondency can be checked by various means while the patient is wearing the attenuator. Bagolini striated lenses are good for this purpose. If, in fact, there is normal correspondence with this type of occluder, the patient is instructed to wear it full-time.

Optical Procedures   Many practitioners are beginning to use prism overcorrections in the treatment of anomalous correspondence. Fleming et al.[3] recommend keeping the patient about 15 p.d. overcorrected to disrupt the A R C and possibly bring about N R C. For example, assume the left eye is esotropic, and the overcorrecting prism is placed (base-out) before the left eye. The fixated object will be imaged on the temporal retina of the left eye, or the opposite side from which it is habitually imaged (i.e., point zero is usually on the nasal retina in case of esotropia). The patient may be thought of as having "sensory exotropia," and A R C may be disrupted sufficiently in this event. If A R C is eliminated by this procedure, a second stage of prismatic correction is applied. The power of the prism is equal to the objective angle of deviation, so the patient can have "sensory orthophoria."

Amigo[4] reports similar means by stating that the recommended

---

[a]Bangerter Graded Occluders, available from Omega Instrument, Co. Inc., 215 East 37th Street, New York, N.Y. 10016. Other filters are available from Eastman Kodak and other sources. These may be either colored (usually red) or grey. For example, the Bagolini bar of red filters may be used for graded occlusion.

overcorrection should be approximately two-and-a-half to three times the magnitude of the objective angle of deviation. The prism power may be gradually reduced after a month or two, to be finally equal to the objective angle of deviation. This is assuming A R C has been disrupted, and N R C is present.

Arruga[5] also recommends a strong overcorrection. The prismatic power should be at least three times angle H in order to keep the deviation from running ahead of the power of the prism. With improvement of correspondency, the overcorrection may later be gradually diminished.

Ludlam[6] uses a randomized approach for disruption of A R C by optical means. He suggests that the stable, full correction of hyperopia is not advisable in cases of esotropia with A R C. He feels that this makes the anomalous correspondence become even more embedded than if the refractive error were less than fully corrected. The angle of deviation would necessarily be more variable if accommodative convergence were activated more, because of the accommodative responses necessary for clear vision.

Whether or not the full refractive correction is worn, Ludlam feels that various combinations of lenses and/or prisms should be worn during the intervals between office training. For instance, one day the patient may wear 20 base-out over the left eye, the next day 20 base-in, then 20 base-up, etc. Fresnel prisms are ideal for this purpose. Various lenses may be used, e.g., minus lens over one eye, and over the other eye on the following day. The same sort of randomized wearing of plus lenses can be applied. Fresnel lenses and prisms are ideal, since they can be re-applied many times.

This type of therapy should precede office visits for orthoptics. In some cases, the A R C may be eliminated completely by optical means, but in the majority of cases, other therapy, including orthoptics and/or surgery, is necessary.

Instrument Training

There may be less chance of A R C responses when testing is done in a reduced environment, rather than in free space. This is one reason for beginning training with instrumentation. Although many instruments and devices have been introduced for A R C therapy, the major amblyoscope is the best single instrument for this purpose.

MAJOR AMBLYOSCOPE

Training procedures on the major amblyoscope are practically the same as those used in testing. In either event, there are numerous combinations of procedures involving real images, Haidinger's brushes, and afterimages. Synoptophores, as well as other modern major amblyoscopes, are equipped with attachments to make these different procedures possible. Table 9A lists them. It should be noted that there is no typical sequence of training that can be strongly recommended when dealing with anomalous correspondence. As a general rule, it is best to begin wherever a normal correspondence response can be elicited. Many of the more elaborate procedures are limited by the patient's lack of maturity, poor cooperation, or perceptual unawareness. The doctor may, therefore, find he is limited to the more simple procedures and must necessarily begin training with some of these, rather than with others that might possibly be more promising.

TABLE 9A. *Procedures for the Major Amblyoscope*

A. Two real images
1. Peripheral targets at angle H
2. Central targets at angle H
3. Peripheral or small targets from overcorrected position
4. Peripheral or small targets from undercorrected position
5. Alternate flashing at angle H
6. Unilateral flashing at angle H
7. Simultaneous flashing at angle H
8. Macular massage of dominant eye
9. Macular massage of non-dominant eye
10. Kinetic bi-retinal stimulation
11. Vertical displacement at angle H
12. Chasing
13. Alternate fixation
14. Binocular triplopia

B. Afterimages
1. Positive
2. Negative
3. Afterimages with real images

C. Haidinger's brushes (superimposition of two H.B.s at angle H)

D. Combinations
1. Non-dominant eye (H.B.) and dominant eye (real image)
2. Nondominant eye (H.B.) and dominant eye (vertical A.I.)
3. Non-dominant eye (H.B. and real image) and dominant eye (vertical A.I. and real image)

E. Major amblyoscope (Stanworth) and free space
1. Blank wall
2. Penlight fixation target

TWO REAL IMAGES   As in testing, the first training usually attempted is the superimposition of two dissimilar peripheral targets at the objective angle. This may be all right for a short while, but it is important that foveal targets should be used as soon as possible for the elimination of A R C. Thus, bifoveal fixation can be monitored more easily than if peripheral targets were used for superimposition.

It is wise to start with an overcorrection of the deviation and then move the target in toward angle H. For example, an esotropic left eye of 15 p.d. of the left eye would require the carriage arm of the Synoptophore to be moved from base-out (e.g., 30 p.d.) to a lesser amount of base-out until angle H is reached.

Suppose the pair of targets is a circle and a star. Since the circle is larger, it is placed before the nondominant left eye in this case, and the star is placed before the dominant right eye.

The size of these first-degree fusion targets should gradually be made smaller, as long as the patient is able to superimpose at the objective angle. There are several reasons why a patient may be able to superimpose large images properly but not small ones. It may be that there is peripheral N R C but central A R C. Foveal or macular images would probably result in the patient insisting on superimposing at his subjective angle rather than at his objective angle. Smaller targets also may be suppressed more readily, or the patient may have horror fusionis in these instances.

When the patient is able to superimpose central targets in going from an overcorrection to angle H, he should attempt to achieve superimposition of the same target by going from an undercorrection to angle H. This is more difficult since in all but certain paradoxical cases of A R C, the dioptric image of the target will pass through point "a." The circle is moved from base-in to a base-out position, and the dioptric image of the circle falls on point "a" before it gets to the fovea (see Figure 9-1). The procedure of going from an undercorrected position to angle H may cause the patient to superimpose at his subjective angle; if so, it should be discontinued until a later time when the patient is able to superimpose at the objective angle. Training from the overcorrected position should be resumed in these instances.

If these procedures do not elicit a normal correspondence response, flashing may be necessary. Targets are locked at the objective angle and alternating flashing is given. This can be done either manually or by an automatic flash unit attachment. After about one minute of flashing, both lights are turned on simultaneously, and the patient is asked to try to see the circle around the star. The patient may report that the circle tends to jump toward the star but then moves away; however, this may not be noticed until quite a few of these exercises have been completed. As training continues, the patient may be able to see the circle around the star for longer periods than before.

The A R C is broken down (at least in this reduced environment) when the patient can hold superimposition for at least one minute of time.

Unilateral flashing should also be tried. It is merely the rapid flashing of the nondominant eye at the objective angle. Stimulation may be varied from slow to rapid, and the light and dark phases can be altered to best promote superimposition in any given case. The goal is to have the patient superimpose the circle and the star at the objective angle when flashing is stopped and the two targets are seen simultaneously.

The patient should next attempt to superimpose both images during

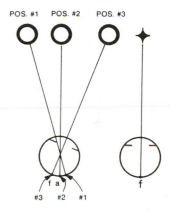

FIGURE 9-1 — Target is moved from base-in position to position that fully compensates the objective angle of deviation

simultaneous flashing and try to maintain superimposition during the moments when flashing is discontinued.

The method of "macular massage" is another traditionally used procedure described in the following example. In the case of an esotropia of 15 p.d. of the left eye with harmonious A R C (subjective angle of zero), the star seen by the right eye would be moved back and forth from approximately 5 p.d. base-out to 25 p.d. base-out. The speed of movement may be varied from slow to fast. Care should be taken to avoid the subjective angle. This is the reason the arm of the major amblyoscope is not moved to a position less than 5 p.d. base-out, assuming this is a case of harmonious A R C with point "a" at point zero. The oscillating image is on the dominant eye, because N R C is more likely to occur when the nondominant eye is fixating.

When the patient is able to report the star passing through the circle as the targets pass the objective angle, a normal correspondence response is being elicited. Angle H may be variable and, therefore, the doctor should not rely completely on the prismatic scale of the major amblyoscope. He should also observe the corneal light reflections to monitor the angle of deviation during these procedures.

If macular massage is effective in breaking down A R C with the nondominant eye fixating, the other eye should fixate. The procedure should be repeated, but with the oscillation of the image of the circle on the nondominant eye. N R C is less likely to occur when the habitually dominant eye is fixating; and consequently, superimposition of the targets at angle H may be more difficult to achieve than when the nondominant eye is fixating.

Gibson[7] describes a procedure called kinetic bi-retinal stimulation. The tubes of the major amblyoscope are locked in place at the objective angle. The patient keeps his gaze in the primary position while the locked tubes are moved laterally from side to side. During the movement of the targets, the patient may report superimposition, but he will probably report separation of the images when the movement is stopped. This procedure is repeated until the patient can maintain superimposition when the movement ceases.

Vertical displacement of the targets may bring about first-degree fusion at the horizontal angle of deviation. For example, the left eye may fixate the circle while the carriage arm of the Synoptophore is elevated to cause a displacement of the star that can be seen above the circle. This procedure is very effective in cases of central A R C with peripheral N R C. The star can be seen directly above the circle, provided enough prismatic displacement is given. The doctor gradually reduces the vertical displacement in an attempt to have the patient superimpose the circle and star. Usually, if there is central A R C, the targets quickly separate as the star invades the central area. This procedure is repeated until the targets jump apart less often. It is also helpful to move the star upward from a lower position. When superimposition is achieved with the left eye fixating, the procedure is repeated with the right eye fixating.

Once superimposition of two real images can be achieved in the primary position, chasing exercises should be given, with the therapist moving one of the targets while the patient moves the other. For instance, the circle may be moved ten degrees to one side. The patient should likewise move his tube with the star ten degrees to the same side and superimpose the two images. The therapist then quickly moves the circle to another position and then another until the patient can consistently superimpose over the entire lateral field.

Alternate fixation is a procedure that may help in breaking down A R C. The targets are set in a position of neither the objective angle nor the subjective angle. The patient is instructed to fixate alternately the star and the circle. At first, the therapist may have to alternately flash the targets to get the patient started. The targets are slowly moved to the subjective angle where superimposition is appreciated by the patient who soon becomes confused because he realizes that eye movements are necessary in order to fixate each target. The targets are then placed at the objective angle, and the patient comes to the realization that eye movements are no longer necessary in order to alternately fixate each target. This kinesthetic feedback tends to help in the elimination of A R C.

Walraven[8] introduced a method of treating A R C by means of binocular triplopia. The occurrence of binocular triplopia is sometimes inappropriately referred to as monocular diplopia. The description of this procedure is best given by the following example: Assume the patient has an esotropia of the left eye of 15 p.d., and the subjective angle is 5 p.d. (a case of typical unharmonious A R C). The larger target (the circle) is placed in the tube for the right eye, and the star is placed so that the left eye can see it. The star is moved to a base-in position, e.g., 5 p.d., as illustrated in Figure 9-2a. The patient is instructed to fixate the star and the circle alternately while the therapist slowly moves the star to the subjective angle (i.e., 5 p.d. base-out).

If there is an underlying N R C as well as an existing A R C, duality of correspondence may occur under these circumstances. Prior extensive orthoptics is usually necessary to elicit this sort of dual response. In this case the perception of binocular triplopia is illustrated in Figure 9-2b. Since the star is imaged on point "a" of the left eye, its ocular image will be superimposed on that of the circle. If there is residual normal correspondence present, the fact that the dioptric image of the star is nasal to the fovea causes it to be seen on the temporal side. It is faint because of the "weakness" of the N R C in relation to the A R C.

The star is next imaged on the fovea, and anti-suppression training is given in order to make the faint foveal ocular image of the star easier to see. This is done by rapidly flashing the star at the objective angle. With

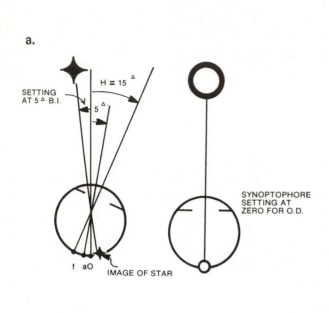

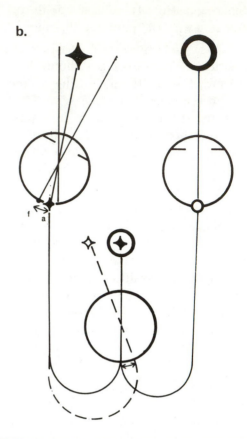

FIGURE 9-2 — Method of Walraven using binocular triplopia. (a) Starting from position of base-in; (b) Illustration of phenomenon of binocular triplopia. The second, non-superimposed star is seen because of duality of correspondence and is faint when this first occurs.

continued training, the superimposed foveal star should become brighter, and the star seen at point "a" should become fainter.

AFTERIMAGES   Most of the newer major amblyoscopes are available with slides and flash units that can generate afterimages. Slides S3 and S4 are used in the Synoptophore. One slide has a light horizontal streak on a dark background, and the other slide has a vertical streak. Each has a central red fixation mark. As with the Hering-Bielschowsky test (Chapter Two), it is customary to first flash the dominant eye with the horizontal streak, and then flash the nondominant eye with the vertical streak. It is important to have the matte surface of each side nearest to the patient for a better lighting effect. Also, the opal diffusing screen should be removed from the optical pathway when each eye is flashed, providing a much stronger afterimage than would otherwise be generated. After each eye has been flashed, the slides are removed, and the diffusing screen is swiveled back into place. Special grey slides may be used, but they are not necessary if the illumination in the

Synoptophore is kept low enough so that the afterimages are not washed out.

The afterimage seen by each eye is sustained by flashing illumination within the instrument. This can be controlled conveniently with the automatic flashing unit, and the rapidity of flashing as well as the timing of light and dark phases can be adjusted as desired.

Positive afterimages are considered less natural than negative; therefore, N R C is more likely to be elicited when positive afterimages are employed. In order to see them, long dark phases should be emphasized initially. If the patient can see a perfect cross with the positive afterimages, the dark phase can be shortened, and the negative afterimage can be made visible more of the time. It is not unusual for the patient to report seeing a cross (N R C) in the dark phase, but seeing a noncross (A R C) in the light phase. In such a case, various adjustments of the automatic flashing unit may help in developing a cross response with the negative afterimages. The goal is to have the patient achieve a perfect cross with both eyes being flashed simultaneously.

When N R C with afterimages is achieved, real images may be incorporated into the training. In the case of esotropia of the left eye, a circle is presented to the left eye, and the patient tries to maintain seeing a perfect cross superimposed on the circle. When this is accomplished, the star is included and presented to the right eye. The patient now tries to superimpose the circle and star while maintaining an A.I. cross that is centered on the superimposed circle and star.

An A R C response is indicated if the A.I. cross comes apart. The doctor should be aware that an A R C also may be present even when there is a perfect cross. This may be because the afterimage is unnatural enough to show N R C, but the real targets may induce A R C at the very same moment. In spite of the duality, the A R C of the real images is easily checked by observing the objective angle by means of corneal reflections, or by dousing the target of the dominant eye and watching for a movement of the other eye, as in the unilateral cover test.

HAIDINGER'S BRUSHES

Many of the Synoptophores come equipped with attachments to produce Haidinger's brushes. The H.B.'s may be for the left eye, the right eye, or for both eyes together. A patient with A R C frequently is unable to superimpose two real images, but may be able to superimpose less natural targets such as Haidinger's brushes. So that superimposition can be monitored, one H.B. should be rotating clockwise; the other, counter-clockwise. Superimposition is indicated when the H.B.'s appear to be together, and when the patient notices fluttering and flapping of the composite image.

The tubes of the Synoptophore should be locked at the objective angle for this procedure. There should be no eccentric fixation, since this ought to have been eliminated prior to A R C therapy. If there is any suspicion of eccentric fixation, visuoscopy or other testing for this anomaly should be performed. Also, the diaphragms in front of both rotating Haidinger's brushes may be closed down to insure bifoveal fixation at the objective angle.

COMBINATIONS OF IMAGES

When test targets are introduced, the Haidinger's brushes are more easily seen if the Synoptophore targets are black and white printed on transparent film.[b] This is more preferable than the colored slides on the translucent film used in most other training procedures.

The following might be a training sequence using combinations of images. First, have the nondominant eye perceive the Haidinger's brushes. Then, introduce a real target to the dominant eye. Have the patient superimpose them. A blue filter (small insertable lens that comes with the Synoptophore) before the dominant eye is used to equalize the light intensities so that the H.B. can be seen by the nondominant eye under binocular conditions. If the patient has trouble superimposing these, the real target is removed and a vertical afterimage is generated on the dominant eye. The patient then attempts to superimpose the H.B. and the A.I. Flashing the instrument lights, either manually or by various settings of the automatic unit, may help the patient achieve superimposition.

When this is done, a real target is placed in the tube for the nondominant eye to fixate. If superimposition of this combination can be maintained, another real target is presented to the dominant eye. Ideally, the patient should have superimposition of the two real images, in conjunction with the superimposed H.B. and the vertical A.I.

These foveal tags are excellent monitors of the state of correspondency. The variations of different combinations are many. It is good to try a number of these on each patient, because some of them might be very effective in helping the patient break down anomalous correspondence.

MAJOR AMBLYOSCOPE
AND FREE SPACE

Although the major amblyoscope is good for training in a reduced environment, the fact remains that the conditions of seeing in such an instrument are very different from those of habitual everyday seeing. Revell[9] describes the Modified Major Amblyoscope of Stanworth as having unsilvered mirrors so that the patient can see in free space, while targets in the instrument can also be seen at the same time. This modification allows the treatment of A R C under slightly more natural conditions than could otherwise be done on the major amblyoscope.

The best initial procedure with the Stanworth instrument is to have the patient view a distant blank wall through the instrument while two dissimilar targets, such as the circle and the star, are superimposed at the objective angle. When this can be done easily, a real target, such as a penlight, can be

---

[b]Slides F 161 and 162, F 163 and 164, and F 165 and 166 are available from Clement Clarke. Similar slides also may be custom-made for use in the Synotophore.

introduced in free space while the patient attempts to maintain superimposition. In the case of esotropia, the target usually must be moved closer and placed at the centration point. Plus lenses may be required for this procedure (refer to Chapter Three for details of determining the centration point). If the penlight and the circle and star are superimposed when the instrument is set at the objective angle, the correspondence appears to be normal. This is verified by shutting off the light for the dominant eye while the doctor watches for any movement of the nondominant eye to fixate. A movement indicates anomalous correspondence, since the patient was superimposing at a subjective angle unequal to the objective angle.

Aside from the major amblyoscope, there are not many instruments designed specifically for the treatment of anomalous correspondence. One particular procedure I use that requires minimal equipment but still retains the qualities of having a reduced environment is the bifoveal test of Cüppers. This involves visuoscopy under binocular conditions (procedure described in Chapter Two). If a flashing unit is attached to the Visuscope, flashing at the objective angle can be given. Furthermore, since the doctor can view the fovea, a procedure similar to macular massage on the major amblyoscope can be administered. With this advantage the doctor can monitor the exact position of the fovea to determine whether or not there is an angle of anomaly.

Vertical displacement exercises also can be done. The doctor merely places the star above (or below) the fovea, and slowly moves the star toward the fovea. The patient is instructed to try to superimpose the fixation red penlight (seen in the mirror) with the star in the Visuscope. As on the major amblyoscope, the patient will at first report the targets jumping apart. The doctor can observe exactly when the movement occurs in this procedure.

Chasing exercises can be done during visuoscopy. The doctor places the star on the retina at some point other than the fovea. In order for the patient to superimpose this with the red light, he will have to appropriately change the angle of the mirror he is holding. When the targets are superimposed, the doctor moves the star to another location, and the procedure is repeated.

This type of training is a transition between having the patient look inside an instrument and having the patient see in free space. The disadvantage of this method is that cooperation must be excellent in order for this to be carried out.

There are very few home training instruments that are good for A R C therapy. The doctor must usually rely on occlusion and/or optical procedures as the out-of-office portion of A R C therapy. Vodnoy[10] recommends the use of the Mirror Stereoscope (see Figure 2-15) for elimination of A R C. He claims that after the Fish-and-Bowl and the Chick-and-Egg Targets can be superimposed at the true angle of strabismus, the FU 3 targets (see Figure 2-16c) are viewed by the patient; and by using the large circles ". . . fusion with normal correspondence is learned far out in the periphery where the patient has not practiced A R C." The appreciation of stereopsis indicates an N R C response.

Unfortunately, with most home training stereoscopes, the patient is tempted to superimpose at the subjective angle rather than at the objective angle. The patient must be monitored very closely. The out-of-office training procedures are not highly recommended unless the patient has learned to achieve first-degree fusion at the objective angle of deviation.

Training in Free Space

Although training for the purpose of eliminating anomalous correspondence may be done with the patient looking in free space, it is generally a good rule to break down A R C by using the major amblyoscope before out-of-instrument training is begun. The reduced environment is used to promote N R C responses. Even when A R C is reported in the major amblyoscope, typical unharmonious A R C is the most frequent response. This is usually easier to disrupt than the condition of harmonious A R C. The chief advantage, however, is that the angles involved (i.e., angles H, S and A) are relatively easy to monitor with the major amblyoscope.

In spite of the advantages offered by the major amblyoscope, some practitioners prefer training to be almost exclusively in free space.

In many respects training in free space is similar to those procedures performed in the Synoptophore. Likewise, many of the procedures are esoteric in nature, difficult to administer in all but the most cooperative patients, and often ineffective. Nevertheless, successful results may be obtained, and various free space procedures may enable the duration of treatment to be shortened.

Categories of free space training include: luster, afterimages, intermittent photic stimulation, real images, entoptic phenomena, Bagolini lenses, and combinations of these.

LUSTER

Ludlam[6] advocates the luster method of training. There are numerous ways to elicit luster, but the best in cases of A R C is to set up conditions to promote red-green color fusion (discussed in Chapter Two). The patient may view a brightly illuminated grey wall, but the illumination should be evenly distributed with no shadows. When the patient is between the source of illumination and the viewing screen, it is difficult to meet these conditions. This is why a retro-illuminated grey screen (see Figure 2-44a) is preferable in this regard.

The esotropic patient may be better able to appreciate luster if plus lenses are used, and the screen is at the centration point. The patient should be able to see luster over the entire surface of the screen. If, instead, the patient reports seeing a split field, no attempt is made for further training because of the poor prognosis indicated by such a response.

The patient tries to maintain luster while a large target, such as the doctor's hand, is placed at the edge of the screen in the peripheral visual field. A split-field response may result because of form perception. If this should happen, the object is removed from the patient's view, and he is instructed to perceive luster in the formless field as before. The process of slowly introducing objects into the periphery is repeated until the patient is able to maintain luster under these circumstances.

When this is accomplished, an object is placed in the central visual field. This may cause a split-field response. This process is repeated until the patient finally is able to maintain the perception of luster when a small fixation target, such as a black dot, is centrally fixated.

It may be necessary to "over-plus" the patient in relation to the fixation distance of the screen. This is for the purpose of blurring the target which may help promote luster easier than when the fixation target is clearly seen. The perception of form with sharp contours is thought to be the triggering mechanism for the A R C split field response.

Under these conditions, the visual axes are at the centration point. The patient is in "sensory orthophoria" in relation to the fixated target, and theoretically, fusion should be possible. This is probably occurring if the patient continually notices luster; however, the N R C could be peripheral, since the patient could still have central A R C and report luster. There is no assurance that central N R C is being developed, and it may well be that only peripheral fusion is being developed at this stage of treatment. This, however, is perfectly acceptable, because some patients with A R C will not get this far along with superimposition training using the major amblyoscope.

The luster method can be refined by projecting red and green targets on the screen to monitor suppression. Brock rings[c] are ideal for testing peripheral fusion. Smaller red and green pictures may be projected to check central fusion.

Motor fusion training is started once sensory fusion can be demonstrated. Too much vergence demand cannot be made at first because the patient's ability to maintain N R C vision is very tenuous, and the A R C response is likely to recur. The best way to induce vergence movements is to have the patient move slowly back and forth (only a few centimeters at first) from the screen and attempt to fuse a target on the screen. Vergences are necessary if binocular fixation is to be maintained in real life. Peripheral fusion targets, e.g., Brock rings, may be required, but eventually, the patient should be able to fuse small targets while he is moving back and forth.

AFTERIMAGES

The procedure with afterimages is similar to the major amblyoscope procedure. The Hering-Bielschowsky test (discussed in Chapter Two) is the recommended procedure for generating afterimages. Positive afterimage training is given first, followed by work with negative afterimages. This is similar to training in the Synoptophore, except that the patient views the

---

[c]Available from Keystone View Division of Mast/Keystone.

afterimages in free space. The goal is to have the patient perceive a perfect cross for both the positive A.I. and the negative A.I. Afterimage therapy may be facilitated by placing the esotropic patient at the centration point. This effectively allows for A.I. training at the objective angle, as when the major amblyoscope is set at the objective angle.

INTERMITTENT PHOTIC STIMULATION

The type of intermittent photic stimulation that has been reported to be the most effective in cases of A R C is alpha rhythm photic driving. Allen[11] claims that 15 minutes of flashing with the Translid Binocular Interaction Trainer (discussed in Chapter Seven) has converted the Hering-Bielschowsky afterimage from a noncross (A R C) to a perfect cross (N R C). This instrument flashes alternately so that impulses of light from the two eyes arrive at the lateral geniculate nucleus asynchronously. Each pulse has a duration of approximately 1/40th second. It is thought that flashing at a rate of 7 to 15 times per second results in the elimination of the mechanisms of anomalous correspondence.

The Translid Binocular Interaction Trainer (T.B.I.) may be used to "normalize" the Hering-Bielschowsky afterimages. Once the cross is perceived, the T.B.I. is held away from the face, and the flashing helps to maintain the afterimages for five to ten minutes. Home training is practical since the T.B.I. is portable, and the patient can monitor his own responses.

Another photic stimulating device that Allen[12] recommends is the Fusion Aider.[d] It is hand-held, and has a rotating sectored disc that provides alpha rhythm stimulation to the eyes. The patient can view real objects in free space through the windows of the device. The eyes can be stimulated alternately or simultaneously, depending on how the device is positioned before the patient's eyes.

A program of home training should include the use of afterimages, the T.B.I. and the Fusion Aider.

OTHER COMBINATIONS

There are many combinations of procedures that can be used in cases of A R C. Real images may be provided by targets such as black dots, anaglyphs, vectographs, a penlight, etc. These may be used together with entoptic phenomena and/or afterimages. Only a few representative procedures can be discussed since the number of possible variations and combinations are legion.

A black dot target is useless in cases of A R C unless some monitoring of the objective angle of deviation can be done while the patient reports superimposition of two targets. This is because the patient is likely to use his subjective rather than his objective angle on a real target in free space.

A practical way to monitor the angle of anomaly is to use Haidinger's

[d]For information on the Fusion Aider, contact Dr. Merrill Allen (Indiana University, School of Optometry, 800 East Atwater, Bloomington, Ind. 47401). This must be custom made, as it is no longer commercially available.

brushes. The Bernell MITT may be set up so that one eye sees the H.B., and the other eye sees a black dot. Assume the patient has an esotropia of the left eye with harmonious A R C. The patient wears a blue filter over the left eye and a dark-green one over the right eye. The MITT is placed at the centration point (see Figure 9-3). The left eye fixates the H.B. and the right eye sees the black dot. Since there is A R C, the fovea of the left eye corresponds to point "a" of the right eye, and cyclopean projection shows the black spot at the left of the H.B. Since the blue filter also allows the black dot to be seen, the left eye may see a dot in the center of the H.B. However, it may appear faded and barely discernible because, most likely, there would be foveal suppression of the nondominant eye in this case. The goal in training is for the patient to superimpose the black spot (seen by the right eye) with the H.B. seen by the left eye.

Changing the dot from black to blue would make this a more reliable procedure allowing only the right eye to see the dot (i.e., blue dot blends in with blue background), and only the left eye to see the H.B. The blue dot can be marked on a clear sheet of plastic with appropriate ink.

The combination of the H.B., a transferred afterimage, and a black dot is sometimes useful in A R C therapy. Suppose the left eye is esotropic, and the anomalous correspondence is harmonious. The patient should see the H.B. on the dot (assuming central fixation) and the H.B. should be to the right of the vertical afterimage (see Figure 9-4). (The details of this as a testing procedure were discussed in Chapter Seven.) The advantage of this method is that eccentric fixation, as well as anomalous correspondence, can be monitored by the patient. The transferred afterimage is greatly reinforced if the right eye is closed, and one of the T.B.I. bulbs is flashed at a close distance from the eye. The patient is instructed to try mentally reducing the angle of anomaly so that all the images are superimposed. The use of a pointer for tactile/kinesthetic stimulation and feedback often helps in this type of training.

The Giessen test (discussed in Chapter Two) is another procedure in which the patient can monitor his own angle of anomaly. This procedure may be used for training purposes by changing the room illumination, having the patient look through the Fusion Aider, alternately occluding, etc.

Ronne and Rindziunski[12] reported a prism-rack afterimage test. This simply involves the placement of a prism bar of horizontal prisms before one eye, while the patient is perceiving afterimages. They found that on the Hering-Bielschowsky test, a noncross may become a cross in some cases, as a result of the introduction of various prisms.

Besides being useful with Hering-Bielschowsky afterimages, the prism-rack procedure can be incorporated with the Giessen test, or for that matter, many of the other afterimage training procedures.

Hugonnier et al.[13] recommend a free space training procedure which they call a "direct attack at the objective angle in space." A target such as a pencil point is placed at the centration point, and the patient attempts to see

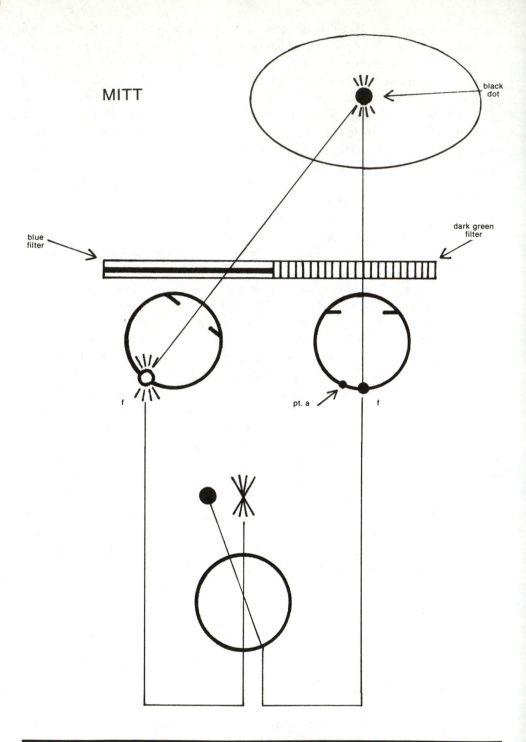

FIGURE 9-3 — Combination of Haidinger's brushes (seen by left eye) and a black dot (seen by right eye) for monitoring the angle of anomaly. The black dot seen by the fovea of the non-dominant left eye is centered in the H.B., but usually is either very faint or not seen at all. Plus lenses may be needed for the black dot to be at the centration point in cases of esotropia.

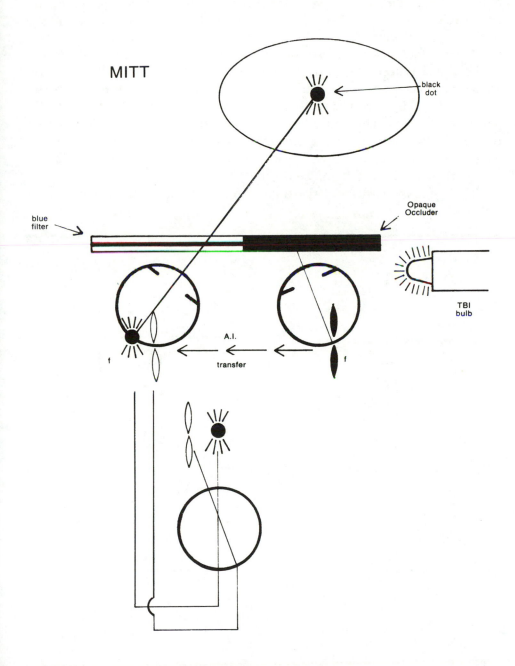

MITT

black dot

Opaque Occluder

blue filter

TBI bulb

A.I.

transfer

f

f

FIGURE 9-4 — Combinations of Haidinger's brushes and black dot (seen by left eye) and the vertical afterimage (also seen by the left eye, but transferred from the right eye). Flashing light near right eye re-inforces the transferred afterimage seen by the left eye.

a Hering-Bielschowsky cross superimposed on the tip of the pencil (see Figure 9-5a). This is an indication of N R C, but notwithstanding, the unilateral cover test should be performed, since the A.I.'s could be seen with N R C, while the pencil tip is seen with A R C. A movement of the uncovered eye on the unilateral cover test would indicate the occurrence of this set of conditions.

Assume the patient has esotropia of the left eye with harmonious A R C. If the pencil is moved slightly beyond the centration point, the tip of the pencil may be seen singly, but there would probably be a noncross (see Figure 9-5b). The presence of H A R C may be confirmed by replacing the pencil with a penlight and having the patient look at the light through Bagolini striated lenses. If the subjective angle is zero, the X and the light would be superimposed (see Figure 9-5c), even though the patient is strabismic in relation to the fixated penlight.

The therapist carries out the training by quickly placing the light (or the

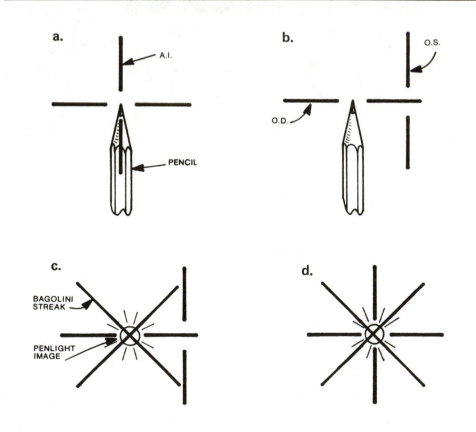

FIGURE 9-5 — The method of direct attack at the objective angle in space. (a) Cross afterimage on pencil tip (probable N R C); (b) Non-cross afterimage on pencil tip (A R C); (c) Bagolini streaks superimposed on light, but with non-cross afterimage (HARC); (d) Superimposition of Bagolini streaks, lights and cross afterimage (N R C if no eye movement on unilateral cover test).

pencil tip) exactly at the centration point and using rapid alternate occlusion. The prism-rack can also be used at the same time, as well as the Fusion Aider, colored filters, etc. With continued repetition, an N R C response may be elicited (see Figure 9-5d). The Bagolini lenses are used mainly for monitoring A R C because the presence of so many images in the field of view is distracting and confusing to the patient during training.

It is hoped that through the use of the myriad combinations of procedures that employ afterimages and entoptic phenomena, the patient will reach a level where anaglyphic and vectographic methods can be used in free space. The many variations of A R C training can be applied to anaglyphs and vectograms, e.g., use of T.B.I., work at centration point, use of Fusion Aider, afterimages, flashing, etc.

Much of the training to eliminate A R C leads to the same procedures used for antisuppression training (to be discussed in Chapter Ten).

Bagolini lenses are used in the last stages of free space training for the elimination of A R C. A response of N R C may be elicited by having the patient look through the Fusion Aider or by reducing the environment in other ways, such as darkening the room, or using colored filters.

Prisms may be used for compensating the strabismic angle of deviation (refer to Figure 9-6). Since most cases of strabismus with A R C show harmonious anomalous correspondence on the Bagolini lenses, the patient sees the "ortho" response with the light centered in the X (see Figure 9-6a).

If the full compensating base-out prism is worn, point zero is now on the fovea of the deviating eye and no longer on point "a." This causes the patient with H A R C to report seeing the lights below the intersection of the streaks (see Figure 9-6b). Since the fovea of the deviating eye is usually suppressed, only one light is seen in most of these cases (see Figure 9-6c).

Rapidly introducing and removing the prism may be sufficient in disrupting the A R C, and an underlying N R C may emerge as a result of extensive training of this nature. The patient should then see the light centered in the cross (see Figure 9-6d) which indicates N R C (providing the strabismic angle is fully compensated by prism).

A bar of graded filters (either grey or red) is useful in eliciting an N R C response on the Bagolini lens test. The attenuators are placed over the dominant eye. The Fusion Aider, alternate occlusion, and various other procedures may be combined with Bagolini lenses for training.

The ultimate procedure in training to eliminate A R C is for the patient to be aware of spontaneous diplopia and to be able to localize the images properly in free space. For instance, if the left eye is 15 p.d. esotropic at a fixation distance of one meter and correspondence is normal, the image of the left eye is seen 15 cm to the left of that seen by the right eye. Any other separation distance indicates A R C. A Maddox scale is used to teach the patient how to properly interpret the separation distance of the images and what they mean. An ordinary yardstick for home training also serves well for this purpose.

a.

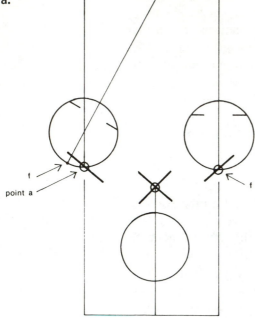

b.

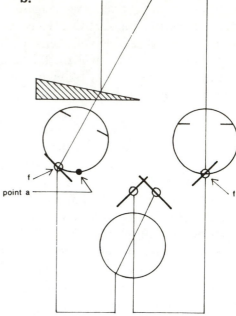

c.

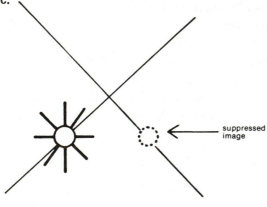

suppressed image

d.

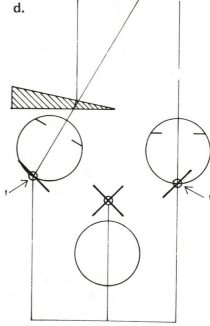

FIGURE 9-6 — Bagolini striated lenses and prisms for treatment of anomalous correspondence. (a) Harmonious A R C response; (b) Harmonious response with compensating prism; (c) Only one light seen because of foveal suppression of the left eye; (d) N R C response after A R C has been eliminated and angle of strabismus fully compensated by prism.

Spontaneous diplopia is not easily seen in free space for the patient who is strabismic; therefore, the environment may have to be slightly less than natural at times. For this purpose, graded occluders, lowered room illumination, vertical dissociating prisms, and other combinations may be helpful.

Exotropia and Anomalous Correspondence

The concern with A R C up to this point has been related to esotropia and not to exotropia. This is because in most cases of exotropia A R C is of little or no significance. Clinical experience and reports in the literature bear this out. Although the effect of A R C on the prognosis for a functional cure is minimal in cases of exotropia, the incidence of A R C associated with exotropia is quite high. Hugonnier and Bernard[14] reported that, in a study of 253 cases of untreated exotropia, 135 had A R C.

Even though many exotropic patients have anomalous correspondence, there are other overriding reasons why there is less concern about A R C in exotropia than in esotropia. It is generally much easier to cure exotropia, regardless of the state of correspondency. The prognosis is better because the age of onset tends to be later for exotropias than for esotropias, and the re-education of fusion is made easier. Fusion had the early opportunity to develop in these cases before an A R C adaptation was made when the exo deviation became manifest.

Many exotropias are intermittent, and the A R C is just as intermittent. The co-variation suggests that there is a strong underlying N R C in these cases of intermittent exotropia. With just a little orthoptic help, N R C may prevail. Most of this type of training to eliminate A R C is in the form of motor fusion training because, when the eyes are straight and the patient is fusing, the A R C disappears. Therefore, training specifically for eliminating A R C can be bypassed in practically all these cases.

Occasionally, an exotropic patient who has A R C may require orthoptics similar to that given in the case of an esotrope with A R C. This is almost always a case of a large-angle constant exotropia with deeply embedded A R C. The main difference in training in free space from that in esotropia is that the centration point may be established through the use of minus lenses, providing the AC/A is sufficiently high to align the visual axes. If that is not feasible, optical alignment by means of base-in prisms is used, but this is not as therapeutic as when the eyes are actually in the ortho position (i.e., with the minus lens method).

Training in a reduced environment, such as with the major amblyoscope, follows the same principles that are applied in cases of esotropia.

Surgical Considerations

The recommendation for surgery in cases of A R C varies according to the individual practitioner's bias. The opinions range from those who believe orthoptics can offer the most hope for functional cure to those who believe surgery is the only solution, with orthoptics of no value whatsoever.

Parks[15] shares the latter view and believes that the esotropic patient should have surgery to align the visual axes. He is of the opinion that orthoptics is of little value for treatment of esotropic patients with A R C, and, therefore, he has abandoned pre-operative and post-operative orthoptics in older children who have anomalous correspondence. Authorities having a moderate opinion believe that presurgical and postsurgical orthoptics may be helpful when a functional cure is sought.

In the final analysis, the need for surgery depends upon the circumstances of the particular case in question. Nonsurgical procedures may be appropriate in some cases, but extraocular muscle surgery may be required in others.

Anti-Suppression Training at the Objective Angle

The lines between therapy for anomalous correspondence and suppression are not clear-cut. The procedures used in treating A R C also tend to reduce suppression. Although antisuppression training is also given when treating cases with A R C, it is important to follow the rule of training at the objective angle.

Divergence Technique

Wick[16] described a divergence technique of Flom and Heath for therapy of small-angle esotropia with A R C. It is thought that co-variation causes A R C to be present when the deviation is manifest but not when there is fusional divergence that places the eyes in the ortho posture. A pair of large peripheral third-degree fusion slides is used in the major amblyoscope and placed at angle S of the patient. Room lights should be dim. Rapid alternate flashing of the targets is continued until some sort of stereopsis is perceived. This process is continued while the targets are slowly moved in the base-in direction, encouraging the patient to have the "feeling" of diverging his eyes. Hopefully, the perceived depth and kinesthetic feeling of divergence remains. If so, the patient is to move away from the instrument, look around the room, and maintain divergence. Supposedly, there is N R C at that moment. When this can be repeated and maintained, the patient is ready for regular sensory and motor fusion training in free space. It is important to note that this technique is applicable only to small-angle esotropia. Therefore, surgery is often not necessary; however, wearing of prism during training sessions may aid the patient in achieving better fusion. Excellent patient cooperation is imperative in order for this technique to be effective. Occlusion between training sessions may be recommended as passive therapy for A R C.

10 | Anti-Suppression Therapy

Patients who have undergone therapy for the elimination of anomalous correspondence have, to a certain extent, also undergone training for antisuppression. Training in cases of A R C is mostly done at the objective angle with the goal of having the objective and subjective angles become the same. It is only after the patient can easily superimpose dissimilar ocular images with normal corresponding points that there can be less concern with the monitoring of these angles. Emphasis can then be placed on the treatment of suppression. In cases that have had extensive training for elimination of anomalous correspondence, the suppression may have been eliminated also. Few, if any, antisuppression procedures may be necessary, and these patients should begin training to develop motor fusion ranges. However, most patients who have had A R C also require certain antisuppression procedures before and during motor fusion training.

Patients who have suppression, but who have always had normal correspondence, can immediately start with traditional antisuppression training. If A R C can be absolutely ruled out, it is all right to stimulate noncorresponding points in order to elicit diplopia, and thus, break down suppression. Procedures designed to make the patient aware of simultaneous perception by stimulation of noncorresponding points constitute the bi-ocular phase of orthoptics.

The next step in treatment is the binocular phase, consisting of superimposition, flat fusion, and stereopsis training. Superimposition training can often be skipped, once A R C has been successfully eliminated. However, the doctor should check carefully for foveal suppression. Flynn et al.[1] recommended using a combination of superimposition targets (e.g., circle and star) with entoptic images. This is ordinarily done in the Synoptophore. As in A R C training (Chapter Nine), there are many possible combinations of various images.

The particular procedures recommended by Flynn et al. are as follows:

Monitoring
Foveal Suppression

Haidinger's brushes are to be seen by only one eye, and each eye is to see a real image. An afterimage (preferably a vertical line) is generated for the eye without the H.B. For example, the slide for the left eye could be a circle. It should be transparent, so that the H.B. can be easily seen by this eye. The right eye, seeing the A.I., is presented with a translucent slide with a star. The patient with normal correspondence and without foveal suppression should be able to superimpose the star, circle, H.B. and A.I. when this is accomplished. As progress is made, the procedure is repeated, but with flat fusion slides rather than superimposition targets. Fusional motor ranges can be developed at this point in time.

The monitoring of bifoveal fixation is made more critical by H.B. substitution for the A.I. Two H.B.'s can cause a fluttering phenomenon, if they are properly superimposed. If the two H.B.'s separate while the flat fusion targets appear to remain fused, A R C with a small angle of anomaly is indicated. Foveal suppression is indicated if the flutter ceases, even though no separation takes place.

If complete functional cure is expected, the patient should be given intensive foveal antisuppression training at some point in therapy. Otherwise, peripheral fusion will continue to mask the presence of foveal suppression. The use of entoptic phenomena for monitoring foveal suppression is important, because practitioners all too often fail to check for this. One reason, perhaps, is that most first- and second-degree fusion slides for the major amblyoscope do not contain critical foveal suppression clues.

Antisuppression Factors   Although elimination of suppression is relatively easy compared to the effort required for eliminating anomalous correspondence, suppression is more variable and, therefore, a rigid structured sequence of antisuppression procedures is not feasible. The therapeutic approach should be varied according to the patient's responses at the moment.

Practitioners have put forth literally hundreds of antisuppression training techniques. In actuality, they are often just variations of tests used to detect suppression. As with testing, the instruments used for training are based on a few basic dissociative methods, e.g., colored filters or septums.

There are 12 antisuppression factors that should always be considered when treating a patient with suppression. They are listed in Table 10A.

PREVENTION OF SUPPRESSION BY OCCLUSION   As in A R C therapy, occlusion between training sessions is generally necessary. Patching is a passive form of therapy, but it does prevent suppression from recurring after it is temporarily broken down during binocular training. This is particularly important in cases of constant strabismus.

If the strabismus is truly intermittent, whereby the patient has bifoveal fusion part of the time, occlusion is contraindicated. Total occlusion may result in an intermittent strabismus becoming constant. This is sometimes referred to as "occlusion strabismus." Compensating prisms, rather than occlusion, may be used in these cases in order to prevent suppression.

Occlusion may also be used in cases of small-angle constant strabismus. They have foveal suppression; yet, there is peripheral fusion that can keep a larger latent deviation from becoming manifest. The use of occlusion must, therefore, be very closely supervised because a small-angle constant strabismus can turn into a large-angle constant strabismus. This is an alarming event unless the patient has been forewarned. A thorough program of strabismus therapy must be anticipated before patching is recommended.

At some point in the therapy program when bifoveal fusion is possible, occlusion antisuppression therapy can be in the form of attenuation of the dominant eye. This requires careful empirical evaluation for determining which filters and/or lenses are best for maintenance of fusion.

TABLE 10A. Factors in Anti-Suppression Training

1. Prevention of suppression by occlusion
2. Naturalness of the environment
3. Attention
4. Brightness
5. Target size
6. Intermittent stimuli
7. Target movement
8. Target contrast
9. Color
10. Tactile and Kinesthetic senses
11. Auditory sense
12. Combinations

The fact of the naturalness of testing conditions was discussed in Chapter Two (see Table 2A). When the intensity of suppression is deep, it is best to begin antisuppression with procedures that are less natural and then proceed to those having more natural seeing conditions.

NATURALNESS OF THE ENVIRONMENT

One of the cardinal rules of orthoptics is that training must be within the patient's capability. If the procedure is so similar to habitual seeing conditions that there is constant suppression, less natural seeing conditions should be used until suppression can be broken. Training should begin with procedures at this level, rather than frustrating the patient by using procedures in which he is unable to appreciate simultaneous perception.

The attention factor is a very important consideration in the treatment of suppression. The therapist should continually remind the patient to be

ATTENTION

attentive of the target presented to the suppressing eye. This can momentarily stop the suppression.

The patient with alternating strabismus sees the target that gets his attention. The ocular image of the other target is suppressed. These patients know how to suppress either one at will. However, in the case of unilateral strabismus, the patient must pay a great amount of attention to the target of the deviating eye in order not to suppress. The patient with unilateral strabismus can use the attention factor to learn how to suppress alternately. This is helpful in disrupting the habitual pattern of suppression being confined to one eye. Since this is only a preliminary step, other antisuppression measures must follow if functional results are to be expected.

BRIGHTNESS   The target before the suppressing eye should be brighter than the target before the nonsuppressing eye. This difference in the level of brightness must be large if suppression is very intense. Even patients who have very deep suppression are unlikely to suppress when the dominant eye has a very dim image and the nondominant eye has a very bright one.

TARGET SIZE   This relates to the size of the suppression zone. Refer to Table 2B in Chapter Two for zone classification and dimensions. Targets larger than the extent of suppression are tried first. For instance, if the patient has parafoveal suppression, training with foveal targets should not be used initially. Paramacular targets are appropriate in this case.

Smaller targets are gradually employed as the suppression zone shrinks as the result of therapy. Rapid progress is made at first, since it is much easier to treat peripheral rather than central suppression. Progress becomes slower as the fovea is approached.

If the deviation is large, point zero may be in the periphery with a large suppression zone. However, eliminating suppression at point zero is relatively easy compared to eliminating it at the fovea.

INTERMITTENT STIMULI   A flashing image of the suppressing eye is very effective in breaking down suppression. This may be done in free space or inside instruments. For example, the flashing of one target of the major amblyoscope works well. This also serves to get the patient's attention. Alpha rhythm flashing is even more effective. Theoretically, suppression does not occur with this type of stimulation. It is good practice to follow up with free space training using the T.B.I. and the Fusion Aider.

TARGET MOVEMENT   This is effective for several reasons. One is that noncorresponding points are being stimulated by the oscillation of the target. These points are less likely to be suppressed than corresponding points. Another possible reason is that retinal receptor fatigue may set in when the same corresponding points are continually stimulated. Movement of the target before one eye prevents this and tends to disrupt suppression. Also, a moving target is apt to draw the patient's attention, tending to keep the target from being suppressed.

Movement of one target under binocular conditions can be brought about in a number of ways. In the office, the major amblyoscope is ideal. For home training, the patient may hold a mirror that is angled before one eye in such a way that he can superimpose two different objects in the room. Getz[2] suggests that a TV can be used for one eye, while the other eye sees an object in the room through the mirror. Jiggling the mirror can create the desired target movement.

TARGET CONTRAST

The contrast between figure and ground is a factor in the treatment of suppression. If the contrast is high, there is less likelihood of suppression. The suppressing eye should be presented with a high-contrast target. This is one of the reasons why suppression is more likely under natural seeing conditions, since figure-ground contrast is relatively low. On the other hand, simplified targets in the major amblyoscope with high contrast are less likely to be suppressed.

COLOR

Certain physiological factors may be involved when color is used, but colored targets hold the patient's attention better than black and white ones. Targets are usually colored for both eyes, but it may be helpful to use a black and white target for the nonsuppressing eye, and one that is colored for the suppressing eye. This is applicable for first-degree targets, but this mixture is generally not feasible for most second- and third-degree targets.

TACTILE AND KINESTHETIC SENSES

Tactile and kinesthetic stimulation can be used for antisuppression purposes. Each practitioner has his own techniques in this regard. Cheiroscopic drawing is the most well-known procedure utilizing the tactile and kinesthetic senses (see Figure 10-1).

Vodnoy[3] reports a chasing technique that can be done with cheiroscopic drawing. He uses the Single Oblique Mirror Stereoscope-Cheiroscope.[a] It is portable, and can be used for home training. A pointer held by the therapist is moved along a printed design. This is seen through the mirror by the patient's dominant eye. The suppressing eye directly views the black surface of the instrument's baseboard. The patient holds a pointer on the baseboard and positions the tip to superimpose with the tip of the therapist's pointer, which is seen in the mirror. The patient attempts to keep the tips superimposed as the therapist's pointer is moved.

Cheiroscopic drawing exercises can be excellent for out-of-office antisuppression exercises. The procedure initially used is for the dominant eye to view a printed design through the mirror. At first, the design should be rather simple. More complex designs can be included as the patient begins to master this procedure. The nondominant eye views a blank white sheet of

[a]Available from Bernell Corp.

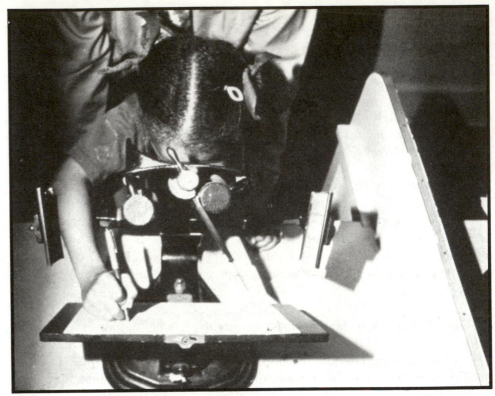

FIGURE 10-1 — An example of a cheiroscope being used for tracing while the tactile and kinesthetic senses aid anti-suppression therapy

paper, on which is seen a pencil tip held by the patient. The patient practices drawing the picture by tracing the design seen in the mirror. There are pitfalls to this training procedure. One is that patients may alternate fixation and, therefore, alternately suppress. Although there may be some benefit in promoting alternate suppression in the case of a unilateral strabismus, cheiroscopic drawing exercises go no further in breaking down suppression if the patient can "cheat" and draw perfectly good pictures. Another reason for contraindicating cheiroscopic drawing is that A R C may be reinforced, since the patient sees at the subjective rather than at the objective angle.

AUDITORY SENSE   Auditory stimulation can be helpful, and is an effective way to motivate the patient and to keep his attention. Therapy time may be reduced when auditory feedback devices are incorporated into the training program.

One such device is the Eye Hand Coordinator[b] (shown in Figure 10-2). The procedure requires the patient to hold two pointers having metallic tips. Proper contact with the targets sets off lights and a buzzer. When one of the

[b] Available from Keystone View, Division of Mast/Keystone.

a.

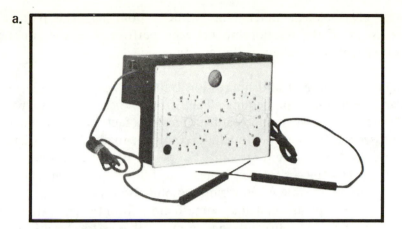

b.

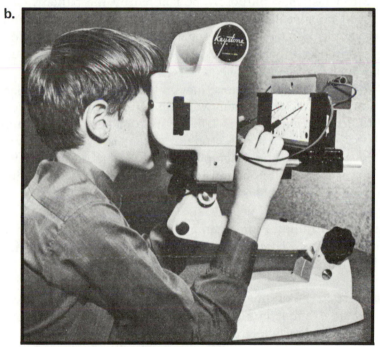

FIGURE 10-2 — The Eye Hand Coordinator can be used to provide auditory feedback in anti-suppression training. (Courtesy of Keystone View, Division of Mast/Keystone)

pointers makes contact with a numbered spot, one of the lights will turn on. When the other pointer also makes contact with the corresponding numbered spot seen by the other eye, the other light turns on, and a buzzer is activated. Once the patient knows what to expect, he is instructed to move both pointers simultaneously toward the target and attempt to touch the corresponding numbered spots at the same time. This is difficult to perform if one eye is suppressing. The involvement of the tactile and kinesthetic senses may help to break down the suppression more quickly than if the patient merely looks at stereograms without pointing. The patient soon becomes aware of the relationship between performance and suppression, and auditory feedback enhances this awareness.

COMBINATIONS

More than one factor of antisuppression training is usually involved in any particular therapeutic procedure. The effectiveness of any particular procedure is greater when more antisuppression factors are included. With the Cheiroscope, for instance, include colored pencils, have patient blink suppressing eye (intermittent stimuli), tap pencil tip for auditory sense, etc. With only a few pieces of equipment, a full scope of antisuppression procedures can be possible when various combinations are used.

It should be kept in mind that some factors in antisuppression training are not always favorable. For instance, a target that is too bright, too large, and moving too fast may purposely be ignored by the patient. Or, certain colors may not be appealing to the patient, and in this regard, color vision deficiencies should also be tested, especially in males. Also, auditory sense can be a hindrance to antisuppression training if there are too many distracting sounds.

Tactile and kinesthetic senses may, at times, cause the patient to suppress. For instance, the patient who tends to suppress one eye may be more apt to do so when trying to balance on a balance board. Suppression may result because the patient's afferent system is overloaded with other stimuli. As antisuppression therapy progresses, more complete multi-sensorial approaches can be incorporated into the training program for the development of good binocularity.

Bi-Ocular Training

This phase of antisuppression training requires the stimulation of non-corresponding points. These procedures are based on the principles of physiological and pathological diplopia.

USE OF PHYSIOLOGICAL DIPLOPIA

This is the normal type of diplopia that occurs for a nonfixated object. Refer to the illustrated example in Figure 1-12 (Chapter One), in which one object is seen diplopically. Physiological diplopia training may be done with either one or two targets for stimulation of noncorresponding points.

TRAINING WITH ONE TARGET

Assume there is an esotropia of the right eye and there is a suppression zone from point zero to the fovea of the right eye. Now, if neither eye is fixating and the object (penlight, for example) is moved closer to the patient, noncorresponding points on the temporal portion of each retina are stimulated (see Figure 10-3).

This bi-ocular procedure is good in cases of esotropia with deep suppression. Because the dioptric image of the right eye is not on the suppression zone, the patient can usually experience diplopia under these conditions, particularly if the room illumination is lowered. Diplopia can almost always be elicited with the inclusion of red-green filters.

Working with targets within the angle of deviation is helpful, not only to arouse the binocular sensorial awareness of simultaneous perception, but also to cause a motor divergence movement of the eyes. This happens as the target is moved farther away, providing the patient can maintain seeing diplopically. If, though, there is no divergence when the target is moved farther away, the dioptric image of the right eye will fall on the suppression zone, and diplopic perception will be gone.

Strong plus lenses may be used in this procedure to aid divergence. The incorporation of several other antisuppression factors (e.g., attention, flashing, etc.) can make this type of physiological diplopia training very effective.

Training with one target may also be done when prisms are used. If there is a strong overcorrection of base-out prism before the esotropic eye, the temporal retina of that eye will be stimulated. The patient is urged to

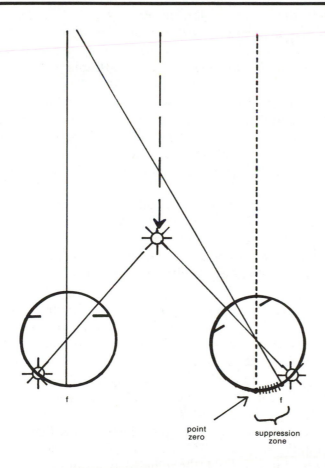

point
zero

suppression
zone

FIGURE 10-3 — Illustration of target being placed within the angle of esotropia to elicit physiological diplopia

maintain diplopia while the prismatic power is gradually reduced. This is the optical equivalent of the previous method of gradually moving the target to a farther distance when it has been placed inside the angle of strabismus.

Inverse prism may be used to elicit diplopia in strabismic patients. In the example of esotropia of the right eye, the prism is placed base-in before the right eye. The use of base-in prism causes the dioptric image to fall on a retinal point outside the suppression zone, and the patient should become aware of homonymous diplopia. If there is convergence of the eyes, the separation distance of the ocular images becomes greater. If, however, the patient diverges by a sufficient amount, the dioptric image of the deviating eye falls on the suppression zone. The disappearance of one of the diplopic images provides feedback and tells the patient that a divergent movement has been made.

The goal of this procedure is for the patient to become aware of diplopia with divergence, indicating a reduction in the size of the suppression zone as well as a lessening of the intensity of the suppression.

The doctor should always be on guard for A R C. This anomaly can eliminate diplopia and mislead the patient into thinking suppression is the sole cause of the disappearance of the diplopic image. Inverse prism procedures are not recommended for antisuppression training when anomalous correspondence is suspected.

Vertical prisms are good for antisuppression training. It is easier to elicit diplopia in the vertical than in the horizontal meridian, because the vertical size of the suppression zone is smaller than the horizontal (refer to Figure 2-1c). This is true for esotropia, but not always for exotropia. Some authorities think that the entire temporal hemi-retina may be suppressed in exotropia.

Alternate fixation and/or accommodative rock exercises may be included once the patient can easily perceive vertical diplopia.

No matter what type of prism procedure is used (i.e., horizontal or vertical), the rapid interposing and removing of a prism before the deviating eye helps the patient in having simultaneous perception.

TRAINING WITH TWO TARGETS

Simultaneous perception training with two targets is done conveniently with instruments, such as the major amblyoscope. For instance, the circle and star can be positioned so noncorresponding points are stimulated. The goal is to have both ocular images seen simultaneously in all base-in and base-out positions. After that achievement, superimposition training is given.

The Bernell Mirror Stereoscope (Figure 2-15) is good for simultaneous perception training at home, and is a substitute for the major amblyoscope.

The Brewster stereoscope (example illustrated in Figure 2-18) may be used for simultaneous perception training. The Keystone Test number 1 (DB-10A), with the dog and the pig, is an example of a simultaneous perception demand. A stereogram such as this lacks some of the advantages of first-degree fusion targets used in the major amblyoscope. The principal disadvantage is the lack of movement. Another is the relatively small base-in to base-out range.

The use of split stereograms may overcome the disadvantage of lack of movement. Also, a greater prismatic range can be effected if the patient wears prisms.

Cantonnet devised a practical bi-ocular test for suppression, described by Cantonnet and Filliozat.[4] A septum is used for dissociation (see Figure 10-4). The next step is to have the patient fixate a bright light with his nondominant eye while the dominant eye is presented with a moving target, such as a hand. This determines whether or not the patient has appreciation of rudimentary simultaneous perception. This procedure should be practiced at home if the patient has trouble seeing both objects. Cantonnet believed that this should be one of the initial steps in deneutralization (i.e., antisuppression training).

USE OF PATHOLOGICAL DIPLOPIA

This type of diplopia occurs when the fixated object appears doubled, owing to a manifest deviation of the visual axes. In order for diplopia to be classified as being pathological, the dioptric image of the fixated image must fall on the fovea of the fixating eye, and the dioptric image of the fixated object must fall on point zero, which is a noncorresponding point. The suppression at point zero of the deviating eye must be broken down before

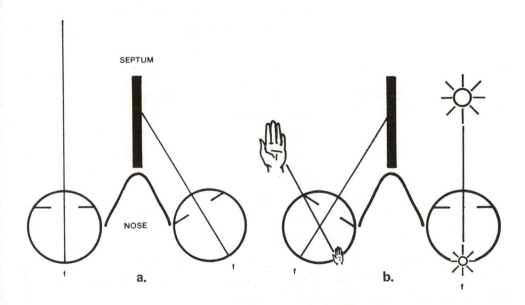

FIGURE 10-4 — The procedure of Cantonnet for testing suppression. (a) Septum is used for dissociation; (b) Physiological diplopia is elicited by stimulation of non-corresponding points.

pathological diplopia is perceived. It is hoped that compensatory motor fusional movements will be stimulated by the desire to eliminate this type of diplopia.

CONTRAINDICATIONS
There are two risks the doctor takes when pathological diplopia is used in strabismus therapy. One bad side effect is that A R C may be produced, or an already existing A R C may be strengthened. There must be a recapitulation of therapy in this event, and those procedures discussed in Chapter Nine pertaining to anomalous correspondence must be used. The other risk is that intractable diplopia may result from the indiscriminate use of pathological diplopia training. The doctor must be prepared to go all the way toward functional cure before this procedure is used.

USEFULNESS
There are two advantages for using pathological diplopia in cases of strabismus. One is that the annoyance of this type of diplopia may motivate the patient to use corresponding points. This works well if the points correspond in a normal manner, but not if there is anomalous correspondence. The awareness of pathological diplopia may cause the patient to make the necessary vergence movement so that bifoveal fixation is attained if correspondence is normal.

Besides helping to straighten the eyes, pathological diplopia is a useful monitoring mechanism for intermittent deviations. The patient should be taught to use the diplopia as a cue to immediately straighten the eyes.

The procedures used to develop awareness of pathological diplopia can

---

TABLE 10B. Typical Sequence of Procedures to Develop Awareness of Pathological Diplopia

1. Penlight fixation with patient wearing red and green filters, in darkened room, and intermittent, rapid occlusion of deviating eye
2. Same, but with red lens over fixating eye (no green lens)
3. Same, but with red lens over deviating eye
4. Same, but without intermittent occlusion
5. Same, but with pink lens over fixating eye
6. Same, but with pink lens over deviating eye
7. Same, but with no lens over either eye
8. Repeat procedures 1-7, but with normal room illumination.
9. Fixation of ordinary object in room while deviating eye is intermittently and rapidly occluded or blinked
10. Same, but without intermittent occlusion or blinking of the deviating eye

be quite simple. Any suppression test in which one target is employed can also be used for training. It is generally best to start with the less natural procedures and work toward the more natural ones. A typical sequence of training procedures that may be used to develop the patient's awareness of pathological diplopia is presented in Table 10B.

Sensory Fusion Training

This phase of antisuppression training is intimately linked to motor fusion training. Consequently, this will be covered along with therapeutic procedures relating to the motoric aspect of vision training.

Several aspects of suppression therapy, however, should be re-emphasized at this time. It is most important for the doctor (and therapist) to monitor suppression during motor fusion training. If, for example, a patient has peripheral suppression, he may not make the requisite vergence movements at all as prismatic demand is increased, e.g., via Risley prisms, vectograms, anaglyphic targets, or stereoscopes. Nothing is being accomplished in such an event. Even if there is peripheral sensory fusion but with central suppression, the patient will make only the necessary vergence movements to keep the target single. Exact vergence alignment will not be maintained.

It may be necessary to incorporate entoptic monitoring methods in order to rule out central suppression and/or small-angle A R C. An interesting case-in-point was a young patient who claimed she could see foveal suppression clues of a flat fusion target in a Brewster stereoscope. The target was a small digit with a dot above, seen only by the right eye, and a dot below, seen only by the left eye. The patient reported seeing both dots simultaneously, even though she had a small-angle constant, unilateral esotropia of the left eye. Very careful A R C testing revealed a small angle of anomaly. Subsequent questioning indicated that the lower dot was "faded but never gone." It is speculated that the lower dot was visualized with point "a" rather than point "f." This case of A R C could mislead an unsuspecting clinician into the conclusion that the patient is bifixating and not suppressing.

It should be noted that patients with heterophoria, as well as those with heterotropia, may have suppression. The heterophore will tend to have only central, rather than peripheral, suppression. Anisometropia is one reason, and vergence stress is the other. Anisometropic suppression is evaluated with an ortho demand. Suppression due to vergence stress is monitored as vergence demands are induced, either directly by prisms or other means, or indirectly via spherical, plus or minus, lenses. This must be monitored during motor fusion training.

11 | Management of Nonconcomitant Deviations

Patients who have nonconcomitant deviations due to extraocular muscle paresis should have all of the necessary professional attention that can be provided, in addition to being treated for their binocular problems. A thorough evaluation of nonconcomitancy (discussed in Chapter One) is necessary for the proper amelioration of the deviation. Management and treatment involve the prevention of secondary contractures, maintenance of fusion, and appropriate referrals.

Prevention of Secondary Contractures

The prognosis for remission of acute extraocular muscle paresis is good. Hugonnier et al.[1] believe that 80 percent of the patients will recover with total function after a waiting time of three to six months. Although waiting is advocated, certain therapeutic and preventive measures should be instituted in the meantime. Occlusion and ocular calisthenics are the principal procedures employed in these cases.

Use of Occlusion

Diplopia is the most pressing problem facing patients with recent onset of extraocular muscle paresis. This annoyance can easily be eliminated by prescribing an occluder to be worn over the affected eye. Although this has been the traditional method in these cases, generally it is better to recommend alternate occlusion rather than confining the patch to the paretic eye.

Occluding the sound eye may provide beneficial stimulation to the paretic eye that can lead to eye movements into the field of action of the paretic muscle. This may reduce the risk of secondary contracture of the homolateral antagonist. For example, if the right lateral rectus is paretic, patching of the left eye might compel the patient to occasionally abduct the right eye in order to see on gaze right. This is true, unless the individual has completely become a head turner. Patching in this manner causes the right medial rectus muscle to relax during abduction of the right eye; and consequently, this may help prevent contracture of the right medial rectus muscle.

Patching the nonparetic eye continuously can lead to trouble, because contracture may develop in the contralateral synergist. In this example where there is a paretic right lateral rectus, the yoke muscle is the left medial rectus, which will overact (because of Hering's law) when abduction is attempted by the right eye.

Alternate occlusion is preferable because of the possibility of contracture of the homolateral antagonist (when the affected eye is occluded) and of the contralateral synergist (when the sound eye is occluded) (see Figure 11-1).

Although alternate occlusion is prescribed, the affected eye should be occluded in order to avoid past pointing and problems of spatial localization when the patient is required to do critical tasks, such as those required on the job or when driving a car.

Proper use of binasal occlusion can also be applied to prevention of contracture in the case of paresis of a lateral rectus muscle. This procedure has the advantage of providing continuous alternate fixation as a stimulus for abduction of each eye. It works well on cooperative adults who understand the importance of alternately abducting each eye as much as possible. The

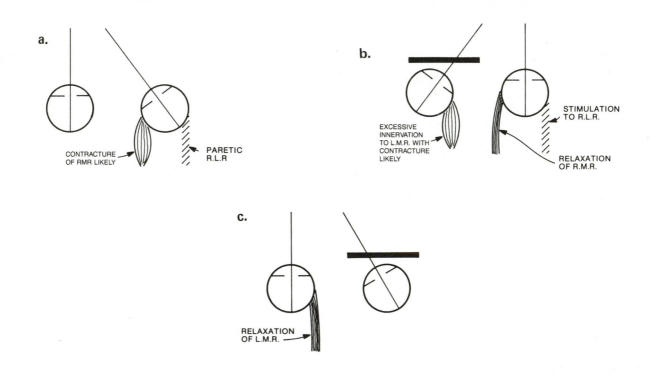

FIGURE 11-1 — Alternate occlusion for prevention of contractures. (a) Paresis of right lateral rectus with development of contracture of the right medial rectus; (b) Occlusion of non-paretic eye to prevent contracture of the right medial rectus; (c) Occlusion of paretic eye to prevent contracture of the left medial rectus.

young child, however, is less apt to cooperate fully. He tends to become a head turner and use only one eye. Full occlusion is recommended in such instances.

Partial occlusion can be used to prevent diplopia when the patch is regionally positioned before one eye. The diplopic patient with right lateral paresis will be relieved by a patch on the temporal portion of the right spectacle lens (see Figure 11-2a). This should be recommended only if the nonconcomitancy is of long duration with no chance of remission, because this procedure does nothing in the way of preventing contracture. It merely serves to prevent diplopia in a particular position of gaze.

If the paresis is of recent onset, the regional application of prism is preferable to prescribing an opaque patch so that fusion can be maintained in all positions of gaze. In the case of RLR paresis, a base-out Fresnel prism is placed on the temporal half of the right spectacle lens (see Figure 11-2b).

Exercises designed to force the paretic eye to move, particularly toward the field of action of the affected muscle, may help in restoring function and preventing contracture.

OCULAR CALISTHENICS

The usual procedure is to occlude the sound eye, while the unoccluded paretic eye attempts to follow a moving target, such as a Marsden ball. In the case of paresis of a lateral rectus, the accommodative rock procedure, using a septum and a laterally swinging ball (see Figure 2-49, Chapter Two), is effective.

Fixation targets may be stationary. The patient makes voluntary saccadic eye movements to various objects around the room; or systematized programs requiring accurate fixations in a predetermined sequence may be employed.

There are many variations of ocular calisthenics. Recommended examples of these are in the monocular training activities that were discussed in Chapter Seven. Although these are used in the treatment of amblyopia, they may also be used in cases of nonconcomitancy (see Table 7A-D for list of these procedures).

Occasionally, there is the functionally monocular patient who has a recent paresis. This may be an individual who has always had poor vision in one eye, or it could be a truly monocular situation in which there is a prosthetic eye. If the good eye becomes paretic, the patient can have problems similar to those of the amblyopic patient who is wearing a patch on the nonamblyopic eye. The patient tends to past point and show signs of faulty spatial localization.

OTHER METHODS

A prism may be tried if the problem is severe. The base of the prism is placed in the direction of the action field of the paretic muscle. If the right lateral rectus is paretic, the patient probably past points on right gaze. A base-out prism worn before the right eye may help the patient in viewing on right gaze. The prism minimizes the need for abduction of the right eye.

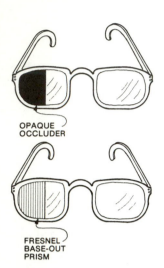

OPAQUE
OCCLUDER

FRESNEL
BASE-OUT
PRISM

FIGURE 11-2 — Partial occlusion for relief of diplopia in
cases of nonconcomitancy. (a)
Occluder on temporal portion
of spectacle lens in case of
right lateral rectus paresis; (b)
Base-Out Fresnel Press-On [T.M.]
prism for paresis of recent
onset when fusion can be
maintained on dextroversion
with the aid of the prism.

Prismatic power must be determined empirically, and much is dependent
upon the severity of the muscle underaction.

Although prism over the paretic eye may at times be helpful in reducing
errors of faulty spatial localization, this procedure is of no help in preventing
contracture.

Hurtt et al.[2] state that wearing of conjugate prisms (i.e., both prisms
either "base-left" or "base-right") may be recommended as a possible means
for prevention of contracture. If the right lateral rectus is paretic, the patient
would wear prism over each eye (i.e., base-out before O.S. and base-in before
O.D.). A dextroversion resulting from the patient's viewing through the
prisms causes stimulation of the paretic right lateral rectus and relaxation of
the right medial rectus.

Burian and Von Noorden[3] list several methods for preventing
contracture, including injection of the homolateral antagonistic muscle with
an anesthetic. Another possible recommendation is very early surgery before
there is time for development of contracture. This is normally a recession of
the homolateral antagonist. They also cite Guibor's method to prevent
contracture by placing a prism before the sound eye. In the case of a right
lateral rectus paresis, for example, the prism is worn base-out before the left
eye, to relax the right medial rectus.

In spite of these preventive measures, Burian and Von Noodren state that
there are no studies available indicating that any of these methods are
effective in preventing contracture of the homolateral antagonist of a paretic
muscle. This pessimism notwithstanding, I feel it behooves the doctor to try
to prevent contracture. Preventive measures are particularly important in the
developmental years of young patients who can develop contractures very
soon after the onset of extraocular muscle paresis.

Maintenance of Fusion

It is important to keep the patient fusing as much of the time as possible
following an acquired extraocular muscle paresis. The majority of patients
have a history of good binocularity prior to the onset of nonconcomitancy.
Since sensory fusion has been good, this type of fusion training may not be
necessary. However, the expansion of the motor fusion range is recommended in practically all cases.

There are a few peculiar instances in which the onset of paresis appears
to be of help to a patient with an existing deviation. For example, if the
patient has a large exotropia and acquires a partial paresis of the right lateral
rectus, the angle of deviation is reduced in the primary position, and greatly
so on dextroversion.

Nevertheless, fusion training should still be recommended, because
nonconcomitancy is not a suitable solution for decreasing the angle of
deviation. If there is no remission and the degree of nonconcomitancy
remains the same, the patient will subsequently be required to have excellent
vergence facility in order to maintain reasonably comfortable binocular
vision in all positions of gaze. However, remission is likely to occur, and the

patient will need to have good fusional vergence when the large magnitude of deviation returns.

Lenses and prisms may be helpful in maintaining fusion in cases of recent onset. Plus lenses may be used to reduce eso deviations at nearpoint. Minus lenses may help the patient with an exodeviation, whether fixation is at far or near.

Compensating prisms, particularly the Fresnels, are good for maintaining fusion. The power should be on the conservative side, with the patient wearing just enough prism to maintain fusion, yet be comfortable at the same time. Weaning the patient from prism is gradual, reducing the powers commensurately with remission of the paresis.

In those cases with a history of poor sensory fusion, prisms are not recommended, because the angle of deviation may increase as a result. Refer to the discussion of the prism adaptation test in Chapter Three. The increase in the angle of deviation tends to exacerbate the condition of contractures.

Extraocular muscle surgery is another possible way of maintaining fusion. However, it is generally wise for surgery to be postponed for three to six months, since the chance of remission is good. In the meantime, lenses and/or prisms are employed to maintain fusion whenever feasible. When surgery is necessary, recession of the homolateral antagonist is the principal procedure for reducing the magnitude of the deviation. Somehow, this may prevent contracture of this muscle. Resection is sometimes used, but only for a temporary straightening effect of the eye. No function is restored to a completely paretic muscle because the muscle has been resected.

Referrals

Patients with acute nonconcomitancy should receive immediate medical attention with neurologists and internists being consulted. There is less urgency in chronic cases of long duration.

Ophthalmological care is required when there is active pathology of the eye, adnexa or the orbit. Evaluation is also recommended in chronic cases, if restricted ocular motility is due to mechanical causes, or if strabismus surgery is contemplated.

The optometrist's role in cases of nonconcomitancy is one of detecting, evaluating and referring. After necessary medical care, the functional aspects of the nonconcomitant deviation may be managed by the use of lenses, prisms, occlusion, calisthenics and other procedures for the maintenance of fusion.

Case Example

An example of the management of a case with a paresis of the left superior oblique is given in Case Number Nine, discussed in Chapters Three and Five.

Assuming the patient has received all necessary medical attention and care, the procedures relating to the management of this case are as follows:

1. Temporarily occlude the left eye to relieve symptoms.
2. Prescribe alternate occlusion as soon as possible.

3. Recommend ocular calisthenics.
4. Discontinue occlusion and prescribe base-down prism before the left eye to maintain fusion. The power should be just enough to allow fusion in the primary position and slightly beyond the midline on dextroversion.
5. If the eso deviation disrupts fusion at near, prescribe necessary plus lenses.
6. Allow the patient to tilt head (to the right shoulder in this case) to compensate for the cyclo deviation. Then have patient try to maintain fusion when head is upright; then, later, when head is tilted toward left shoulder.
7. Conjugate prisms may be tried if the patient can maintain fusion in the primary position without compensating vertical prism. In this case, an equal amount of base-up prism is worn over each eye. This forces the left eye to move downward (approaching the field of action of the affected superior oblique).
8. Assuming the patient has good sensory fusion, the ranges of motor fusion are expanded, i.e., horizontal, vertical, and torsional.
9. The patient attempts to maintain fusion in all positions of gaze without the aid of prisms.
10. Assuming spontaneous remission of the superior oblique paresis, no further treatment is necessary. If remission does not occur, extraocular muscle surgery may be required.

Most of the procedures listed above are carried out away from the office. The patient may be advised to follow specific instructions during each of the procedures. For example, when the right eye is occluded, the patient should be encouraged to sit to the left of the television so that the left eye will have to adduct, to help stimulate the left superior oblique and relax its homolateral antagonist, the left inferior oblique.

Treatment for the above case is merely representative, and in no way is this meant to be applicable to all cases of superior oblique paresis. No two cases are identical, even though the same muscle, or muscles, may be involved. Therefore, management and treatment will vary with each case.

12 | Training Procedures for Eso Deviations

The diagnostic variables of a deviation were discussed in Chapter One. They relate to the motoric aspect of the binocular problem, and play an important part in the determination of the prognosis in any given case of esotropia or esophoria.

Many clinicians find it convenient to put the classification of eso deviations into three main categories of divergence insufficiency, basic eso, and convergence excess. This is a convenient way of expressing the type of esophoria or esotropia for a particular case. It must be remembered, however, that only two of the nine variables are taken into account. They are the magnitude of the eso deviation at far and near, and the AC/A ratio.

This method of classification is more applicable to heterophoria than to strabismus, because other variables, such as cosmesis, are usually not significant. Nevertheless, it has been customary to use this scheme in cases of heterotropia when a quick summary of the vergence problem is needed. Also, the use of only two categories avoids the hundreds of possible permutations that could be listed when the nine variables are considered.

For this reason, the discussion in this chapter will follow this simplified classification of eso deviations, because otherwise, it would be impossible to mention the countless number of diagnoses. It should be remembered, however, that a complete diagnosis for any one patient should include all nine variables, and the diagnosis is far from being complete when it is superficially summarized as being either divergence insufficiency, basic eso, or convergence excess.

The patient with an eso deviation must be sensorily ready for flat fusion demands before motor fusion training is given. It is logical to assume that, with intensive therapy for A R C and suppression, the patient should have developed an acute awareness of simultaneous perception, as well as having fairly good first-degree fusion (superimposition). Refer to Chapters Nine and Ten for suppression and A R C procedures.

General Approach

In addition to sensory fusion development, ocular motility must be relatively normal (refer to Chapter Eleven). It is usually helpful to include duction and version motility training prior to and during the early part of the motor fusion training program for eso deviations. Even in cases of concomitant eso deviations, each eye may have limited abduction. This is particularly so for the nondominant eye. Figure 12-1 shows a patient doing motility training requiring saccadic versions.

Motor fusion training begins with second-degree sensory fusion targets. Third-degree fusion targets are introduced as suppression is further reduced with binocular therapy.

The patient should be kept fusing as much of the time as possible. Prisms and/or lenses may be needed for this purpose. Very large angles may require surgery for reduction in magnitude, if optical means are inadequate.

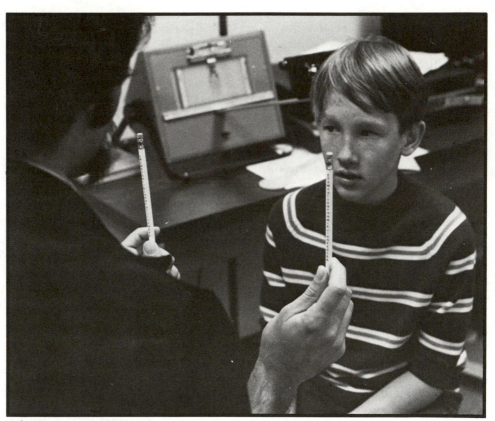

FIGURE 12-1 — Motility training with the use of two Alphabet Pencils

Foveal suppression should be monitored periodically, and the patient should not be discouraged too quickly if a persistent central suppression remains. This may be improved with time, and good binocular motor coordination is of great help in breaking down foveal suppression.

Flat fusion training is started at the objective angle of deviation in the case of constant esotropia. If the deviation is latent or if the manifest deviation is intermittent, it is better to start with an ortho vergence demand, if the patient can manage this.

Various combinations of antisuppression factors for reducing suppression and enhancing the fusion percept may be required for the constant esotrope. These procedures may use flashing, large target size, brightness, etc. As soon as flat fusion is steady and consistent for a particular pair of targets, the vergence demand should be changed slightly from the position of no demand (i.e., targets at objective angle of deviation for cases of constant E.T.) to a new position of base-out demand.

If, for example, angle H is 15 p.d., the tubes of the major amblyoscope

---

TABLE 12A. Methods for Changing Prismatic Demand

A. Prisms
  1. Risley
  2. Loose prisms
  3. Prism bar
      a. Conventional
      b. Wick's Fresnel bar

B. Use of Septums
  1. Brewster Stereoscope (increase separation distance on stereogram for B.I. effect and decrease for B.O. effect)
  2. Wheatstone Stereoscope (change angle of mirror(s) for B.I. or B.O. effect)
  3. Remy Separator (produces base-in demand, but this may be reduced by decreasing the separation distance of the two targets)

C. Vectographics and colored filters (lateral separation determines prismatic demand)

D. Plus and minus spherical lenses
  1. Plus creates a base-out demand (for fusional vergence).
  2. Minus creates a base-in demand (for fusional vergence).

E. Chiastopic (crossed) and orthopic (uncrossed)
  1. Chiastopic creates a base-out demand.
  2. Orthopic creates a base-in demand.

F. Changing fixation distance
  1. Inside instruments (e.g., Telebinocular from far to near setting and vice versa)
  2. In free space (e.g., Bagolini lenses and penlight at far and near)

---

are slowly moved from the 15 p.d. base-out setting to 20 p.d. base-out setting. The patient attempts to maintain fusion during this gradual change in vergence demand. If the patient is able to converge 5 p.d., the tubes are reset at 15, and then 5 p.d. base-in demand is introduced to the patient; that is, the base-out setting on the instrument scale is reduced to the 10 p.d. base-out position.

Base-out and base-in demand procedures are repeated until the patient's fusion range, with clear vision, is at least ten p.d. Accommodative changes will blur the fused image; blur indicates pure fusional vergences are not in play. In other words, when the target becomes blurred, the patient is using changes in accommodative vergence in order to maintain single vision.

As a rule, most patients with eso deviations are ready for free space training when the horizontal motor fusion range is 10 p.d. or more. There are numerous methods for changing prismatic vergence demand. A list is presented in Table 12A.

Prisms are practical for creating vergence demands in free space. They can be hand-held by the patient. A Risley prism before the nondominant eye produces a gradually changing demand, and this may be desirable when the patient's ability to fuse is equivocal. This simulates the smoothness of movement afforded by the major amblyoscope. However, the patient should soon try to learn to perform with discrete changes of prism, as with loose prisms of various power, because everyday seeing involves step vergences more often than non-step, or "sliding," vergences.

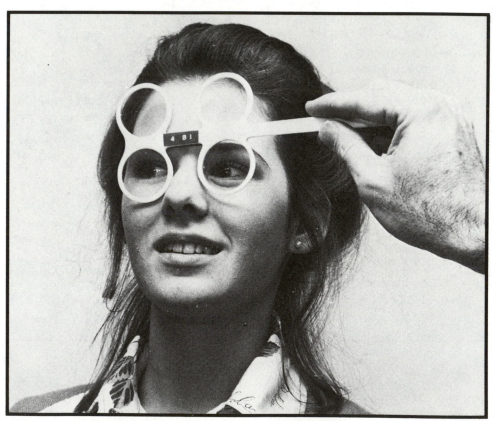

FIGURE 12-2 — Flip prisms for expanding range of motor fusion

Rapid changes in vergence demand are conveniently done with the use of a prism bar. Wick[1] describes the fabrication of an inexpensive prism bar made with Fresnel Press-On™ prisms. This has the advantage of less weight and bulkiness as compared to conventional glass or plastic prism bars.

Flip prisms are also very good for step vergence training (see Figure 12-2). Only base-out prisms may have to be used at first, until the patient can begin to fuse when base-in prisms are flipped in front of the eyes. The important rule to remember is that the demand must be within the patient's ability. As the motor range expands, the difference in prisms can be made greater. The range is eventually expanded to include an adequate base-in vergence. The goal is to have the patient fuse, with clear vision, a base-in demand that is twice the magnitude of the eso deviation. This is Sheard's traditionally used criterion.

Instruments with septums are used for changing prismatic demand. The most obvious examples are the incorporation of septums into stereoscopes, such as the Wheatstone or the Brewster. The Bernell Mirror Stereoscope (Figure 2-15) is an example of a Wheatstone instrument that is good for home training. The Stori-View Stereoscope (Figure 2-19) is an example of a Brewster stereoscope incorporating prisms for vergence demand changes. Prismatic changes can be made as required, which is ideal for home training in cases of eso deviations.

The Remy Separator is an excellent, but infrequently used, home training device that utilizes a septum. It is useful for eso therapy since this presents a base-in demand (see Figure 12-3). Since there is no optical system involved in the Remy Separator, the vergence demand can be figured quite simply. Suppose the fixation distance to the F and the L is 40 cm. If the separation between the F and the L is 6 cm, the demand for divergence is 15 p.d. base-in. This is calculated as follows:

1. At 40 cm, every 4 mm equals 1 p.d.
2. Convert 6 cm to 60 mm.
3. To find prism diopters, divide 60 by 4.
4. Therefore, the demand is 15 p.d.

The base-in demand can be increased by making the target separation greater. Similarly, the base-in demand can be decreased by making the separation less. It should be noted that the eso deviation must be overcome by the patient, in addition to the base-in demand from the ortho position. If the patient has 10 p.d. of esophoria at 40 cm fixation distance, he would have to diverge a total of 25 p.d. in order to fuse the F and L.

Most esophoric or esotropic patients cannot perform on this test at first, without either the aid of plus lenses (to reduce the accommodative convergence) or without base-out prisms. These optical aids are useful in the beginning, but the patient should be weaned away from them as soon as possible. Any set of fusion targets, either second degree or third degree, can be used with the Remy Separator, depending on what the patient prefers.

Other methods for creating vergence demands include the use of

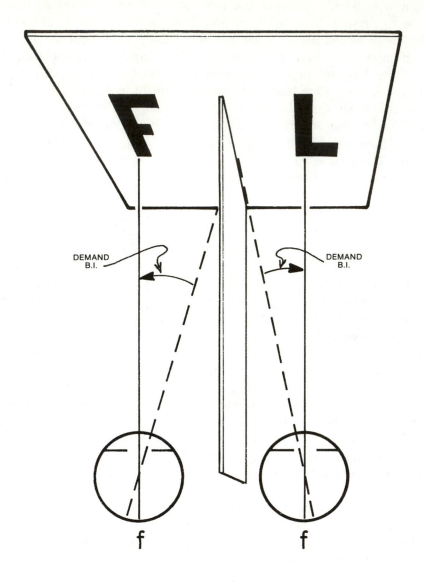

FIGURE 12-3 — Top view drawing of the Remy Separator, illustrating the principle of base-in vergence demand with this instrument

vectographics, colored filters, lenses (binocular accommodative rock), and free space fusion exercises.

Farpoint Eso Problems   The eso deviations considered to be farpoint eso problems include the categories of divergence insufficiency and basic eso. The category of convergence excess is classically considered to be one that causes a nearpoint problem because of the high AC/A ratio. There are, however, some cases of convergence excess exotropia in which the far eso deviation is so large that the farpoint deviation requires attention, as do those cases of basic eso and divergence insufficiency.

If the patient has an esotropia of 15 p.d. at far and 15 p.d. at near, he is considered to have a basic eso deviation. If, however, he had 15 p.d. at far but only 5 p.d. at near, he would be considered to have divergence insufficiency.

In the case of the basic eso, the AC/A is normal. Therefore, the esotropic (or esophoric) patient with a large farpoint deviation has approximately the same large deviation at near as well as at far. Thus, the prognosis may be poorer in this type of case as compared to one with divergence insufficiency.

The patient with divergence insufficiency has a low AC/A ratio, which causes the eso to be less at near than at far. This may allow fusion at near, and intermittency greatly improves the chance for the functional improvement in cases of strabismus (either eso or exo).

In cases with constant esotropia at both far and at near, the prognosis is probably no better for one category than for the other. In general, constant esotropia is difficult to cure by orthoptics or, for that matter, by any means.

Procedures for basic eso and divergence insufficiency are not too different in many respects. The main difference in treatment programs for patients is not based on this simplified classification system, but rather, on the fact that each patient is different. Different training procedures are required for each patient, and therefore, only broad generalizations can be made in regard to the treatment of all farpoint eso deviations.

Esophorias of the basic eso or divergence insufficiency types are effectively treated by using many of the same procedures as recommended for these types of esotropia. Treatment is much easier, and functional improvement or cure is brought about much more quickly than in the strabismic cases.

USE OF BASE-OUT PRISM

Plus lens additions are not too effective in reducing the angle of esotropia if the AC/A ratio is low. Consequently, base-out prism may be the necessary optical procedure to keep the patient fusing and, therefore, prevent the recurrence of sensorial anomalies. The importance of developing and maintaining good sensory fusion should always be stressed in cases of esotropia.

The difficulty with the patient's wearing base-out prism is that sensory fusion must usually be fairly good before this can be beneficial. If there is A.R.C. or deep suppression, the angle of deviation is very likely to increase. Refer to the prism adaptation test discussed in **Chapter Three.**

Base-out prism can be an ideal way to maintain fusion if sensory fusion is good. Prisms are sometimes used on a permanent basis in this regard, but most often, the power can either be reduced considerably or totally removed.

> *TABLE 12B. Recommended Instrumentation and Targets for Training Procedures in Cases of Divergence Insufficiency*

A. Stereoscopes
    1. Wheatstone
        a. Office (e.g., Synoptophore)
        b. Out-of-office (e.g., Bernell Mirror Stereoscope)
    2. Brewster
        a. Office (e.g., Telebinocular for "tromboning")
        b. Out-of-office (e.g., Stori-View Stereoscope)

B. Vectographics (in-office or out-of-office)
    1. Pola-Mirror
    2. Vis-A-Vis
    3. Vectograms
    4. Titmus Stereo Tests
    5. A.O. Vectographic Slide
    6. T.V. Trainer

C. Colored Filters (in-office or out-of-office)
    1. Worth lights (4-dot test)
    2. Anaglyphics (e.g., Keystone Basic Binocular Test Set)
    3. Root Rings

D. Septums (Turville Septum or vertical bar on window)

E. Directly Viewed Instruments
    1. Penlight push-aways
    2. Penlight and Bagolini striated lenses
    3. Penlight with flip prisms
    4. Brock String
    5. T.B.I.
        a. Chiastopic (crossed) fusion
        b. Orthopic (uncrossed) fusion
    6. Eccentric Circles (Keystone transparent acetate)
    7. Two thumbs

F. Combinations

CENTRATION POINT

Vodnoy[2] points out the importance of finding a fixation distance in which fusion can be made possible. He believes that the nearpoint is the place to begin, since it has the greatest potential for achieving binocularity.

It is logical to put fusion targets at the centration point. Calculation of the centration point was discussed in Chapter Three. If, for example, the esotropia is 15 p.d. at far and near, the patient should wear ∤ 2.50 diopter spherical lens additions while fixating a target 40 cm away. This should put the patient into a condition of sensorial orthophoria relative to the fixated target. Hopefully, the patient can fuse under these conditions.

The magnitude of the AC/A ratio has no influence on this procedure, since testing is done at optical infinity. Accommodative stimulus is zero because of the plus lenses.

As progress is made, the fixation distance is gradually increased. Instrument training is often necessary before the patient is ready for free space training, and the major amblyoscope is probably the best instrument with which to begin fusion training in cases of esotropia.

Additional instruments and targets recommended in cases of farpoint esotropia include vectographics, colored filters, septums, and other directly viewed targets (refer to Table 12B). Most of these procedures can be done at the centration point.

The patient is encouraged to maintain fusion at the centration point, and then slowly walk backward while keeping fusion. The power of the plus lenses will have to be reduced accordingly so that the patient's vision is not blurred as the fixation distance is increased.

Split vectograms are particularly helpful for the patient who loses fusion as the fixation distance is increased. A good pair of targets is the #12 slides (see Figure 12-4). The reason for its effectiveness is that as the fixation distance increases, the prismatic demand decreases. Suppose, for instance, that the patient is able to maintain fusion at 40 cm with the vectograms set at 4 p.d. base-in. As the patient moves back, the base-in mathematically becomes less. At 80 cm the demand is only 2 p.d. base-in. The patient thinks he is meeting the same base-in demand that he had at the closer distance. This encourages him to try fusing at farther distances. Along with this gain in confidence, the patient is also instructed to use mental effort to promote divergence.

Pola-Mirror training commences with the patient getting close enough to the mirror so that both eyes can be seen (see Figure 12-5). The patient is fusing with little, if any, foveal suppression when both eyes are seen simultaneously. He then backs away from the mirror and tries to keep seeing with both eyes. The loss of fusion is indicated by the blacking out of one of the polarizing lenses. The procedure is repeated, with the patient trying to increase the fixation distance each time. The goal is for the patient to be able to see both eyes at a distance of approximately 150 cm, a total distance of 3 meters when looking through the mirror.

The Vis-A-Vis procedure can be used in a similar manner, and hopefully, the patient will see both of the therapist's eyes from a distance of 3 meters.

The Titmus Stereo Tests are introduced to determine if stereopsis can be maintained as the distance is increased (see Figure 12-6a). Flip prisms may be introduced for jump fusional vergence training (see Figure 12-6b).

The patient may require training in a reduced environment if stereoacuity is very poor. Wick[3] writes that rapid alternate flashing in the major amblyoscope can improve stereopsis, using third-degree fusion slides. Good vergence ability in free space is important in the development of

FUSION WITH INCREASED FIXATION DISTANCE

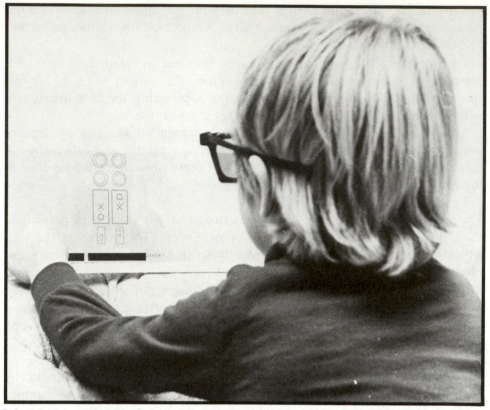

FIGURE 12-4 — Split vectograms used for development of negative fusional vergence

stereopsis. If motor control can be improved so that bifixation is possible, stereoacuity usually improves rapidly.

The A.O. Vectographic slide is used by having the patient maintain fusion while walking from near to far. The bull's-eye target is a good flat fusion demand (Figures 2-9 and 2-52). The stereoscopic rings, also on this slide, can be used for fusion walk-away exercises when the patient is ready for a third-degree fusion demand.

The T.V. trainer[a] is effective for home use. See Figure 12-7 showing the Polaroid[R] T.V. Kit of Bernell. A similar procedure is possible with colored filters, and this is sometimes better than a polarizing unit, if suppression is a great problem. Esotropic patients tend to suppress less with red-green television units than with ones that are polarized, probably because dissociation by polarization simulates natural seeing conditions more closely than by red-green filters. The patient should switch to a polarized unit as soon as possible, so that he can transfer to fusing under more natural conditions.

Although procedures using anaglyphs are less natural than those with

---

[a]This may be either the A.O. Polaroid[R] Television Trainer or the Polaroid[R] T.V. Kit of Bernell.

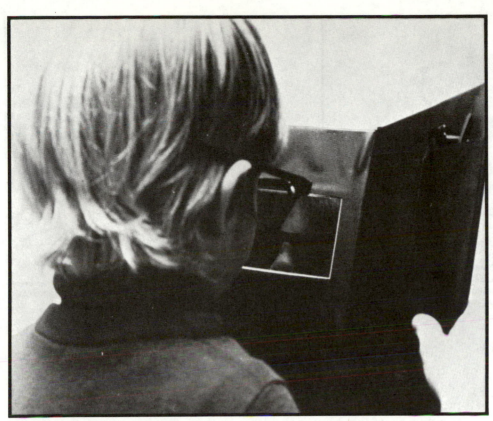

FIGURE 12-5 — Pola-Mirror training

vectograms, they can be performed in a similar manner. The Keystone Basic Binocular Test Set contains several good targets for peripheral stereopsis. The goal is for the patient to move away from the target while maintaining the stereo effect. The floating of the target indicates peripheral fusion is being maintained. The Root rings procedure is especially good for this type of training (see Figure 2-10).

Some of the recommended directly-viewed procedures include the many variations of training that can be done with a penlight. The patient is to maintain fixation on the light while the fixation distance is slowly increased. Suppression should be monitored from time to time, unless spontaneous diplopia is reliably reported whenever fusion is lost. There are many means to monitor suppression; for example, with the Bagolini striated lenses (see Figure 12-8).

Flip prisms can be used for vergence demand changes, using the penlight as the fixation target. The Bagolini lenses may be combined to monitor suppression during flip lens or prism training.

Training to achieve a functional cure in cases of eso deviations can take considerable time, possibly a year or more in some cases of esotropia.

OUT-OF-OFFICE PROCEDURES

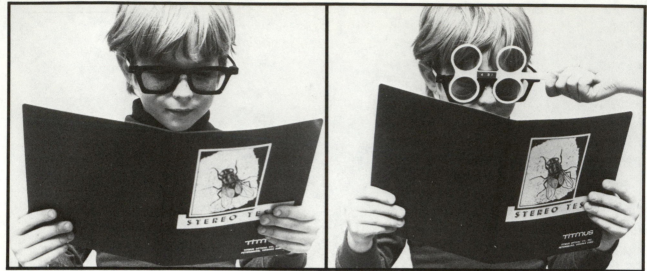

FIGURE 12-6 — The Titmus Stereo Tests for sensory and motor fusion development. (a) Motor fusion being trained by varying fixation distance; (b) Jump fusional vergence demands introduced with flip prisms.

Cooperative patients may reduce this time by faithfully doing all of the home training that is prescribed. Some patients, however, are not motivated to undergo office procedures, much less home training, which requires self-motivation to a large extent. In young patients, the degree of cooperation that can be expected from the parents is another factor to consider in any prognosis. If cooperation and enthusiasm are lacking from either the patient or the parents, then the home training program is unlikely to lead to significant functional improvement.

Most practitioners recommend the use of home training for patients who may be helped by orthoptic training. However, there is a minority view in opposition to out-of-office training. Sharing this opinion is Smith[4], who feels that the doctor is unable to enforce strict home training schedules. He believes the training is of low quality when parents are used as therapists. It is my opinion that unless intensive everyday office therapy can be given (as is done in certain clinics in Europe), home training is essential in most orthoptic cases.

Table 12C lists a typical sequence of out-of-office procedures that might be recommended for a patient who has a farpoint eso problem. This represents an overall plan of attack, and substantial modification of any list such as this is required in each individual case. This merely serves as a guide for organizing a program for out-of-office therapy.

Duction and version rotations can be performed in many ways. The target may either be a Marsden ball or a pencil with letters on it[b]. The target

[b]Lettered pencils, known as Alphabet Pencils, are available from Creative Associates, Aptos, CA 95003.

may be moved to stimulate pursuit movements. Two pencils make excellent alternate fixation targets for saccadic versions (see Figure 12-1).

Pencil push-aways are the opposite from the frequently used pencil push-up exercises. Instead of the target being advanced, it is slowly moved away. Starting from within the angle of the esotropia is advised.

A penlight is probably a better target than a pencil if suppression is recurrent. Red-green lenses and/or darkening the room may be required in this event. A lettered pencil can be used after suppression becomes insignificant as a result of antisuppression therapy.

The patient should progress to the point where step vergences, with the awareness of physiological diplopia, can be performed with ease (see Figure 12-9). Some clinicians have erroneously referred to these jump vergence exercises as "jump ductions." This type of training aids the patient in learning voluntary vergence control. It is hoped that by continued training, reflexive motor fusional (disparity) vergences will be developed.

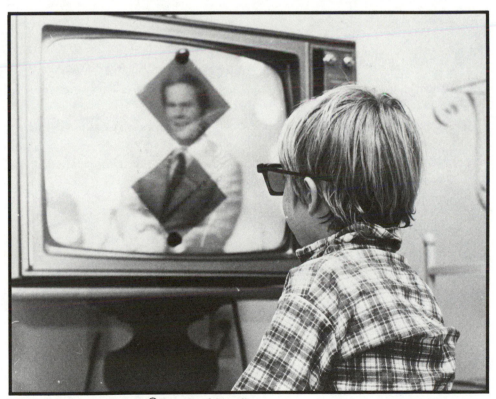

FIGURE 12-7 — The Polaroid® T.V. Kit of Bernell

There are several good home training devices for enhancement of peripheral fusion; e.g., Root rings. The Bernell Mirror Stereoscope (Figure 2-15) is good for home training, and paramacular targets are recommended until fusion with good ranges can be attained with smaller ones.

Hand-held stereoscopes of the Brewster type are useful for monitoring suppression. Variations in vergence demand can be produced either by changing the separation between homologous points or by altering the fixation distance. The latter method may be used for "tromboning." As the stereogram is brought closer to the patient, the reduced fixation distance produces a base-in effect. This is very different from ordinary seeing, since divergence must accompany positive accommodation. Likewise, as the

---

TABLE 12C. Typical Sequence of Out-of-Office Procedures Recommended for Eso Problems at the Farpoint

1. Ductions and versions for motility
2. Pencil push-aways
3. Base-out prism in spectacles
4. Peripheral fusion training
    a.   Keystone anaglyphs
    b.   Root Rings
    c.   Wheatstone stereoscopes with para-macular targets (e.g., mirror stereoscope)
5. Hand-held stereoscopes (e.g., Stori-View, G.A.F. Viewmaster or other Brewster stereoscopes)
6. Brock string techniques (e.g., red-green filters, minus lenses, nine positions of gaze, pursuit vergences, saccadic vergences)
7. Prism demand flippers (base-out and base-in; e.g., those using Bausch and Lomb Comparators)
8. T.V. Trainer
    a.   Red-green (custom-made or Bernell)
    b.   Polaroid (A.O. or Bernell)
9. Fusion walk-aways
    a.   Worth lights (viewed through red-green spectacles)
    b.   Bagolini striated lenses
10. Reduction of power of base-out prism in spectacles
11. Supplemental procedures (e.g., hole-in-hand game, Tranaglyphs, T.B.I., Eccentric Circles — Keystone Transparent acetate, flannel board training, etc.)
12. Combinations

---

stereogram is moved away, the base-in demand is lessened along with the decreased accommodative stimulus. This is contrary to the ordinary accommodative-convergence relationship in free space, but is useful for the development of good negative fusional vergence. Some clinicians refer to this procedure as "shaking up" accommodation and convergence.

Slides for the Stori-View Stereoscope and the G.A.F. Viewmaster must

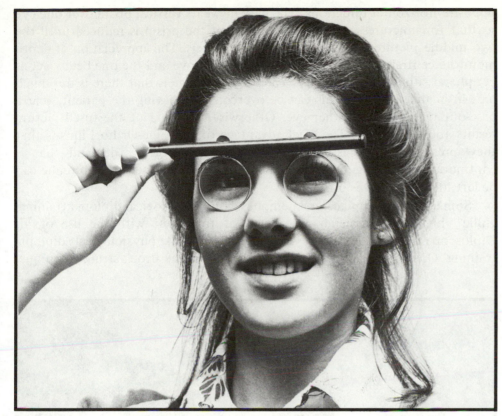

FIGURE 12-8 — Bagolini striated lenses being used to monitor suppression, as fixation distance of the penlight is increased

be custom-made at the present time. This may be accomplished by using the commercially available film transparencies and putting on ink spots or lines, or punching pinholes to act as suppression clues. Several different models of conventional Brewster stereoscopes are available from Keystone View Co. A multitude of different stereograms can be used in these instruments for home training. A recommended stereogram is the Test 4 (DB-4K). This is a flat fusion demand and is included in the Keystone Visual Skills Profile. The vergence demand can be varied by the patient's wearing different prisms, and fusion is indicated when three discs are seen. Keystone has available a series of similar stereograms called the Progress of Fusion Test set (see Figure 12-10). The size of the disc diameter ranges from 20 mm to 1 mm to allow for various sizes of the suppression zone. The series is also available in split stereograms to allow vergence demand changes.

Oakley[5] has devised an ingenious training procedure in which a moving picture in color is shown to the patient. Two similar pictures are seen, one above the other. As the movie film[c] is run, the two pictures move in

---

[c]Cine-Ortho Films available from Keystone View, Division of Mast/Keystone, 2212 E. Twelfth St., Davenport, Iowa 52803.

opposite horizontal directions. The patient wears vertical prism over one eye so that four pictures are seen. The power of the prism is reduced until the two middle pictures can be fused with stereopsis. The appreciation of depth monitors central suppression, and the picture above and the one below act as peripheral suppression clues. The chief disadvantage is that there is too much base-in in the films, but this can be overcome by having the patient wear a base-out prism on the other eye. Otherwise, diplopia of the fused picture results too frequently. The chief advantage of the Cine-Ortho Films is that they present an interesting farpoint, fusional vergence demand that is continuously changing. Once the patient knows the proper procedure, he can be left to do this on his own.

Some authorities place great emphasis on physiological diplopia training. Gillie[6] highly recommends this form of treatment with the use of his Diploscope. There are many ways to go about physiological diplopia training. One of the simplest for home training is the Brock string technique,

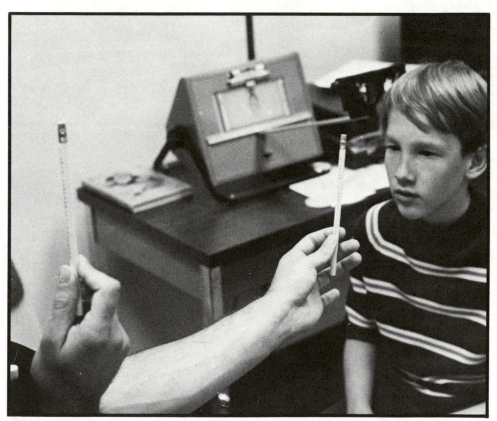

FIGURE 12-9 — Two Alphabet Pencils being used for physiological diplopia and jump vergences

in which the patient holds one end of a string to the tip of his nose, with the other end of the string tied to a distant object, such as a door knob. The patient should be able to see two strings apparently intersecting wherever the

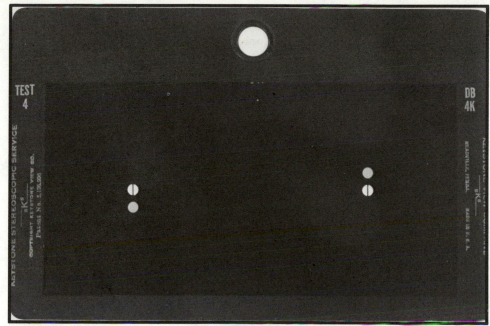

FIGURE 12-10 — Illustration of a stereogram of the Keystone Progress of Fusion Test set

horizontal component of the visual axes meet. If suppression is a problem, the patient may wear red-green spectacles in order to see both strings.

A small fixation target (such as a bead, paper clip, or piece of paper) is placed on the string at approximately the patient's centration point. If the patient is bifixating properly, the perceived apparent intersection of the strings will be exactly at the position where the fixation target is located, but if the strings cross in front of the fixated bead, the eyes are esotropic in relation to the fixated bead. The patient should then move the bead closer until bifixation can be achieved. Plus lenses may be helpful in getting the patient started on this procedure. The eventual goal is to have the patient fixate the bead as far away as two or three meters while maintaining accurate bifixation. The presence of the diplopic strings serves to act as suppression clues, as well as monitoring the exactness of bifixation. It should be noted that the diplopic perception of the strings is homonymous for that portion of the string in back of the fixated bead. The diplopia is heteronymous for that closer portion of string. In other words, if the patient wore a red filter over the right eye, the near portion of the red string would appear to be on the left side, and the far portion of the red string would appear to be on the right side.

The patient should try to maintain bifixation while minus lenses are worn. The effect of the lenses is the stimulation of accommodative convergence, and there must be sufficient fusional divergence in order to maintain bifixation.

The bead can be removed for practicing voluntary vergences. The patient looks at various portions of the string, and everywhere the visual axes cross, the patient should see the strings appearing to intersect. Voluntary control of vergences can be learned with this type of exercise.

Several beads may be used on one string for jump vergences. A string with three beads that is commercially available is the Physiological Diplopia String[d] (see Figure 12-11a showing this in use). When one bead is fixated, the other two should be seen diplopically.

The Brock String Technique is applicable to training in all nine positions of gaze (see Figure 12-11b). The string may be tied to a stationary object or one that moves (e.g., Keystone Rotator), so that bifixation can be trained during versions.

The patient with divergence insufficiency or basic eso should attempt to do fusion walk-aways. The T.V. Trainers are good for this type of home training. Also, the Worth four dot test serves to monitor suppression while the patient is moving from a near to a farpoint fixation distance. The Bagolini striated lenses provide a more natural set of conditions for this type of training, and should be recommended as soon as the patient is ready.

If compensatory base-out prisms are used, power should be reduced as conditions warrant. It is a mistake to remove, or to reduce too soon, the power of the prism. This could result in the loss of fusion. The power of the prism can be reduced as the fusional divergence ability improves. There are numerous supplemental home training exercises the patient may want to try for relief of boredom. One of these is the hole-in-hand game (see Figure 12-12). Another is the Eccentric Circle (Keystone transparent acetate) fusion exercises (see Figure 12-13).

The esotropic patient can use chiastopic (crossed) fusion to fuse the Eccentric Circles. For instance, if the patient's centration point is at 20 cm, the two cards are held 40 cm away. The right eye sees the left card, and the left eye sees the one on the right (see Figure 12-14). If the patient can fuse these, he will see one card having two eccentric circles with the word "CLEAR" in the center of the smaller circle. The larger circle should appear to float forward if the patient has a fair degree of stereopsis. This is so if the "A's" on the cards are matched near each other.

Divergence demand may be stimulated in this case by the patient's moving the cards closer together. Conversely, positive fusional vergence is stimulated by the cards being moved farther apart.

Eccentric circles may be used in orthopic[e] (uncrossed) fusion exercises. This is the opposite of chiastopic fusion; the visual axes are uncrossed relative to the fixation distance of the two cards. This procedure requires the patient to look beyond the plane of regard while trying to fuse. The cards may have to be moved close to each other in order for the eso patient to fuse them. Plus lenses may also be necessary. The same percept as with chiastopic

---

[d]Available from Bernell Corp., 422 East Monroe St., South Bend, Indiana 46601.

[e]Spelled orthopic, not to be confused with the word, orthoptic.

fusion will result with orthopic fusion, except that the smaller circle rather than the larger one will float forward. It should be noted that each picture is seen diplopically. Therefore, there are four ocular images involved. If two are fused, and the other two remain unfused, the patient is left with a total of

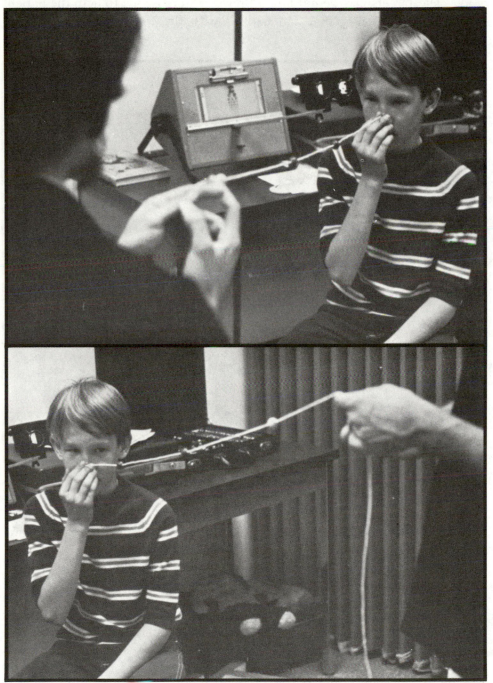

FIGURE 12-11 — Beads on a Brock string for physiological diplopia training. (a) Training in the primary position of gaze; (b) Training in a secondary position of gaze.

three ocular images. The fused image is seen straight ahead, with an unfused image on either side.

In most cases of esotropia, the patient is not ready for orthopic fusion exercises until a much later time when negative fusional vergence is very good. The targets may be put into a Brewster stereoscope to help the patient fuse them, and to become familiarized with the concept of this type of

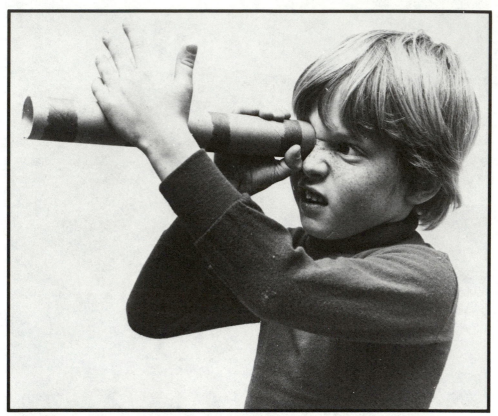

FIGURE 12-12 — The hole-in-hand game for anti-suppression training and promotion of voluntary vergence

training. This is also useful for making the patient aware of the depth effect of the fused images.

The patient should work toward achieving orthopic fusion with ease. He should be able to do this while the cards are moving (or while the head is moving, with stationary targets) so that versions are in play. He should be able to fuse these as the target separation is increased. It should be noted that the target separation is relatively small, as compared to the wide separation possible with chiastopic fusion. This value is similar to that found with the Remy Separator. Six centimeters represents 15 p.d. base-in at 40 cm fixation distance, and the eso patient is doing very well if he can fuse when the target separation is this amount.

Other targets, such as two thumbs or two coins, can be used for either chiastopic or orthopic fusion exercises. Orthopic fusion is more easily done if the viewing surface is transparent. Two similar objects can be glued to a clear sheet of plastic for this purpose.

The T.B.I. is useful as a directly-viewed fusion training instrument (see Figure 12-15). Note: the doctor should rule out photoconvulsive reactions before this instrument is taken home (refer to the discussion in Chapter Seven).

Alpha rhythm photic stimulation with the eyelids closed helps in the initial stages of antisuppression training (Figure 12-15a).

Physiological diplopia exercises can also be done with the instrument

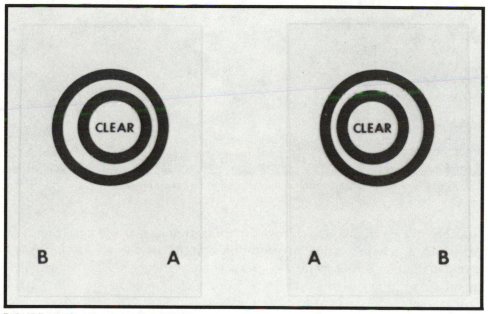

FIGURE 12-13 — Keystone Eccentric Circles

held a short distance away from the eyes (Figure 12-15c). Jump vergences can be made while physiological diplopia is used to monitor suppression.

The T.B.I. can be oriented so that each bulb is directly in front of each eye (checked by centering pupillary light reflections) and placed about 5 cm away from the face (Figure 12-15b). This allows the patient to have orthopic fusion while receiving alpha rhythm stimuli.

Before attempting orthopic fusion, the patient may find it easier to begin with chiastopic fusion (Figure 12-15d). As with the Eccentric Circles, the separation distance of the lights can be increased or decreased for variable vergence demands.

There are too many different out-of-office training procedures to

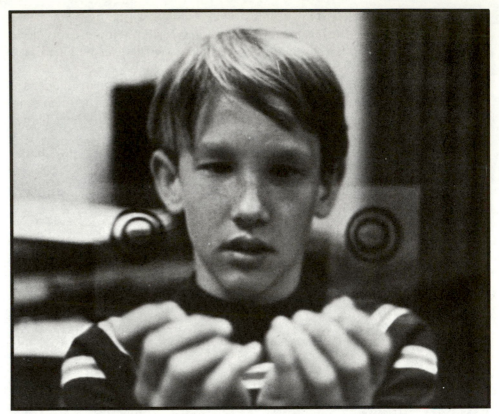

FIGURE 12-14 — Patient practicing chiastopic fusion with the Eccentric Circles

possibly discuss in one book. Their hybridization can lead to even more. An example of a combination of procedures would be the use of the Brock string with flip prisms while red-green filters are worn. Another example might be wearing red-green glasses and doing chiastopic fusion with a T.B.I. bulb directly behind each Eccentric Circle.

The permutations of training procedures are almost limitless. The doctor, therapist and patient can all contribute in the creation and selection of those that are most effective for the patient.

CASE EXAMPLE OF DIVERGENCE INSUFFICIENCY

Case Number Six, discussed in Chapters Three and Five, is an example of a patient with divergence insufficiency. There is a constant esotropia of 15 p.d. at far. At near, it is only 4 p.d. with intermittent strabismus. Extensive pleoptics is not indicated since the amblyopia is shallow, and total occlusion would disrupt whatever fusion the patient has.

A brief outline for therapy in this case might proceed as follows:
1. Treat amblyopia under binocular conditions rather than monocularly.
2. Use binasal occlusion in a manner similar to that advocated by Greenwald (Chapter Nine) to eliminate A R C and help fixation to

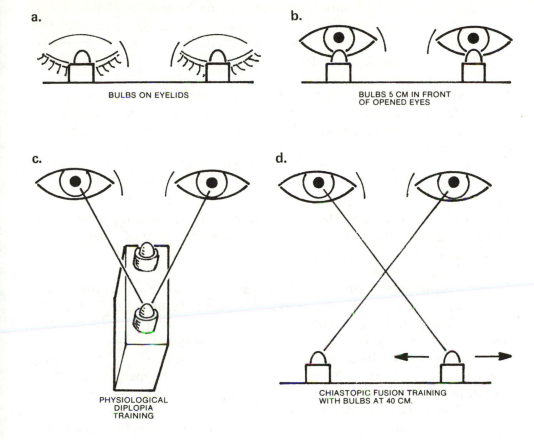

a.

BULBS ON EYELIDS

b.

BULBS 5 CM IN FRONT
OF OPENED EYES

c.

PHYSIOLOGICAL
DIPLOPIA
TRAINING

d.

CHIASTOPIC FUSION TRAINING
WITH BULBS AT 40 CM.

FIGURE 12-15 — Procedures with the T.B.I. (Translid Binocular Interaction) Trainer. (a) Bulbs placed on eyelids; (b) Bulbs placed five cm away in front of open eyes; (c) Physiological diplopia training with the T.B.I.; (d) Chiastopic fusion training with bulbs 40 cm away. Various spacing of bulbs is afforded by sliding one of them — variable from 35 to 88 mm. Vergence demand changes can also be affected by increasing or decreasing the fixation distance.

become alternating rather than unilateral.

3. Prescribe base-out prism with an overcorrection according to the method of Fleming et al. (Chapter Nine). When A R C is eliminated, reduce power to exactly compensate the angle of deviation.

4. Give antisuppression training with major amblyoscope at objective angle. Use antisuppression factors presented in Chapter Ten.

5. Apply intermittent photic stimulation in free space; e.g., uses of T.B.I.

6. Give physiological diplopia training with fixation being at the centration point.

7. Teach the patient to become aware of pathological diplopia.

8. Use second-degree fusion demand to develop limited vergence range.

9. Use third-degree fusion demand to establish stereopsis and develop

limited motor fusion range while maintaining stereopsis.

10. Intensify central antisuppression training to establish bifoveal fixation. Work on improving visual acuity of poorer eye under binocular conditions. Some temporary form of attenuation may be necessary.

11. Recommend fusion walk-aways and other vergence exercises in free space.

12. Reduce base-out prism when good fusional vergences can be demonstrated in all positions of gaze. Finally, there should be no evidence of suppression during gross motor activity; e.g., balance board.

The above outline is representative of cases similar to the example given. The details of any treatment plan often need to be modified considerably during the course of therapy, but it is always wise to have an overall treatment plan. This helps the doctor prescribe the appropriate procedures, as well as making the therapist, parent, and patient aware of what needs to be accomplished.

OTHER CONSIDERATIONS

There is an unusual form of esotropia referred to as cyclic esotropia. The strabismus is periodic; the deviation is regularly manifest in a clock-like fashion. Burian and von Noorden[7] believe the mechanism usually follows a 48-hour rhythmic cycle. There is good binocularity for a 24-hour period, with no significant latent deviation that can be found. This is followed by another period of 24 hours in which there is a large manifest esotropic deviation. Greene[8] reported a case of cyclic esotropia that was given orthoptics, but no progress could be made.

Most authorities agree that after several years from the time of onset of this mysterious type of esotropia, the deviation becomes constant. Surgery must be considered in these cases.

Vertical and torsional deviations must be considered in cases of eso deviations. It is thought that a purposive esotropia can result from a vertical deviation.

If the hyper or hypo deviation is 10 p.d. or less, vertical prism compensation is generally the first procedure to be considered. Prism therapy may be combined with vertical vergence training. Crone[9] states that a vertical divergence of 5 degrees (9 p.d.) can be achieved. Therefore, this type of motor fusion training should also be given consideration if the vertical deviation is small. For very large manifest vertical deviations, however, surgery may be necessary. Orthoptics to improve horizontal motor ranges may aid the patient with latent vertical deviations. The horizontal control in some ways helps to control the vertical component.

Crone[9] also states that a cyclovergence of 8 degrees can be achieved. Since there is no ophthalmic prism[f], as yet, that can be used for

---

[f]A double dove prism can be fabricated to rotate an image, but this is not feasible for ophthalmic use at the present time.

compensating this type of deviation, the expansion of the torsional fusion range should be considered in cases of cyclophoria. If that fails, cyclovertical muscle surgery may have to be attempted.

Unlike cases of basic eso and divergency insufficiency, which are eso problems at the farpoint, convergence excess is considered to be primarily a nearpoint problem.

NEARPOINT
ESO PROBLEMS

This is the type of heterotropia or heterophoria in which the eso deviation is larger at near than at far. This is attributed to a high AC/A ratio. The severity of binocular problems due to convergence excess may be great if there is constant esotropia at far and near. In such cases, therapeutic procedures similar to those used in cases of basic eso and divergence insufficiency may be required. For instance, it may be necessary to use base-out prism therapy, centration point training, and many of the other elaborate procedures required for treating farpoint eso problems. The doctor, however, has the one important advantage, in cases of convergence excess, of being able to reduce the deviation by means of plus lenses. This is the most important reason why these prognoses are generally better than in cases of basic eso and divergence insufficiency.

CONVERGENCE EXCESS

The effect of plus lenses can be remarkable in cases with a high AC/A ratio. For example, suppose a patient with a 60 mm I.P.D. has 6 p.d. of esotropia at far, and 16 at a near fixation distance of 40 cm. The AC/A is calculated to be 10/1. This implies that for every diopter of plus lens addition that is worn, the eso deviation is reduced by 10 p.d. Therefore, a $+$ 1.00 addition would cause the deviation at near to be reduced to 6 eso; and, a $+$ 1.50 would cause the reduction to 1 eso. A $+$ 2.00 addition would cause the deviation to become 4 p.d. in the exo direction. These are theoretical values, since the esotropic patient does not always respond at first to the plus additions in a mechanistic manner. This notwithstanding, sufficient training usually results in the theoretical relationship holding fairly true. Plus addition lenses can be of great help in time.

USE OF PLUS LENSES

Accommodative esotropia is typically of the convergence excess type. Besides the high AC/A ratio causing the eso to become prominent, many of these patients have a significant amount of hyperopia. This refractive error should be corrected as soon as possible to prevent an excessive amount of eso deviation from becoming constantly manifest.

Cases in which corrective lenses have not been prescribed often become those referred to as "deteriorated accommodative esotropias." For all intents and purposes, these secondary cases of esotropia have the same characteristics as those with primary (nonaccommodative) esotropia. They can be equally difficult to treat successfully.

Although full plus correction is generally advocated in cases of convergence excess, the doctor should be aware of any sensorial anomalies that can possibly result when the strabismic angle becomes stabilized due to the wearing of lenses. This is one of the reasons why orthoptics must necessarily be included in the treatment of convergence excess.

FUSION WITH DECREASED
FIXATION DISTANCE

The mechanism of training in cases of convergence excess is different from that used for eso problems at far. The patient attempts to maintain fusion while the fixation distance is decreased, rather than when it is increased, as in divergence insufficiency. The goal of treatment is to develop strong negative fusional vergence. This can be developed by the patient's maintaining bifixation as the fixated object is brought nearer. The demand on negative fusional vergence becomes greater as the target comes closer (refer to Figure 12-16 for an illustration of this). If the eso deviation is 6 p.d. at far, the patient is required to diverge by this amount. At a fixation distance of 40 cm, the patient must exert considerable effort to keep fusing, since the base-in demand is now 16 p.d. The demand is 26 p.d. at the 20 cm fixation distance, and even greater effort is required. Fusion can be monitored by many of the various sensory fusion tests; e.g., Worth lights or Bagolini lenses.

Blurring is a characteristic response that most patients give as the target draws near. This is because the accommodative response is reduced in order to reduce the accommodative-convergence, allowing the target to remain single but out of focus.

Fusion walk-ups (as opposed to fusion walk-aways, used for divergence insufficiency) are prescribed for home training. They are repeated until the target can be seen clearly at a close fixation distance. Ultimately, the patient should have a normal nearpoint of convergence (N P C̆) without the advancing fixation target inducing an esotropia.

OUT-OF-OFFICE PROCEDURES

The less severe cases of convergence excess are amenable to home training. Table 12D lists a sequence of out-of-office procedures typically used in these cases.

Pencil push-ups are performed in the traditional manner; the patient follows the tip of a pencil that is moving slowly from arm's length to his nose. He should be able to perform these pursuit vergences to a distance of 10 cm before there is blurring. This blur-point represents the limit of the relative fusional vergence (or accommodative amplitude), and in the cases of convergence excess, it represents the negative relative fusional vergence.

The target continues to advance, and the pursuit vergence should be maintained (with blurring allowed) to a normal N P C of 3 cm. One of two things will happen if bifixation is lost. Either the target will be seen diplopically (indication of nonsuppression), or it will continue to be seen singly (indication of suppression).

When suppression is suspected, the doctor should do a nearpoint Hirschberg test using a penlight to monitor vergence movements. Note that the doctor's sighting eye must be closely behind the penlight. If suppression is a problem, antisuppression training, particularly that for the awareness of pathological diplopia, should be re-emphasized.

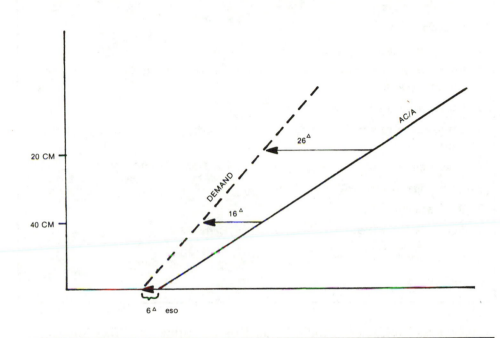

FIGURE 12-16 — Graphical illustration of convergence excess

When the patient is able to perform well with a penlight fixation target, a pencil can be substituted. An alphabet pencil is excellent for this purpose, because the clarity of a letter provides feedback as to accommodative response. The patient can look at different letters during the exercise to relieve boredom. This also promotes learning the alphabet for very young children doing this type of home training.

Binocular rock procedures according to Pierce and Greenspan's method (Chapter Two) are recommended for improving fusional vergence. Patients with convergence excess generally have difficulty in clearing the minus lens accommodative stimulus under these binocular conditions. Figure 2-50 illustrates two devices used for home training. Office procedures are easily performed by using the Van Orden Trainer attachment[g] for the Correct-Eye-Scope (further discussed in Chapter Fifteen).

Pola-Mirror home training is done in a similar manner, as in cases of divergence insufficiency, except that walk-ups are stressed rather than

[g]Available from Keystone View, Division of Mast/Keystone, 2212 E. Twelfth St., Davenport, Iowa 52803.

TABLE 12D. *Typical Sequence of Out-of-Office Procedures Recommended for Eso Problems at the Nearpoint*

1. Ductions and versions for motility

2. Bifocals

3. Pencil push-ups

4. Binocular accommodative rock (Van Orden Trainer used with Correct-Eye-Scope or custom-made devices)

5. Pola-Mirror with decreasing fixation distance

6. Orthopic (uncrossed) fusion with acetate rings (Eccentric Circles on transparent acetate)

7. Polachrome Orthoptic Trainer (Vectograms and Tranaglyphs)

8. Titmus Stereo Tests with flip prisms

9. Bar reading

10. Remy Separator (Septum Orthoptic Trainer, Bernell)

11. Supplemental Procedures

12. Combinations

walk-aways. The patient should be able to see both eyes as fixation distance is reduced.

Orthopic (uncrossed) fusion is practiced in the same way as in other types of eso deviations. Plus lenses are of great help in getting the patient started.

The Titmus Stereo Tests can be used to arouse the patient's awareness of stereopsis at the nearpoint. Fusional vergences can be developed by using flip prisms. Loss of stereopsis is feedback to the patient when there is suppression.

Bar reading can be carried out in a number of ways. Refer to discussion in Chapter Two regarding the use of septums. A form of bar reading may be done, without using opaque septums, by anaglyphics. The most popular method is to blot out certain words or lines of ordinary print with red ink, and other portions of the print with green ink. The commercially available felt-tip pens are good for this purpose. The patient wears red-green spectacles. The eye with the red filter can see only the words covered over with the red ink. Likewise, the eye with the green filter can see only the words covered with green ink. Central suppression can be monitored while the patient is reading. It is important to have the patient read something of interest.

Base-in fusional vergence demands can be introduced by having the patient read through minus addition lenses and/or by wearing base-in prisms with the red-green spectacles. Fresnel lenses and prisms are good for these purposes.

Small strips of red and green plastic may be used for dissociation during reading. Bernell T.V. kits come with a transparent plastic card, having vertically oriented red and green strips interspersed by clear spaces to allow fusion. The Polaroid[R] T.V. kit has a similar card based on the light polarization principle.

The Remy Separator provides an excellent means of producing base-in demand at the nearpoint. Home training can be done with a commercially-available device, such as the septum Orthoptic Trainer[h]. There are also ways to do this at home with custom-made devices. For example, the Keystone Colored Circles[i], commonly referred to as the "lifesaver" card, can be used with a septum (see Figure 12-17). The base-in demand is calculated in the same way as with the Remy Separator.

Plus addition lenses are almost always required at first, until the patient can learn to fuse the red and green circles. Some are for flat fusion, with letters acting as suppression clues, and others are for stereopsis.

Supplemental home training procedures for convergence excess may include the Brock Posture Board, Ortho-Fusor, Vodnoy Aperture Rule Trainer, and many more.

Brock and Folsom[10] described a nearpoint procedure using red-green filters for dissociation with tactile and kinesthetic senses used in the training program. The instrument required for this procedure is known as the Brock Posture Board.

A modified version of the Posture Board can be custom-made and used for home training purposes. The necessary components include red-green spectacles, 8½ x 11 inch sheet of transparent or translucent red plastic, same size sheet of white paper, red drawing pencil, and a penlight (see Figure 12-18).

The patient draws red visual tracing lines on the white paper. The sheet of paper is placed on the plastic sheet, and is held by the patient with one hand. The penlight is held in the other hand, and moved to trace the lines on the white sheet. The eye with the red filter can see the red light (shining brightly through the plastic and the paper), but the light cannot be seen by the other eye with the green filter. The red-filtered eye, however, cannot see the red lines (blending with perceived red background), as these lines are seen only by the green-filtered eye. It should be noted that the same procedure can be performed without a red plastic plate, if a clear plate with a red light-bulb is used instead.

Brock and Folsom reported that this procedure "reveals a latent posture deficiency which is normally concealed by the fusion compulsion . . ." It

---

[h]Bernell Corp., 422 East Monroe St., Southbend, Indiana 46601.

[i]A white card with four pairs of circles (red ones on the right, and green ones on the left), number BO8-1.

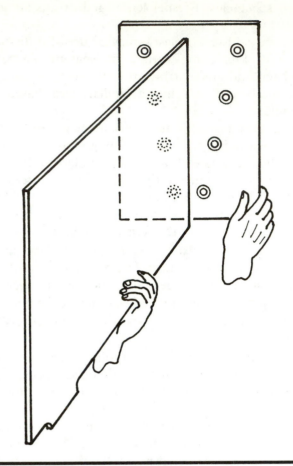

FIGURE 12-17 — Illustration of a home training procedure based on the principle of the Remy Separator

should be noted that binocular vision is not fully dissociated, because peripheral borders of the paper can be fused. The procedure can, therefore, be used to monitor central suppression while motor training (to encourage bifixation) is given. The patient is instructed to follow a red drawn line to its end, and then remove the red-green viewers. The inaccuracy of fixation under these slightly dissociated conditions can be checked by determining how far off the light is from the line. The procedure can be repeated and checked after minus lenses and/or base-in prisms are worn. This is done to stimulate negative fusional vergence while central suppression is being monitored.

The Ortho-Fusor[j] is a small compact vectographic kit that holds the interest of the adult patient and the older child who performs fairly well on

[j]Manufactured by Bausch and Lomb Optical Co. The original sets have been discontinued and replaced by a set having only one target.

the other stereoscopic demands. The original kit is described below.

Set No. 1 is recommended over the other two available kits, as it includes both base-in and base-out demands. Base-out targets help to encourage the patient with convergence excess to begin fusing and gain confidence. Set No. 3 has only base-in demands, and is generally too difficult for most of these patients to use until a much later time in therapy. This kit may be used when there is adequate fusional divergence.

The Ortho-Fusor Set No. 2 has only base-out demands, and is designed for use with exo deviations. For the patient with an eso deviation, this should be used only as a starter, in the event the patient is unable to fuse

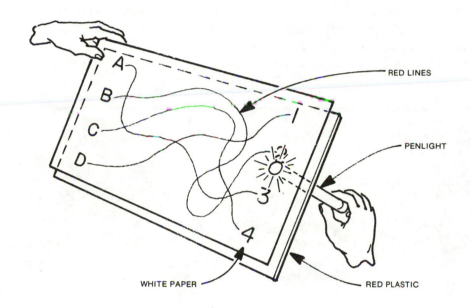

FIGURE 12-18 — Illustration of a training procedure with a modified Brock Posture Board

Sets No. 1 or 3. The patient may be able to appreciate stereopsis with this set and not the others because the base-out targets of the Ortho-Fusor act as compensatory prisms for the eso deviation.

The Vodnoy Aperture-Rule Orthoptic Trainer[k] may be used for the patient with convergence excess. It is a good home training device for patients who have achieved a good motor range with second- and third-degree fusion targets. This procedure is very difficult for most patients who have nearpoint eso deviations. A double aperture must be used to create a base-in demand (see Figure 12-19).

[k]Available from the Bernell Corp., 422 E. Monroe St., So. Bend, IN 46601.

The septum between the two apertures acts to dissociate vision in the same manner as the septum of the Remy Separator, and the prismatic demand can be calculated in the same way. The manufacturer of the Aperture Rule Trainer has provided a very simple and convenient method of determining the prismatic vergence demand. This is done by multiplying the number of the test card by 2½, to find the base-in demand; e.g., card number one has a base-in demand of 2½ p.d.

If the single aperture is used, instead of the double aperture, the patient must use chiastopic (crossed) fusion, and the demand becomes base-out rather than base-in. The magnitude of the base-out demand is determined by multiplying the card number by 2½ p.d., just as with the double aperture.

It may be necessary to start the esotropic or esophoric patient with the single aperture for base-out targets, until he becomes sufficiently familiar with this procedure to progress to base-in training. Targets for the Aperture-Rule Orthoptic Trainer have both second- and third-degree fusion targets with ample suppression clues.

There are many possible combinations of procedures that may be used

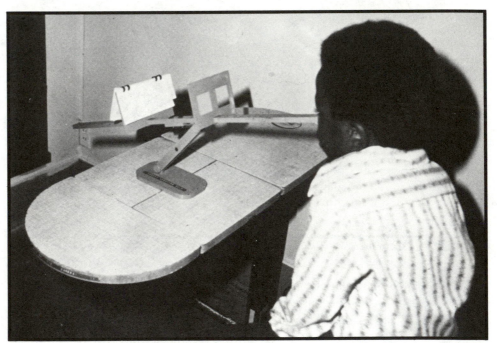

FIGURE 12-19 — Double aperture used on the Aperture-Rule Orthoptic trainer to create base-in demands

for home training. For instance, the patient can do push-ups with the Ortho-Fusor while using flip prisms. Another example might be the use of flip prisms with bar reading. The number of possibilities is limited only by the imagination of the doctor, therapist and patient.

Refer to Case Number Ten in Chapters Three and Five. This case of convergence excess can be managed principally with the use of plus addition lenses in the form of bifocals, and with home training to improve sensory and motor fusion. The initial bifocal segment power should be approximately $+$ 1.00 diopter. Theoretically, the deviation would be reduced to 6 p.d. at near, equal to the magnitude of the deviation at far. The patient is now more likely to fuse with the AC/A line equalized in relation to the vergence demand line. Central antisuppression training (Chapter Ten) should be emphasized along with motor fusion training. All the home training procedures listed in Table 12D can be used.

CASE EXAMPLE OF CONVERGENCE EXCESS

There is no possible way to cover the myriad considerations in cases of eso deviations. However, one that should be mentioned is the case of very small-angle esotropias with peripheral fusion (monofixation pattern). This problem may occur with any of the three categories of eso deviations. It is probably less commonly found in those cases of convergence excess in which there is true intermittency.

OTHER CONSIDERATIONS

Most authorities believe that the chance for complete functional cure in the case of monofixation pattern is poor. Christian[11] recommends reinforcing an existing A R C in these small strabismic angles on the ground that the patient will be provided with a "link between the two eyes" for some form of useful binocular vision.

It is sometimes more practical for the patient with monofixation strabismus to discontinue functional therapy and be content with the condition he has, or with the progress that had been made previously. There are cases, however, in which a complete functional cure is possible, provided the patient is sufficiently motivated to undergo intensive therapy for a relatively long period of time. The patient should be forewarned of the poor prognosis in these cases, and no guarantees of success can be made.

Surgery is rarely warranted in cases of eso deviations of small magnitude. If the angle is moderately large, surgery may or may not be needed, depending upon the case. However, surgery is frequently necessary when the angle is greater than 20 p.d. When the patient is of the appropriate age for orthoptics, it is wise to consider the inclusion of pre- and post-surgical orthoptics, if a functional cure is sought. Surgery alone is the treatment of choice in cases with a strictly cosmetic problem. Refer to Chapter Four for discussion on extraocular muscle surgery.

13 | Training Procedures for Exo Deviations

Cases of exo deviations can be categorized into three types. They are divergence excess, basic exo, and convergence insufficiency. The first two are considered farpoint exo problems, and convergence insufficiency is thought of as mainly a nearpoint problem.[a] Cases of either exotropia or exophoria are included in this system of classifying exo deviations.

Many of the same procedures used in treating patients with farpoint esotropia are used in the treatment of divergence excess and basic exo cases when there is constant exotropia (refer to Tables 12A, B, and C in Chapter Twelve). Patients who have constant exotropia (i.e., constant strabismus at far and near) often have associated conditions, such as amblyopia, suppression and A R C, as does the patient with constant esotropia. These anomalies must be cared for in a similar manner.

General Approach

Pleoptic procedures presented in Chapter Seven are applicable to the treatment of amblyopia in the cases of exotropia.

Anomalous correspondence is usually not considered a great deterrent to the successful treatment of patients with exotropia. Perhaps this is because most cases of exotropia have a duality of A R C (sometimes referred to as co-variable A R C). The anomaly is intermittent in respect to N R C occurring when the visual axes are aligned in the ortho posture, and A R C being present when the deviation is manifest.

Duality of A R C is more frequently found in exotropia than in esotropia. The factor of intermittency may be a reason for this difference. Clinical experience shows that a history (past or present) of true intermittency is more common in cases of exotropia.

An important key to eliminating A R C in the exotrope is to get him to fuse at the centration point. The necessary convergence to put the visual

---

[a]As in cases of eso deviations, the "problem" is in terms of the status of sensory and motor fusion. Cosmesis may be either good or poor.

axes at the centration point can usually be brought about with the help of minus addition lenses. For instance, suppose the patient has an exotropia of 20 p.d. at far and 10 p.d. at 40 cm. Assume the I.P.D. is 60 mm. The AC/A ratio is calculated (not a "true" AC/A) as follows:

$$AC/A = 6 + .4 (-10 - (-20))$$
$$= 6 + .4 (+10)$$
$$= 6 + 4$$
$$= 10$$

Since the calculated AC/A ratio is 10/1, the deviation at the far point can be reduced to ortho by an accommodative response of two diopters. Therefore, a minus over-correction of two diopters is prescribed for temporary wear, but only at the farpoint.

Farpoint A R C and antisuppression training can be given at the distance centration point, but cases of divergence excess or basic exo respond better when training is begun at a near centration point. When the patient fixates an object at 40 cm in this particular case, the accommodative stimulus is 2.50 diopters. Multiplying this by the 10/1 ratio theoretically produces an accommodative-convergence of 25 p.d. Since the ortho demand at 40 cm is only 15 p.d.[b], and the visual axes converge 25 p.d. from the ortho posture at far, the result is an eso deviation of 10 p.d. at near. In order to have the eyes in an ortho posture at this distance, the -2.00 diopter overcorrection should be reduced by one diopter.[c] Once the centration point is found, the patient is ready for peripheral fusion training similar to that used in training the esotropic patient.

When sensory fusion is well established, motor fusion demands can be presented. Refer to Table 12A listing the various methods for changing prismatic demand. Most of the equipment used for vergence improvement for eso deviations can also be applied to training in cases of exo deviations; but instead of the emphasis being placed on development of negative fusional vergence as in eso cases (with base-in training), the patient with an exo deviation works to improve positive fusional vergence by means of base-out training.

The association of horror fusionis with exotropia seems to be less than with esotropia. If a patient with exotropia is found to have horror fusionis, appropriate therapy should be considered (refer to discussion in Chapter Eight). Bitemporal occlusion may be recommended in the case of an exotropia rather than binasal occlusion used with esotropia. Otherwise, the investigation of aniseikonia and training of peripheral fusion should be carried out in a similar fashion.

---

[b]Calculated by multiplying the I.P.D. times meter-angles.

[c]The above relationships between accommodation and convergence are not always mathematically exact for a number of reasons, principally because accommodative response and stimulus are seldom exactly the same. Also, other purposive types of vergence may occur (either under- or over-converging) because of A R C and/or suppression zones. Calculation of the centration point is supplemented by clinical empirical findings.

It is fortunate that the majority of exotropic patients have a history of intermittency. If the exotropia is now, or has been, intermittent, the prognosis may not be poor.

The standard approach to therapy of intermittent exotropia at far is, first, a temporary overcorrection of minus lenses. Then the monocular phase is begun, to improve accommodation facility and fixations. This is followed by the bi-ocular phase to promote diplopia awareness. The sequence of training in the binocular phase is to improve superimposition, flat fusion, stereopsis, and motor fusion. Refer to Table 6B for a more detailed outline of the standard orthoptic philosophy for functional cure.

Practitioners who tend to follow Brock's philosophy do not adhere to the standard approach in cases of farpoint intermittent exotropia. Their recommended sequence is somewhat the reverse: training for stereopsis comes first, then flat fusion and superimposition. Motor fusion is worked on as soon as stereopsis can be appreciated. Training is done first in free space, and only much later, instrument training is recommended. Flax[1] follows this approach in treating patients with divergence excess who have intermittent exotropia at the farpoint. He reports the distance deviation is usually between 18 to 25 p.d. in these cases, and the near deviation may be much less: ortho, or maybe eso in some cases if the AC/A ratio is very high. He does not recommend base-in prism. Plus adds (bifocals), however, may be prescribed.

Effective motor fusion training is the key to successful treatment of divergence excess and basic exo types of intermittent exotropia. Training is essentially the same in case of exophoria, but treatment of heterophoria is much easier and faster. The main difference is that training for elimination of A R C and suppression is unnecessary.

Farpoint Exo Problems

These procedures include the use of base-in prism, minus lens overcorrection, and plus lens additions. The minus lens approach is only on a temporary basis during training, and is usually in the initial stages of treatment of exotropia to aid convergence at far.

OPTICAL PROCEDURES

Long[2] recommends using minus overcorrections in the training program for a particular purpose. He encourages the deviation to become manifest by unilaterally occluding the patient for a moment to determine if fusion recovery is either lacking or slow when the occluder is removed. If so, minus trial lenses are momentarily worn by the patient to aid convergence. The strength of the minus power is increased to the point where the patient can begin to show normal recoveries, i.e., immediate and swift refusional eye movements when the cover is removed.

The patient with farpoint intermittent exotropia tends to have deep suppression when the deviation is manifest. This is the principal reason training is not always successful when the patient's eyes are deviated in the exo posture. Base-in prism compensation may be given in a variety of ways (e.g., ophthalmic prisms or positioning the tubes of the major amblyoscope to a base-in position), but they do not help the eyes to converge to the ortho posture. The patient tends to suppress, in spite of the fact that "sensory orthophoria" is attained by optical means. Furthermore, many practitioners feel that if fusion training is given when the eyes are in the exo posture, the strabismic condition is reinforced, which tends to make the deviation become manifest more frequently.

Base-in prism is not highly recommended in cases of farpoint exotropia, but it may be tried in cases of constant exotropia to allow sensory fusion training at the objective angle. This approach may have to be taken, if minus lenses are not effective in reducing the angle of deviation. The combination of base-in prism and minus lenses may be tried in some cases of constant exotropia in the hope of developing sensory fusion.

There are patients with exophoria who require base-in prism compensation for relief of subjective symptoms. This form of therapy is commonly used when there are symptoms associated with heterophoria and fixation disparity (to be discussed in Chapter Fourteen).

In cases of intermittent farpoint exotropia, overcorrection with minus lenses is preferable to base-in prism compensation. This is only temporary, and is for the purpose of having the eyes in the ortho posture for centration point training. It should be noted that some patients who have divergence excess have very high AC/A ratios. Minus overcorrections may not be needed if the AC/A line meets the ortho vergence demand line at a convenient nearpoint fixation distance.

Because the AC/A ratio is relatively high in these cases, plus additions in the form of bifocal lenses are recommended to equalize the AC/A line and the ortho vergence demand line. If, for example, the patient is 10 exo at near and 20 exo at far, he is very likely not to make the extra effort required to fuse 10 more prism diopters in the distance as he looks from near to far. The bifocals cause the patient to have an equal demand at near and far. This reduces the chance of farpoint strabismus, and also provides positive fusional vergence training when the patient is looking through the bifocal segment.

FUSION WITH INCREASED FIXATION DISTANCE

Great emphasis must be placed on the patient's ability to transfer nearpoint binocular skills to the farpoint. The patient should attempt to fuse in free space as much as possible, starting at the nearpoint initially. The fixation distance should gradually be increased to the intermediate distance, and as progress is made, to the farpoint. Positive fusional vergence is being strengthened while the patient maintains fusion as the fixation distance is increased.

It is important to check frequently for the presence of suppression. If it is found, many of the antisuppression procedures discussed in Chapter Ten should be recommended.

Suppression is apt to occur as the target is moved farther away, because the magnitude of the exo deviation becomes larger at far in cases of divergence excess. Suppression is likely in cases of basic exotropia, even though the near and far deviations are approximately the same. The reasons for this may include less interest in the farpoint objects, smaller images to allow peripheral fusion, less stereopsis at far to serve as a fusion lock, and the lack of proximal convergence.

If the exo deviation becomes manifest for just a brief moment, suppression may occur. Point zero is on the temporal retina, which is on the side of the retina of the deviating eye that is habitually suppressed. The temporal retina seems to be more susceptible to suppression than the nasal. Fleeting foveal suppression may occur in exophoria, probably due to stress on the vergence system.

The major portion of motor fusion training can be done at home, if there is good cooperation. Office visits should be used primarily for teaching the patient new procedures and evaluating the progress made with the old ones.

There are literally hundreds of various techniques for motor fusion training advocated by practitioners in the field. For the sake of brevity, only a limited selection of recommended techniques will be discussed. They are listed in Table 13A.

OUT-OF-OFFICE PROCEDURES

Voluntary convergence is the willful crossing of the eyes. The definition implies the lack of any visual stimulus. Most exotropic patients can be taught voluntary convergence. The mechanism each patient uses is not always known, but it is important to note that it is learned, regardless of how it is brought about. If visual stimuli help, this is fine. Some patients imagine seeing visual objects (such as a bug flying near the nose) to trigger the convergence response.

After sufficient repetitive exercises, the patient begins to be aware of the proprioceptive feeling of his eyes being converged, as opposed to being in the fusion-free exo deviated posture. The doctor and therapist can monitor the extent of the convergence by using the Hirschberg test, and giving the patient feedback as to when the eyes are in the ortho posture. The "feeling" the patient has at that moment should be remembered and be recaptured every time the eyes assume the ortho position. Once the patient knows this feeling and can bring it about at will, he can practice this at home.

Voluntary convergence can also be aided by awareness of diplopia. The exotropic patient may have trouble noticing pathological diplopia, because point zero is on the temporal retina. If the patient is unable to perceive pathological diplopia, procedures designed to promote the awareness of physiological diplopia should be given. Some examples of these are the use of diploscopes, framing, bar readers, and the Brock string. The latter is versatile and ideal for out-of-office therapy. Refer to the discussion of the Brock string techniques in Chapter Twelve.

Push-away exercises are used to train positive fusional vergence when the AC/A is greater than the patient's I.P.D. That is, if the patient's I.P.D. is 60 mm, an AC/A of 6/1 would keep the AC/A line and the ortho demand line parallel to each other. No base-out demand would be created by moving the target (either closer or farther). However, positive fusional vergence is required to maintain fusion if the AC/A ratio is higher than 6/1, if the target is moved farther away. This is because there is less accommodation as the fixation distance is increased, and therefore, less accommodative-convergence to help the patient cross his eyes. The target used for push-aways may be a penlight or any object of interest. An Alphabet pencil is a good target.

TABLE 13A. Typical Sequence of Out-of-Office Training Procedures Recommended for Exo Problems at the Farpoint

1. Voluntary convergence (use of mental effort and learning to tell the difference between the proprioceptive feeling of the eyes being converged or deviated to the exo posture)

2. Brock string techniques (for awareness of physiological diplopia)

3. Pencil push-aways

4. Peripheral stereopsis (Root Rings or Keystone Basic Binocular Test Set)

5. Binocular accommodative rock

6. Hand-held Brewster stereoscopes

7. Television trainer
   a. Red-green
   b. Polarizing

8. Prism demand flippers

9. Chiastopic fusion at far (after mastering Eccentric Circles procedure at nearpoint)

10. Fusion walk-aways
    a. Worth four dot
    b. Bagolini striated lenses

11. Combinations

12. Supplemental procedures
    a. Duction and version rotations
    b. Risley prism for pursuit vergences
    c. Prism bar for saccadic vergences
    d. Split Vectograms
    e. Pola-Mirror training with afterimages
    f. Pola-Mirror training with two mirrors at different distances
    g. Vis-A-Vis walk-aways
    h. T.B.I.
    i. Intermittent flashing
    j. Cine-Ortho Films
    k. Framing

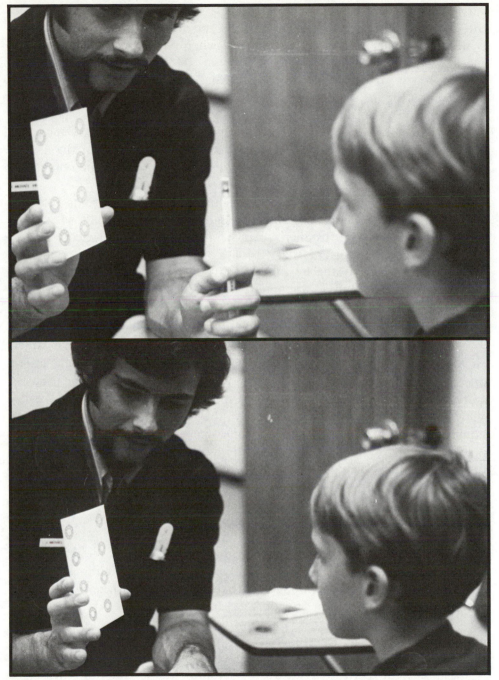

FIGURE 13-1 — Chiastopic fusion training with the use of Keystone Colored Circles ("Lifesaver" card). (a) Use of pencil to aid convergence and teach patient to cross-fuse; (b) Chiastopic fusion without the use of pencil as aid to convergence.

The method of pencil push-ups is contraindicated in the beginning stages of training in cases of divergence excess because of the great amount of accommodative-convergence. This causes the eyes to be in an eso posture at very near fixation distances. See Figure 3-1b for a graphical illustration of the exo at far becoming eso at near. The type of motor fusion being trained is negative, rather than positive, vergence when pencil push-ups are used in these cases.

Awareness of peripheral stereopsis can be promoted by training with Root rings (Figure 2-10) or other large third-degree fusion targets, such as the Titmus Fly or the Keystone Basic Binocular Test Set. As peripheral stereopsis is improved, training for the improvement of central stereoacuity should be started with smaller targets such as the Wirt rings of the Titmus Stereo Tests. Push-aways with third-degree fusion targets are then practiced, with suppression indicated by the loss of stereopsis.

Binocular accommodative rock procedures are given according to Pierce and Greenspan's recommendations discussed in Chapter Two. Plus lens additions stimulate positive fusional vergence, since accommodative-convergence is reduced. It is important that fusion be maintained, otherwise fusional vergences are not activated by this procedure, and the only things changing are accommodation and accommodative vergences. Using a second- or third-degree fusion target; e.g., Wirt rings, while plus and minus lenses are interchanged, can inform the patient that he is fusing.

Hand-held Brewster stereoscopes are recommended because the targets are at optical infinity, which aids the patient in transferring farpoint instrument fusion skills to farpoint free space skills. Positive fusional vergence demands can be introduced by incorporating Fresnel prisms in the Stori-View Stereoscope, or by decreasing the separation distance of the homologous points in the Keystone stereoscopes. When a good motor range is achieved in the stereoscope, the patient is ready for free space positive fusional vergence training at far. Television Trainers are excellent for this purpose.

Prism demand flippers can be used in conjunction with the Television Trainers to stimulate both positive and negative vergence while suppression is being monitored. It should be noted that motor fusion in both directions should be full, in order for the patient to have good vergence facility.

Chiastopic fusion at far is particularly good for home training, as it is in free space, and very little equipment is required. Two identical pictures, each with a suppression clue, can provide a flat fusion demand at far.

The patient usually has to learn chiastopic fusion at near before proceeding to far. The Keystone Colored Circles ("lifesaver" card) is a good flat fusion demand for this (see Figure 13-1). Once the nearpoint procedure is mastered, the patient can begin chiastopic fusion with farpoint targets (Figure 13-2).

Fusion walk-aways should be repeated frequently during home training. The target may be varied for interest. It can be an ordinary object in the room (without suppression clues) or, preferably, a dissociative one, such as a Television Trainer (with suppression clues). In this regard, the Worth four dot test is useful. It is very dissociative, and helps the patient who tends to

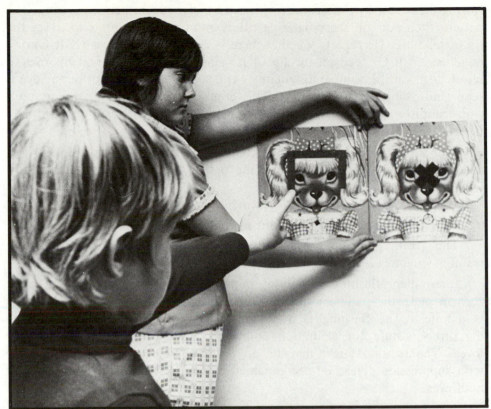

FIGURE 13-2 — Chiastopic fusion training at far. Two similar pictures are cross-fused. The special markings act as suppression clues.

suppress, but it makes motor fusion difficult because of the high degree of dissociation. The Bagolini striated lenses provide more natural seeing conditions because they are less dissociative. Therefore, motor fusion may be easier, but suppression and/or A R C are more likely to occur. Each target has certain advantages, and it is recommended that both be used for fusion walk-aways.

There are many combinations of motor fusion training procedures. An example would be to have the patient practice the Brock string techniques while using prism demand flippers. Another would be alternately fusing with hand-held stereoscopes and a Television Trainer. The patient would wear polarizing filters when looking in the stereoscope as well as when looking at the T.V.

There are numerous supplemental training procedures that are applicable for exo problems at the farpoint. Pola-Mirror push-aways are good for checking on suppression (if one eye appears black) when the fixation distance is increased. See Figure 12-5 showing a patient with the Pola-Mirror. The patient can use the Pola-Mirror with afterimages to monitor A R C. He is first exposed to afterimages prior to his putting on the polarizing filters. The

Hering-Bielschowsky afterimage procedure is recommended here. The patient then puts on the polarizing filters and looks in the mirror to see the tip of his nose. He reports whether there is an afterimage cross (N R C) or a noncross (A R C) seen on the tip of his nose. He then looks at his eyes to see if both can be seen simultaneously (no suppression) or if only one eye is seen (indication of suppression). This combination of A R C and suppression monitoring is useful in cases of exotropia with suppression and intermittent A R C.

Pola-Mirror training with two mirrors at different fixation distances can be used for step vergences, giving the patient feedback as to suppression status.

Vis-A-Vis walk-aways are useful for non-step ("sliding") vergence training, and are similar to Pola-Mirror push-aways.

The T.B.I. can be used for antisuppression and chiastopic motor fusion training (Figure 12-15). Refer to discussion in Chapter Twelve.

Intermittent flashing is helpful in breaking down suppression at point zero to make the patient aware of pathological diplopia when the deviation is manifest. The flashing is more importantly used when the eyes are in the ortho posture (or centration point) for eliminating suppression at the fovea. The fixation target may be an ordinary object in the room or one with suppression clues and accompanied by rapid on-off occlusion of one or both eyes.

The orthoptic exercise referred to as "framing" is simply a form of farpoint bar reading. The patient is instructed to look at a distance object (e.g., a letter on a sign) and hold a pencil (or finger) vertically in the midline about 40 cm away. The pencil should be seen diplopically. Since the pencil is closer to the patient than the fixated object, its dioptric images fall on the temporal side of the retina of each eye. This causes the physiological diplopia to be of the heteronymous (crossed) type. The patient is instructed to bracket the two pencils around the fixated object. He can then look at other objects while keeping it centered between the two pencils.

The exercise is particularly useful because the temporal area of the exotropic eye is the habitually suppressed portion of the retina. Framing promotes bifixation at the farpoint while enhancing the awareness of physiological diplopia.

CASE EXAMPLE OF
DIVERGENCE EXCESS

Case Number Seven discussed in Chapters Three and Five is an example of an exotropic patient of the divergence excess type. A logical approach to therapy is the following:

1. Amblyopic therapy can be used to equalize the visual acuity of each eye. Direct patching with monocular training activities (Table 7B) is probably all that is required in the way of training.
2. Minus overcorrection should be worn during office visits to achieve a nearpoint centration point, and sensory fusion can be developed.

3. As progress is made, sensory fusion training can be given at far with minus overcorrection being worn, if necessary.
4. When there is sensory fusion at far, the minus lenses may be reduced or removed to encourage positive fusional vergence.
5. Bifocals are prescribed to equalize the AC/A ratio and promote positive fusional vergence while doing nearpoint tasks.
6. Prescribe out-of-office training procedures for motor fusion training (Table 13A).
7. Teach the patient to develop a large motor fusion range, both base-in and base-out; e.g., with the major amblyoscope. Start with third degree and proceed to second and then first degree fusion targets. The goal is for the patient to have a good motor range with super-imposition targets. This requires excellent motor control of the eyes, and considerable voluntary vergence must be in play.
8. Teach the patient to be aware of the deviation when it is manifest. This may be done by the patient's learning the "feeling" of converging.
9. Increase the awareness of pathological diplopia, or more subtle clues to exotropia being manifest, such as the loss of stereopsis.
10. With enough repetition, voluntary vergence will hopefully become automatically reflexive and habitual.

Nearpoint Exo Problems

Convergence insufficiency is generally thought to be associated with symptoms rather than poor cosmesis. This is because the majority of cases classified as convergence insufficiency are typically the kind of exotropia that is intermittent at near with full-time fusion at far.

The magnitude of the strabismus at far is usually not large, and the intermittent exotropia or high exophoria at near is due to a low AC/A ratio. Minus overcorrections are of little help in reducing the angle of deviation because the AC/A ratio is low. Similarly, binocular accommodative rock exercises are not very effective in expanding the horizontal fusional vergence range.

Some cases of constant exotropia are necessarily classified as convergence insufficiency because of the relationship between the near and far deviations. In these cases, the patient must be treated as though he had constant farpoint exotropia (basic exo or divergence excess).

FUSION WITH DECREASED FIXATION DISTANCE

Because the AC/A ratio is low, positive fusional vergence is stimulated when the fixated target is brought nearer to the patient. Graphical plotting of the near and far deviations shows the AC/A line getting farther away from the ortho demand line as the fixation distance is decreased (refer to Figure 3-1c). Therefore, positive fusional vergence can be stimulated by moving the target closer to the patient.

OUT-OF-OFFICE PROCEDURES

Positive fusional vergence training will suffice in most instances of convergence insufficiency. This is often referred to as "base-out" training. Although therapy is predominantly motor, there should be monitoring of sensorial anomalies, particularly of suppression during training sessions. A typical sequence of recommended out-of-office training procedures is listed in Table 13B.

Pencil push-ups are generally effective in stimulating positive fusional vergence. Any small fixation object is suitable, but it is better to have accommodative response controls incorporated into the target. An alphabet pencil is a good target. If the patient has trouble attaining a normal N P C (2 to 3 cm) he should touch the pencil. Tactile/kinesthetic stimuli often help in this regard.

A three-dot convergence card, such as the one printed by Allbee[d], is an excellent convergence stimulus for the patient with convergence insufficiency. It has the same principle as the Brock string with three beads. The dots represent the beads, and the patient should appreciate physiological diplopia of the nonfixated dots when one pair is fused. Since one side of the card has red dots and the other has blue, the one fused dot should be

---

TABLE 13B. *Typical Sequence of Out-of-Office Training Procedures Recommended for Exo Problems at the Nearpoint*

1. Pencil push-ups

2. Three-dot card

3. Pola-Mirror push-ups

4. Keystone Colored Circles

5. Eccentric Circles for chiastopic fusion with stereopsis

6. Polachrome Orthoptic Trainer (Vectograms and Tranaglyphs for sliding vergences and jump vergences)

7. Nearpoint chiastopic (crossed) fusion with ordinary objects (e.g., two coins and thumbs)

8. Bar reading (custom-made)

9. Bar reading with base-out demand

10. Aperture-Rule Trainer (single aperture)

11. Combinations

12. Supplemental procedures
    a. Anaglyphic reading
    b. Mirror Stereoscope
    c. Brock posture board
    d. Three-eye mirror method
    e. Numerous other procedures

---

[d]Allbee and Son Co., Waterloo, Iowa 50704.

perceived as a blend of purple. Figure 13-3 shows a patient doing this procedure.

Because the septum is dissociative, the patient may have trouble converging. There are two things that may help. First, let the patient practice on the beads and strings. This should be relatively easy since the beads can be moved farther away and there is no septum involved. Another way to get the patient started on the Three-dot Card is to effectively remove the septum. This is done by cutting off the top portion of the card, down to the

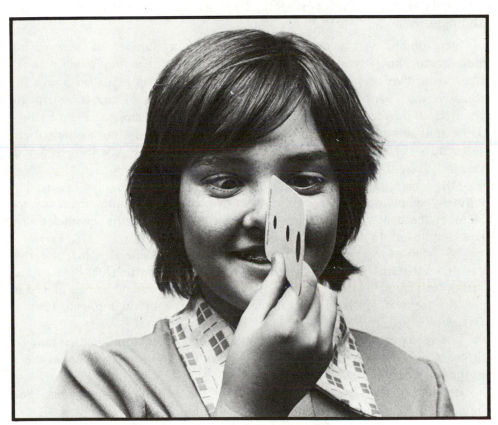

FIGURE 13-3 — Nearpoint convergence training with a three-dot card

top of the dots. The patient can then look directly at the dots without dissociation. When the patient can quickly change fixation from one dot (fused pair) to another while appreciating physiological diplopia, the regular card is substituted for the one that has been cut off at the top. The patient works at this until it is mastered. It may be necessary to move the card a few centimeters away from the face to achieve fusion, even for the most remote dot. Once this is done, the card is brought in to touch the nose, and fusion of the closer dots is attempted.

Pola-Mirror push-ups are good for monitoring suppression while developing positive fusional vergence. The mirror is moved from arm's length to a distance of approximately 10 cm from the eyes. Both eyes should be seen during this procedure.

The Keystone Colored Circles provide excellent chiastopic fusion demands. Similarly, the patient should be able to fuse the Eccentric Circles (Figure 12-13) with appreciation of stereopsis. Eccentric Circles are also printed on opaque card stock[e] and are less expensive than the ones on transparent acetate. These are perfectly fine for chiastopic fusion exercises.

Split vectograms, such as the Quoits (Figure 2-5), Mother Goose (Figure 2-6) and the Basic Fusion (Figure 2-7) slides are excellent for non-step (sliding) vergences.

Step (jump) vergences can be trained in a number of ways using these vectograms. Ryan and Pronchick[3] suggest using a "reversible viewer" made from two rectangular polarizing strips. One strip is placed above the other in the fashion of a Franklin bifocal. The axes of the top strip are oriented 90 degrees away from those of the bottom strip (see Figure 13-4). If the split vectograms are set, for example, at 5 p.d. base-out as the patient looks through the top strip, the demand can be quickly changed to 5 p.d. base-in if the patient looks through the bottom strip.

This same change in direction of vergence demand can also be brought about by simply turning regular viewers over so that the non-ocular surface becomes the ocular surface. This works if crossed polarizing spectacles have axes oriented at 45 and 135 degrees.

To create jump vergence demands without spectacle flipping, use two sets of vectograms. One set is placed above the other in the Dual Polachrome Orthoptic Trainer[f]. The desired amount of vergence demand can be placed in each of the two levels. For example, 5 p.d. base-in on top and 15 p.d. base-out on bottom.

The vectograms may be the same at the top and bottom, or they may be different; for instance, the Quoits could be on top and the Basic fusion slides on the bottom.

Jump vergences can be practiced with the Bernell Tranaglyphs. (See Figure 13-5, showing an example of Tranaglyphic training.)

Another interesting way to create jump vergence demands is to use vectograms on one level and Tranaglyphs on the other. This necessitates wearing red-green over the polarizing filters, and is used mainly for the sake of variety, but may have some advantage if the colored slides help reduce suppression at a certain vergence demand better than the black and white vectographic slides.

The patient should now be ready for nearpoint chiastopic training with ordinary identical objects: two thumbs, two hands, two coins, two buttons,

[e]Available from Keystone View Co., Division of Mast Development Co., 2212 E. 12th St., Davenport, Iowa 52803.

[f]Available from Bernell Corp., 422 E. Monroe St., S. Bend, Indiana 46601.

etc. The sensory demand is flat fusion and the suppression clues are in the periphery.

Bar reading can provide flat fusion demands with foveal suppression clues. Refer to discussion of bar reading in Chapter Two.

Incorporation of base-out prisms (e.g., Fresnels) and bar reading may be useful for improving fusional convergence while suppression is monitored. There may be fleeting central suppression when the vergence system is stressed via the base-out demand during this task.

The Aperture-Rule Orthoptic Trainer contains both second- and third-degree fusion targets. The single aperture is used for positive fusional

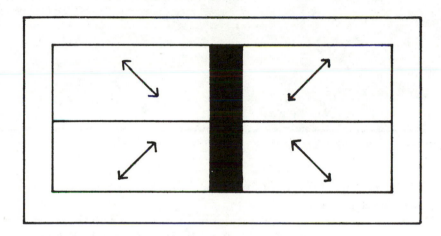

FIGURE 13-4 — Illustration of a "reversible viewer," useful for vectographic jump vergences

vergence training. This is very effective if the patient looks over the device onto a distance object and then looks into the aperture to fuse (jump vergences). This procedure is shown in Figure 13-6.

Vodnoy[4] advises that patients who have trouble fusing can hold a pointer in the aperture. Since this is really chiastopic fusion, the pointer works in the same way as holding a pencil between the Keystone Colored Circles when assisting chiastopic fusion in free space (as shown in Figure 13-1a).

There are very many combinations of procedures. One example could be jump vergences by fusing two thumbs (chiastopic fusion for base-out demand) and quickly looking at vectograms with a base-in demand. Polarizing viewers are worn during the entire procedure.

There are numerous supplemental training procedures that can be used for convergence insufficiency. Four of them worth mentioning are

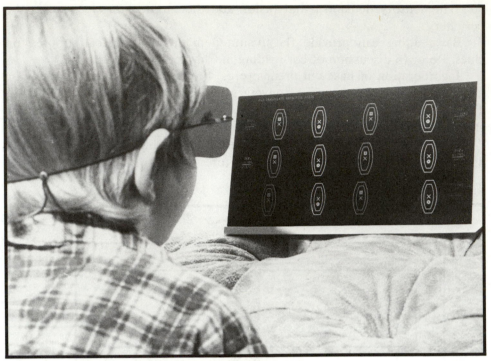

FIGURE 13-5 — Fusion training with the Bernell Tranaglyphs

anaglyphic reading, Mirror Stereoscope, Brock posture board, and the three-eye mirror method.

There are several forms of anaglyphic reading. Vertical red and green strips of plastic that come with the Bernell Red-Green T.V. Kit can be used as a Javal grid (discussed in Chapter Two) for bar reading. See Figure 13-7 showing a patient wearing red-green filters and reading through the vertical red and green strips.

Red and green ink can be used to block out selected words for anaglyphic reading (refer to discussion of this procedure in Chapter Twelve).

Red reading has been a traditional method for fusion training. The patient wears a red filter over the dominant eye with no filter over the nondominant eye. The writing is in red ink (e.g., red typewriter ink). Only the nondominant eye can see the red writing. The red filter also acts as an attenuator and is helpful for antisuppression purposes. Words printed in black ink should be interspersed occasionally for fusion locks. Motor fusion demands can be changed by means of loose prisms or flip prisms while reading.

Tsukomoto[5] advocates using a procedure called the three-eye mirror method. The instructions to the patient are as follows:

1. With a felt pen, draw a 12 mm diameter circle on a mirror.
2. Looking at the center of the circle with both eyes, try to see your "one-fused-eye."

3. Also, try to see your right eye and left eye simultaneously to see a total of three eyes.
4. The fixation distance can vary from arm's length to 5 or 10 cm from the face.

This procedure, which can be made readily available, holds the patient's interest where others may fail. The three-eye-mirror method is useful to introduce the principle of chiastopic fusion in free space, making this an excellent out-of-office training procedure for the patient who is learning to do chiastopic fusion.

Case Number Eleven, discussed in Chapters Three and Five, is an example of a patient with convergence insufficiency. Training procedures can follow the dispensing of the correction lenses for the myopic anisometropia. These procedures should emphasize the improvement of positive fusional vergence. Therapy can consist mainly of out-of-office procedures. The sequence listed in Table 13B is a logical program to recommend in this case.

CASE EXAMPLE OF CONVERGENCE INSUFFICIENCY

Hopefully, the training to expand the motor fusion range will result in the patient's ability to fuse all of the time at near and far. Stereoacuity may also be improved as a result of vision training.

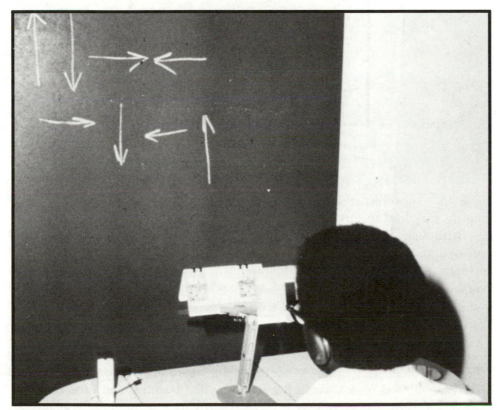

FIGURE 13-6 — The single aperture is used with the Aperture-Rule Orthoptic Trainer for nearpoint fusion training. Fixation targets at far can be included for jump vergence training.

CHAPTER 13
332

Other Considerations

The magnitude of an exo deviation is large if it is greater than 20 p.d. Surgery in these instances becomes a consideration, either for cosmetic or functional reasons. However, there should be no definite set of rules that weds the need for surgery to magnitudes of deviation, because each case is different. What can be said in this regard is that, in general, the need for surgery is more likely when the magnitude is large.

Crone[6] points out a possible contraindication of pre-operative orthoptics in cases of exotropia, particularly those of the divergence excess type. He

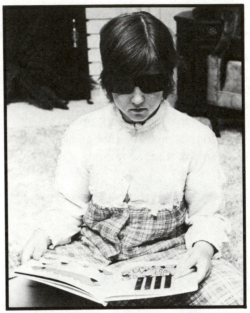

FIGURE 13-7 — Anaglyphic bar reading with the use of vertical red and green strips of transparent plastic

feels that convergence exercises should be discouraged because convergence spasms may lead to surgical overcorrection.

Although some surgeons have expressed this concern, I recommend pre-operative orthoptics; and the problem of convergence spasms can be effectively managed by developing both positive and negative fusional vergences. Otherwise, a one-sided approach to motor fusion training (with only positive vergence being worked on) can possibly lead to poor post-operative results.

The possibility of vertical deviations should be looked for in all cases of exophoria or exotropia. Refer to discussion of vertical deviation testing in Chapter Three. The available methods of treatment listed in preferential order are vertical prisms, vertical vergence fusion training, and surgery.

If a torsional deviation is present, the treatment methods available are cyclo fusional vergence training and surgery. I personally have seldom been able to develop a cyclo vergence motor range in patients who are significantly cyclotropic (i.e., incyclotropia or excyclotropia). However, I have had considerable success in expanding the range in cases of cyclophoria.

Exotropia is frequently associated with myopic anisometropia. Because of the possibility of aniseikonic problems with spectacle correction, contact lenses may be prescribed in conjunction with training procedures to bring about a functional cure. Ellin[7] reports a case of high degree of myopic anisometropia in a young adult with exotropia. Onset of the strabismus was at age five. Contact lenses and orthoptics were prescribed and resulted in a functional cure.

The prognosis for a complete functional cure is usually poor when there is lack of bifoveal fusion of long duration. However, there are some heartening exceptions to this generalization. Wick[8] reports a well documented case of a 13-year-old patient who had constant exotropia since the age of four. The magnitude of the deviation was 45 p.d. at far and 50 p.d. at near. Also, there was harmonious anomalous correspondence. As a result of orthoptics and surgery, the patient had normal correspondence, no suppression, fusion 100 percent of the time, 40 seconds of arc stereoacuity, and a nearpoint of convergence of 3 cm. In spite of there being a constant strabismus of long duration, vision therapy resulted in a functional cure.

Horopter

The horopter in esotropia was discussed as an explanation of horror fusionis in Chapter Eight. An interesting speculation about a possible etiology for exo deviations that involves the horopter was advanced by Flom.[9] If the identical visual direction horopter happens to have a very sharp curvature so it lies inside the Vieth-Müller circle (horopter being concave toward the patient), it will cause the patient to perceive peripheral objects in homonymous (eso) diplopia when bifixating a central target. Conceivably, peripheral diplopia could produce an exo deviation because of the divergence demand being met. An exotropia would allow haplopia of the peripheral visual field, but diplopia in the central field. There would be an exotropia of the visual axes so that heteronymous (exo) diplopia would be perceived centrally, unless central suppression (or A R C) occurred. Suppression could become larger, as necessary, for the patient to control the problem of diplopia in his central field of view. This seems to have all the earmarks of frank exotropia. Understanding the horopter in this way can provide a logical explanation for exotropia, co-variation of A R C, why suppression may be so deep in many cases of exotropia, and why some exotropic patients (particularly farpoint exotropic problem cases) are very difficult to treat successfully.

14 | Management of Fixation Disparity

Evaluation of fixation disparity was discussed in Chapter Two. The management of fixation disparity involves several methods, including lenses, prisms, motor fusion training, and surgery. Since there is usually no great sensory fusion problem in cases of fixation disparity, except possibly foveal suppression and reduced stereoacuity, emphasis of therapy is motoric. In many cases, stereopsis is improved as a result of the binocular motor therapy.

The weight of modern authority is shifting toward associating binocular symptoms with fixation disparity. Symptoms are of more concern to the patient than a reduction of stereoacuity.

Lenses are useful in caring for patients with fixation disparity, particularly plus lenses in the form of bifocals. They may be recommended in cases of convergence excess. A tentative prescription is determined by increasing the lens power until the angle of fixation disparity is reduced to zero. Other factors may have to be considered before deciding upon a final prescription.

Lenses

A tentative prismatic prescription in cases of fixation disparity is determined by varying the power until the associated phoria (not the dissociated phoria) is measured. This power of prism reduces angle F to zero (refer to discussion in Chapter Two). The versatility of prisms lies in the fact that horizontal and/or vertical fixation disparities can be neutralized in many cases by means of prisms.

Prisms

Convergence insufficiency is thought to be a factor in symptomatic complaints during reading and nearpoint tasks. Since there is a dissociated exophoria in these cases, there is often an exo fixation disparity. Base-in prism compensation may neutralize the exo fixation disparity. A final prescription is often that amount of base-in prismatic power required to neutralize angle F.

Payne et al.[1] evaluated nine patients who had nearpoint exo fixation disparity and symptoms. The Mallett unit was used in this study. One of the conclusions was that, "Non-presbyopic patients with near exo fixation disparity and symptoms prefer a prescription with the prism that reduces their near fixation disparity to zero."

Mallett's method for prismatic prescriptions was discussed in Chapter Four. The important recommendation to remember is that more power should be placed before the nondominant eye and less for the dominant.

Some practitioners fear the angle of heterophoria will increase if compensatory prism is worn. The prevailing evidence at present is that this will not happen, if neutralizing prisms are prescribed for those patients who have fixation disparity with symptoms (refer to the study of Carter, discussed in Chapter Three).

Motor Fusion Training

Orthoptics can be very helpful in cases of fixation disparity. Training procedures in cases of heterophoria have pertained to the improvement of motor fusion ranges. Results have often been successful with symptomatic complaints being relieved, but the doctor has not always known why. Understanding the status of the patient's fixation disparity can now provide an answer to this question.

Borish[2] summarized the extensive work that has been done regarding the graphical analysis approach to evaluating binocular problems. This has been used by many for plotting dissociated phorias and vergence measurements on a graph. Hofstetter[3,4] codified the use of binocular motoric clinical data for purposes of graphical analysis.

Refer to Figure 14-1 for an illustration of a graphical plot of clinical data. By convention, letter X is a symbol for the angle of deviation of the visual axes. In this example, assume the patient is orthophoric at near and far. Therefore, the AC/A line and the demand line coincide. Refer to Figures 3-1 and 3-2 for examples of different relationships between the AC/A and demand lines. Circles represent blur points, and squares symbolize break (diplopia) points.

A zone of *clear* single binocular vision can be plotted. This enclosure is formed by connecting the blur points (and also the line of blur represented by the amplitude of accommodation). See Figure 14-2a. It should be noted that the plotted accommodation line represents the maximum amplitude determined under monocular conditions, usually by the push-up test. This should not be confused with positive relative accommodation and negative relative accommodation, done under binocular conditions.

The zone of *single* binocular vision can be plotted, and is represented by the enclosure formed by connecting the break points (see Figure 14-2b). Because accommodative vergence may enter into the picture, the zone for break points is larger than the one of plotted blur points. Positive vergence, for instance, can be increased by combining accommodative convergence with positive fusional vergence. This enables the patient to maintain singleness, but at the expense of clearness.

Understanding these concepts helps to explain why binocular problems

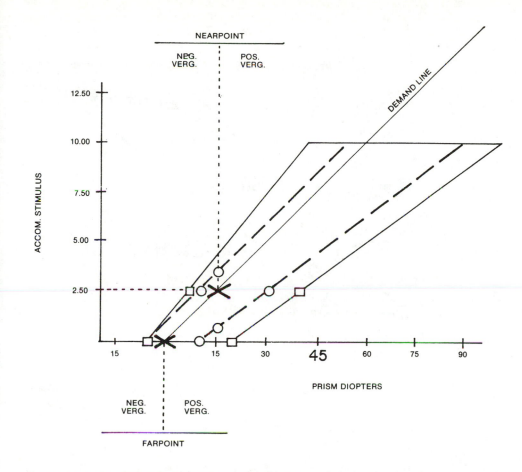

FIGURE 14-1 — Plotting of blur and break points on a two dimensional graph. Circles represent blur, and squares represent diplopia. The letter X represents the angle of deviation; and in this example, it is on the demand line at both the near and far fixation distances. This indicates the visual axes are in the horizontal ortho position at both distances.

can cause blurring of vision when the patient is unable to properly meet vergence demands.

A new dimension can be added to the graphical approach to possibly account for binocular symptoms. Ogle and Prangen[5] introduced a three-dimensional model depicting the relationship of fixation disparity to the zone of single binocular vision. A modified drawing of this model is shown in Figure 14-3. The sigmoid fixation disparity curves (discussed in Chapter Two and illustrated in Figure 2-53) are combined with the plotted zone of single binocular vision (example illustrated in Figure 14-2b).

The axis running through the three-dimensional drawing represents the locus of points at which the angle of fixation disparity is zero. According to current clinical thinking, points on the sigmoid curve located anywhere other

a.

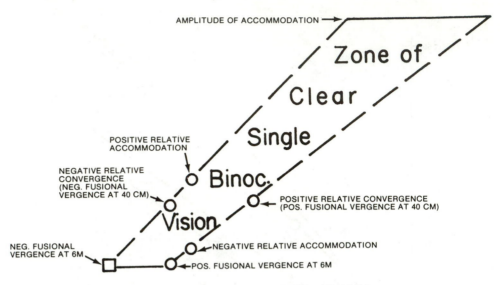

NO BASE-IN BLUR POINT EXPECTED IF MAX. PLUS CORRECTIVE LENSES WORN AT FAR

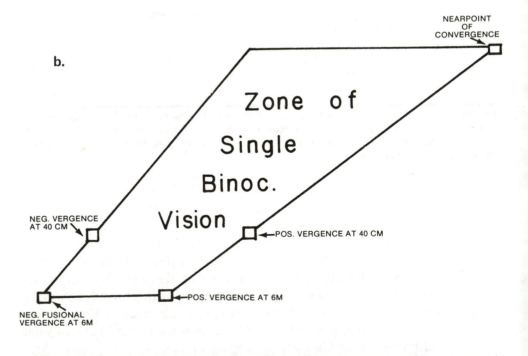

FIGURE 14-2 — Graphical zones of Figure 14-1 shown in isolation. (a) The blur points represent the zone of clear, single, binocular vision; (b) The break points represent the zone of single, binocular vision.

than at zero are representative of vergence demands that cannot be sufficiently met; and consequently, there may be symptoms (e.g., blur, fatigue,
headaches, etc.). Motor fusion therapy is indicated in this case, in order to
try to flatten the steep sigmoid fixation disparity curves (refer to Figure 2-53
for comparison of flat and steep curves).

The purpose of presenting this figure is for instructional purposes only,
and the clinician is not expected to draw them. However, the revisualization
of this figure may be of help in organizing clinical data into a meaningful
composite for cases in general.

The consideration of the third dimension of fixation disparity relating to
the two-dimensional approach of standard graphical analysis may help
answer some of the questions as to the cause of binocular symptoms.

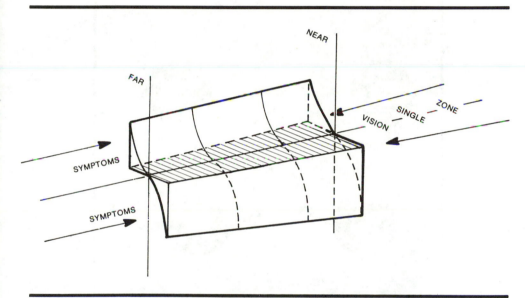

FIGURE 14-3 — A three-dimensional approach to graphical analysis showing the zone of single,
binocular vision in the horizontal plane and fixation disparity in the vertical plane

The understanding of fixation disparity related to asthenopia has helped
shorten the time required for orthoptic therapy in many cases. The doctor
has a more definite way of assessing the patient's heterophoric problem than
before. Be that as it may, the procedures used for motor fusion training have
remained basically the same as before.

Training consists essentially of developing motor fusion ranges with
sliding vergences and improving vergence facility with step vergence
exercises. Procedures listed in Table 12 A-D, and 13 A-B are applicable for
these purposes.

The Mallett Unit is ideal for use as the fixation target because of the
vernier lines that monitor fixation disparity. Likewise, the A.O. vectographic

slide can be used in training. Targets, such as the Keystone Eccentric Circles or Colored Circles, can be marked with appropriate vernier clues which allow the patient to monitor fixation disparity while doing chiastopic or orthopic fusion exercises. See Figure 14-4 showing vertical pencil markings on the Colored Circles for monitoring either exo or eso fixation disparities. Horizontal vernier marks can also be added for cases of vertical fixation disparity.

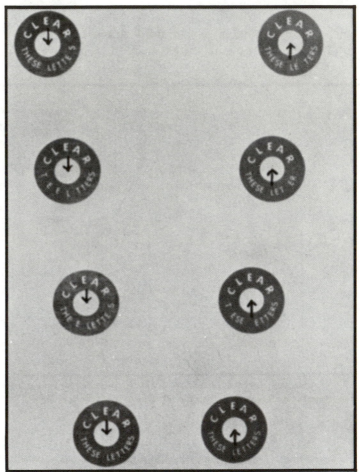

FIGURE 14-4 — Modification of the Keystone Colored Circles for monitoring fixation disparity during motor fusion training

Case Number Twelve discussed in Chapters Three and Five may be treated successfully through the use of motor fusion training procedures.

Surgery   Surgical treatment of fixation disparity is relatively infrequent, as extra-ocular muscle surgery is usually uncalled for in cases of heterophoria, unless the magnitude of the deviation is large.

Methods for the management of vertical fixation disparity include motor fusion training, vertical prism compensation, and surgery. Of the three methods, prisms are most commonly used. Prisms, however, are not helpful in compensating torsional fixation disparities. The method of therapy in these cases is either motor fusion training to improve cyclovergence, or surgery for reduction of the torsional deviation.

Carter[6] pointed out that the magnitude of the angle of fixation disparity is found to be smaller if a foveal target is fused than if nonfoveal contours are fused. The same principle applies when using targets for training purposes, and the doctor must keep this in mind when progress evaluations are being made. The doctor can be misled if nonfoveal contours are used initially, and foveal ones are used for retesting. The erroneous assumption might be made that the problem of fixation disparity is less severe than before.

Other Considerations

Management of fixation disparity is no panacea, and it must be remembered that there are causes for visual symptoms other than fixation disparity. They may be binocular in nature (e.g., diplopia or aniseikonia) or nonbinocular (e.g., astigmatism). Furthermore, psychogenic problems may simulate those that are binocular, and this possibility should be given consideration. In all cases, systemic and ocular diseases must be ruled out.

Clinical determination of fixation disparity curves by the use of the Disparometer™ is advocated by Sheedy.[7] This instrument[a] has pre-set vernier misaligned stimuli (see Figure 14-5) that allow estimation of angle F for either the ortho demand or vergence stress demands. The Disparometer can be attached to the nearpoint rod of a phoropter. Crossed polarizing filters are used in the phoropter. Horizontal angle F is measured by the examiner's dialing in the particular vertical vernier lines that create the patient's perception of the top line being exactly above the bottom line. Angle F can be determined to within 2 minutes of arc via bracketing the stimuli between eso and exo responses.

Forced-vergence fixation disparity curves are plotted by knowing the magnitude of angle F that corresponds with varying amounts of base-in and base-out prism. Base-in measurements are made first; then base-out measurements can commence, once the ortho-demand angle F is approximately the same as it originally was when testing began. Risley prism increments of 3 p.d. are advised to produce clinically reliable fixation disparity curves. Although this testing is done at 40 cm, special slides are available for far-point fixation disparity testing.

The four basic *types* of fixation disparity curves are shown in Figure 14-6. Sheedy and Saladin[7, 8] associated symptoms with types II, III, and IV curves, but found that symptoms did not tend to be associated with type I curves. However, type I curves that are steep (around the ortho demand area)

---

[a] Available from Vision Analysis, Columbus, Ohio.

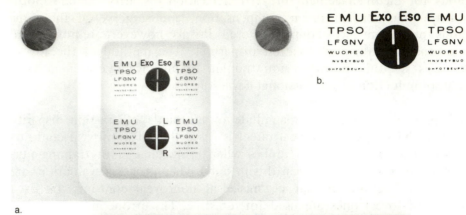

a.

b.

c.

FIGURE 14-5 — Disparometer™ (Courtesy, Vision Analysis). (a) Front view for testing horizontal and vertical fixation disparity. A penlight shone into a circular space illuminates the vernier lines via fiber optics; (b) Vernier offset in measurement of the angle of fixation disparity (angle F); (c) Back view showing fiber optics, which are illuminated from the front of the instrument, the knob to dial varying pre-set disparities, and the dials for reading magnitudes of angle F (in minutes of arc).

are associated with symptoms. Fortunately, fusional vergence training often can flatten out this portion of the fixation disparity curve and abate patients' symptoms. Prismatic prescriptions may be considered if steep type I curves cannot be flattened through functional training procedures. Prismatic prescriptions may also be necessary for patients who have types II, III, and IV curves. The *steepness* of the curve is apparently second in importance to the *type* of fixation disparity curve in regard to symptoms. The third factor is the *y-intercept*, which is the magnitude of angle F with an ortho demand. Sheedy and Saladin found this factor of the *y-intercept* to be more applicable to exophores than to esophores. In either case, vergence training should be attempted before prisms are prescribed.

The least important factor found by Sheedy and Saladin was the traditionally measured *x-intercept* (the associated phoria). This points out the potential usefulness of measuring angle F with an instrument such as the Disparometer for clinical purposes to effect clear, single, *comfortable,* binocular vision.

Sheedy and Saladin[8, 9] indicated that at least two mechanisms are operating in horizontal oculomotor imbalances. They found statistical argument for their clinical impression that in exophores, poor motor fusion definitely should be treated, and in esophores, sensory fusion should receive the most attention. They pointed out that Ogle-type I, III, and IV curves have been successfully treated with functional training procedures. The slopes flatten out, and types III and IV have a tendency to become type I curves with vision training. Type II curves, however, have not generally been amenable to change through orthoptic techniques. It should be noted that all fixation disparity curves should be plotted from "break to break" so a sharp downturn on the base-out side just before the break will not be missed. Many patients have been incorrectly labeled as type II when they really were type I. This is a critical point, because the prognosis for complete cure is much better for type I patients.[10]

In a study of 11 clinical indicators, but not including fixation disparity curve *types,* Sheedy and Saladin[8] found Sheard's criterion[b] to be the best discriminator for symptoms versus non-symptoms for exophoric subjects. The amount of heterophoria, on the other hand, was the best discriminator for esophoric subjects. Fixation disparity (slope and magnitude) was the next effective discriminator for both groups. Sheedy and Saladin reported, however, that Percival's criterion (demand in the middle third of the fusional vergence amplitude) showed very little discriminating power in exophoria, but it was somewhat better in esophoria. Nevertheless, each patient's symptoms must be assessed in concert with various clinical variables without reliance on any one test result or criterion.

---

[b]Sheard chose a 2/1 ratio between fusional vergence (blur point) and magnitude of opposing heterophoria as a criterion for separating symptomatic from non-symptomatic populations; Sheedy and Saladin found a 2.1/1 ratio, which is evidence for the efficacy of Sheard's criterion for exophoric patients.

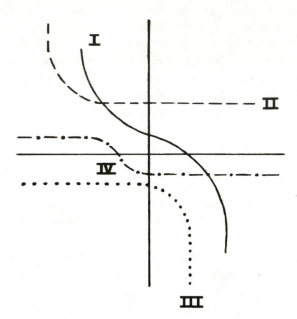

FIGURE 14-6 — Four basic types of fixation disparity curves. The position of each, relative to the abscissa and ordinate, may be different (up, down, right, or left) from that shown in this example.

15 | Efficient Visual Skills

The ultimate goal for any patient, and particularly one who is being treated for binocular anomalies, is the achievement of clear, single, comfortable, and *efficient* binocular vision. This applies in cases of either heterotropia or heterophoria. In the treatment of strabismus, the accomplishment of clear, single, comfortable, efficient binocular vision is the finishing process of therapy after the heterotropia is cured. In the case of heterophoria, the goal is comfortable and efficient visual skills, and therapy may begin immediately.

Practitioners in the 19th century were concerned almost exclusively with clearness of eyesight. They concerned themselves with lenses that would optimally reduce or eliminate blurred vision. Clearness and singleness of binocular vision became the issue with the advent of orthoptics. Effective therapeutic regimens for strabismus were introduced by Javel and, later, by others. (Refer to Chapter Six.)

Astute clinicians in the first half of the 20th century became aware of the relationship between accommodation and vergence. Knowledge of the zone of clear, single, *comfortable,* binocular vision was gained through various models of vision, such as the graphical analysis approach, and especially through an understanding of fixation disparity (see Chapter Fourteen).

There has been more and more emphasis on *efficiency* of vision in the latter half of the 20th century. This implies that efficient visual skills are related to good scholastic learning abilities *(school)* and occupational production *(work),* and to achievement in sports and hobbies *(play).* As a result, lenses and/or functional training procedures are frequently applied in clinical practice to help patients attain efficient binocular vision in these activities. (Surgery, drugs, and occlusion are not modes of therapy commonly associated with vision efficiency therapy.)

This chapter deals with the following topics: saccadic eye movements, pursuit eye movements, nonoptic eye movements, position maintenance of fixation, accommodation efficiency, various ranges of vergence, sensory fusion status, visual developmental-perceptual evaluation, and finally, the situations that may arise when strabismus is not completely cured; nevertheless, clear, single, comfortable, efficient, "monocular" vision is the goal of therapy.

Saccadic Eye Movements

There are four separate eye movement systems from a neurological point of view. These include the saccadic, pursuit, nonoptic, and vergence eye movement systems. The saccadic eye movements are abrupt shifts in fixation and are classified as *fast,* with the other three eye movement systems being classified as *slow.*

The velocity of saccades may be very high and is necessary if eye movements must exceed 40 degrees per second.[1] A good clinical average velocity to consider would be about 300 degrees per second as contrasted with movements of about 30 degrees per second. Therefore, saccades may be thought of as having velocities approximately 10 times greater than pursuits, vergences, and nonoptic-induced eye movements. According to Gay et al.,[2] saccadic eye movements are mainly voluntary, with the others being mainly involuntary. The duration and velocity of a saccade are proportional to the magnitude of the eye movement. A 40-degree sweep would have a greater velocity and a longer duration than would a 5-degree sweep.

The velocity of eye movement during a saccade changes, being fast at the beginning and slower toward the end of the sweep. Although this may be shown in the laboratory, it is difficult to observe clinically, even with recording instruments such as the Eye-Trac®.[a] (See Figure 15-1 showing the instrument, Figure 15-2 showing the five-dot test for saccades, and Figure 15-3 showing the Eye-Trac recording tape readout of the results of the five-dot test.)

SACCADIC SUPPRESSION

Javal may have been among the first to note that vision turns off as a saccadic eye movement is occurring. This makes sense; otherwise, the world would appear to be a swimming, blurry mess. This perceptual inhibition has been referred to as saccadic "blindness." It is more appropriate, however, to refer to this phenomenon as saccadic *suppression.* According to Solomons,[3] each saccadic eye movement is preceded by a latent period of about 120 to 180 milliseconds before the eye movement actually begins, and saccadic suppression begins to occur about 40 milliseconds before the movement commences. The inhibition increases until visual perception is almost zero during the first part of the movement. It is probably not until after the saccadic movement has ended that the saccadic suppression completely ceases.

NEUROLOGICAL PATHWAYS

Keep in mind that supranuclear lesions may cause limitations in eye movements, but deviations of the visual axes that may occur will be *concomitant.* On the other hand, infranuclear lesions will cause nonconcomitant deviations of the visual axes. (Refer to Chapter One for review of nonconcomitant deviations.) Saccades are presumed to be mediated via the fronto-

---

[a]Available from G&W Applied Science Laboratories.

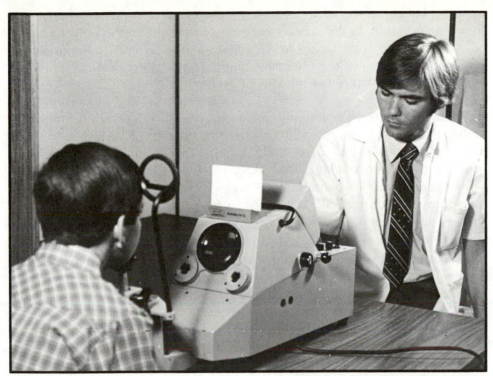

FIGURE 15-1 — Eye-Trac.®

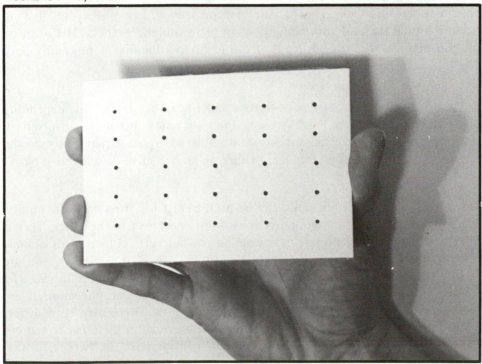

FIGURE 15-2 — The five-dot reading test used to evaluate reading saccades without cognitive demands from reading of words or from reading for comprehension. This was devised by Howard Walton, O.D., of the Southern California College of Optometry.

mesencephalic pathway. For example, stimulation from area 8 in the left frontal lobe results in conjugate movement of the eyes to the right side. The neural pathway is from area 8 to the conjugate gaze centers in the midbrain-pons and on to the nuclei of the third, fourth, and sixth cranial nerves, which innervate the six extraocular muscles of each eye.

SIGNS AND SYMPTOMS

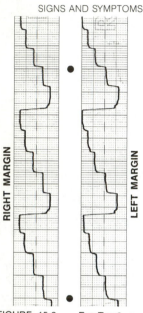

RIGHT MARGIN   LEFT MARGIN

FIGURE 15-3 — Eye-Trac® recording graph of normal saccadic eye movements made during the five-dot test.

If voluntary versions are severely restricted, you should suspect neurological problems affecting the saccadic neural pathway, e.g., myasthenia, vascular disease, or tumors that may affect supranuclear control. Other signs of neurological dysfunctioning would likely be evident in such cases. However, many times there may be only "soft" signs, with the patient appearing to be normal in all other respects. Many patients have *functional* saccadic problems, such as those from poor attention, hyperkinesis, and poor visual acuity due to uncorrected refractive errors.

What are the symptoms of either organic soft-sign or functional saccadic dysfunctioning? A patient may have several performance problems if saccadic eye movements are poor, even though he cannot otherwise be considered neurologically abnormal. Inefficiency in reading is a major problem and a frequent complaint in such cases. Words may be omitted, lines may be skipped, or a frequent loss of place when reading may be evident. Finger reading may indicate the need for hand "support" due to poor eye movements when reading. Head movement when reading is also a common sign attributable to poor saccades. The patient may present with a history of "having trouble hitting the ball" or "being poor in many athletic events." His work on the job may be affected adversely if eye-hand coordination is unusually poor due to saccadic eye movement problems.

TESTING FOR SACCADIC SKILLS

There are two types of saccades—gross and fine—that are tested, depending upon the magnitude of each sweep. Fine saccades are those involved in reading. Larger saccades than these are considered gross. A patient's saccadic eye movement skill can be evaluated either on an objective or subjective basis.

Any target, such as two pencils, can be used to test for gross saccadic ability. Merely have the patient voluntarily look from one target to the other. This is usually done in right and left gaze orientation, but vertical as well as oblique orientations can be tested. If one of the patient's eyes is occluded, you are testing saccadic ductions. If both eyes are open, you are checking for saccadic versions. It should be noted that even under the occluder, the covered eye moves conjugately with the uncovered, fixating eye. There may be a difference, however, in the performance of one tested eye from the other tested eye during duction testing. This is an important consideration in therapy, in that you want the patient to have (if possible) an equal saccadic skill with each eye. (Refer to Figure 12-1, illustrating the use of two pencils for testing of saccades.)

A quick and simple routine used at the Southern California College of Optometry (SCCO) for testing horizontal saccadic eye movements is as follows. A target with a letter printed on it that is approximately equivalent to 20/80 acuity demand is placed to the patient's right side. A similar target is placed to his left. The targets are separated approximately 25 cm and held at a distance of 40 cm from the patient. The patient is asked to move his eyes back and forth to each target approximately 10 times. The practitioner should look for inaccuracies—either undershooting or overshooting. Scoring of the results of observation is on a 4+ basis and is as follows: 4+ if movements are accurate, 3+ if there is one inaccuracy, 2+ if there are two inaccuracies, and 1+ if there are more than two inaccuracies.

SCCO SYSTEM

A score of 2+ or less is considered failure, as would be any head movement that could not be controlled. Hoffman and Rouse[4] consider a failure on this basis as a need for referral for vision therapy for saccadic dysfunctioning.

I like to use two Alphabet Pencils in the manner described above. These are the same targets as those used for physiological diplopia and jump vergences. (Refer to Figure 12-9 in Chapter Twelve.) Do not expect the young child to go all the way down the alphabet, but merely let him read the "A" on each pencil. For the adult, a sequence of "A" to "Z," "B" to "Y," "C" to "X," and so on is demanding and checks for false saccadic responses.

A five-point scoring system was proposed by Marcus.[5] It is similar to the previously mentioned procedures with two pencils, except that Marcus includes jump vergences in his saccadic evaluation, so that x-, y-, and z-axis evaluations are made. Again, Alphabet Pencils are suitable for this purpose. Five points are given if saccades are "accurate in all meridians tested." Four points are given if there are "fair landings but slight corrective movements"; three points are given if there are "accurate fixations in the X and Y axis but 'break down' on Z axis." Two points are scored if fixational performance is "different between right and left eyes." A score of one is made if "head or hand reinforcement is necessary for landings." No point is given if there is "no rapport with target."

MARCUS SYSTEM

A ten-point scale is another system that is recommended by Heinsen and Schrock[6] of San Jose and San Diego (California), respectively. It can be performed with pencils or similarly lettered targets, as previously described. For example, the patient can get 3 points if there is no head movement, 2 points if saccades are accurate, 2 points if saccades are automated (that is, occurring normally and simultaneously with simple cognitive demands), 2 points if eye movements are stable for 20 seconds of time, and 1 point if there is adequate stamina. Thus, 10 possible points can be given using this procedure. (Refer to Table 15A for clarification.)

HEINSEN-SCHROCK SYSTEM

TABLE 15A. Heinsen-Schrock System for Testing and Rating Saccadic Eye Movements[6]

A		B		C	
No head movement	(3)	Accuracies	(2)	Automated saccades	(2)
Head movement, but can inhibit	(2)	Slight inaccuracies	(1)	Reduced automation	(1)
Slight head movement persists	(1)				

D		E	
Stable saccades for 20 seconds	(2)	Adequate stamina	(1)
Stable saccades for 10 seconds	(1)		

With regard to automated saccades, I ask the person a simple question that is appropriate for his cognitive abilities under such circumstances. For example, I may ask a 5-year-old patient to tell me his name as he is looking from one target to the other. A 7-year-old patient could be expected to count from 1 to 10 while maintaining accurate saccades. A 9-year-old patient should be able to count backward from 10 to 1. An 11-year-old patient should be able to count backward from 100 on down. A 13-year-old patient can normally be expected to count backward from 100 by intervals of 2; a high school or college student should be able to do it in intervals of 3. This is what I believe Heinsen and Schrock mean by "automated." It stands to reason that the individual will be a poor performer in school, work, or play if his saccadic eye movements are not automatic. It is somewhat like the driving of a motor vehicle. The eye movements, even though saccades are mainly voluntary, must become almost reflexive in order for the motorist to be an efficient driver. The same holds true for reading. Unless the reader can automatically make the reading saccades, he is unlikely to be able to visualize and concentrate on the contents of the reading material. It often happens, when testing patients who have saccadic eye movement problems, that a cognitive demand will cause patients to look in the wrong direction of the test target and fail to make an accurate saccadic eye movement. In other words, the cognitive demand can make the saccadic movements poor (and poor saccades even poorer) unless automation is achieved. It is conversely presumed that poor saccadic eye movements have an adverse effect on reading (cognitive) skills.

OPHTHALMOGRAPHY

The best clinical ophthalmographic test for recording saccades in reading is the Eye-Trac (Figure 15-1). The most ideal target is the five-dot card (Figure 15-2) designed by Walton and tested by Griffin et al.[7] They analyzed the eye movements during reading and fixation tasks by using the Reading Eye

Camera. The subjects included 12 adequate readers and 13 inadequate ones. They concluded that "inadequate readers seem to have less efficient saccadic eye movements regardless of the type of material used." Besides using words for fixation material, rows of dots were also used, so that the lack of comprehension of certain words would not be an intervening factor. The five-dot card was adapted to the Eye-Trac instrument, which has an advantage over the Reading Eye Camera in that an instantaneous printout of the results is available for analysis. Refer to the example of a fairly normal saccadic pattern in five-dot testing shown on the Eye-Trac recording strip in Figure 15-3. Note that five fixations were made for each row of dots and they were spaced fairly equally, but there was a slight problem of undershooting on some of the return sweeps. Figure 15-4 shows an example of obvious problems with saccades on this test.

Another reading saccade test that is objective but much less sensitive than the Eye-Trac is the use of printed cards, such as the five-dot test, where the practitioner directly observes the patient's eye movements when looking from dot to dot. These sequential fixations tests come in a variety of forms. The dots (or other symbols such as asterisks, stars, numbers, letters, and words) may be printed on a clear acetate sheet so that the practitioner can look directly at the patient's eyes through the printed sheet and look for any inaccuracies or head movements (see Figure 15-5). Another variation is an opaque card on which the symbols are printed; there is a hole in the center for the tester to look through to observe the patient's eye movements. (see Figure 15-6). Obviously, assessment of saccadic ability must be made quickly and on

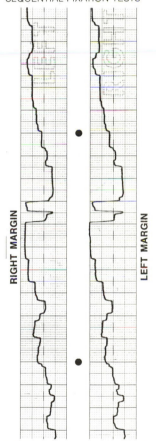

SEQUENTIAL FIXATION TESTS

RIGHT MARGIN   LEFT MARGIN

FIGURE 15-4 — Poor saccadic responses on the five-dot test as graphically shown on the readout ecording tape of the Eye-Trac.

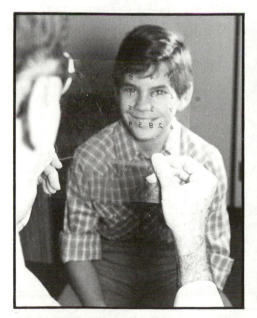

FIGURE 15-5 — Sequential fixation device. A clear acetate sheet has numbers for saccadic eye movement testing/training.

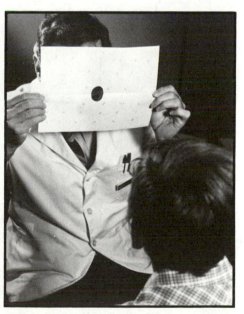

FIGURE 15-6 — Sequential fixation device. This is a hole in a card with numbers for saccadic eye movement testing/training.

the spot, so to speak, as there is no permanent readout to analyze later on. Furthermore, judgments are strictly qualitative and lack precision. Notwithstanding these drawbacks, experience goes a long way in making this procedure useful in the event the Eye-Trac is not available at the time of testing. Sequential fixation tests are referred to as a "poor person's Eye-Trac." It is very helpful to see the same patients for both the Eye-Trac and the sequential fixation testing; thus, the practitioner can increase his clinical acumen with this simple testing procedure.

Unfortunately, with sequential fixation testing without a recording instrument, the doctor can only speculate on what he saw, without the aid of the permanent recording that is afforded with the Eye-Trac. Whether the Eye-Trac is used or not, the patient should be tested on the reading of sentences and paragraphs in addition to the five-dot test. (See Figures 15-7 for Eye-Trac recording examples of poor and good reading saccades. This patient was more efficient in reading after saccadic training.) By testing with cognitive (paragraph) and noncognitive (five-dot) visual stimuli, a differential diagnosis can

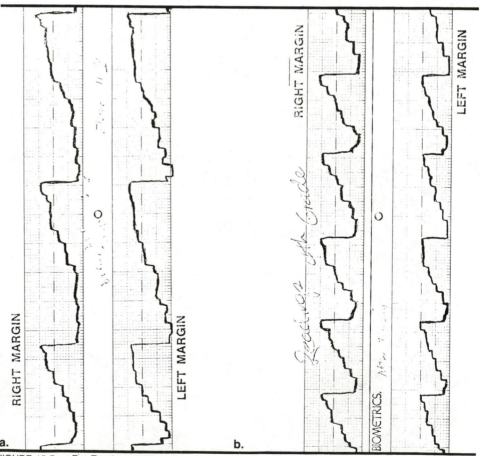

FIGURE 15-7 — Eye-Trac® recordings of an 11-year-old girl reading material of a fourth-grade level. (a) Before vision therapy for saccadic eye movement problems; (b) After 5 weeks of training (five visits in the office with daily out-of-office training). Note the increased rate of reading after therapy (about twice the number of lines of similar reading material of the same grade level).

be made between purely saccadic problems and cognitive problems (e.g., dyslexia, poor comprehension, and unfamiliarity with certain words).

Saccades are evaluated indirectly by subjective means rather than by direct, objective observations in the following tests.

The most popular normed subjective test for saccadic abilities is the Pierce Saccade Test.[b] This test was designed to evaluate (indirectly) the patient's gross saccadic eye movement development according to age expectancies. It consists of three subtests, each of which is a series of two laterally displaced numbers (see Figure 15-8). The patient is asked to hold the demonstration card at his normal reading distance and read each number aloud, from side to side. (Note: Holding the card too close would invalidate the test, as very large saccades would be demanded, e.g., over 30 degrees beyond the midline. Thus, accuracy of saccades would not be expected, even by a normal patient taking this test. Therefore, it is wise to have the patient hold the card at a distance approaching 40 cm, if possible.) A demonstration is given initially so the patient can start with the number at the top left corner of the page and follow the arrow to the number on the top right corner, then follow the arrow for the return sweep to the number on the left-hand side of the page, and so forth. The room should be well illuminated for testing purposes.

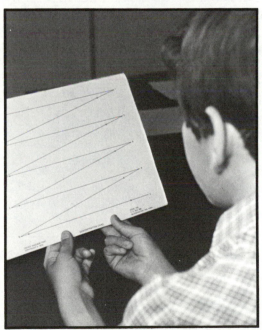

FIGURE 15-8 — Patient being tested on the demonstration card of the Pierce Saccade Test.

Once the demonstration is completed, the first subtest is begun. Explain to the patient that he should try to read the numbers as quickly as he can in the

[b] Available from Cook Inc.

same manner as the demonstration. However, he should also try to read the numbers accurately. This is a timed test, and thus one supposedly intended for determining saccadic efficiency. Each of the three subtests is timed, and errors are recorded. For each subtest, calculate the corrected score using the following formula for each subtest:

$$\text{Corrected time score} = \frac{30}{30 - \text{errors}} \times \text{Time in seconds.}$$

For example, suppose the patient takes 45 seconds to complete the first subtest, but there were no errors. The corrected score for this subtest would be 45 seconds. But what if there had been 10 errors? The corrected score of this subtest would be 67 seconds. The total of the three corrected scores is determined and compared with the norms for the Pierce Saccade Test to judge the patient's chronological age equivalence. (See Table 15B for a sample of norms.) In using the Pierce Saccade Test, the doctor has an idea if the patient's saccadic ability is above, below, or normal for his age. This subjective assessment, together with objective testing of saccades, can give the doctor evidence of whether the patient does or does not have problems with saccadic eye movements. One possible drawback to the Pierce test is that the saccades being tested are gross and do not necessarily represent the fine saccades that occur in the act of reading.

TABLE 15B. *Sample of Normative Values for the Pierce Saccade Test*

Chronological Age (Years)	Corrected Time Scores Expected (seconds)
6	150
7	125
8	100
9	82
10	70
11	65
12	59
13	55

KING-DEVICK TEST

The King-Devick Test[8] was devised with fine saccades in mind. It contains several numbers per line (five numbers in each line). The numbers are randomly spaced to supposedly simulate saccades that would occur in a reading situation. (See Figures 15-9a through 15-9d, showing the 8½-×-11-inch pages of the King-Devick Test.) Scores are evaluated in terms of errors and time; they are then compared with normed scores according to chronological age in a manner similar to that in the Pierce Saccade Test. Normative values are given in Table 15C.

Samples of approximate norms determined by Cohen and Lieberman (in a study in cooperation with a New York Optometric Association team) are given in Table 15D.[9] Subjects consisted of 1,202 students in regular public schools. They found that subtests II and III were too difficult for many 6-year-old

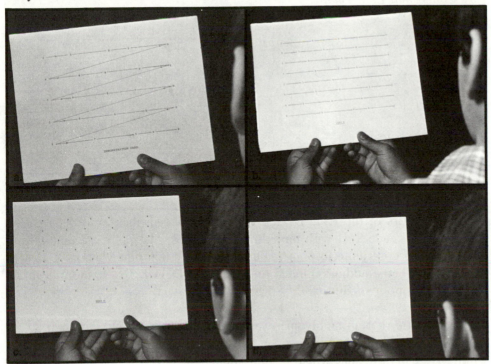

FIGURE 15-9 — King-Devick Test. (a) Demonstration card; (b) Subtest I; (c) Subtest II; (d) Subtest III.

children and do not recommend all three subtests at the 6-year-old level. Instead, use only subtest number I, which was found to have norms of 30.98 seconds with 1.32 errors for children aged 6. The King-Devick Test includes a demonstration card (Figure 15-9a) and three test cards (Figures 15-9b through 15-9d). Each test card has eight rows of 5 numbers, for a total of 40 numbers per card (as opposed to 30 per card in the Pierce Saccade Test). The numbers are sized to approximate 20/100 reduced Snellen acuity. Testing is done in the same manner as the Pierce test.

TABLE 15C. Normative Values of Two Saccadic Tests As Found by King-Devick[8]

Age	Pierce Test	King-Devick Test
6	119	116
7	122	103
8	102	85
9	92	77
10	82	69
11	71	64
12	71	63

TABLE 15D. Samples of Norms for the King-Devick Test As Determined by Cohen and Lieberman[9]

Age	Time in Seconds (Total of 3 Subtests)	Number of Errors (Total of 3 Subtests)
6	119	17
7	101	12
8	79	3
9	73	3
10	68	2
11	57	1
12	54	1
13	52	1
14	50	0

The authors of the King-Devick Test concluded in their study comparing the Pierce Saccade Test with the King-Devick Test that poor saccadic ability does seem to contribute to poor reading ability. When other factors are ruled out (e.g., IQ), the authors implied that the King-Devick Test is more accurate in predicting poor reading ability than the Pierce test.

FUNCTIONAL TRAINING PROCEDURES

It is axiomatic that an amblyopic eye tends to show poor eye movements, for example, saccades. Therefore, poor performance, as in reading, may result. Similarly, I believe that when an individual reads with a nonamblyopic eye, but with an eye that shows poor saccadic ability, there will be poor reading performance. Consequently, the training in monocular saccadic dysfunction and the monocular occlusion training methods in cases of amblyopia parallel each other very closely. In fact, following the procedures outlined in Chapter Seven for the therapy for amblyopia will yield a reasonably good regimen for saccadic therapy for nonamblyopic eyes. (Refer to Tables 7A through 7E.)

However, let us list some sequences that apply only to saccadic therapy, and exclude the issue of amblyopia. It is best to begin with monocular training, right eye or left eye alone. After each eye is shown to perform equally well, proceed to binocular training. Table 15E lists general approaches to training for saccadic eye movement dysfunction.

STEP ONE

Position maintenance probably involves all four of the eye movement systems, i.e., saccades, pursuits, vergences, and nonoptic. (This will be discussed later.) If position maintenance ability is reasonably good, then move on to step two for saccadic training. Remember that in the case of amblyopia, this anomaly would need to be attacked before finishing the patient training with efficient skills discussed in this chapter. As is customary, binocular saccadic training would be started after the improvement of amblyopia. However, if there is no amblyopia and position maintenance is good, proceed with saccadic therapy. Saccades are voluntary, and a principle of vision therapy is to go from voluntary actions to reflexive ones that are automatic.

TABLE 15E. Approaches to Training for Saccadic Eye Movement Dysfunction

1. Ensure good position maintenance (steady fixation on a stationary target)
2. Go from gross (large) saccades to fine (small) saccades, as in reading
3. Go from slow to fast (timing of several cycles)
4. Develop good eye-hand coordination during saccadic demands, and then go without hand as support (e.g., no finger reading)
5. Train eye equalness (so O.D. and O.S. have equal facility)
6. Go from monocular (duction) to binocular (version) saccades
7. Eliminate any head movement
8. Introduce motor sequencing with metronome (auditory-visual integration) and ensure good left-to-right sequencing of saccades, as in reading the English language.
9. Develop automated saccades (simple cognitive demands during saccades should not have an adverse effect on the quality of eye movements)
10. Eliminate (if possible) any significant overshoots, undershoots, regressions, or inefficient return sweeps

---

TABLE 15F. Specific Training Procedures for Saccadic Dysfunction

1. Picking up objects on a table (e.g., raisins, peanuts, and candy)
2. Visual-motor bat and Marsden ball (different colored portions of the bat are to hit a swinging ball upon varying commands; see Figure 7-3)
3. Toothpick in soda straw (patient's other hand is used to locate the straw if the hole is missed when therapist is holding the straw)
4. Pegboard games (e.g., Lite-Brite, as in Figure 15-12, or other commercially available toys) and LaBarge Electro Therapist, Figure 15-10 (with auditory-visual integrative sequencing)
5. Wall fixations (e.g., randomly placed animal pictures on a wall, with the patient being asked to look at a particular one on command; a baseball diamond can be used in a similar fashion to "play" a ball game)
6. Wall fixations with an afterimage (patient has good feedback as to accuracy of eye movement and fixation)
7. Fixation of numbers with eye-hand training (numbers 1 through 15 are randomly displayed on a page, and the patient has to find and mark each number in ascending order upon command); a continuous motion type of training can be used by having the patient draw lines to each corrective number (Figure 15-14)
8. Loose prism jumps (patient eventually learns to perceive image jumps when making saccades as small as 0.5 p.d.); note that this is done monocularly (ductions), with the other eye being occluded
9. Tic-tac-toe game (therapist or home "helper" and patient are players)
10. Dot-to-dot games; the pegboard demands, such as those of the Rosner TVAS (Figure 15-13), are good for this activity
11. Filling Os (filling in each letter "O" in newspaper printing)
12. Sequentially marking alphabetical letters (e.g., Michigan Tracking, as in Figure 15-20)
13. Sequential fixation sheet (marks not involving cognition, such as dots, dashes, and asterisks)
14. Modified sequential fixation sheet (symbols demanding cognition, e.g., Bs, Ds, Ps, Qs, numbers, and words; see Figure 15-5)
15. Other. Haidinger's brushes may be used as a foveal tag; also afterimages and Maxwell's spot. Red-green or polarizing filters may be used to monitor suppression when binocular saccadic training is given. Stereoscopes may be used in this regard; for example, refer to Figure 10-2.

STEP TWO

In step two, the patient practices making accurate, large saccades until he can make smaller saccades that are accurate. The large saccades are mostly voluntary and can generally be improved with concentrated effort on the part of the patient. Fine saccades involved in reading are somewhat less voluntary than the gross saccades and are more difficult to train early on. Training procedures would go, for example, from the patient doing wall fixations (gross) to Michigan Tracking[c] (fine). Table 15F lists many specific training procedures that are arranged in an easy-to-difficult progressive sequence. Most of these can be performed at home, where the principles listed in table 15E can be applied.

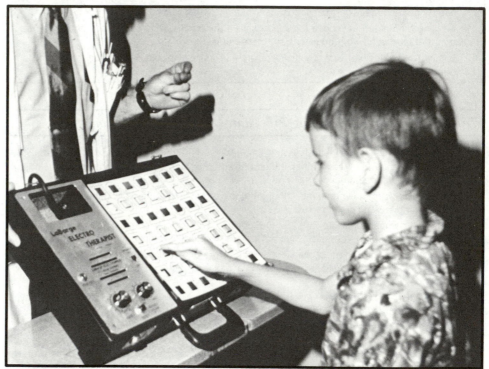

FIGURE 15-10 — LaBarge Electro Therapist.

STEP THREE

Step three makes the patient more efficient in saccades as to time. The Pierce Saccade Test is ideal for testing and retesting for efficiency of gross saccades, and the King-Devick Test for fine reading saccades. Also, timing on the sequential fixation tests can be compared from the beginning to end of this phase of therapy. Various metronome devices can be used in this training. The LaBarge Electro Therapist[d] is excellent for saccadic therapy (see Figure 15-10). Another useful instrument is the Saccadic Fixator[e] (Figure 15-11). Most children enjoy playing games on this instrument to see if their speed (efficiency) can be improved.

[c]Ann Arbor Publishers Inc. Note that ordinary newsprint is suitable for home training. Ask the patient to circle each letter of the alphabet in sequence (starting with the letter "a" and ending with the letter "z").

[d]Distributed by Rader Child Development Products.

[e]Manufactured by Wayne Engineering.

Step four is to ensure good eye-hand coordination during saccadic demands. Any of the pointing procedures discussed in Chapter Seven for amblyopia apply here, as well as the LaBarge Electro Therapist or the Saccadic Fixator. Figure 7-3 shows a patient using the visual motor bat and the Marsden ball, which may be used in saccadic (as well as in pursuit) training.

STEP FOUR

The purpose in this phase, once good eye-hand coordination is achieved, is to drop the hand as a support. (It is very interesting to see how the finger is used, even by adults, as a "support" under certain stressful situations, such as reading through a legal document on which a signature is required.)

Usually, the patient with poor saccadic ability may be performing better if he can point to the numbers, letters, or words, than if he has to locate them accurately by visual means alone. Since it is inefficient to have to point to each fixated object of regard, the hand/finger support must be discouraged as soon as possible in the therapy program.

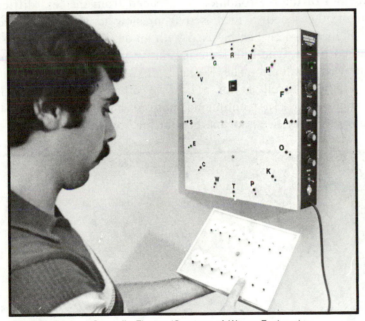

FIGURE 15-11 — Saccadic Fixator (Courtesy of Wayne Engineering, Orthoptic Division).

Training should be given for each eye until the saccadic ability is approximately equal. Therefore, duction (monocular) training has been emphasized up to this point in therapy of saccades.

STEP FIVE

When the eyes are approximately equal in ability, proceed to binocular conjugate movements (versions).

STEP SIX

This upward step in therapy is for the purpose of eliminating any head movement during saccades. The finely turned extraocular muscles are much more efficient and accurate in aiming fixation than are the relatively gross

STEP SEVEN

neck and body muscles. Most patients (even those with neurological soft signs) can voluntarily learn to control their head movements when making saccadic eye movements. Their reading efficiency is expected to improve as a result.

STEP EIGHT   It is time to introduce auditory stimuli into the saccadic visual task and ensure that the patient is able to motorically sequence in a good left-to-right fashion (that is, if English is his written language). The LaBarge Electro Therapist is ideal for this, as it contains a metronome and is designed to use letters and words that can be put in a left-to-right sequence. The introduction of the auditory stimuli sets the stage for the patient's being able to integrate the visual, kinesthetic, tactile, and auditory stimuli. The patient should be able to take control of this so that he can hit each target with his finger in time to the beat of the metronome. He should be able to develop the ability to keep up with the rhythm of the metronome. To proceed from the less difficult to the more difficult, the speed is increased from slow to fast. Toys, such as the Lite-Brite (Figure 15-12), can be used with an auxiliary metronome for many of the same purposes. The Lite-Brite is relatively inexpensive and suitable for home training of children. The Rosner[10] TVAS activity is also useful for saccadic therapy, as well as for a host of other developmental-perceptual skills (see Figure 15-13). Continuous motion games (Figure 15-14) can be custom made to fit the needs of the patient for home therapy.

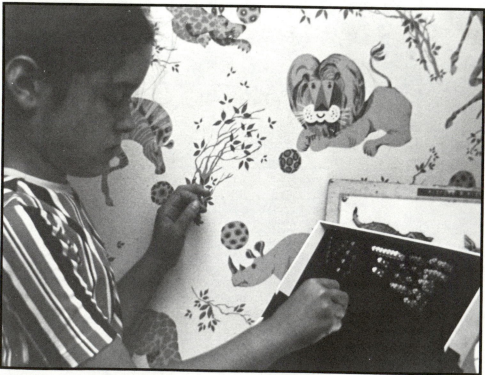

FIGURE 15-12 — Lite-Brite toy used for saccadic eye movement therapy. This is ideal for out-of-office therapy.

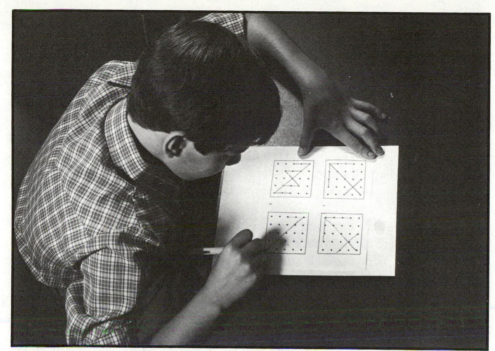

FIGURE 15-13 — Sample page of Rosner TVAS.

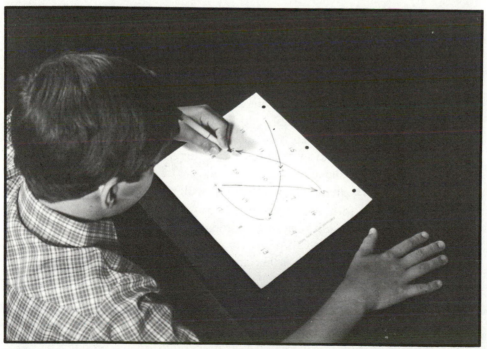

FIGURE 15-14 — Continuous motion game. This can be custom made and varied for out-of-office therapy. The patient is instructed to draw a continuous line to connect the numbers in proper sequence.

STEP NINE

The development of automated saccades is involved in this step. As in the testing described earlier, the patient should be able to cope with cognitive demands (commensurate with his mental ability) during training so he is not distracted from making accurate eye movements. This is absolutely essential for good reading ability, good work performance, or effective and enjoyable play. Much of this type of training can be done at home and, it is hoped, at school. However, close supervision must be provided to ensure proper saccadic responses in order for vision therapy to be successful. Moreover, unless the patient is able to get through step nine, he will not be much better off than if no saccadic vision therapy were done at all. The importance of establishing automated responses cannot be overemphasized.

STEP TEN

The final step is the finishing process in which any significant overshoots, undershoots, regressions, or inefficient return sweeps are eliminated. If there are subclinical neurological soft signs, the patient may not be able to completely overcome these inaccurate eye movements. However, I have been amazed at what progress can be made in many cases in which the saccades were very inaccurate at the beginning of therapy. If speed can be increased, and good left-to-right sequencing, motor planning with rhythm, and elimination of head movement can be achieved, the patient is better off as a result of vision therapy for poor saccadic eye movement skills than he was before, the soft signs notwithstanding. Practically all saccadic eye movement problems can be helped if there are functional causes for the poor saccadic skills.

Pursuit Eye Movements

A pursuit eye movement is defined as a "movement of an eye fixating a moving object."[11]

CHARACTERISTICS

According to Michaels,[12] pursuits are unlike saccades in that they are tracking responses and vision is present (without suppression as in saccades) throughout their excursions. The speed of pursuits is limited to about 30 degrees per second. They may be considerably slower, but not much faster. If the target velocity is too high, the pursuits break down into a cogwheel, jerky motion. The attempt to keep tracking requires the faster saccadic responses to come into play in order for the patient to keep his eye on the target. Furthermore, pursuits are relatively involuntary compared with saccades.

Pursuits are a form of duction when only one eye is being tested (monocular viewing conditions), but binocular viewing conditions allow for testing a form of version. (Versions may be either saccades, pursuits, or nonoptic.) Regardless of the fact that an eye may be occluded, the covered eye moves conjugately with the fixating eye under most normal circumstances. But this would be duction (rather than version) testing, because the patient is under monocular viewing conditions.

NEUROLOGICAL PATHWAYS

Pursuit eye movements are mediated via the occipito-mesencephalic pathway. Impulses travel from the occipital lobes (presumably from area 19) to the midbrain and pontine gaze centers, and on to the nuclei of the third, fourth, and sixth cranial nerves to innervate the extraocular muscles of the eyes. Current thinking is that each occipital lobe is involved in the pursuit of a target, in both directions, horizontally or vertically.[13] The assumption is that the right and left occipital area is connected to each right and left pontine gaze center so that, for example, stimulation from the left occipital lobe may stimulate both the left and right pontine gaze centers, for left or right pursuit movement. Because of this double coverage, pursuits may sometimes be intact in spite of an extensive lesion in one hemisphere of the brain that could concomitantly cause a visual field loss.

A notable exception to this is in the asymmetric optokinetic nystagmus (OKN) response when there is a deep parietal lobe lesion. The amplitude of the fast saccadic portion of the OKN response is reduced. This may be due to the fact that the pursuit is limited by such a lesion. For example, if a lesion of the left parietal lobe is very deep, it could cause a right homonymous hemianoptic visual field defect along with a decreased optokinetic nystagmus response when the OKN stimuli (e.g., vertical stripes) are moving toward the patient's left. Anatomically, the fibers of the pursuit pathway from the left and right occipital lobes join in the internal sagittal stratum. If there is a lesion in the left parietal lobe such that the joined fibers are affected, this would disrupt a pursuit movement to the patient's left and cause a decreased OKN response when the OKN stimuli are moving to his left. Saccades to the right may be affected also because of a "disconnection syndrome" to the frontal lobe.[14] However, pursuits to the patient's right would be unaffected, and optokinetic nystagmus would be normal when the OKN stripes were moved toward his right side. OKN testing gives an estimation of visual acuity (Chapter Two), in addition to providing a quick neurological screening test for pursuit and saccadic pathway involvements.

There may be soft signs neurologically in the case of jerky pursuits. Problems may be so subtle that no lesion can be found (by radiology or other means) along the occipito-mesencephalic pathway. Nevertheless, evidence of pursuit dysfunctioning should always be questioned. In some cases, functional training procedures may help. In many others, however, not much can be done to improve pursuits when these soft signs are present.

Differential diagnostic testing should be considered in any event. For example, suppose a patient has voluntary versions (saccades) that are normal, but following (pursuit) movements are significantly restricted and jerky. A supranuclear lesion affecting the occipito-mesencephalic pathway would be suspected. On the other hand, if saccades were inaccurate and restricted but pursuits were normal, a fronto-mesencephalic pathway lesion would be suspected. It is always wise to check both pursuits and saccades on a routine basis, not only to determine gross organic defects but to detect subtle problems that can also handicap individuals because of resulting visual inefficiencies. Additionally, keep in mind that the effects of drugs, fatigue, and emotional stress may adversely affect pursuit performance.

TESTING OF PURSUIT SKILLS

Four objective and two subjective testing procedures will be discussed. Without doubt, many others could be listed, but time does not permit. They are all basically the same in that the principal point of all these tests is to allow monitoring for accuracy of pursuit eye movements.

SCCO SYSTEM

A quick and convenient testing and rating system for pursuits on a 4+ scale is used at the Southern California College of Optometry (SCCO).[15] A fixation target approximately the size of a 20/80 letter is moved in front of the patient at a distance of about 40 cm in left-right-left, up-down-up, and diagonal orientations, with the patient's being instructed to track the target. A 4+ is given if pursuits are smooth and fixation is always accurate, 3+ if there is one fixation loss, 2+ if there are two fixation losses, and 1+ if there are more than two fixation losses. The patient is considered to have pursuit problems if the score is less than 3+ using this system.

If there should be any head movements during testing after the patient has been instructed not to move his head, performance is considered to be inadequate. I believe that the right eye, the left eye, and then both eyes should routinely be tested, whether this or any other method of testing pursuits is used.

H-S SCALE

Heinsen and Schrock[16] use a rating system (H-S Scale) for pursuits similar to the one they use for evaluating saccades (discussed previously). This is on a 10-point scale and is shown in Table 15G. The advantage of the Heinsen-

---

TABLE 15G. *Heinsen-Schrock System for Testing and Rating Pursuit Eye Movements*[16]

A	
Smooth, always on target	(3)
Smooth, sometimes off target	(2)
Jerky, generally on target	(1)
B	
Free of head movement	(3)
Head movement, but can inhibit	(2)
Slight head movement persists	(1)
C	
Automated pursuits	(3)
Reduced automation	(2)
Much reduced automation	(1)
D	
Adequate stamina	(1)

Schrock system over the SCCO 4+ system is that not only are head movements, smoothness, and accuracy taken into account, but also automation and stamina. Either a Marsden ball (see Figure 7-3 in Chapter Seven) or an instrument such as the Keystone Rotator (Figure 15-15) would be ideal for this type of testing, although a hand-held penlight that is moved smoothly and evenly will suffice. Whatever target is used, smoothness, accuracy, head movement, automation, and stamina are to be evaluated. Using the same cognitive demands as in saccadic testing (discussed previously) and continuing the pursuits for about 1 minute of time will allow a judgment of automation and stamina, respectively.

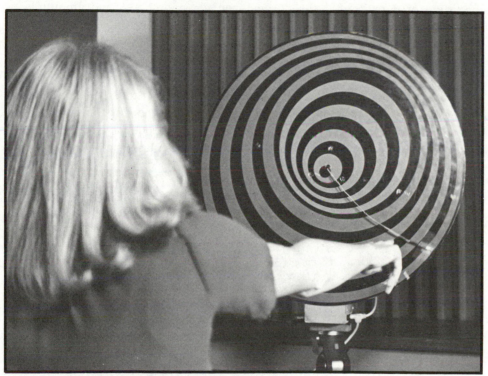

FIGURE 15-15 — Keystone Rotator for testing pursuit eye movements.

A five-point scale for rating pursuits was presented by Marcus[17] (see Table 15H). Both horizontal meridians can be judged, presumably by using a target such as a hand-held penlight. The qualities of accuracy, smoothness, effort, and head movements are implied in this system of evaluation.

MARCUS SYSTEM

The Eye-Trac is one of the best ophthalmographic clinical methods to measure and evaluate pursuit movements. (There are excellent experimental laboratory-like instruments for eye tracking that are not discussed in this text; only the readily available clinical methods are covered.) The rotating optokinetic nystagmus (OKN) drum attachment to the Eye-Trac can be modified to make a tracking target. (See Figure 15-16 showing the modified target using a pencil tip as a fixation target for tracking.) This allows a permanent graphical

OPHTHALMOGRAPH

TABLE 15H. Marcus Scoring System for Pursuit Eye Movements[17]

Smooth and effortless in both meridians	(5 points)
Smooth, with effort, in both meridians	(4 points)
Smooth in horizontal meridian, but jerky in vertical	(3 points)
Jerky in both meridians	(2 points)
Head turning for support	(1 point)
No rapport with target	(no point)

recording of pursuits that can be analyzed for smoothness and amplitude by studying the printouts of the Eye-Trac instruments (see Figures 15-17a and 15-17b). The sensitivity of testing is much greater than with those methods having no graphical recording of eye movements.

FLICKER METHOD   The aforementioned testing methods are objective in nature. A very sensitive subjective method is an illuminated wand attached to the Keystone Rotator that pulses at a rate above the critical flicker fusion frequency. The flicker is obliterated as long as the patient is fixating the moving target. However, when

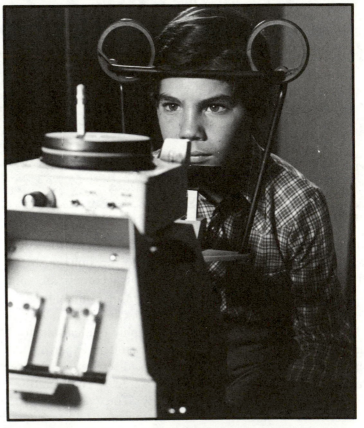

FIGURE 15-16 — Modified rotating drum for pursuit testing with the Eye-Trac.

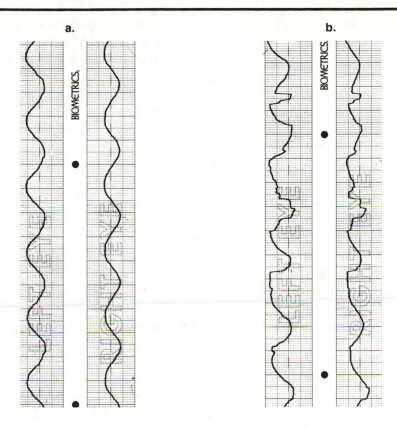

FIGURE 15-17 — Recordings from Eye-Trac®. (a) Smooth pursuits; (b) Jerky pursuits.

fixation is lost momentarily, the pulsing light moves across different retinal receptors, so that the continuous light sensation is lost and a flicker is perceived. This happens when the smooth pursuit breaks down and the saccades are called into play in order to maintain fixation on the moving light. It provides good feedback in the process of training pursuit skills, and it is used as a subjective testing method for smoothness and accuracy of pursuits. The speed of the moving light can be varied on the instrument. The amplitude of pursuits can be changed by having the patient move closer (for larger excursions) or farther away (for smaller excursions).

Afterimages can also be used in conjunction with a moving target to provide visual feedback for the patient to see if tracking is accurate with fixation always being on the target. This is useful in both testing and training.

AFTERIMAGES

Patients who have poor pursuit skills may also have histories of various visual inefficiencies. I have found that many poor readers have poor pursuits, although the cause and effect is not as easy to comprehend as in the relation of saccadic dysfunction and poor reading. Patients with poor pursuit eye

SIGNS AND SYMPTOMS

movements also tend to have significant problems in sports. It is conceivable, for example, that it would be much more difficult to accurately track a tennis ball if head movements are necessary, because the gross neck muscles are not as efficient as the finely tuned extraocular muscles. However, I saw a patient who had Duane's syndrome of each eye, which severely restricted ocular activity, who reported being able to play tennis "fairly well." This was in spite of head turning being necessary to see the approaching ball. Therefore, statements relating to pursuit skills and athletic skills must be made with caution and with other factors kept in mind.

It is natural to expect a patient with nuclear or infranuclear lesions affecting the extraocular muscles to have many signs and symptoms. Pursuits would likely be inaccurate and jerky in the diagnostic action field of the affected muscle (refer to Chapter One, regarding nonconcomitancy). However, the infranuclear "hard" signs are relatively easy to detect, explain, and understand in contrast to supranuclear soft signs, in which the only sign may be a slight problem in pursuits. In either case, the patient with pursuit problems will possibly have symptoms of vertigo, nausea, asthenopia, and inefficient vision for moving objects, as well as a host of other complaints.

Since pursuits are mainly involuntary and many of the neurological soft signs are incurable, one must ask what functional training procedures can do to help patients with pursuit problems. There are some voluntary aspects in the testing procedures of pursuits mentioned previously, e.g., head movement, automation, and stamina. These aspects can be worked on and made more reflexive, starting from volition to automation. In many cases, accuracy and smoothness are improved as a result of functional training procedures.

FUNCTIONAL TRAINING
PROCEDURES FOR PURSUITS

Like the patient with amblyopia who has poor saccadic skills, the patient viewing through his amblyopic eye is likely to have poor pursuit skills.[18] Accommodation inefficiency also is common for the amblyopic eye. It is interesting to observe the similarity between a patient who is "learning disabled" and an amblyopic individual (one who is not learning disabled) who nevertheless tries to perform well using the amblyopic eye, for example, in reading or playing tennis. The amblyopic eye is visually inefficient, with resulting performance being poor, the same as in a patient with learning disabilities.

Many practitioners realize the close correlation between poor pursuits and poor performance in school, work, and play. Yet there is not a great deal of study that deals with *therapy* and what positive results can be obtained via therapy. Suggested approaches following an easy-to-difficult format have been published[19] and will be elaborated on at this point.

Pursuit training is frequently used in therapy to attempt to increase excursions when there is restricted motility in cases of nonconcomitancy. This is also done in amblyopia therapy to promote foveal fixation. However, the degree to which only pursuit therapy for vision efficiency is emphasized varies among practitioners. Some advocate pursuit training for all patients who show signs of or have symptoms of poor pursuits. Others, however, seldom recommend therapy for pursuit improvement. Perhaps if this function were evaluated thoroughly, the need for therapy would be realized by more practitioners than at present. (Refer to Table 15I for strategies in training to improve pursuit eye movements.)

TABLE 15I. Approaches to Improvement of Pursuit Eye Movements

1. Steady position maintenance of stationary target
2. Voluntary to reflexive responses
3. Eye-hand coordination to no eye-hand support
4. Small to large excursions
5. Slow to fast speed of pursuits
6. Jerky to smooth movements
7. Head movement to no head movement
8. Unequalness to equalness of right eye and left eye
9. Monocular to binocular pursuits
10. Simple to complex cognitive demands
11. Sitting to standing position
12. No vergence demand to prismatic demands
13. Combinations of less stress to more stress

Equipment for pursuit training can be quite simple, and most training consists of out-of-office procedures. A partial list of instrumentation for pursuit training is given in Table 15J. With the exception of large automatic rotating devices, all the equipment can be taken home for training.

INSTRUMENTATION

TABLE 15J. Instrumentation for Pursuit Training; Corresponding Therapy Applies to Home As Well As Office Procedures

Office	Home
1. Automatic rotating device (e.g., Keystone Rotator)	Pie pan rotations (marble rolling)
2. Marsden ball	Suspended ball
3. Penlight (hand held)	Penlight (hand held)
4. Spot flashlight (chasing on wall)	Spot flashlight (chasing on wall)

The patient in therapy must become aware of his errors during the practice of a given task. Otherwise, mere practice alone possibly can hinder rather than help if the person is making incorrect responses. This principle applies to pursuit therapy as well as all phases of vision therapy. There are three

PRINCIPLES

convenient ways in which the patient can have this necessary feedback during pursuit practice: (1) objectively watch the patient and tell him when he is making incorrect responses; (2) have him report flicker on the light of the Keystone Rotator as an indicator that pursuits are breaking down; and (3) generate an afterimage on the macula so monitoring of correct fixation during pursuits can be maintained by the patient.

Another principle of vision therapy is to make the patient aware of what he is doing. An effective way to make the patient aware of his eye movements is to ask him to follow his thumb. Then have him try to do this with closed eyes. This accentuates proprioceptiveness and feeling of the movement of his eyes.

Another principle to follow is to have the patient aware of his peripheral field of vision. When training with the Keystone Rotator, for example, have him attend the total field of view with his eyes stationary so that he will be aware of the moving target in his periphery. Otherwise, his visual field may become "restricted" as stress is added in the therapy sessions later on, which would only exacerbate already deficient pursuit skills. This is particularly true in young children and even teenagers, who frequently show signs of hysterical visual fields (tubular responses).

POSITION MAINTENANCE

Step one in Table 15I is to ensure that the patient has adequate position maintenance of a stationary target. Position maintenance is probably the combined involvement of all four eye movement systems (i.e., saccades, pursuits, nonoptic, and vergence). Refer to Figure 15-18 showing Eye-Trac recordings.

True position maintenance is actually a misnomer in that there are very small movements occurring all the time during so-called steady fixation. The eyes are not motionless during fixation. According to Gay et al.,[20] the "micro" eye movements consist of rapid flicks (probably of the saccadic system) and slow drifts (probably of the pursuit system) of a very small amplitude not observable without special equipment. These small movements are thought to be useful and for the purpose of correcting fixational errors to keep the fixated target precisely on the fovea, and yet possibly preventing retinal adaptation (fatigue). These small movements in position maintenance may also be stimulated by vergence errors. Gay et al. classify these coordinated eye movements as the "position maintenance system" and state, "It is the ultimate monitor of the eye movements, coordinating all the other eye movement systems and determining the precise position of the eye with respect to the target as well as to the head and body." Position maintenance must be the first step in evaluating pursuits; moreover, it should be the primary step when evaluating any of the eye movement systems.

According to Gay et al., position maintenance can be examined by asking the patient to fixate (monocularly) on a nearpoint target (about 40 cm away) for at least 5 seconds. This is also done at a farpoint fixation distance of 6 meters. There should be no noticeable drifting or eye movement from the

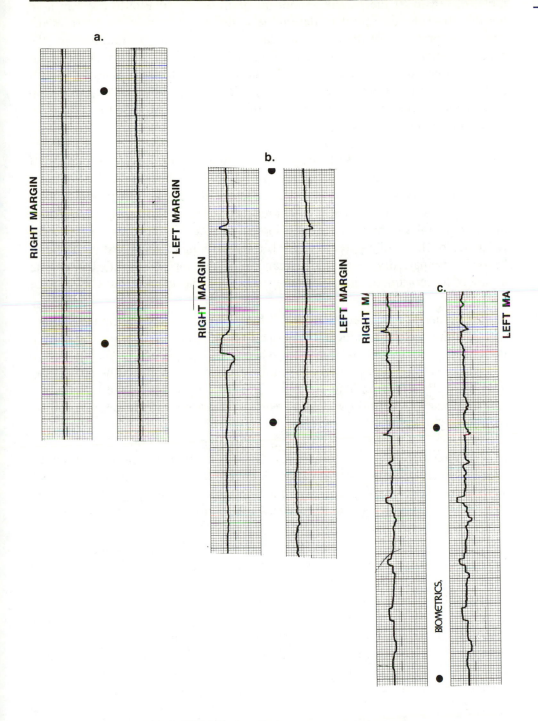

FIGURE 15-18 — Recordings from Eye-Trac℠ on position maintenance testing. (a) Patient was considered to have normal fixation; (b) Drifts would cause fixation maintenance to be borderline normal; (c) Example of poor position maintenance.

target of regard. If the patient cannot maintain steady fixation, have him hold his thumb at the nearpoint to determine if the proprioceptive input from the "hand support" is of help in maintaining steady eye positioning. If the problem persists (e.g., in nystagmus) and psychological (e.g., lack of attention) or other known causes (e.g., fatigue or drug effects) can be ruled out, pathological causes must be considered. Barring pathological causes, improvement of position maintenance is often possible through the efforts of functional training procedures.

VOLITION

Step two in Table 15I is to proceed from voluntary to reflexive responses. If volition helps in establishing steady positioning of the eye on a stationary target, the use of saccades to help pursuits may also apply. For instance, even a person with the best pursuits will break down and begin using saccades as the velocity of the target is greatly increased (over 30 degrees per second). Evidence of this is the percept of flicker of the light on the Keystone Rotator. In order to partially meet the demand of following the light, the patient attempts to coordinate saccadic movements with the moving light as best he can.

If the demand of speed is reduced by slowing the rotating light, continuous pursuits may be regained. It is hoped that higher speeds will be achieved with repeated training and practice. Therefore, the patient is encouraged to use all the volition he can muster to follow the target, whether it be a swinging Marsden ball, a moving hand-held penlight, an afterimage on the hubcap of a car, or whatever. Volition will be important in the rest of the steps to follow, particularly in controlling head movement.

EYE-HAND COORDINATION

In step three, eye-hand coordination may be poor at first. The patient should practice correctly pointing to the moving target. The act of pointing serves as a support mechanism for proper eye fixation. The rotating peg board (Figure 7-2) as well as many other procedures for amblyopia presented in Chapter Seven apply here.

In time, after good eye-hand coordination is achieved, pointing should be discontinued so that pursuits can be practiced and improved without this support.

Additional procedures may be introduced for variety. One that most children are fond of is the Perceptuometor Pen[f] (see Figure 15-19). The pencillike device has an infrared light sensor in its tip. Color and amount of light control the frequency of an audio-oscillator. When the tip of the pen is exactly on a dark line, there is no sound emitted from the hookup sounding system, but when the tip is off the dark line and on the brighter paper, a buzzing sound is heard. The sound is louder and higher in pitch as the tip moves from a darker to lighter area, as when moving off the black line.

---

[f]Manufactured by Wayne Engineering, 4120 Greenwood, Skokie, IL 60076.

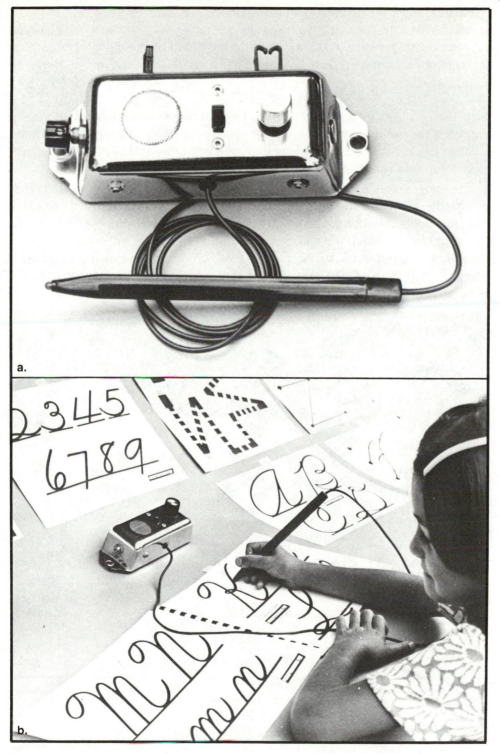

FIGURE 15-19 — The Perceptuomotor Pen. (a) The apparatus; (b) Example of its use in therapy. (Courtesy of Wayne Engineering, Orthoptic Division.)

Later on, when corrections via auditory feedback are not as essential, strictly visual tracing can be used in pursuits. A good way to combine saccades with pursuits and train the child on letters of the alphabet is to have the patient perform Michigan Tracking by using a continuous line, as shown in Figure 15-20.

EXCURSION RANGE

Step four involves going from small to large excursions. This range should be extended as much as possible. (Note that in saccadic therapy, the training went from gross to fine movements in that larger, gross saccades are more easy to control than smaller, fine ones, as in reading.)

Pursuit excursions should begin within a range where success comes easily; then progress to larger amplitudes. The range of movement is naturally limited, being smaller for supraduction (about 30 degrees) but greater for infraduction, levoduction, and dextroduction. The angle of rotation can be increased by simply having the patient move closer to the moving target. If a Marsden ball is used, the arc of the angular swing can be increased as the need arises.

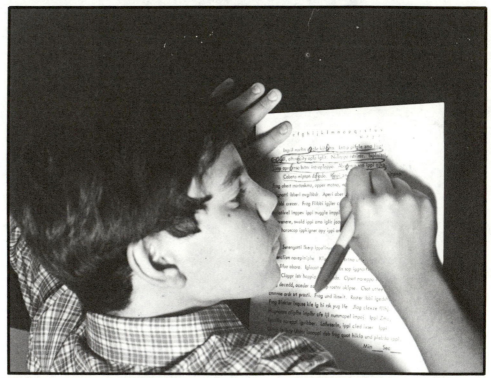

FIGURE 15-20 — Michigan Tracking type of activity for pursuits combined with saccades. Patient makes saccades to find letters but is to follow the pencil tip in a continuous motion.

SPEED

As mentioned earlier, fast pursuits are normally more difficult to perform well than slow pursuits. Therefore, it is best to start pursuit training with the Keystone Rotator, for example, set at a slow speed within the patient's ability to perform.

Gay et al.[21] point out an irony in that pursuits may be higher in velocity via peripheral retinal stimulation when there is a case of a dense central scotoma. Presumably, the normal-eyed person would notice the target slipping from foveal fixation and resort to a faster saccadic movement to regain fixation. This would not be perceived if there were an absence of the fovea. Pursuits would not be interrupted centrally, which would allow the attainment of higher velocities (up to 90 degrees per second). Clinical evidence corroborates in that "peripheral awareness" training sometimes helps accomplish higher velocities for the patient who has normal foveas but poor pursuit skills.

SMOOTHNESS

Smooth movements can be strived for, in step six, by giving the patient as much feedback as possible (e.g., flicker). This step is the most difficult to successfully achieve, because neurological defects cannot always be worked around, even in soft signs of jerky pursuits. Nystagmus presents a formidable obstacle in this regard. However, if jerky pursuits are due to functional causes, the prognosis to achieve smoothness of pursuits via functional training procedures is good.

The practitioner should pass through this step as quickly as possible and hope for the best after all 13 steps are completed. I have seen patients with jerky pursuits improve as a result of much and varied training (e.g., training that involves the reduction of nystagmus through vergence training, better saccades, and accommodation facility improvement).

HEAD MOVEMENT

In step seven the patient must become aware of head movement during pursuits and exert voluntary control to stop it. Again, positive feedback to the patient is important. A convenient adjunct in out-of-office therapy is to have the patient "wear a book" on his head. When it falls off, he knows head motion was the cause. (A bean bag or eraser will also work well for this purpose.)

EYE EQUALNESS

If monocular training of each eye has been effective up to this point, the pursuit skill of the right and left eyes should be approximately the same. If not, further training for the deficient eye may be called for in step eight. On occasion, it is impossible to achieve equalness, e.g., a case of organic amblyopia.

One necessary principle in vision therapy is that each eye has been optically corrected to the status of emmetropia. Obviously, an ametropic eye may be at a disadvantage with respect to the fellow emmetropic eye.

A caveat regarding the wearing of spectacles is that excursions of pursuits may exceed the limits of the eyesize of the spectacle frame, forcing the patient to make head movements in order to keep his eye on the target. The office therapist, the helper-at-home therapist, and the doctor must keep this in mind.

BINOCULAR PURSUITS

When equalness is accomplished to the highest degree possible, binocular pursuits should be trained and practiced in step nine. These should be developed to become as good as monocular pursuits. Usually the patient has no problem making the transition from ductions to versions. An exception occurs when there is a vergence anomaly. For example, an intermittent exotropic patient may have difficulty in going from monocular to binocular pursuit training because of the voluntary effort required to maintain bifixation on the target; this is much more difficult than monofixation with one eye closed under these circumstances.

Another consideration to be made in the transition from monocular to binocular pursuits is the phase of therapy referred to as "bi-ocular." This is when noncorresponding points are stimulated to give rise to diplopia. A large base-down prism can be placed before one eye to create the perception of two moving targets (e.g., Keystone Rotator light). The patient is asked to switch fixation from the top to the bottom target to be aware of simultaneous perception involving each eye.

COGNITIVE DEMANDS

The cognitive demands for training in step ten are similar to those in testing, as in the Heinsen-Schrock system of testing saccades and pursuits. These should proceed from simple (or hardly any) to more complex demands. Some adults can perform long division, after much practice, while maintaining fixation on the moving target. However, such complex tasks exceed what is normally expected of patients in vision therapy.

NONOPTIC SYSTEMS

Step eleven involves the nonoptic eye movement system. This reflex system involves the otolith organs, semicircular canals, and neck receptors. According to Gay et al.,[22] the nonoptic system integrates eye movements and body movements. Discussion of neurological pathways of the nonoptic system is beyond the scope of this text.

The nonoptic system is more involved when the patient changes from a sitting to a standing position in training. Even more reflexive demands are created when the patient is asked to stand on a balance board (Figure 7-1 in Chapter Seven) or to move forward and backward on a walking rail. The goal, in regard to the nonoptic system, is for the patient to be able to pursue the target accurately and smoothly while standing, and preferably while balancing, on a balance board. At first, there is an "overloading" for the patient; he will not be able to balance and maintain good pursuit eye movements as well as he could when in a sitting position. Providing there are no lesions involving the nonoptic system, most patients eventually learn to cope with these demands while performing pursuits well.

VERGENCES AND PURSUITS

Step twelve "overloads" the patient even more by bringing in another eye movement system—the vergence system (refer to Chapters Twelve, Thirteen, and Fourteen). Base-out loose prisms can be placed before the patient's eyes to create a convergence demand while the patient views a Marsden ball, a target on the automatic rotating device, a hand-held moving penlight, etc. Conversely, a divergence demand can be created by placing base-in loose prism before the patient's eyes. If a patient can overcome the prismatic demand and continue to perform pursuits well, he is ready to go on to more stressful demands.

More stress and "overloading" the patient can be accomplished in many ways. The permutations and variations using the previously discussed 12 steps are countless. For example, the patient may be asked to follow a target while balancing a book on the top of his head (i.e., no head movement is allowed) while counting backward by 3s from 100 (complex cognitive demand) and balancing on the balance board (nonoptic system in play to a great extent), while wearing 15 p.d. base-out (convergence demand).

The purpose of such combinations is to proceed from little or no stress to more and more stress. This should always go just to the point where the patient can achieve. Success breeds success, and failure has the opposite effect. The patient must not be threatened by seemingly impossible demands early in vision therapy. He must learn to go through the steps successfully.

The most important vision therapy principle is having the patient know *why* he is in vision therapy. Treatment is doomed to failure unless the patient can answer the question, What am I doing here? Goals must be specified and put into behavioral terms.

The patient should understand *what* he will be able to do as a result of therapy. For example, he may work toward achieving pursuit eye movements without head movement, counting backward from 100 in intervals of 2, while standing on a balance board and facing a target on the Keystone Rotator that is moving at a moderate speed.

Also, the patient should learn to perceive exactly *how* the proper response is made and how to make it. Feedback and operant conditioning (see Chapter Sixteen) are needed for this learning process. Success breeds success.

The patient should know *when* to do training, and the doctor should know when it should not be done. Instructions may be, for example, "Practice pie pan rotations and suspended ball pursuits for 10 minutes every afternoon right after school." The doctor should know when it is time to discontinue a certain procedure, either because the patient is bored or because success is not attainable at that particular time for one reason or another. This principle applies to the overall regimen as well as to specific steps in therapy. Sometimes it is wise to dismiss the patient for a while and let him continue after a period of time, e.g., for a family vacation, Little League playoffs, or change of job (adult patient or parent of a young patient).

Other principles the doctor should follow include the following. (1) Always *ask* the patient to do something, rather than tell him to do it. (2) Make sure the best possible *refraction* has been made and the patient is wearing his ametropic corrective lenses for testing and training. (3) At the beginning of therapy, consider having *short* training sessions in the office, and ones that are *enjoyable* to the patient. (4) Proceed from *less* difficult to *more* difficult demands for the patient. (5) Help the patient learn *voluntary* control and the realization of visual functions becoming *reflexive,* automated responses. (6) Go from *monocular,* to *bi-ocular* (when appropriate), to *binocular* therapy. (7) Have the patient learn to be aware of objects in his peripheral visual field and to use *peripheral vision* in mastering tasks in therapy and in real life. (8) To the extent possible, ensure that the visual functioning of each eye is *equal*. (9) Make sure the patient knows *who* is to do what in therapy. He is to do most of it, but others are involved, including the doctor, therapist, helper at home, and special resource teacher, among others. (10) Keep in mind that vision therapy is an educational process, and learning theories (Chapter Sixteen) that apply to the particular patient must be used in order for therapy to be successful.

Accommodation Efficiency

Dysfunctions of accommodation can be separated into four types of problems: insufficiency, excess, infacility of accommodation, and ill-sustained accommodation. A brief review of these conditions and appropriate therapy follow.

INSUFFICIENCY OF ACCOMMODATION

This is defined by Cline et al.[23] as "insufficient amplitude of accommodation to afford clear imagery of a stimulus object at a specified distance, usually the normal or desired reading distance." This is a common problem in prepresbyopic and presbyopic patients but is not too frequent in younger patients. Of course, pathological conditions affecting the third cranial nerve, the ciliary muscle, or the crystalline lens itself can result in paresis or paralysis of accommodation. Furthermore, the use of sympathomimetic and parasympatholytic drugs can result in lowered amplitudes of accommodation. However, true, isolated accommodation insufficiency in young patients is relatively rare. (I have seen three patients with isolated accommodation insufficiency within a 1-month period, however. All had a history of having been in the tropics and had tropical illnesses of some kind. They had to wear bifocals in order to read clearly. I happened to see them after they had been to other practitioners who insisted they did not need to wear bifocals. The accommodative amplitude in each of the three patients was practically zero, but I doubt if that had been tested. The resumption of wearing plus addition bifocals solved their problems, and no further treatment was necessary.) Even though accommodative insufficiency is relatively rare, its possible existence should be noted. Bifocals are usually indicated in such cases.

Semantic confusion often arises with the term *accommodation insufficiency*. Some sources (inappropriately, in my opinion) refer to "accommodation deficiency" or "insufficiency" when they are really talking about *accommodation infacility*.[24] (Accommodation infacility will be discussed later.)

Although a lag of accommodation does not necessarily imply an insufficient amplitude of accommodation, it can be thought of as a clinical form of accommodation insufficiency for a particular nearpoint target, and it is a common finding in clinical practice. There are several ways to measure the lag of accommodation, but two of the most popular and reliable ways are included here.

The Nott dynamic retinoscopy method, based on the linear difference between the fixation distance (usually 40 cm) and the distance of the retinoscope from the patient, is converted into diopters to determine the accommodative lag.[25] The patient fixates reading material at 40 cm (2.50D) while retinoscopy, performed through a hole in a card, shows a neutral reflex at, say, 67 cm (1.50D). (Refer to Figure 15-21.) The accommodative lag, according to the Nott method, would be 1.00D in this example. The fact that this can be done while the patient is behind the refractor, and lenses can be presented in the lens wells to correct an existing ametropia, makes the Nott method very convenient. Another desirable feature is that once there is optical emmetropia (i.e., farpoint correction), lenses do not have to be introduced that could possibly vitiate the reliability of testing.

NOTT METHOD

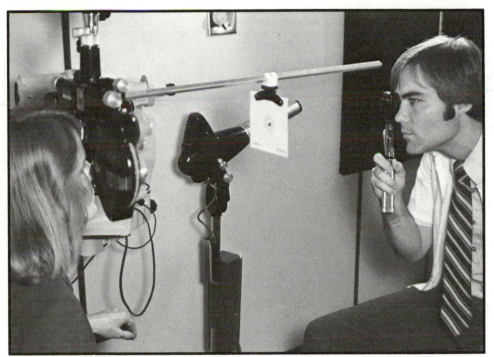

FIGURE 15-21 — Nott method of dynamic retinoscopy. If, for example, the patient is viewing a reading card at 2.50D distance and the doctor's retinoscope is at true conjugate focus of the patient's eye(s) at a distance of 1.50D, then the lag of accommodation would be 1.00D.

The accommodation stimulus does not change, because the testing distance is kept constant, and no dioptric changes are made by the intervention of additional lenses. The nearpoint rod of the refractor can be used to measure directly the dioptric distance between the fixation distance and the retinoscopic neutralization distance, i.e., the distance representing the accommodative lag.

When testing is done outside the refractor, monocular estimate method (MEM) retinoscopy is more convenient. The monocular estimate method of Haynes[26] is similar to the Nott method, except that the retinoscopic distance is

MEM RETINOSCOPY

kept constant. This is often at the Harmon distance, but distances may be varied (e.g., the patient's customary working or reading distance may be used). The patient is to read appropriate reading material (for his age or cognitive level) mounted on the retinoscope. A trial lens is interposed in the spectacle plane of the patient to neutralize the reflex. (See Figure 15-22 showing MEM retinoscopy.) The lens is removed from the eye within a split second, because latency of accommodation response is short. Tucker and Charman[27] found a mean reaction (latency) time of 0.28 second for one subject and 0.29 second for another. Therefore, the neutralizing lens must be quickly removed once it is introduced before an eye. The stimulus to accommodation possibly could be changed if the lens were before the eye for a longer duration. Of course, the other eye is not receiving lenses, and it is presumed to maintain a stable accommodative response.

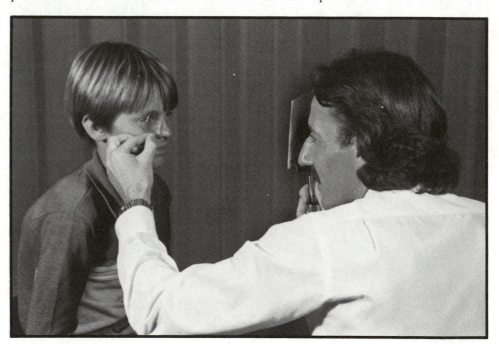

FIGURE 15-22 — The monocular estimate method (MEM) of dynamic retinoscopy for determining the lag of accommodation. The retinoscope is held at the patient's customary reading distance while various trial lenses are quickly introduced and removed. The lens power that neutralizes the retinoscopic reflex represents the amount of accommodative lag.

This assumption may not always hold true, and the possibility of changing accommodative responses by changing accommodative stimuli must always be kept in mind when doing the MEM test.

The lens power (addition of plus) necessary to achieve retinoscopic neutralization is the estimated accommodative lag of the eye being tested at the moment. If minus power should be required for neutralization, accommodation excess would be indicated.

The MEM is called "monocular" although the patient has both eyes open and testing is under binocular viewing conditions. Using the Nott or MEM procedures, I believe an accommodative lag of 1.00D or greater is cause for further investigation. This concern was shared by Bieber.[28] A high lag of accommodation suggests the possibility of the accommodation anomalies of infacility of accommodation, ill-sustained accommodation, and insufficiency of accommodation, any of which can be significant factors in visual efficiency.

Lenses are the principal means to help patients who have accommodative insufficiency. Presbyopia (physiological) in adults must, of course, be ruled out when pathological etiologies are suspected. Knowing the patient's exact age, therefore, is necessary. (Remember that many patients look younger than their chronological age, due to good nutrition and cosmetic care.)

THERAPY

Low-plus addition lenses are sometimes prescribed for children and young adults. This procedure is not without controversy.[29,30,31] However, there are times when prescribing a low plus addition (either single vision reading lenses or bifocals) appears to help the patient perform efficiently in reading and other nearpoint tasks. In many cases, the lenses are worn on a temporary basis; usually less than 1 year is necessary.

Functional training procedures are prescribed in many cases of accommodative insufficiency for children and nonpresbyopic adults. These are accommodative rock procedures and are essentially the same as if the patient had accommodation infacility (to be discussed later). Accommodative rock training is preferable to having the patient wear low plus spectacles, but occasionally both modes of therapy are beneficial.

Accommodation may be excessive in focusing on a stimulus object. Accommodative excess is considered to be an anomaly, sometimes referred to as spasm of accommodation, hyperaccommodation, hypertonic accommodation, or pseudomyopia.[32] Causes may be overstimulation of the accommodative system as a result of prolonged near work, emotional problems, or focal infections. Numerous symptoms may be associated with accommodative excess, such as asthenopia, blurring of distance vision, headaches, diplopia (if excessive accommodative convergence is brought into play), and inefficient performance at nearpoint (e.g., the person may hold reading material at an exceptionally close range).

EXCESS OF ACCOMMODATION

Maintaining or sustaining accommodation in the absence of a dioptric stimulus is another form of accommodative excess.[33] This form is physiological in that it is not abnormal for accommodation of about 1.00D to be in play in a formless field, as in night myopia. There is no effective therapy for this condition except the individual's becoming familiar with the set of circumstances in which it occurs and/or making appropriate adjustments to it (e.g., temporarily wearing minus overcorrections, if necessary, for nighttime driving). Retinoscopy is necessary in the diagnosis of accommodative excess.

Static retinoscopy with the aid of cycloplegia is helpful to determine ametropia at farpoint. For nearpoint, dynamic retinoscopy is important; however, cycloplegia must not be used in nearpoint testing. Either Nott or

MEM dynamic retinoscopy can be used to determine if there is a lag (i.e., insufficiency) or lead (i.e., excess) of accommodation. If accommodative response leads the accommodative stimulus by more than 0.25D, I believe accommodative excess exists at that moment of testing. This should be verified on repeated testing.

Accommodative excess can also occur when excessive accommodative convergence is required to maintain fusion, as in cases of large exophoria in which positive fusional convergence is insufficient.

THERAPY   The cause of accommodative excess must be sought. If the etiology is nonpathological, then functional training procedures may be attempted in the form of the accommodative rock procedures that would be used in the case of accommodative infacility (to be discussed). Plus acceptance training in the form of wearing spectacles on a temporary basis may be encouraged. I have seen patients with pseudomyopia gradually accept more plus (or less minus) in time and lose their apparent myopic refractive error. The wearing of spectacles helps the patient with accommodative excess at farpoint. However, accommodative rock procedures are necessary if accommodative excess persists at nearpoint.

TABLE 15K. Norms for Accommodation Facility

Investigations	Results	Comments
Alpert and Zellers[39]	± 2.00D, 11 cycles per minute, monocular 8 cycles per minute, binocular, with suppression being monitored	Young adults
Borish[34]	Range of + 1.50 to − 2.00D, clearing in less than 5 seconds	Young adults
Burge[38]	± 2.00D, 12 cycles per minute, monocular 10 cycles per minute, binocular 7 cycles per minute, binocular, with suppression being monitored	Children and Young adults
Griffin et al.[36]	± 2.00D, 17 cycles per minute, monocular	Young adults
Griffin et al.[37]	± 2.00D, 17 cycles per minute, monocular 13 cycles per minute, binocular 6 cycles per minute, binocular, with suppression being monitored	Young adults
Hoffman et al.[41]	± 2.50D, approximately 3 cycles per minute	Children 6 to 12 years
Liu et al.[35]	± 1.50D, 20 cycles per 90 seconds (1.5 minutes)	Suggested criteria in general
Schlange et al.[40]	± 2.00D, 7 cycles per minute, binocular	Children

Testing for facility of accommodation was covered in Chapter Two. A summary of norms of facility by several investigators is included in Table 15K for reference.

Borish[34] states that monocular accommodative facility when tested at the patient's habitual nearpoint distance should have a range of lenses from +1.50 to −2.00D with clear vision, with the normal response time being less than 5 seconds. Also, there should be less than 0.5 seconds difference between facility of each eye.

Liu et al.[35] suggest that "a normal subject can perform 20 flipper cycles of ±1.50D within 4.5 seconds." This probably is meant as 20 cycles per 90 seconds, with each cycle being 4.5 seconds or each flip being 2.25 seconds.

Griffin et al.[36] studied monocular accommodative facility on 14 subjects ranging in age form 20 to 35 years. They found ±2.00D rock to have an average value of 17 cycles per minute. The average response time to clear the minus lens was 2 seconds, and to clear the plus lens, 1.4 seconds.

Griffin et al.[37] made a study to determine monocular facility compared with binocular facility. They wanted to eliminate the possibility of guessing and ensure that patients were actually seeing clearly rather than reporting "clear" with each flipping of lenses. Instead of changing targets (double-digit numbers) manually, an electrical mechanism introduced random numbers (of 6-point type size at a distance of 40 cm) in synchrony with the lens-flipper mechanism. Rock of ±2.00D was done for 1 minute to determine the average number of cycles in a young adult population, ages 20 to 23 years. Monocular facility was approximately 17 cycles per minute. Binocular facility was approximately 13 cycles per minute, without suppression being monitored. To monitor suppression, a vectographic plate was arranged so that the leftward (first) digit was seen only by the left eye, and the right eye saw only the second digit. For example, the number *53* that appeared with the new lens change would be presented so that only the number *5* could be seen by the left eye and the number *3* by the right eye. There were only 6 cycles per minute as an average for this group of subjects when suppression was monitored and guessing of numbers was absent. The investigators reviewed the 27 records of complete vision examinations and selected 16 subjects who showed evidence of poor visual skills and 11 who showed normal visual skills. (All subjects wore lens correction for any existing ametropia during the time of testing.) Monocular rock for the "normal" subjects averaged 18 cycles per minute compared with 15 cycles per minute for the subjects having poor visual skills. Binocular rock without suppression monitoring gave averages of 17 and 9 cycles per minute for the same two groups, respectively. When binocular rock was tested using suppression, monitoring gave an average of 9 cycles per minute for the "normal" subjects, but only 4 cycles per minute for those having poor visual skills. The authors concluded that binocular accommodative facility testing can be definitive in the assessment of a patient's binocular status.

Burge[38] used a more clinical method than that just described to study binocular facility using suppression monitoring. He used a Spriangle vectogram target[g] with cross-polarizing viewers and ±2.00D lens flippers. The results were similar to those of Griffin et al. just described: approximately 12 cycles per minute monocularly, 10 cycles per minute binocularly without suppression monitoring, and 7 cycles per minute with suppression monitoring via the vectogram. Burge's values tended to be slightly lower than those just described of Griffin et al. He included children rather than adults only as subjects (ranging from 6 to 30 years).

Alpert and Zellers[39] carried out a study similar to that of Burge on 100 young adults (18 to 30 years) and found similar results: approximately 11 cycles per minute monocularly and approximately 8 cycles per minute binocularly. There was no significant difference between the right eye and the left eye, or between males and females.

Schlange et al.[40] did a normative study on 266 subjects, ages 6 to 11 years. They were tested with ±2.00D while viewing a 20/30 line of letters at a 40 cm distance. The binocular accommodative facility averaged 7 cycles per minute. However, refractive status and other anomalies were not accounted for in this sample.

Hoffman et al.[41] tested 80 children with ages ranging from 6 to 12 years using ±2.50D rock. Refractive errors were corrected, and none of the children were reported to have visual or academic handicaps. These criteria notwithstanding, the investigators found the median accommodative facility monocularly to be only 2 to 4 cycles per minute, and binocularly, only 1 to 2 cycles per minute. If the children had had suppression monitoring, perhaps the cycles per minute would have even been lower.

It is not clear why children did so poorly on accommodative facility testing. It may be that ±2.50D is too great a demand for them. Also, the initial testing procedure may not reflect their true facility. I have seen many such examples of 2 cycles per minute in children in which facilities can be increased through training to well over the ideals of Pierce and Greenspan (±2.50D of 20 cycles per minute; see Chapter Two). It may be wise to retest children several times before concluding that accommodation is poor and referral for functional training is recommended.

There is no consensus on developmental norms from childhood to adulthood for accommodative facility. We do know that the ideal of Pierce and Greenspan can be met via functional training procedures in the majority of patients, and this should be strived for in most cases. As to referral criteria for facility, Hoffman and Rouse[42] recommended the following: flipper test of ±2.00D monocularly and binocularly showing less than 12 cycles per minute, with the patient viewing a 20/30 line at 40 cm, or a difference of more than 2 cycles per minute between the two eyes. In light of the results shown in Table

[g] Available from the Bernell Corp.

15K, these referral criteria may be too stringent, especially for young children. Retesting and/or lowered initial standards should be considered during the routine testing of new patients.

THERAPY

Symptoms of accommodation infacility are legion and may include blurring at far or near, fatigue while doing close work, slow reading speed, unusual working distance, and asthenopia, among other complaints. As in all evaluations, it is important to have the maximum visual acuity with the most plus lens correction in place during testing. For example, a hyperopic individual without his corrective lenses may complain of intermittent blurring at nearpoint. Conversely, a slightly myopic patient not wearing his spectacles may notice that distance vision blur is exceptionally greater when looking out at a distance after reading at nearpoint for a prolonged period. Such problems of blurring are exacerbated when accommodative infacility is compounded by the refractive error.

Once patients are shown how many cycles per minute they can achieve compared with the ideal cycles per minute, they know what their goal is and understand why they need therapy. Approaches to therapy for accommodative infacility are listed in Table 15L.

TABLE 15L. Approaches to Therapy for Accommodative Infacility
1. Achieve sufficient accommodative amplitude, monocularly
2. Monocularly, achieve a range of ± 2.50D, untimed; proceed from small to large ranges
3. Achieve 20 cycles per minute, monocularly; proceed from slow to fast
4. Stimulatory and inhibitory phases should be quick
5. Facility of the right eye and left eye should be equal
6. Introduce bi-ocular rock
7. Introduce binocular rock, achieving goals in steps one through four
8. Introduce base-in and base-out prism demands during binocular rock

STEP ONE

Unless a sufficient amplitude of accommodation is present, there is no point in prescribing accommodative facility training. A presbyopic patient, or a prepresbyopic patient with a very reduced amplitude, would be excluded from this type of therapy.

Refer to Donder's values[43] (Table 15M) or to Hofstetter's amplitude formula[44] for age and amplitude expectancies. The Hofstetter formula for amplitude of accommodation is as follows: $A = 18.5 - 0.3Y$, where A is the average amplitude of accommodation and Y is the age in years. For example, a patient 30 years old would be expected to have an amplitude of 9.50D; a 40 year old, 6.50D; and so on, using this formula.

As mentioned earlier in the discussion on accommodative insufficiency, plus addition lens prescription is the usual choice of treatment for such conditions. If and when accommodative amplitude is sufficient, therapy can proceed to step two.

TABLE 15M. Donder's Table of Amplitude of Accommodation, Abridged from Borish.[43]	
Age (Years)	Amplitude (Diopters)
10	14
20	10
30	7
40	4.5
50	2.5

STEP TWO   Monocular accommodative rock exercises can be used in a variety of ways. The testing procedures described in Chapter Two are appropriate. These can be done as out-of-office training procedures, because very little equipment is necessary. Procedures in the office can utilize more elaborate equipment, such as the Van Orden attachment to the Keystone Correct-Eye-Scope. Figure 15-23a shows monocular rock training in which minus and plus lenses are placed before one eye while the other eye is occluded. It may be wise to introduce both the stimulatory and inhibitory phases of training to the same eye in the early part of training, rather than initially using alternate occlusion rock procedures as shown in Figure 2-48 of Chapter Two. Once it has been established that good monocular facility is achieved for the plus and minus lens in each eye, alternate occlusion procedures can be employed, which may be more convenient for prolonged exercises at home.

Whether strictly monocular rock or alternate monocular rock is used, it may be necessary to begin with ± 0.50D lenses and then proceed to larger powers as the patient gains success and confidence. Remember, each eye should be optically emmetropic. For example, an uncorrected myopic eye of 0.50D will not be able to see clearly at 40 cm through a +2.50D lens. The patient will be blurred by 0.50D at this distance. The target will have to be moved in to 33 cm for clear vision. If the myopia is corrected with a −0.50D lens, there should be no problem, assuming the patient eventually learns to relax accommodation the full amount to clear the target with a +2.50D lens in place. Because of the problem of blurring, the therapist initially may have to use a target with large print, and then proceed with smaller and smaller print (to the patient's threshold, e.g., 20/20 equivalent at near). When a range of ± 2.50D is achieved for each eye (regardless of the time per cycle), go to step three.

STEP THREE   Step three involves speed rather than the amplitude that was accomplished in step two. Some patients may have such great difficulty in achieving the full amplitude that step two will have to be curtailed somewhat. In this event, go on to step three.

The goal is to have the patient achieve 20 cycles per minute on accommodative rock. Start with small lens powers in the beginning, even if only ±0.50D is used. Once adequate speed is achieved, use larger lens powers until the ideal range of clear vision (if possible for a particular patient) of ±2.50D is achieved with a speed of 20 cycles per minute.

Step four is the same as step three, but with careful monitoring of the stimulatory and inhibitory phases. These phases should be fairly equal and quick. If, for example, the patient has trouble clearing the target through plus lenses, this problem should be worked on both in the office and in home training. When quickness of clearing is achieved for plus and minus lenses, move on to the next step.

Step five is a repetition of the previous steps, except that careful monitoring of each eye's performance is important. The right and left eye should be approximately equal. Sometimes this is not possible for many reasons, e.g., ocular pathology or incurable amblyopia. However, most patients are able to achieve good monocular accommodative facility in each eye. Proceed to the next step when this is accomplished.

Bi-ocular rock is a transition phase between monocular and binocular training. The most practical way to set this up is to introduce a vertical dissociating prism before one eye of the patient. The Van Orden apparatus (Figure 15-23a through 15-23d) is suitable for this purpose. Simply remove the occluder that was used in monocular rock and replace it with a 10 p.d. prism, base-down. This will cause the patient to see one target above the other. If the base-down prism is placed before the left eye and that eye views through a minus lens, the image will be higher and will be an accommodative stimulus. The right eye will be viewing the lower image through a plus lens, which requires inhibition of accommodation for clarity. The stimulation of noncorresponding points should result in diplopia, so that the patient can be aware of simultaneous perception (without suppression) with no demands on fusional vergence being made.

Bi-ocular accommodative rock may be discontinued after a brief training period once it has been established that the patient can do the best he can; it is hoped he can achieve ±2.50D with 20 cycles per minute.

The same goals of range and speed in the first six steps also apply to binocular rock. The Van Orden attachment (Figures 15-23b and 15-23c) for binocular training is good as an office procedure. For example, +2.50D lenses can be put into the right and left lens wells with two −5.00D lenses in the flipper attachment. The patient would have a zero accommodation stimulus with the +2.50D lenses when viewing a target at 40 cm; when the −5.00D lenses are superimposed, the patient views through a −2.50D lens combination (−5.00D + 2.50D) along with the 2.50D accommodative demand of the

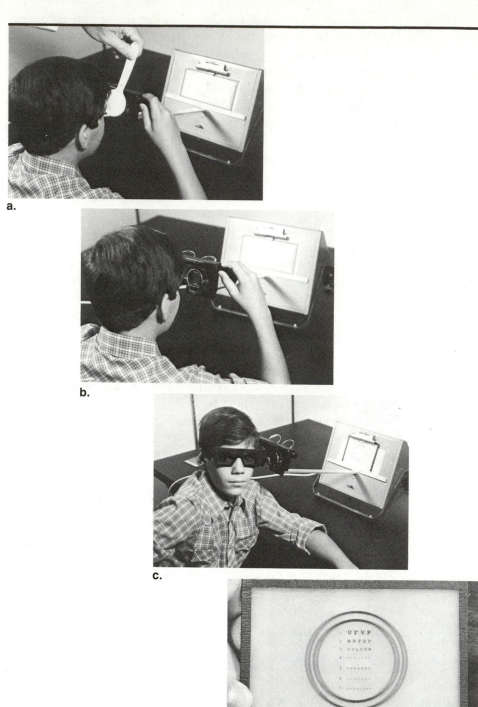

FIGURE 15-23 — Van Orden attachment to the Keystone Correct-Eye-Scope for accommodative rock. (a) Monocular rock setup; (b) Binocular rock setup; (c) Setup for monitoring suppression during accommodative rock; (d) Vectographic target (Bernell Vectogram #9).

40 cm distance. This provides a total change of 5.00D with a flip of the lenses. This is ±2.50D rock via the Van Orden method. Lesser lens powers can be arranged similarly. For example, place +1.00D lenses in the lens wells with −2.00D lenses in the holders of the flipper attachment for ±1.00D rock.

A more convenient way for the patient to practice binocular rock at home it to use the Bausch and Lomb Demonstrator (Figure 2-50 in Chapter Two) or similar flipper devices.

As was pointed out earlier in the normative studies of several investigators, vergence problems can have a profound effect on binocular accommodative facility. Plotting blur and break points in the graphical analysis approach can explain why this is so. (Refer to Chapter Fourteen for a discussion of graphical analysis.)

Take, for example, an esophoric patient. When minus lenses are introduced binocularly, accommodation causes accommodative convergence to be increased. The patient must offset this increased convergence by exerting extra fusional divergence. If he has a sufficiently large fusional divergence range (negative relative convergence), he may be able to keep the target clear and single. But suppose his fusional divergence is less than adequate for this particular demand. In order to diverge his eyes enough to keep the target single, he will have to give up some accommodative convergence. In doing so, some accommodative response is released, thus causing blurring of the target.

A similar explanation can be made for the exophoric patient who has trouble keeping the target clear and single when plus lenses are introduced binocularly. Plus lenses would cause a decrease in accommodative response, thus causing a reduction in accommodative convergence. This results in greater exophoria in relation to the target. In order to converge his eye sufficiently to keep the target single, the patient may need to accommodate excessively to increase accommodative convergence. This would be so if his fusional convergence were less than sufficient for this particular demand, i.e., poor positive fusional vergence. The accommodative excess results in blurring of the target.

Most patients during binocular accommodative rock will resort to this and have blur, because the desire to keep the target single is so great that they will sacrifice clarity for singleness. It is good for patients to realize how accommodation and/or vergence problems can result in blurring of vision even though they may have 20/20 acuity at farpoint, and why vision therapy may be indicated in such cases.

In binocular rock, the patient should achieve quickness with full ranges for both the minus and the plus lenses. Sometimes it is impossible to achieve the ideal of ±2.50D with 20 cycles per minute because of vergence anomalies. In cases of vergence anomalies, complete success may depend on vergence therapy (Chapters Thirteen and Fourteen) to achieve ideal binocular accommodative facility.

Step eight is more for the training of horizontal fusional vergence abilities than for accommodation facility. It is a finishing process for the patient in that binocular rock can be given, with horizontal prismatic demands on vergence incorporated. For office training, loose prisms can be mounted in the Van Orden attachment. For home training, the patient could wear loaner spectacles with 4p.d. base-in as the plus-minus lens flipper is used for binocular accommodative rock. The combination of minus lenses and base-in prisms can create a large demand on fusional divergence. Similarly, the combination of plus lenses and base-out prisms can produce a large demand on fusional convergence.

This is similar to insufficiency of accommodation except that ill-sustained accommodation shows up after a period of time when accommodation is active. Amplitude may be normal in the beginning, but it is maintained only with effort, and it decreases with time.[45] The time during which the amplitude decreases may be short, often within 1 minute.

Ill-sustained accommodation relates to stamina, or the power to endure fatigue. It is easily detected in most routine accommodative facility testing. This is why clinicians carry out facility testing over a period of at least 1 minute. For example, a patient with ill-sustained accommodation may begin $\pm 2.50D$ lens rock quickly and sufficiently, but the responses may become inadequate after a few flips of the lenses. If the doctor tests only one or two cycles, the patient's lack of accommodative stamina will possibly not be discovered. Ill-sustained accommodation can definitely have an effect on performance as well as result in various visual symptoms. Individuals vary in their ability to meet and sustain accommodative demands. It is not known why some have very good stamina while others do not. Clinical experience has shown, however, that stamina can be improved in most cases where the cause of ill-sustained accommodation is functional in nonpresbyopic patients. Therapy is the same as for accommodative infacility. Monocular, bi-ocular, and binocular accommodative rock procedures are performed in the office and at home. The only difference is that sustaining ability is emphasized to a greater extent than otherwise.

There are two principal ways to have demand changes for accommodative rock: by different dioptric spherical lens powers or by changing fixation distance. When lenses are not available, as in certain instances of out-of-office training, a near-far-near rock sequence may be effective. A procedure referred to as "calendar rock" is good for this purpose. The patient is instructed to look at newsprint at nearpoint, then to focus on a number on a calendar hanging on a wall, then back to the newsprint, and so on. This can be done in 1-to-2-minute intervals several times a day. One eye is occluded for monocular rock, and both eyes can be open for binocular rock once the patient has achieved satisfactory results monocularly.

The same principles as in monocular training in amblyopia (Chapter Seven) apply to near-far-near monocular accommodative rock for the nonamblyopic patient. Many of the same procedures can be used, such as the Marsden ball or the Hart chart. (The Hart chart is illustrated in Figure 15-24.)

There are many variations on the same theme for near-far-near rock. For example, newspaper headlines can be used at farpoint, with newsprint at nearpoint, for accommodative rock. For novelty, alternate up-and-down fixation by vertically displaced apertures (Manas mask) can be used in monocular training (illustrated in Figure 2-48c in Chapter Two). A creative therapist can think of many more ways to interest the patient in accommodative rock.

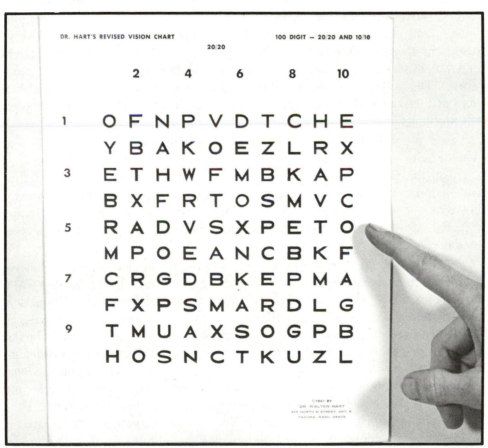

FIGURE 15-24 — The Hart Distance Motivation Chart. A similar chart of random letters is used for nearpoint, with the patient being instructed to clear each successive letter before changing fixation from one chart to the other. Saccadic eye movement training is thus combined with accommodative rock in this procedure.

OTHER ACCOMMODATION CONSIDERATIONS

A modified Updegrave method may be used in therapy to increase plus lens acceptance. Intermittently illuminated reading material is fixated through a specific lens power, and an attempt is made to keep the print clear as the fixation distance is increased.[46] The Hart chart is appropriate for this type of training. The procedure can be helpful when the patient is unable to fully relax accommodation at the farpoint, a form of accommodative excess that may result in pseudomyopia. The modified Updegrave method along with accommodative facility training (rock) will usually help the patient overcome this problem.

Another condition in which there is an apparent accommodative dysfunctioning is the Streff ("non-malingering") syndrome.[47] Young children are usually involved, and typical findings are as follows: slightly reduced distance visual acuity not attributable to refractive error, usually significantly reduced nearpoint visual acuity, very close reading posture, reduced stereopsis, and a large accommodative lag on dynamic retinoscopy. Gilman[48] reported a case of an 8-year-old female who had signs and symptoms of the Streff syndrome. Accommodative facility was poor—worse than ±0.50D on 20/30 letters. Vision therapy including accommodative rock, wearing of low plus lenses, and other procedures relieved the symptoms and "produced positive results as the accommodative system regained its flexibility." It was thought that the syndrome was due to "an accommodative stress response to close work." The author believed that this was not a variation of hysterical amblyopia but that visual skills inefficiencies may have caused overlying psychological problems, rather than vice versa.

In a study by Hoffman,[49] there was an association between accommodative deficits and visual perceptual development, e.g., in visual-motor tests such as the Bender-Gestalt. Vision therapy, including accommodative rock and fusional vergence training, resulted in changes in perceptual development, but only for the age group of 5 to 7 years, with older age groups not being affected. This report emphasized the importance of "remediation of accommodative stress."

Mention should be made of positive relative accommodation and negative relative accommodation. Normally, each value should be at least 1.75D. Positive relative accommodation is tested by introducing minus spherical powers binocularly when the patient's fixation is at nearpoint. This is an indirect means of assessing fusional divergence, because as the accommodative response increases, so does the accommodative convergence. In order for the patient to keep the fixated target single, he must call upon fusional divergence to combat the excess of accommodative convergence brought into play by the increased accommodative response. The blur occurs when the limit of fusional divergence is reached. This causes the patient to decrease his accommodative convergence so diplopia will be prevented. In order to decrease the accommodative convergence, the accommodative response (or at least the patient's accommodative effort) must be reduced. The decrease in accommodation response for that particular fixation distance causes a blurring of the target. Note that the blur point (indicated by a circle in Figure 14-2) is on the left-hand (negative) side of the zone of clear, single, binocular vision. Therefore, a lower-than-normal (i.e., below 1.75D of minus lens stimulation), positive relative accommodation is not so much a condition of accommodative insufficiency as it is one of insufficiency of fusional divergence.

Negative relative accommodation is tested by binocularly introducing plus lenses. An insufficiency of fusional convergence is suspected if values are less than +1.75D, which occurs when the limit of positive fusional vergence is reached. This point is indicated by a circle on the right-hand (positive) side of the zone of clear, single, binocular vision. Because there can be no more fusional convergence brought into play in this situation, the patient elects to call upon more accommodative convergence to prevent diplopia and keep the target single. Since the increased accommodative convergence is brought about by an increased accommodative response (or at least by an increased accommodative effort), blurring of the fixated target will occur with an increased accommodative response because of the excess of accommodation.

Another suspicious negative relative accommodation finding is one that exceeds +2.50D. Latent hyperopia may be indicated. This is because testing is done at 40 cm (2.50D accommodative demand), and the introduction of +2.50D lenses should simulate optical infinity for the patient. If greater plus powers are accepted, the patient was either overminused in the farpoint refraction or underplussed (as may occur in latent hyperopia). This mistake can occur unless an accurate refraction is performed. Again, it must be emphasized that all testing must be done through the maximum vision, most plus, farpoint corrective lenses. This is particularly evident in testing of negative relative accommodation. It does not mean, however, that the doctor cannot perform any testing without the patient's corrective spectacles (or contact lenses) being worn. It only means that all baseline data must be determined through the corrective lenses in order for the analysis of clinical data to be reliable. (If the patient is emmetropic in each eye, no lenses are required.) Valuable impressions, however, can be made by testing under the patient's habitual seeing conditions.

Vergence Efficiency

Vergences are disjunctive eye movements (rather than conjugate movements, as in the three other movement systems). The occipito-mesencephalic neural pathway for vergences, at least as far as convergence is concerned, is probably from area 19 to the third nerve nuclei. Vergence movements are slow (compared with saccades) and mainly involuntary.

COMPONENTS

There are four components of convergence, according to Maddox: tonic, fusional (disparity vergence), proximal, and accommodative. Although authorities may disagree on this classification, the consensus is that the Maddox concept has stood the test of time. (Refer to the Appendix for elaboration on the components.)

EFFECTS OF TRAINING

It is doubtful that much permanent change in accommodative convergence takes place as a result of functional training procedures. This issue was debated extensively by Manas[50] and Flom.[51] Both researchers found a small increase in the AC/A ratio following training. For Manas, the change was from 4.4/1 to 4.9/1. For Flom, the increase was an average of 0.66/1 during training, but it was reported to be lost upon retesting a year later.

Grosvenor[52] pointed out the importance of distinguishing between stimulus (clinical) AC/A ratios and response (research) AC/A ratios. An increase in accommodative convergence may be due merely to an increase in accommodative response rather than to an actual higher AC/A ratio. This may lead the clinician to erroneously assume a change has occurred in the ratio (as a result of training) when measuring a stimulus AC/A ratio.

The effect of functional training on tonic convergence is not certain. While it is true that training may result in an apparent decrease in the deviation of the visual axes, it is probable that the basic deviation, as it was before training, will be revealed once again upon prolonged occlusion. (Refer to the discussion of prolonged occlusion in Chapter Three.) For example, suppose a constant strabismic patient has 25 p.d. of exo deviation at far and near (basic exo case); after 10 weeks of functional training, the exotropia is cured, and the latent deviation on alternate cover testing (with prism) shows an exo deviation of only 10 p.d. The clinician may jump to the conclusion that the low tonic convergence was changed by 15 p.d. Almost invariably, however, the full 25 p.d. will become manifest upon prolonged occlusion testing.

To obtain similar results, the time of occlusion may need to be longer for cases of eso deviations than exo deviations. For hyper deviations, the required time may be the longest in order to bring out the full amount of deviation of the visual axes.

Bergin et al.[53] reported a patient with 52 p.d. of left hyperphoria that was totally revealed only upon prolonged occlusion of approximately 1 hour (Figure 15-25). This patient had fairly normal fusion at all times and was not strabismic except for a few minutes following prolonged occlusion. The patient had fusion in the primary position of gaze as well as in all other positions almost all the time under normal binocular viewing conditions.

The effect of functional training procedures on *proximal* convergence is not clear. However, familiarity with the testing environment causes the sophisticated examinee to have a reduction of proximal convergence as compared with the novice who is being tested in a "reduced environment" for the first time. This can be an important consideration for applicants undergoing visual screening procedures to qualify for special occupations, such as aviation and military service.

The one component that has been shown to be trainable during the past century is fusional (disparity) vergence. The greatest changes are in positive fusional vergence; changes are less for negative fusional vergence, and least for vertical vergences. Torsional fusional vergences may be increased with variable results, depending on the particular patient. At any rate, in functional training procedures for the amelioration of vergence anomalies, concentration is on disparity vergence (whether horizontal, vertical, or torsional). The goal is to achieve efficient vergences. Efficiency of the disparity vergence system depends on ranges and speed. These relate to quantity and quality, with the goal of sufficient amplitudes and velocities.

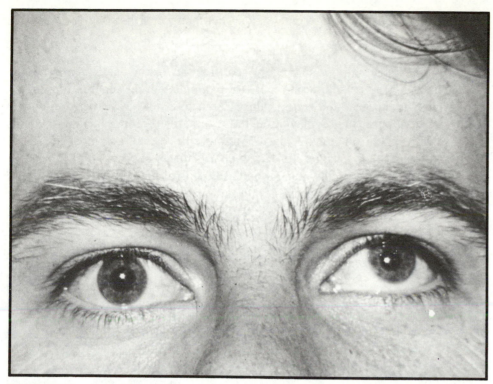

FIGURE 15-25 — Hyperphoria of large magnitude: hyper deviation of the left eye of 52 p.d., manifest after prolonged occlusion of the left eye for about 1 hour. (Note: It is always important to occlude each eye to determine if a hyper deviation is produced for either eye. However, this patient's right eye had a hypo deviation following prolonged occlusion.)

QUANTITY

The amplitude of vergence has been extensively studied. The classic values are those of Morgan[54] and are presented in Table 15N. These are statistical norms and are not meant to apply to any particular patient. However, the values are useful in clinical decisions to show what is expected to be normal or abnormal for base-in and base-out ranges. Blur and break points can be plotted on a two-dimensional graph to determine the zone of clear, single, binocular vision and the zone of single binocular vision, respectively (see Chapter Fourteen). Referral for vision therapy possibly should be considered if a patient has any blur, break, or recovery findings that are significantly lower than the normative values of Morgan. Similarly, the analysis of a graphical plotting of these data can lead to professional judgment on the need for vision therapy to improve fusional convergence and divergence. It should be noted that vertical divergences and torsional vergences cannot be represented in the standard graphical analysis approach. The factor of *time* also cannot be represented in this form of graphical analysis. (The factor of time will be discussed later, with facility and stamina of vergence.)

RANGES AND QUALITY

There are 10 important ranges to consider in the evaluation and treatment of horizontal vergences. They are listed in Table 15O. There are numerous methods in which prismatic demands can be changed; a list is given in Table 12A.

The first and most important range to consider in testing and therapy is the vergence range free of suppression. If, for example, foveal suppression occurs during base-in and base-out testing, the patient does not have bifixation during that time. Peripheral fusion may allow the disjunctive eye movements to occur, but foveal fusion is not taking place. Suppression, therefore, must be monitored and treated (see Chapter Ten). The goal is for *no* suppression to occur all the way to the break points and beyond. Flat fusion targets with suppression clues are used in this testing. Sliding (nonstep) vergence demands may be induced either by Risley prisms or by variable split targets, e.g., vectograms.

TABLE 15N. Norms of Morgan (Partial List), with Values in Prism Diopters[54]

Test	Farpoint	Nearpoint
Blur, B.I.	—	13
Break, B.I.	7	21
Recovery, B.I.	4	13
Blur, B.O.	9	17
Break, B.O.	19	21
Recovery, B.O.	10	11

TABLE 15O. Various Ranges in Vergence Evaluation

1. Fusion without suppression
2. Fusion without blur of flat fusion target (second-degree fusion)
3. Fusion without break (diplopia) of flat fusion target
4. Recovery of fusion to singleness
5. Recovery of fusion to singleness and clearness
6. Fusion without loss of stereopsis (third-degree fusion)
7. Fusion without fixation disparity
8. Fusion without discomfort
9. Adequate fusion with fullness and quickness (facility)
10. Adequate fusion with repeated testing (stamina)

The second range to consider is fusion without blur. Flat fusion (second-degree) targets are used for this purpose. Therapeutic goals should be meeting or exceeding Morgan's values.

BLUR

The third range is fusion without diplopia. Break points are recorded at the point at which diplopia first occurs. These values should at least be in accord with those of Morgan. Flat fusion targets are used in this testing.

DIPLOPIA

The fourth range is the recovery of fusion to singleness. Magnitudes should be at least as large as the blur point findings (which also should be normal) for a particular patient. Flat fusion targets are used.

RECOVERY

The fifth range is the recovery of singleness *and* clearness of a flat fusion target. Values may be slightly lower than the blur point findings for a particular patient and yet be considered normal, assuming the blur point findings are normal for that patient. Recovery points tend to represent the *quality* of fusion, and the blur and break points tend to represent the *quantity* of fusion. Recovery abilities tend to correlate with those of facility and stamina of vergence.

RECOVERY WITH CLEARNESS

The sixth range to consider is fusion without loss or reduction of stereopsis. Most third-degree fusion tests (e.g., Fly, Reindeer, or Randot) may be suitable for such purposes. A mini-vectogram or mini-Tranaglyph (Figure 15-26) is very convenient for this type of out-of-office training. With successful therapy, the patient should be able to maintain good stereoacuity without reduction or loss of stereopsis, and with the vergence amplitudes being almost as large as the extent of the blur point ranges.

STEREOPSIS

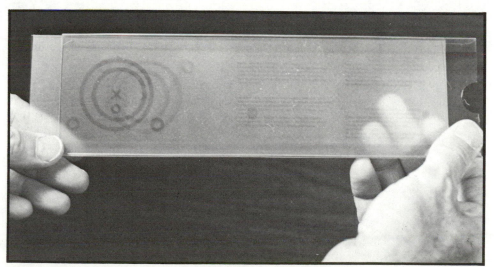

FIGURE 15-26 — Mini-Tranaglyph. Sensory fusion can be monitored while base-in and base-out motor fusion demands are introduced. This is a good device for home training. Minivectograms are available in similar designs, requiring cross-polarizing viewers. Tranaglyphs require red-green viewers (available from the Bernell Corp.).

The seventh range in vergence testing and therapy pertains to fixation disparity. Ideally, there should be no fixation disparity between blur points for base-in and base-out demands, but this is usually not possible to achieve. Moreover, some patients have fixation disparity even at the ortho demand point (the y-intercept). However, functional training procedures, lenses, and prisms (or combinations of these) may reduce the fixation disparity to zero at the ortho demand point in most cases. It is hoped that the angle of fixation disparity will remain zero (the x-intercept) throughout a reasonable vergence range. Reasonable base-in and base-out ranges are not known at present. As Grisham[55] pointed out, the ordinary Risley prism technique used by clinicians suffers may drawbacks in regard to reliability: "Test results are markedly influenced by such procedural factors as speed and smoothness of prism power induction, amount of contour in the fixation target, and phrasing of patient instructions. . . . As with most subjective techniques, a subject's attentional or arousal level can influence the test endpoints, as can other intangible factors, such as toleration of discomfort and precision of observation."

It is no wonder that firm data are lacking for normal vergence ranges free of fixation disparity. As a clinical guide, I believe the fixation disparity-free range should be at least 75 percent as large as the blur point range for a particular patient. This, of course, is what may be expected after therapy, but not necessarily before. (Refer to Chapters Two and Fourteen for further discussion of fixation disparity.)

The eighth range in vergence testing and therapy is the range that is free of discomfort. Clinicians and researchers believe that fixation disparity is related to symptoms.[56,57] Whether it is the only reason or just a part of the cause of symptoms is not certain. It is reasonable to assume there are other causes of symptoms resulting from vergence stress. At any rate, a comfort range for vergences should be determined. Newman[58] suggests that the "effortless" quality be considered when testing patients, particularly when evaluation of vergence ranges are being made. He stated, "Although the practitioner measures low phorias and finds high blur, break, and recovery at both far and near, the patient may still have a history of pain, headaches and discomfort. These symptoms often occur in patients who experience varying degrees of eye discomfort or a sensation of muscle pulling during all phases of ophthalmic testing." Newman instructs the patient to indicate any pulling sensation or pain during any phorometry tests. The magnitude of prism required to cause an uncomfortable sensation is noted and recorded along with the other range values (blur, break, etc.). The exact words of the patient are recorded, e.g., "pain," "strain," or "bothers." Functional training procedures are prescribed in many cases. The range of fusion without discomfort thus can be evaluated—another verification of the patient's binocular status before and after therapy.

Note that it is advisable to take the symptoms of patients into account when testing as well as when taking a case history during the initial interview.

The ninth range in vergence testing concerns vergence facility. This depends upon both amplitude and speed of vergence movements. The quantity and quality of disparity vergences can be judged. It is desirable to have flexible and fluent vergences that are done with ease. (Discussion will be limited to horizontal vergence facility of positive and negative disparity vergence at farpoint and nearpoint.) Grisham[59] studied the vergence tracking rate, using 2 p.d. jump-vergence steps in eight subjects, four of whom had "normal vergence characteristics" and four who had "abnormal" heterophoric or vergence characteristics, based upon clinical data. He found that the normal group had an average minimum stimulus duration of 0.84 seconds per step, and the abnormal group had a significantly longer duration of 1.67 seconds per step. Grisham cited the observation of Rashbass and Westheimer "that normal disparity vergence eye movements take on the order of 1 sec to complete independent of step stimulus amplitude" and said that his study "compares well with the observation of Rashbass and Westheimer." Grisham also found that the normal and abnormal groups could be differentiated according to other dynamic properties of fusional vergence response, including percentage of completion of step responses, response velocity, and divergence latency (but not convergence latency).

Kenyon et al.[60] studied "dynamic" vergence responses to stimuli at two different distances, 25 and 50 cm. They actually tested fusional facility of vergence, because disparity vergence was being tested (the author preferred the term *disparity* over *fusional*). While Grisham found distinguishingly poorer responses in heterophoric subjects, an absence of disparity vergence was found by Kenyon et al. in all strabismic individuals and in some who had amblyopia with no strabismus. Accommodative convergence, rather than fusional (disparity) vergences, was used to foveate the target.

From the literature and clinical experience, I believe clinical testing of vergence facility can be useful in evaluating the quality of a patient's binocular status and possibly his developmental-perceptual status. Pierce[61] reported a difference in vergence facility between normal and learning-disabled children. Other studies[62,63] reported developmental differences between schoolchildren in the third and sixth grades being around 5 and 7 cycles per minute, respectively, using ±8 p.d. (Refer to Table 15P.) Moser and Atkinson[64] found an average of 8.14 cycles per minute in young adults using ±8 p.d. in vergence facility testing. Rosner[65] stated criteria of 4 p.d. base-in and 12 p.d. base-out for farpoint and 12 p.d. base-in and 14 p.d. base-out for nearpoint, with fusion expected to occur within 3 seconds. Rosner[66] later stated criteria for screening (for referral) and for ultimate goals as follows: Screening at 6 meters is 6 p.d. base-in and 12 p.d. base-out and at 40 cm, 12 p.d. base-in and 14 p.d. base-out, with 3 cycles per 30 seconds for each distance. Rosner's ultimate goals are 6 p.d. base-in and 12 p.d. base-out at farpoint and 12 p.d. base-in and 14 p.d. base-out at nearpoint. These amplitudes are the same as in screening, but the speed is twice as fast and the number of cycles is greater. The goal of at least 18 cycles in 90 seconds is desired at farpoint and nearpoint

TABLE 15P. Summary of Studies on Vergence Facility

Investigators	Fusional (Disparity) Vergence Facility (c/min. = Cycles per Minute)	Comments
1. Kenyon et al.[60]	None in strabismics	Also none in some amblyopic subjects without strabismus
2. Pierce[61]	8 B.I. and 8 B.O., 10 c/min. (median); screening criterion of 7.5 c/min.	Median for children; 7.5 c/min. recommended as cutoff for "normal" versus "learning-disabled" children
3. Stuckle and Rouse[62]	8 B.I. and 8 B.O., approx. 7 c/min. 8 B.I. and 8 B.O., approx. 5 c/min.	Mean for 6th graders Mean for 3rd graders
4. Mitchell et al.[63]	8 B.I. and 8 B.O., 6.53 c/min. 8 B.I. and 8 B.O., 5.05 c/min.	Mean for 6th graders Mean for 3rd graders (cutoff criterion of 3 c/min. recommended)
5. Moser and Atkinson[64]	8 B.I. and 8 B.O., 8.14 c/min.	Young adults
6. Rosner[65]	4 B.I. and 12 B.O., fuse within 3 seconds 12 B.I. and 14 B.O., fuse within 3 seconds	At farpoint At nearpoint (vertically oriented 20/30 line of letters)
7. Rosner[66]	Screening: 6 B.I. and 12 B.O., 3 c/0.5 min. 12 B.I. and 14 B.O., 3 c/0.5 min. Goals: 6 B.I. and 12 B.O., 18 c/1.5 min. 12 B.I. and 14 B.O., 18 c/1.5 min.	At farpoint At nearpoint At farpoint At nearpoint
8. Jacobson et al.[67]	5 B.I. and 15 B.O. in relation to the phoric position of each subject, 8.6 c/min.	Young adults with no visual problems; jump vergences with two sets of vectographic targets
9. Griffin[68]	Goals: 5 B.I. and 15 B.O., 20 c/min. 5 B.I. and 15 B.O., 20 c/min.	At farpoint At nearpoint (Either with or without instrumentation)

using free space orthopic and chiastopic fusion without instrumentation or filters.

Jacobson et al.[67] studied vergence facility in 41 young adults with no referable visual problems or significant binocular problems. Two sets of Quoits vectographic targets (Figure 2-5 in Chapter Two) were used, the upper pair having a base-in demand, and the lower pair a base-out demand. Testing was done at 40 cm. A 5 p.d. base-in demand was presented relative to the patient's nearpoint heterophoric eye positioning. (A nearpoint phoria is also referred to as *fusional supplementary convergence (FSC) value*.) For example, if the patient had an esophoria of 4 p.d. at nearpoint, only 1 p.d. base-in was set in the upper Quoits slides. Similarly, a 15 p.d. base-out demand relative to the near phoria was set in the lower Quoits slides, or in this example, the setting would be at 19 p.d. base-out. The investigators found it necessary to make these adjustments for the heterophoria because many subjects could not perform a range of 20 p.d. using absolute 5 p.d. base-in and 15 p.d. base-out. The principal problem for many subjects was with base-in demands, particularly if the subjects were esophoric at near. A mean of 8.6 cycles per minute was found. This would indicate a rather low recommended number for screening and referral purposes. If absolute base-in and base-out powers of 5 p.d. and 15 p.d., respectively, are used, I believe a screening criterion of 4 cycles per minute is useful as a cutoff value, particularly for children. The ultimate goal, however, would be much larger.

Griffin[68] advocates a goal for vergence facility referred to as the *20/20 vergence rock rule*. This means it is desirable to have a range of 20 p.d. magnitude with a speed of 20 cycles per minute. Absolute 5 p.d. base-in and 15 p.d. base-out demands are recommended. These powers seem reasonable in light of the results of the study of Jacobson et al. This rule applies to farpoint and nearpoint for both esophoric and exophoric patients. The rationale is that esophoric patients should be expected to meet the 15 p.d. base-out demand with quickness and ease but will need intensive divergence training to meet the base-in demand efficiently. Even the small power of 5 p.d. is difficult to overcome, especially when springing back from the converged posture caused by the 15 p.d. base-out demand. It would be unreasonable to expect the esophoric patient to go more than 5 p.d. beyond the ortho demand point, whether at 6 meters or 40 cm.

An exophoric patient, on the other hand, should have no difficulty with the 5 p.d. base-in, but he needs training to go from the base-in to the 15 p.d. base-out demand with quickness and ease. Although the other studies[61-66] have lesser base-out demands, it is reasonable for patients (even those with exophoria) to have 15 p.d. base-out as a goal in facility and to meet the 20/20 vergence rock criteria if training is done faithfully.

In step ten it is important to find out if a patient has adequate fusion with repeated testing. Stamina is tested when vergence facility is tested over a period of time rather than when testing involves just one or two vergence changes. This is why practitioners test for 1 minute or longer during facility evaluations. (The same applies to stamina testing in accommodation.)

STAMINA OF VERGENCE

Testing for stamina is the same as for facility of vergence, and the criteria are the same. However, it is important not to forget about testing for a patient's sustaining ability, or ability to endure vergence demands. It is one thing to meet the demand briefly, but another to continue it for an extended period of time (which is necessary in the real world). Not to test for stamina is being artificial and neglecting to check the patient's ability to cope with vergence demands in life's study, work, and play.

The equipment used in vergence facility testing can be used here. Prism flippers (Figure 12-2 in Chapter Twelve) can be used while viewing a single object, e.g., a doorknob. Better yet, use a second- or third-degree fusion target, e.g., a Reindeer with filters. Vectographic and anaglyphic split targets can be used to create base-in and base-out demands for jump vergences if flip prisms are not used. Orthopic-chiastopic vergence rock is very convenient, as no equipment is required other than common objects like two pencils, thumbs, lifesavers, etc.

Several ranges of vergence can be assessed when doing nearpoint of convergence (NPC) testing. Keep in mind that more than disparity vergence is in play (including accommodative and proximal convergence). However, useful information can be derived from NPC results when testing is done in the following manner. Have the patient fixate a letter on the Alphabet Pencil, and slowly move it toward him in the midline until he reports blurring of the fixated letter. Keep moving it closer until the break point. Then slowly move the pencil away until there is recovery of fusion (but not necessarily clearness).

A remote distance blurring would provide an obvious explanation of visual symptoms associated with near work, in spite of the patient's having good monocular accommodative amplitude and 20/20 acuity of each eye.

Screening criteria for break and recovery distances are 5 and 8 cm, respectively.[69] Ideally, the break point should be trained to be about 2 to 3 cm from the bridge of the nose. It is impressive to consider how many prism diopters a distance of 2 cm represents. The calculation is as follows:

$$\Delta = IPD \times \frac{100}{2 + 2.7}.$$

Assume interpupilary distance is 6 cm, and 2.7 cm is the distance from the bridge of nose (roughly the spectacle plan) to the center of rotation of the eyes. Therefore,

$$\Delta = 6 \left(\frac{100}{2 + 2.7} \right) = 128.$$

The magnitude of 128 p.d. seems extraordinary, but remember, the combination of fusional, accommodative, and proximal convergence may be working together in this task.

It is good to repeat the NPC testing five times to determine stamina. Therefore, sustaining ability of convergence can be evaluated along with blur, break, and recoveries.

Efficiency depends on how well the patient reaches his goals for the ranges of vergence listed in Table 15O. Therapy for horizontal vergence anomalies are covered in detail in Chapters Twelve and Thirteen. Tables 12C, 12D, 13A, and 13B provide logical sequences of training for vergence anomalies associated with esophoria and exophoria. A finishing process of having the patient achieve the 20/20 vergence rock (20 p.d. with 20 cycles per minute) would ensure adequate facility and stamina. Unless the patient can develop efficient vergences, he may be left with blurring, slow reading, and other signs and symptoms, such as those listed in Table 3E. Practically all the instruments referred to in Chapters Twelve and Thirteen for horizontal training can be used for vertical vergence therapy. During chiastopic fusion, for example, the Keystone Eccentric Circles can be separated vertically a slight amount to induce disparity stimuli for fusion.

A Tranaglyph with vertical disparity[h] is available for training with the hyperphoric patient (Figure 15-27). I recommend rotating the Tranaglyph 90 degrees so there is no demand on vertical vergence. When the red and green images are fused, slowly rotate the Tranaglyph to its original position of maximum vertical demand on vergence. A very gradual increase in vertical demand can be smoothly made to the maximum limit of fusion. This is possible since red and green filters are used rather than a vectographic system, which would not allow for rotation of the target.

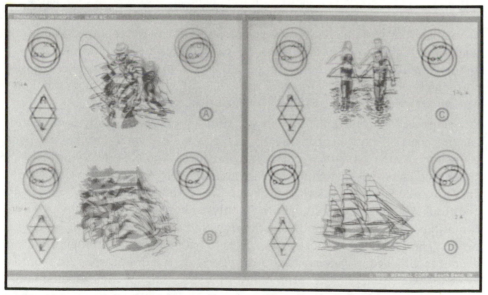

FIGURE 15-27 — Vertical Tranaglyph for the training of vertical vergence skills in cases of hyperphoria.

When vertical disparities cannot be induced through target separation, the doctor can use a base-up or base-down prism (whichever is appropriate for the patient) to create a vertical fusion demand. Clip-ons or Fresnel prisms can be

---

[h] Available from Bernell Corp.

placed on the patient's spectacle lenses. For a momentary stimulus, a loose prism in vertical orientation can be held before the patient's eye. Most fixation disparity targets are excellent for training vertical vergences. As vertical prism is increased, suppression, break ranges, and fixation disparity can be evaluated. If the prism is quickly changed from base-up to base-down, facility and stamina can be assessed. The ultimate ranges may be quite small—only several prism diopters. Nevertheless, training may help the patient cope with a problem caused by hyperphoria.

The improvement of horizontal vergence efficiency usually helps the patient cope with a vertical deviation. Once the horizontal ranges begin to expand, introduce a vertical demand, e.g., via a loose base-down prism, along with the base-in and base-out demands. Vertical vergence training has limits, and the doctor may have to call upon the compensatory effects of prescribed vertical prism. This is particularly true when a prism neutralizes a vertical fixation disparity. It is likely that only when a vertical deviation of the visual axes is large (i.e., over 10 p.d.) that extraocular muscle surgery should be considered at all.

Much of what was said for functional training for vertical deviations can be said for cyclotorsional deviations. (Prism compensation is not feasible for cyclophoria.) For instance, the Keystone Eccentric Circles can be rotated during orthopic or chiastopic fusion to stimulate incyclovergence or excyclovergence. Many targets can be used in this manner, but the major amblyoscope is the most ideal instrument for this type of training. Torsional amplitudes can be increased in most patients with excyclophoria or incyclophoria. Aside from functional training procedures, surgery is the only other method of treatment for these problems. However, it is not advisable in most heterophoric cases. Fortunately, cyclophoric problems are often alleviated after horizontal and vertical vergences become efficient by means of vision therapy.

Vergence efficiency therapy is sometimes important for the orthophoric patient. This is particularly true if vergence facility and stamina are poor. Clinicians in the past have wondered why a patient who is perfectly orthophoric at far and near has symptoms pathognomonic of vergence anomalies. The kinetic cover test (discussed in Chapter Three) helps answer this enigmatic question. The so-called orthophore is only orthophoric under static viewing conditions. However, people live under dynamic viewing conditions in the real world. The kinetic cover test reveals how a patient who is orthophoric at all distances will become momentarily exophoric as fixation is changed from far to near. Conversely, the orthophoric patient will become momentarily esophoric as fixation is changed from near to far. Such a patient may have binocular problems unless he has adequate vergence efficiency, his orthophoria notwithstanding. If so, general vergence therapy (as described in Chapters Twelve and Thirteen) would be recommended. The patient would be treated as though he had both an eso and an exo problem.

The patient with this type of vergence anomaly would fit the category of the ninth basic vergence problem of Schapero.[70] According to Schapero, the narrow zone of clear, single, binocular vision could be caused by poor sensory fusion, uncorrected refractive errors, aniseikonia, uncorrected vertical phoria, disuse of motor fusion, and systemic disturbances. All these possibilities should be checked and accounted for. If the narrow zone continues to exist, the patient will likely have a vergence problem causing signs and symptoms of inefficiency and asthenopia. Functional training procedures to improve the fusional (disparity) vergence ranges most always alleviate the problem, providing the patient is cooperative and faithful in doing the office and home training. Figures 15-28 through 15-37 graphically illustrate the ten basic types of vergence problems according to Schapero.

The vergence anomalies depicted in Figures 15-28 through 15-37 represent cases of nonstrabismus, or at most, intermittent strabismus. It is not customary to use graphical analysis in cases of constant strabismus; graphical analysis applies to accommodation and vergence relationships in heterophoria. Bear in mind that what is shown are *clinical* sketchings of the phoria lines, and the blur/break lines for base-in and for base-out—not the research-like, haploscopically derived lines that would be found in laboratory experiments. After all, we seek the clinical usefulness of the graphical analysis.

The first type of basic problem is convergence insufficiency that would cause a patient to have nearpoint exo problems (Figure 15-28). Therapy would be that of nearpoint exo problems as outlined and discussed in Chapter Thirteen.

THERAPY FOR THE
TEN BASIC TYPES OF
VERGENCE ANOMALIES

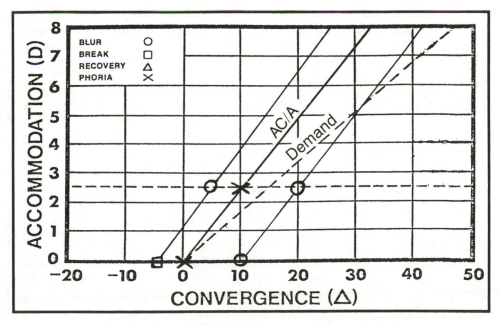

FIGURE 15-28 — First basic problem of vergence anomalies according to Schapero. There is normal tonic convergence (approximately orthophoria), low fusional convergence, and a low AC/A ratio. This nearpoint exo problem is a classic example of convergence insufficiency.

The second type of basic problem is convergence excess that would cause a patient to have nearpoint eso problems (Figure 15-29). Therapy would be that of nearpoint eso problems as outlined and discussed in Chapter Twelve. Plus addition lenses in the form of bifocals may be required in this type of case.

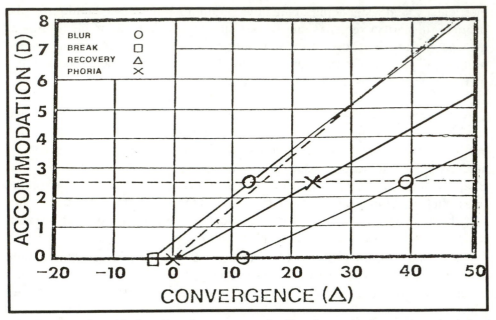

FIGURE 15-29 — Second basic problem of vergence anomalies. There is normal tonic convergence, low fusional divergence, and a high AC/A ratio. This nearpoint eso problem is a classic example of convergence excess.

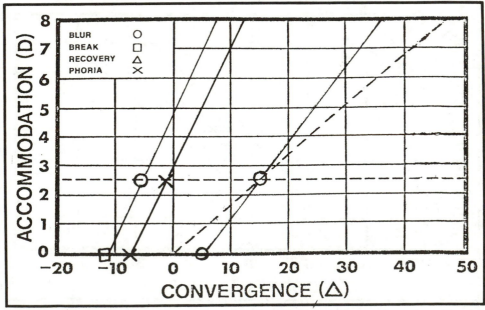

FIGURE 15-30 — Third basic problem of vergence anomalies. There is low tonic convergence (exo at farpoint), low fusional convergence, and a low AC/A ratio. This is a case of convergence insufficiency with a nearpoint exo problem and an exo farpoint problem.

The third type of basic problem is convergence insufficiency combined with a farpoint exo problem due to the combination of low tonic convergence and a low AC/A ratio along with positive fusional vergence being less than adequate (Figure 15-30). It is likely that intermittent exotropia will occur at very close viewing distances. Note that the demand line is to the right of the base-out-to-blur line when the fixation distance is closer than 40 cm (2.50D). Base-in prism may be considered along with functional training procedures to increase the fusional convergence ranges at near and far.

The fourth type of basic problem is called *basic exo* and would cause a patient to have problems at farpoint and nearpoint (Figure 15-31). As in the third type of vergence problem, both farpoint and nearpoint exo therapy would apply (Chapter Thirteen). However, the emphasis would be on farpoint therapy as outlined in Table 13A. Base-in prisms would not be considered unless necessary, e.g., for neutralization of fixation disparity, relief of symptoms, or prevention of exotropia.

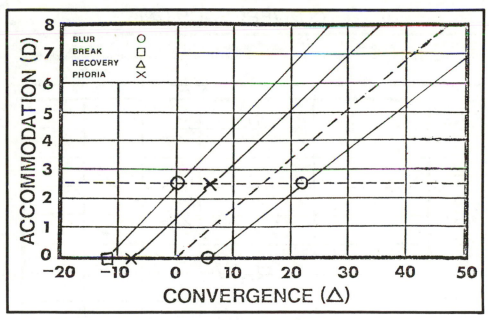

FIGURE 15-31 — Fourth basic problem of vergence anomalies. There is low tonic convergence, low fusional convergence, and a normal AC/A ratio. This is a classic example of a basic exo problem (at far and near).

The fifth type of basic problem is divergence excess, and it would cause the patient to have exo problems at farpoint (Figure 15-32). Treatment would follow the outline in Table 13A for farpoint exo problems. Plus addition lenses in the form of bifocals might be considered to help "harmonize" the AC/A ratio line with the demand. (Refer to the discussion in Chapter Thirteen.)

The sixth type of basic problem is divergence insufficiency, and it would cause a patient to have eso problems at farpoint (Figure 15-33). Base-out prism prescription may have to be considered, particularly if esotropia becomes manifest at farpoint. The goal of functional training would be to

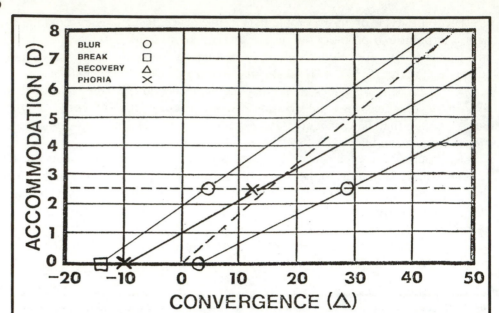

FIGURE 15-32 — Fifth basic problem of vergence anomalies. There is low tonic convergence, low fusional convergence, and a high AC/A ratio. This is a classic example of divergence excess (farpoint exo problem).

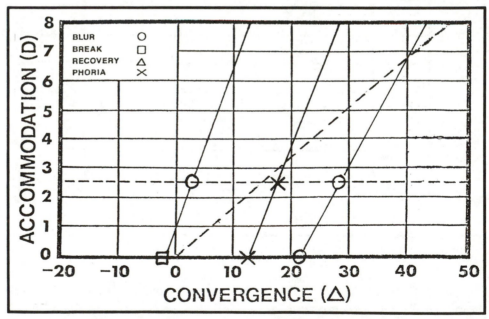

FIGURE 15-33 — Sixth basic problem of vergence anomalies. There is high tonic convergence (eso at farpoint), low fusional divergence, and a low AC/A ratio.This is a classic example of divergence insufficiency (farpoint eso problem).

improve fusional divergence, as listed in Table 12C. Note that too much base-out prism would cause a convergent stimulus at nearpoint (the demand line being shifted to the right of the phoria, or AC/A, line). Therefore, great caution must be exercised if any base-out prism is to be considered in a case of divergence insufficiency. Preferably, no prism will be used in most of these cases, as it could exacerbate the eso problem rather than help the patient.

The seventh type of basic problem is called *basic eso* and would cause a patient to have problems at farpoint and nearpoint (Figure 15-34). It would be safer to consider base-out prisms in this type of case than in divergence insufficiency, because the AC/A line (phoria line) and the ortho demand line are in "harmony" by being parallel to one another. In other words, the eso at far is approximately equal to the eso at near. Training would be for farpoint eso problems as listed in Table 12C.

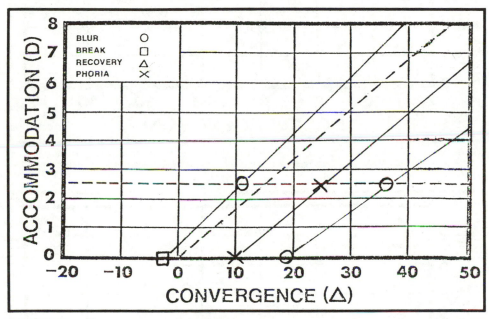

FIGURE 15-34 — Seventh basic problem of vergence anomalies. There is high tonic convergence, low fusional divergence, and a normal AC/A ratio. This is a classic example of a basic eso problem (at far and near).

The eighth type of basic problem is convergence excess combined with a farpoint eso problem due to the combination of high tonic convergence and a high AC/A ratio along with negative fusional vergence being less than adequate (Figure 15-35). It is likely that intermittent esotropia will occur at very close viewing distances. Note the eso deviation becoming larger as the fixation distance is decreased. The practitioner must be careful when testing the NPC, because the NPC appears to be more than adequate, and in fact may overshoot the fixation target due to the excessive convergence. A "nearpoint Hirschberg" test may help detect this loss of bifixation in such cases. Plus addition lenses in the form of bifocals and possibly base-out prism compensation should be considered. Functional training procedures would follow the outline in Table 12D for nearpoint eso problems.

The ninth type of basic problem is *basic ortho* with poor fusional vergences (Figure 15-36). Functional training procedures would include all those for the improvement of fusional convergence and divergence at farpoint

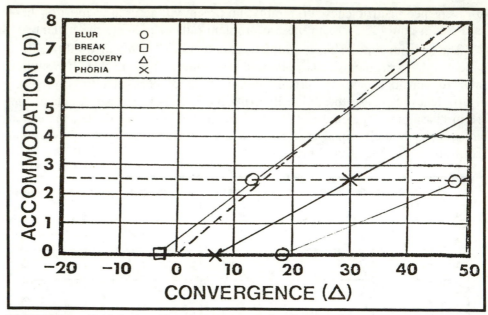

FIGURE 15-35 — Eighth basic problem of vergence anomalies. There is high tonic convergence, low fusional divergence, and a high AC/A ratio. This is a case of convergence excess with a nearpoint eso problem as well as an eso farpoint problem.

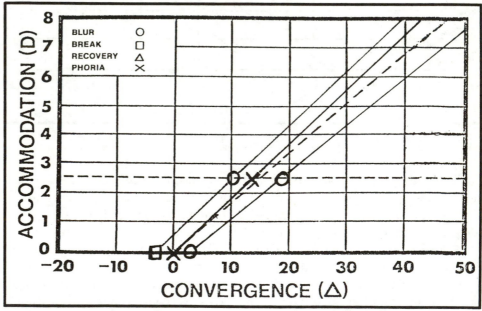

FIGURE 15-36 — Ninth basic problem of vergence anomalies. There is normal tonic convergence, low fusional convergence and low fusional divergence, and a normal AC/A ratio. This is a case of basic ortho with vergence problems at far and near.

and nearpoint. Reasons for the poor fusional vergences should be sought. (Refer to the previous discussion in this chapter.)

The tenth type of basic problem has symptoms typical of those found in vergence anomalies (Figure 15-37). Further testing reveals other problems,

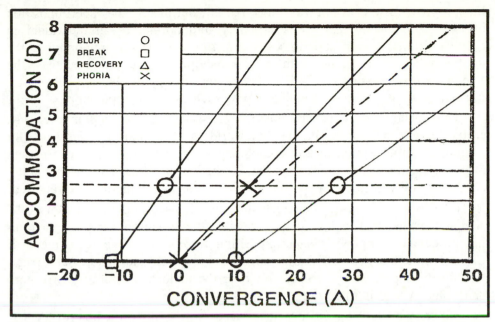

FIGURE 15-37 — Tenth basic problem of vergence anomalies. There is apparently normal tonic convergence, normal fusional vergences, and a normal AC/A ratio. Schapero[70] speculated that visual symptoms could be due to psychosomatic problems, systemic or ocular pathology, aniseikonia, uncorrected refractive errors, vertical phorias, disguised high exophoria (due to persistence of fusional convergence during testing), and fatigue (lack of stamina). Poor vergence facility could also be a factor.

such as poor stamina, poor facility, or latent heterophoric conditions not apparent until prolonged occlusion is done. If, for instance, a basic exo problem is found, the patient would be treated as though he had a case resembling type four. In any event, the underlying etiology must be looked for and the problem corrected. Note that the graphical analysis approach has many limitations. Figure 15-37 is what the ideal graph should look like; yet a patient with a graph of this type may or may not have problems. The graphical approach to analysis is valuable, but it can only tell the doctor so much. All possible causes of symptoms and visual inefficiencies must be considered.

Sensory Fusion Systems

The systems of saccades, pursuits, accommodation, and vergences are principally motoric from a clinical perspective. However, there must be sensory (and probably perceptual) input so visual functioning can occur. Clinical testing of sensory fusion also involves a motoric component. Nevertheless, for pedagogic purposes it is convenient to deal with motor fusion and sensory fusion as though they were separate, but keep in mind that this distinction is artificial, and they are really not dissoluble.

On a clinical basis, motor fusion can be considered as basically involving the amplitude and speed of various ranges of vergences. On the other hand, the clinical concern in sensory fusion is with the question of suppression. Sensory fusion is classified according to the Worth taxonomy into three categories—first-, second-, and third-degree fusion. (Refer to Chapter Two for a detailed discussion of testing of these degrees of sensory fusion.)

First-degree "fusion" is not truly fusion at all, but merely the superimposition of two dissimilar images. It is probably unimportant to an individual in everyday life. However, superimposition *testing* may be very important to the doctor when it is done with a stereoscopic instrument such as the Synoptophore. Testing of A R C relies heavily upon the use of super-imposition targets in major amblyoscopes, such as the Synoptophore.

The counterpart to superimposition (first-degree "fusion") in everyday, casual, seeing conditions in the real world in strabismus is *confusion* (for example, the perception of a doorknob superimposed on a vase). The patient may complain of symptoms because of this visual nuisance. At any rate, confusion leads to foveal suppression, whether or not symptoms are reported.

It follows that first-degree targets may also be used in the evaluation of the size and intensity of suppression. Likewise, functional antisuppression train-ing procedures employing superimposition targets are often recommended. Cheiroscopic drawings (dissimilar targets being a pen and picture) are excel-lent for antisuppression therapy, providing the patient has normal correspon-dence and A R C is ruled out.

Superimposition targets are also used in *therapy* in cases of A R C (Chapter Nine). Other than that, there is not much else to say about first-degree "fusion" in regard to efficient visual skills except that the phenomenon of confusion in everyday seeing could have an adverse effect on a person's efficiency in school, work, and play. Fortunately (or unfortunately, as the case may be), suppression usually solves that dilemma for the individual, and the report of "confusion" is seldom the presenting complaint of patients who have binocular problems.

Second-degree fusion and *flat fusion* are synonymous. There is a theoretical debate on whether true fusion really is a phenomenon or if it is only rapid rivalry of two uniocular images giving the apparent perception of fusion. For clinical purposes, however, let us consider that there is true sensory fusion. Most ranges of vergence are measured by the use of flat fusion targets (e.g., blur, break, recovery, and fixation disparity). Refer to Chapter Two for a discussion on testing for flat fusion. Functional training procedures are practically the same as testing procedures. (Refer to Chapters Twelve and Thirteen for therapy for eso and exo deviations, respectively.)

Michaels[71] pointed out the peculiarity of flat fusion in that "there is no way to prove that it is taking place when the two uniocular images are exactly alike." This is why suppression clues must be added for clinical testing in order for flat fusion targets to provide information as to whether the patient has flat fusion or not. (Refer to examples of targets in Figure 2-2 in Chapter Two.) Examples of second-degree fusion tests are the Worth four-dot test, red lens test, vectographic Snellen charts, bar reading, Turville infinity balance test, etc. Flat fusion targets have all homologous points that are equally separated on a stereogram. This makes a "pure" clinical test for vergence ranges, as base-in or base-out demands are the same for all homologous points on a particular stereogram. This is not true for third-degree fusion targets, which have homologous points that are unequally spaced.

Stereopsis is synonymous with *third-degree fusion* for purposes of this discussion. Although it is probable that infants have some stereopsis, it is difficult to test for it by clinical means in patients under the age of 2 years. Simons[72] reported on various stereoacuity tests and believed that binocular visual development is not complete by the age of 5 years. Cooper et al.[73] studied young children using several tests of stereopsis and stated that "results indicated that stereoacuity scores improved with age and that performance variability decreased with age. Normal adult findings were achieved by age 7." This would concur with the study of Hofstetter and Bertsch,[74] who determined thresholds of stereoacuity on 242 subjects with normal visual acuity, ranging in age from 8 to 46 years. No trend was found for age, and there was no significant sex difference.

Cooper and Feldman[75] found stereoacuity improving from the age of 2 to 5 years. Operant conditioning was given in children aged 2 to 5 years. They found that this type of approach yielded superior stereoacuities which were more reliable in the assessment of stereopsis than the traditional approach of testing. However, they found no stereoscopic responses, by any method, for most of the children in the 2-year-old group, in spite of there being a remarkable increase in stereoacuity levels for children aged 3 and up. They stated the opinion that operant conditioning is important in testing to account for factors of problems with attention, motivation, and language ability that may give falsely poor stereoacuity test scores otherwise.

A popular vectographic contoured test of stereopsis is the Stereo Reindeer test.[i] Unlike most stereo tests, the stereoacuity values are expressed in percentages rather than in seconds of arc disparity. The test is keyed for a fixation distance of 14 inches (35.6 cm). Fagin and Griffin[76] calculated values for the Reindeer test in seconds of arc for this and other distances (see Table 15Q). Traditionally used stereopsis tests are discussed in Chapter Two.

THIRD DEGREE

NEW TESTS

TABLE 15Q. Key for the Stereo Reindeer Test				
Target	Answer	Testing Distance and Seconds of Arc		
Row	No.	35.6 cm	40 cm	100 cm
A	4	592	526	211
B	2	256	227	91
C	5	143	128	51
D	3	74	66	26
E	4	45	41	16
F	2	31	28	11

[i]Available from the Bernell Corp.

Random dot stereograms are not new in principle, but their clinical use has become very widespread only relatively recently. The first random dot stereogram was made in 1954.[77] In 1960 Julesz[78] used computer-generated patterns to produce random dot stereograms. These were anaglyphic targets using red and green filters. Later on, vectographic random dot stereograms became available.

The TNO test[j] was developed in The Netherlands and uses a red-green anaglyphic system in the random dot stereograms. At the recommended 40 cm testing distance, the range of disparities is from 15 to 1,980 seconds of arc, making this an extensive testing procedure for stereoacuity.

The Random Dot E Stereotest[k] is a vectographic test employing the Julesz design. It has a demonstrator that simulates a random dot stereoscopic view of an "E" that would be seen floating in front of the plane of a hand-held card (see Figure 15-38). The test consists of asking the patient to choose between a blank card and one which presents an "E" produced by stereofusion. This forced-choice testing is done with the same two cards at various distances, providing a range of 42 to 1,261 seconds of arc, based on a 20 cm to 6 meter testing distance range.

The Randot Stereotest[l] is bound in a small booklet similar to that of the Titmus Fly test. The values for each Randot circle target in the test when used at 16 inches (40.64 cm) are as follows: one, 400 seconds of arc; two, 200 seconds of arc; three, 100 seconds of arc; four, 70 seconds of arc; five, 50 seconds of arc; six, 40 seconds of arc; seven, 30 seconds of arc; and eight, 20 seconds of arc. The advantages the Randot test has over the Titmus Fly test are that the targets are not contoured (preventing guessing), and testing is more sensitive (Titmus Fly stops at 40 seconds of arc, with a fixation distance of 16 inches).

The Frisby Stereo test[m] is also based on the Julesz random dot design, but it has randomized patterns on each side of a clear plate to produce retinal disparity. Four plates are available to produce levels of stereoacuity demand ranging from approximately 880 to 20 seconds of arc by viewing the targets from various distances. Cooper and Feldman[79] concluded that the Frisby Stereo test is a fairly effective stereopsis test for adults. Although it has the advantage of not requiring the patient to wear filters (e.g., cross-polarizing or red-green filters), as do many other tests of stereopsis, testing could be invalidated by head movement causing motion-parallax clues, a likelihood in young children.

---

[j] Available from Alfred P. Poll, Inc.

[k] Available from Stereo Optical Company, Inc.

[l] Available from Stereo Optical Company, Inc.

[m] Available from Clement-Clark Ltd.

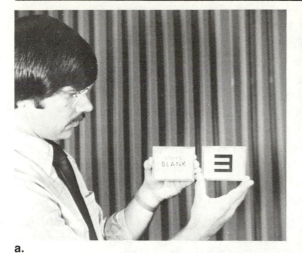

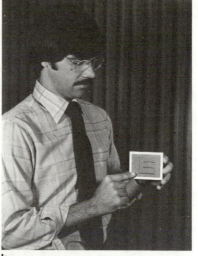

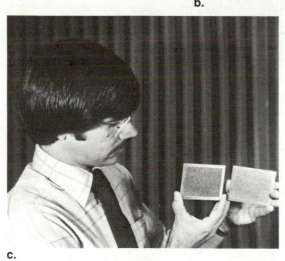

FIGURE 15-38 — The Random Dot E Stereotest. (a) Back side for examiner's view; (b) Demonstration card; (c) Examinee's view of testing cards, one being blank.

The level of stereopsis determines the level of binocular status in most cases. According to Vodnoy,[80] stereopsis is the "barometer" of binocularity. If stereopsis is good, the binocular status is good. But the opposite cannot be said with certainty. That is, a patient may be found to have no stereopsis but have normal sensory and motor fusion in all other respects. Some individuals may lack cortical binocular disparity cells. Hine[81] cited a study of Richards[82] that reported that 30 percent of subjects showed inabilities to detect disparity, comparing crossed and uncrossed disparity processing. It was implied that such stereoanomalies are genetic in origin. If lack of both types of disparity detectors (i.e., crossed and uncrossed) are inherited, an individual may lack normal binocular vision and be at risk for strabismus. Hine stated, "It is

SCREENING FOR
BINOCULAR PROBLEMS

feasible then, that by screening parents for stereoanomalies it may be possible to identify those off-spring at risk earlier."

Cooper and Warshowsky[83] found that monocular lateral displacement on a vectographic stereoacuity test was used by subjects as a clue to identifying the correct answer. They placed the axis of the polarizing viewer at 135 degrees for the lens of both eyes to remove binocular retinal image disparity as a depth clue. They concluded that the first four or more of the nine modified Wirt circles of the Titmus Stereo test (Figure 2-8 in Chapter Two) should be used and interpreted with caution, as a person with suppression of an eye could possibly pass those by looking for monocular displacement clues. However, they found that the "speed and confidence of the responses are less for suppressing subjects than for normal binocular individuals."

Recent studies have tended to utilize random dot testing because of the criticism that contoured targets may allow guessing. Walraven[84] tested 81 patients, aged 2 to 7 years, with known visual health records, using the TNO test. As to screening for amblyopia, it was concluded that "failure to pass this test at the 240 seconds of arc disparity level yielded an excellent screening criterion."

Rosner[85] reported that the Random Dot E test is effective in detecting young children (3 to 6 years) with binocular anomalies.

Cooper and Feldman[86] used a special random dot stereogram of 660 seconds of arc disparity to determine the effectiveness of screening for binocular anomalies. They found that passing this particular testing situation depended upon good binocularity and was not directly related to visual acuity. For example, some subjects with 20/20 right eye and 20/80 left eye could "pass" the test, while some with 20/20 right eye and 20/15 left eye failed to appreciate the random dot stereoscopic form. The investigators concluded that "all the normal (control group) subjects passed the test, and none of the microtropes, constant strabismics, or amblyopic strabismics did."

I summarize the use of stereopsis testing for screening for binocular anomalies by saying that even a gross random dot stereogram target is good, but a fine target is needed when using contoured stereograms. The value of 67 seconds of arc for the contoured stereograms (e.g., Fly or Reindeer) remains a reliable cutoff criterion. (Refer to the discussion in Chapter Five.)

Stereopsis tests will show poor stereoacuity in monofixating patients (e.g., strabismics, or amblyopes with central suppression). However, peripheral (extramacular) stereopsis tests may reveal the presence of gross stereopsis in many of these patients. Birnbaum[87] found that "a large number of strabismics (47.5%) exhibited peripheral stereopsis on some tests or test distances, but not others" and that "strabismics with A R C or amblyopia were unlikely to exhibit good peripheral stereo responses to all tests and distances; however, the presence of amblyopia, eccentric fixation, or A R C did not preclude good peripheral stereo responses on some tests or at some test distances in space."

It is important to test for peripheral stereopsis, as this can be very important in developing and improving motor fusion ranges. This is particularly so in small-angle strabismics, who can develop good fusional amplitudes but yet may have a poor prognosis for developing bifixation (with central, fine stereopsis).

In light of this discussion, one may wonder why random dot stereo tests, even gross ones, apparently seem to be effective in identifying the binocular anomalies of suppression, A R C, amblyopia, etc. Conversely, the stereo tests with contoured patterns must be within relatively sensitive criteria, e.g., 67 seconds of arc, to be effective in this regard. The difference in criteria between the two types of stereopsis tests may have something to do with "local" versus "global" stereopsis. Cline et al.[88] define *local stereopsis* as a "very simple disparity stimulus pattern such as, for example, a stereogram with two parallel vertical line segments seen by each eye with slightly differing lateral separations." On the other hand, they define *global stereopsis* as that "elicited by the disparity of portions and/or clusters within relatively large stereogram patterns, involving complex textured surfaces and repetitive elements for which many disparately paired details might provide ambiguous or even conflicting stereopsis clues without destroying the overlying percept of depth, believed by Julesz to represent a perceptual interpretation process differentiable from local stereopsis."

Hamsher[89] confirmed the hypothesis that "the right hemisphere is dominant for global stereopsis but not local stereopsis. The additional mechanism(s) needed to achieve global stereopsis, while working with stereoscopic mechanisms, may not be of a strictly stereoscopic but of a more general visuoperceptive nature, perhaps those involved in utilizing subtle cues to achieve form recognition."

There may be two different types of stereopsis, global requiring more "visual perception" than local. It may be that people with poor binocularity have a lack of development in this regard. This could be the reason they do relatively poorly on random dot types of stereo tests.

THERAPY

There is little doubt in the minds of experienced clinicians that stereoacuity can be improved by vision therapy. Improvement could be due to the results of antisuppression training, cure of amblyopia, elimination of A R C, reduction or elimination of fixation disparity, increased perceptual awareness of binocular depth, practice, and so forth. At any rate, clinical evidence is overwhelming that poor stereoacuities can be made better, in many cases, as a result of vision therapy. Wittenberg[90] reported on a study done with Dr. Frederick Brock (Brock's treatment philosophy is discussed in Chapter Six) a number of years ago and indicated that "stereoscopic acuity had definitely improved in the trained group."

There is really no specific regimen of training procedures that can be prescribed for improving stereoacuity. Better stereoacuity is usually a result when sensory and motor fusion have been improved through therapy. All treatment procedures in the previous chapters should be considered. There is no question about good stereoacuity being an indicator of success in therapy, at least for persons with binocular anomalies. Poor stereoacuity (or possibly none) in the strabismic patient may be transformed into good stereoacuity when the strabismus is cured. Furthermore, fair stereoacuity may be made good in the heterophoric patient when efficient visual skills have been achieved.

Does having better stereopsis necessarily mean that people are more efficient in real life? I am unable to answer this question at the present time, but I can say that good stereopsis is an index to good efficient binocular vision.

Monovision and Efficiency

Some patients may not achieve bifixation, and, consequently, they may not achieve a high level of stereopsis. If a person does not have bifixation, he is classified as having monofixation. Many practitioners refer to this condition as *monovision*. Monofixation is found in varying degrees, from the patient with constant, large-angle strabismus with A R C to the otherwise normal binocular patient who is a presbyopic contact lens wearer and has an ametropic correction for the dominant eye for distance seeing and a plus addition lens for the nondominant eye for near seeing. If such a contact lens-wearing patient is carefully tested, foveal suppression will be found. Monofixation is the case, albeit artificially induced.

To date, it is difficult to find hard evidence that monofixators present a threat on the highways, or that they necessarily have reading difficulties or other problems in school, work, or play. Many of them do have symptoms, but many do not. Research is needed to determine those who have symptoms and visual inefficiencies, and why, and how debilitated they may be. This points out the importance of helping all patients in need of vision therapy, including monofixators and bifixators, to become as visually efficient as they possibly can. For example, a patient may not achieve a functional cure of strabismus; nevertheless, saccades, pursuits, and accommodation can be worked on and, it is hoped, improved when there are visual efficiency problems in these "monocular" skills.

16 | Other Considerations in Evaluation and Therapy

A brief overview of some important considerations—some old and some new—includes such topics as the prevalence of problems, functional training for the elderly, reading problems related to binocular vision, nystagmus, auditory biofeedback in strabismus therapy, amblyopia methods, special uses of the cover test, learning theories applied to binocular therapy, an aniseikonia summary, and some things to consider and remember. Several texts would be required in order to delve into each of these topics adequately. Therefore, the intention here is to highlight only a few topics pertaining to this text.

Unilateral functional amblyopia is found in approximately 3 percent of the general population. Refer to the discussion of amblyopia in Chapter Two.

Prevalence of Problems

Scobee[1] stated that the prevalence of all types of strabismus was estimated to be 1.5 percent. Hugonnier et al.[2] said that "strabismus is found in about 2–4 percent of the general population."

Michaels[3] presented a table indicating a range of 1.3 to 5.4 percent for the prevalence of strabismus in children, but citing 9.0 percent for a sample of retardates. It is well known that strabismus is common in persons with Down's syndrome and other similar severe affections. This association does not imply that strabismics are likely to be mentally retarded, but only that children with severe developmental disorders are more likely to be strabismic than those who are considered to be developmentally normal. The question of whether or not strabismus is a factor in otherwise normal children who have learning disabilities remains to be settled.

It is generally recognized that esotropia occurs more frequently than exotropia in children in a roughly estimated ratio of about 3 to 1. This ratio decreases, however, with age to what I would judge to be approximately 1.5 to 1 in adults. Influences of the effects of vision therapy (e.g., surgery, lenses, and orthoptics) must be considered before predicting prevalences that would occur naturally in the absence of any treatment.

A problem in determining the frequency of strabismus in a population is that the diagnosis may be loose or strict. For example, an eso deviation that is intermittently manifest only 1 percent of the time is technically heterotropic, in my opinion. Some reporters may not agree with this, however. Consider also that very small angles of strabismus (microtropia) are not cosmetically noticeable and may not necessarily be included as heterotropic in statistical accounting. In general, I believe 4 percent is a rough approximation of the prevalence of strabismus in the general population. Therefore, approximately 7% have either strabismus or amblyopia, but I would estimate about 5 percent have amblyopia *and* strabismus.

Estimation of the prevalence of strabismus may vary from one authority to another, but the variation is much greater for heterophoria. However, most practitioners do agree that there are more cases of heterophoria (implying symptomatic problems) than heterotropia. Note that heterophoria is not a problem per se, but the problems associated with it are. Vodnoy[4] commented that "of the total orthoptic case load, the vast majority are nonstrabismic." He also indicated that the percentage of cases of constant strabismus is less than that of intermittent strabismus.

I estimate that approximately 10 percent of the population need and could benefit from nonstrabismic vision therapy (as discussed in Chapter Fifteen). An additional 5 to 10 percent (mainly children) could probably benefit from vision therapy involving visual perception and/or visual motor dysfunctions (not discussed in this text).

Functional Training for the Elderly

Motor fusion training may help older patients with convergence insufficiency to improve positive fusional (disparity) vergence. Sensory fusion training, however, is usually reserved for the younger patient. Vodnoy[5] stated: "Prism base-out training may be prescribed for patients in their sixties and even seventies. The success with these patients is 90 to 100 percent in the training of convergence insufficiencies, just as it is with the pre- or non-presbyopes."

Wick[6] provided functional training procedures for 161 symptomatic patients with an age range of 45 to 89 years, of whom the majority had convergence insufficiency. Therapy goals and the elimination of symptoms were achieved in 92 percent of the patients. Home training was emphasized, and most patients required only about five office visits. The more elderly, however, tended to require follow-up training to maintain the initial level of success.

When functional training may not be effective, other methods of therapy, such as compensatory prisms, may be necessary.

Reading Problems Related to Binocular Vision

There is considerable controversy as to the effect of binocular status on reading ability. The typical example for the primary eye care practitioner is that of a third or fourth grade child who is underachieving in school (i.e., who has a learning disability), notwithstanding normal intelligence, good educational opportunities, etc. A *learning disability* is usually defined as a student's performing, particularly in reading, 2 years or more below the expected level for his grade. A child's learning disability often is not fully realized until the third or fourth grade. This may be because the child is "learning to read" in the first 2 years of school, whereas later he is "reading to learn."

Many authorities claim there is little or no relationship between binocular vision status and reading ability. Other authorities[7-10] among many holding the opposite view contend there is a positive correlation between poor reading ability and such binocular problems as poor fusion, heterophoria, and remote nearpoint of convergence. When the other skills pertaining to visual efficiency are included (refer to Chapter Fifteen), their argument becomes more convincing. This dilemma is analogous to the reported negative correlation between good visual acuity and safe automobile driving.[11] It is common sense that reasonably good acuity is necessary for motorists; however, because of many intervening variables, statistics do not support common sense here. This also seems to be the case when attempting to relate visual skills efficiency to reading ability. There is no way to quickly and validly settle this complex issue. A few excerpts from literature, however, may provide some direction in exploring this question.

Brod and Hamilton[12] studied a sample of 162 fifth grade students and found that "binocular instabilities are a more serious obstacle to learning than is the lack of binocularity." They conclude by stating that "the study demonstrates that a disturbance in binocular functioning results in a highly significant decrement in reading performance."

Flax[13] concluded that "binocular fusion problems are more apt to interfere with sustaining accuracy and comprehension than they are with fundamental word recognition facility." His feeling was that fusion (i.e., binocular vision) problems may not show up until the third or fourth grade, when reading demands (i.e., reading to learn) become much greater. Seemingly in agreement with Brod and Hamilton, Flax summarized by saying that "it is apparently better to be completely one-eyed than to be inefficiently two-eyed." The condition of being "one-eyed" refers to strabismus.

As previously mentioned, visual skills other than the strictly binocular may play important roles in reading efficiency. In a study of saccadic eye movements, Griffin et al.[14] analyzed eye movements during reading and fixation tasks by ophthalmography. Subjects included 12 "adequate" readers and 13 "inadequate" ones. The researchers concluded that "inadequate readers seem to have less efficient saccadic eye movements regardless of the type of material used." Besides words, rows of dots were also used for fixation material, so that the lack of comprehension of certain words would not be a factor. It should be noted that the investigators did not determine which, if any, of the "inadequate" readers were *dyslexic* and which were nondyslexic but nevertheless poor readers possibly due to various other reasons.

The term *dyslexia* has been misused because of its general catchall meaning of "reading disabilities." Saying someone has dyslexia without identifying the specific reading problem is like saying "I'm in poor health" without specifying the specific health problem. Fortunately, dyslexia now can be specified by new testing methodology.

Griffin and Walton[15] advocate determining if a patient has one of seven specific dyslexic patterns; this helps avoid situations in which extensive visual and/or perceptual training programs have been pursued by patients, only to find that reading, writing, and spelling difficulties persist. If a specific dyslexic pattern is found, special approaches to *educational* therapy are definitely called for. Of course, *vision* therapy is recommended when dyslexic patients also have certain visual perception dysfunctions and/or visual skills inefficiencies, such as poor saccades or accommodation and vergence infacilities (see Chapter Fifteen).

Norn et al.[16] concluded that "visual defects bear no causal relation to *specific dyslexia*." It should be noted that their specific dyslexia had not been determined in the same way as that of Griffin and Walton. The same holds for Adler-Grinberg and Stark,[17] who found that two groups of children, one "dyslexic" and the other "normal," the groups being age-matched, could not be differentiated when they were required to follow a meaningless target or to solve pictorial tasks. Furthermore, "the dyslexic's characteristic deficit seems to involve the integration of visual input into the language-acquisition function." These conclusions would concur with those of Griffin and Walton in that dyslexia may be independent of visual skills dysfunctions. Be that as it may, a dyslexic individual, as determined through special testing, would be more handicapped if he had visual skills inefficiencies and/or visual-motor perceptual dysfunctions than if he did not have these added burdens affecting his reading.

Interdisciplinary evaluations are necessary for all learning-disabled children, but eye/vision care practitioners can evaluate relevant problem areas in their domain. I recommend visual skills testing as well as visual perceptual and visual motor functions evaluation; this is similar to the recommendations of Hoffman.[18-20] I like to use a profile scoring form to facilitate organization of the testing sequence and explanation to patients (or parents of young patients). The "Evaluation for Visually Related Learning Difficulties" form is shown in the Appendix. This is a modification of a profile sheet used in the Vision Therapy Clinic of the Southern California College of Optometry.

Getz[21] commented that "current research concerning the success of vision training for students is contradictory in its findings. Both significant positive results, and no correlation between reading and visual perception, have been reported by researchers!" Nevertheless, he found in a 4-month vision training program of 70 children compared with a control group, reading scores of children in the program were significantly improved on the California Cooperative Primary Test and the reading section of the Wide Range Achievement Test. Visual skills and visual-motor perceptual training were included; this combination of therapy appeared to have positive results in this instance. More definitive conclusions as to the role of binocular and other visual skills in relation to reading abilities must await further studies.

Nystagmus   There are some cases of nystagmus in which movement is reduced in certain fields of gaze. Conjugate prism therapy (e.g., base-left before each eye) may be used in certain instances to alleviate head turning (e.g., to the left; in this case the prisms would be used for the patient whose nystagmus is reduced on dextroversion).

Burian and von Noorden[22] reported on the treatment of nystagmus by means of extraocular muscle surgery. According to the Kestenbaum technique, the patient who looks to the right side in order to minimize nystagmus would have an equal amount of surgery on four muscles: a recession of the right lateral rectus and resection of the right medial rectus. At a later time, the left medial rectus would be recessed and the left lateral rectus resected.

Nystagmus is sometimes reduced through the use of lenses, usually in the case of convergence excess with plus addition lenses reducing the nearpoint eso deviation and improving the patient's fusional ability. The result may be a reduction in the nystagmic movements. Occasionally, nystagmic movements can be reduced in cases of divergence excess exotropia by the addition of minus lens overcorrections. Base-out prisms may be used in cases of exophoria with nystagmus in order to force convergence. The *nystagmus blockage syndrome*[23] is thought to be a cause of esotropia in which excessive convergence is brought into play to reduce nystagmus. Such a patient will show a marked head turn when using the fixating eye to see clearly.

Ciuffreda et al.[24] reported using auditory biofeedback to reduce nystagmus in a young adult whose nystagmus was presumably congenital. Photoelectronically monitored changes in eye position produced audio changes so the subject could "hear" when his nystagmus was better or worse, and thus attempt to "hold command" of the steadiness of his eyes. However, his nystagmus was also "markedly reduced with strong convergence." Moreover, the visual acuity in each eye was better than 20/25, so what improvement was made in acuity by the auditory feedback method was minimal. Nevertheless, the reporters stated their belief that "use of auditory biofeedback appears to provide hope in the noninvasive treatment of nystagmus." I believe this is true, but this method is still in the research phase and not widely used effectively for clinical purposes.

Van Brocklin et al.[25] studied the use of *auditory* biofeedback in strabismus therapy using infrared emitters and detectors in the lens cells of a trial frame to produce auditory tones dependent upon eye positioning. A low-frequency tone was heard when the eyes were in the ortho posture; its frequency increased with increasing magnitude of the deviation of the visual axes. Seven strabismics, four of whom were exotropic and three esotropic, were studied. All four exotropes achieved success, whereas one of the three esotropes reached the objective of therapy. Patients reportedly learned to develop the "feeling" of being able to control their eye positions. The investigators felt that future clinical application of auditory biofeedback may help speed up the training process if it is used initially to allow ortho posturing, which can then be followed by traditional sensory and motor fusional training. It should be

Auditory Biofeedback in Strabismus Therapy

noted that *feedback* has been the mainstay in traditional procedures, e.g., suppression clues, location of Haidinger's brushes, float of stereoscopic ring, blur, and diplopia.

Amblyopia Methods

The psychometric visual acuity chart of Flom (see Figure 2-21 in Chapter Two) is helpful in determining the visual acuity of an amblyopic eye.[26] It is more reliable than the conventional Snellen chart, mainly because it accounts for contour interaction effects. A series of 21 slides of psychometric visual acuity charts comes in graduated sizes from 20/277 to 20/9 acuity demands.[a] A quick process for determining the 50 percent cutoff criterion for visual acuity was described in Chapter Two.

PSYCHOMETRIC INTERPRETATION

Another name for the Flom psychometric chart is the *S-chart*. Clinical data produce a sigmoid graph when plotted on special x-y coordinates. (See Figure 16-1, which shows a recording sheet.) The percentage of vision[b] is given an x value, and the number of correct C responses is given a y value.

An example of psychometric visual acuity results is shown for a myopic patient in Figure 16-2. The acuity can be seen to be somewhere between 20/137 and 20/155, and approximately 33 percent. The testing procedure is similar to that described in Chapter Two, but it is important to have at least two y values of 8 on the lower end and at least two on the higher end. This is so a sigmoid with straight lines on either extreme can be drawn, and it is also important for computer calculations. As to the y value of 2, responses of 0, 1, and 2 for a chart of a given size are recorded in the same way, always as a "2." The correct responses are "slashed," and incorrect ones are labeled as to the patient's report of "left," "up," "right," or "down," in case this might add useful clinical information.

Dr. David Kirschen of the Southern California College of Optometry has developed a computerized program to aid in this method. The computer calculations are helpful in teaching the practitioner more reliable S-curve drawings, and they are mathematically precise for research purposes. This can be important for determining acuity before and after vision therapy, and it sometimes is helpful in legal cases where exact percentages of vision are requested.

A legal case for which I was a consultant involved determining the visual efficiency of an amblyopic eye with the aid of a computer. The right eye x, y values for this amblyopic patient are shown in Figure 16-3, and the graphs of the right and left eyes are shown in Figure 16-4. Computerized printouts of the figures as well as plottings are shown in Figures 16-5 and 16-6.

---

[a]Psychometric charts are available in 35 mm black and white slides from the Multimedia Center of the Optometry School of the University of California, Berkeley. A modified S-chart series is also available from The Ohio State University College of Optometry, Columbus, Ohio.

[b]Snell-Sterling vision efficiency scale. *Snell, A.C., and S. Sterling: The Percentage Evaluation of Macular Vision. Arch. Ophth., 54(5), pp. 443-461, 1925.*

Name _____   OD   OS   OU   Date _____

Eccentricity _____   w/ Rx

Duration _____   w/o Rx

	A									**B** 0	1	2	3	4	5	6	7	8
1.	9	L	D	R	D	U	D	R	U	110								
2.	15	D	U	L	D	R	U	L	U	105								
3.	20	R	L	U	L	D	R	U	L	100								
4.	26	U	L	D	R	L	R	D	R	95								
5.	32	L	D	R	U	L	D	U	D	90								
6.	38	D	U	L	D	R	U	L	U	85								
7.	45	U	R	L	R	U	L	D	R	80								
8.	52	U	L	D	R	L	R	D	R	75								
9.	60	L	D	R	U	L	D	U	D	70								
10.	68	R	U	D	U	R	U	L	D	65								
11.	77	U	R	L	R	U	L	D	R	60								
12.	87	D	R	U	L	D	L	R	L	55								
13.	97	L	D	R	D	U	D	R	U	50								
14.	109	U	R	L	R	U	L	D	R	45								
15.	122	D	U	L	D	R	U	L	U	40								
16.	137	D	R	U	L	D	L	R	L	35								
17.	155	R	U	D	U	R	U	L	D	30								
18.	175	L	D	R	U	L	D	U	D	25								
19.	200	R	L	U	L	D	R	U	L	20								
20.	232	U	L	D	R	L	R	D	R	15								
21.	277	D	R	U	L	D	L	R	L	10								

FIGURE 16-1 — Recording page used at the Southern California College of Optometry for Flom psychometric analysis. For each chart, (1) Column A has the Snellen, 20/9 to 20/277, acuities, and (2) Column B has the percentages of vision (x values) from 110 to 10 percent. The row of numbers (y values) from 0 to 8 represents the number of correct responses to the eight Landolt Cs for each chart.

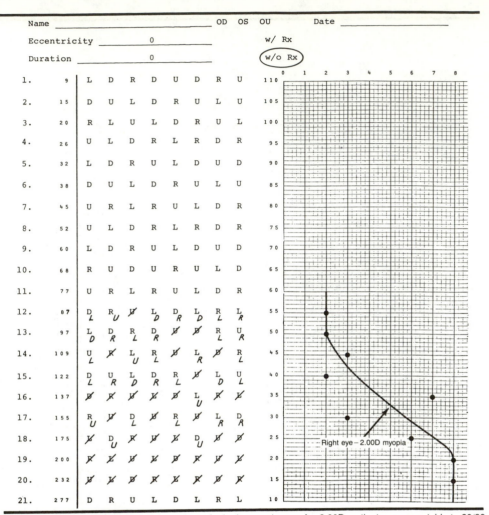

Name _____ OD OS OU   Date _____

Eccentricity _____ 0 _____   w/ Rx

Duration _____ 0 _____   (w/o Rx)

1.	9	L	D	R	D	U	D	R	U	110
2.	15	D	U	L	D	R	U	L	U	105
3.	20	R	L	U	L	D	R	U	L	100
4.	26	U	L	D	R	L	R	D	R	95
5.	32	L	D	R	U	L	D	U	D	90
6.	38	D	U	L	D	R	U	L	U	85
7.	45	U	R	L	R	U	L	D	R	80
8.	52	U	L	D	R	L	R	D	R	75
9.	60	L	D	R	U	L	D	U	D	70
10.	68	R	U	D	U	R	U	L	D	65
11.	77	U	R	L	R	U	L	D	R	60
12.	87	D/L	R/U	ø	L/D	D/R	L/D	R/L	L/R	55
13.	97	L/D	D/R	R/L	D/R	ø	ø	R/L	U/R	50
14.	109	U/L	ø	L/U	R/L	ø	L/R	ø	R/L	45
15.	122	D/L	U/R	L/D	D/R	R/L	ø	U/D	U/L	40
16.	137	ø	ø	ø	ø	ø	L/U	ø	ø	35
17.	155	R/U	ø	D/L	ø	R/L	ø	L/R	D/R	30
18.	175	ø	D/U	ø	ø	ø	D/U	ø	ø	25
19.	200	ø	ø	ø	ø	ø	ø	ø	ø	20
20.	232	ø	ø	ø	ø	ø	ø	ø	ø	15
21.	277	D	R	U	L	D	L	R	L	10

Right eye – 2.00D myopia

FIGURE 16-2 — Graphical results of a patient who had a myopic eye of −2.00D; patient was correctable to 20/20 with lens.

```
Name? AMBLYOPIA RIGHT EYE
Date? 4/16/82
Comment? 0

Enter X,Y Pairs <EG: 80,8   insert COMMA between X and Y>
 1)? 15,8
 2)? 20,8
 3)? 25,7
 4)? 30,8
 5)? 35,7
 6)? 40,7
 7)? 45,5
 8)? 50,5
 9)? 55,2
10)? 60,2
11)?
Enter the number to be changed or <CR>? 0
```

FIGURE 16-3 — Data for computer analysis for determining visual efficiency of an amblyopic patient.

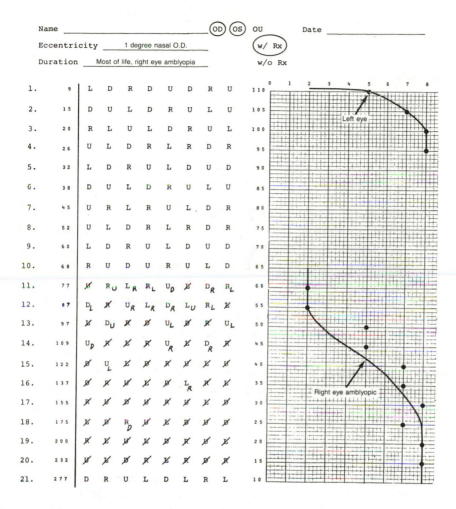

FIGURE 16-4 — Graphical results for an amblyopic patient who had reduced vision in the amblyopic right eye and normal vision in the nonamblyopic left eye.

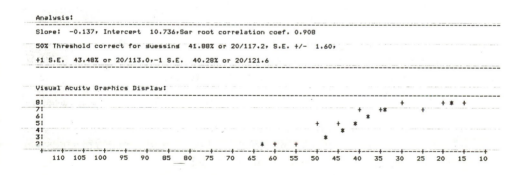

FIGURE 16-5 — Computer printout for amblyopic patient, right eye.

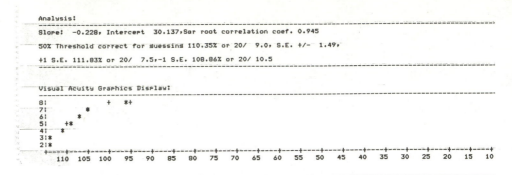

```
Analysis:
-------------------------------------------------------------------------------
Slope:  -0.228,  Intercept  30.137,Sqr root correlation coef. 0.945
-------------------------------------------------------------------------------
50% Threshold correct for guessing 110.35% or 20/  9.0, S.E. +/-  1.49,
-------------------------------------------------------------------------------
+1 S.E. 111.83% or 20/  7.5,-1 S.E. 108.86% or 20/ 10.5
-------------------------------------------------------------------------------

Visual Acuity Graphics Display:
-------------------------------------------------------------------------------
 8|              +    *+
 7|            *
 6|         *
 5|      +*
 4|   *
 3|*
 2|*
  +----+----+----+----+----+----+----+----+----+----+----+----+----+----+----+----+----+----+----+----+----+
    110 105 100  95  90  85  80  75  70  65  60  55  50  45  40  35  30  25  20  15  10
```

FIGURE 16-6 — Computer printout for amblyopic patient, nonamblyopic left eye.

The use of the Flom psychometric chart along with graphical evaluation is probably the most reliable psycho-physical method for determining visual acuity, especially for the amblyopic eye. Computerized calculated results probably make this more precise, but I do not believe computers are absolutely necessary. With practice, the clinician can reliably plot data and determine acuities. However, the nature of sigmoid curves may shed light on the different causes of reduced vision. Furthermore, exact gains in visual acuity resulting from vision therapy can be assessed.

Kirschen[27] reported the successful treatment in a case of anisometropic, strabismic amblyopia in a 10-year-old male who had an exotropia of the right eye manifest before 6 months of age (according to a parent's report). No patching or exercises were tried on this patient before the age of 8 (according to documented medical and optometric records). Acuity of the left eye was 20/20, and acuity of the right eye improved from 20/120 to 20/20 in 11 weeks as a result of constant, alternate patching (amblyopic eye patched at school, dominant eye patched the remainder of the time) along with active monocular training procedures (as described in Chapter Seven). Before- and after-treatment results are shown in S-chart form in Figure 16-7. These curves were drawn from values found by computerized probit analysis;[c] however, according to Kirschen (personal communication), a best-fit curve can be fitted by eye with sufficient experience, ultimately eliminating reliance by the clinician on the computer for this purpose.

Davidson and Eskridge[28] modified the S-chart test (and made it easier to use with young children) by removing the Landolt Cs but leaving eight Es with contour interaction, as in the Flom design. They reported this to be reliable in the assessment of visual acuity. (An example is shown in Figure 16-8.)

TREATMENT WITH
ROTATING GRATINGS

A treatment method for amblyopia was introduced by Banks et al.[29] They claimed a high degree of success by direct occlusion with only 7 minutes per treatment and after only a few sessions in which the patient performed

---

[c]Developed by Dr. David Kirschen of the Southern California College of Optometry.

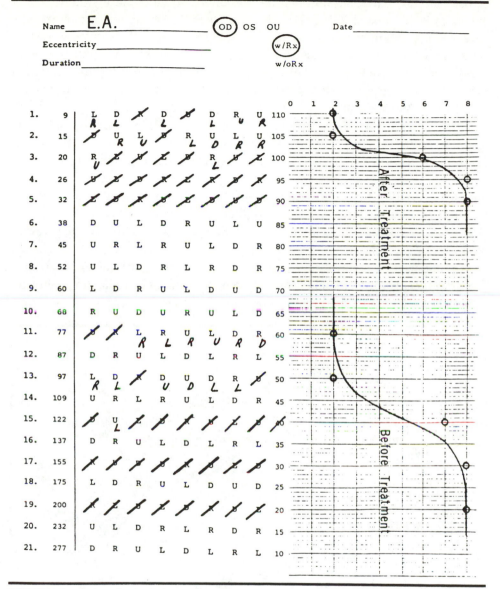

FIGURE 16-7 — S-chart showing before and after results of treatment for a patient of Dr. David Kirschen who had amblyopia of the right eye.[27]

monocular training activities (as in Chapter Seven) on a transparent plate through which could be viewed a high-contrast bar pattern (square wave grating) that rotated at the rate of 1 revolution per minute. Various grating sizes (spatial frequencies) are available in commercially produced instruments for this type of treatment, which is also referred to as "CAM therapy." An example of one such instrument is shown in Figure 16-9.

The principle of CAM therapy is based upon relatively recent research findings that various cells in the visual cortex respond to various spatial frequencies and orientations. It was reasoned that employing a series of sizes of bar patterns that rotate through all meridians would achieve stimulation of the majority of visual cells. This is good in theory, but in practice, results have been questionable. The weight of authority holds that improvement in acuity of an amblyopic eye does not seem to be attributable to rotating grating stimuli per se. Schor et al.[30] used psychometric S-chart testing to compare a CAM treatment group with a control group; they found no significant change of acuity in either group.

Proven methods of amblyopia treatment generally require considerable patching in the training regimen. Occasionally, short-term occlusion is successful. Griffin et al.[31] reported a cure of a refractive amblyopic eye of a 4-year-old male from 20/40 to 20/20 via direct patching approximately 15 minutes every day for a little more than a month. No rotating grating (CAM therapy) was used in this case. Similarly, Dalziel[32] effected a cure of strabismic amblyopia in a 5-year-old male by "occasional" (all day, every other day) direct patching.

In summary, I believe the merits of CAM therapy have yet to be proved. The traditionally used methods for the treatment of amblyopia should not be discarded for a new method that has not yet been proved effective. If, however,

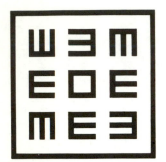

FIGURE 16-8 — Psychometric acuity test of Davidson and Eskridge.

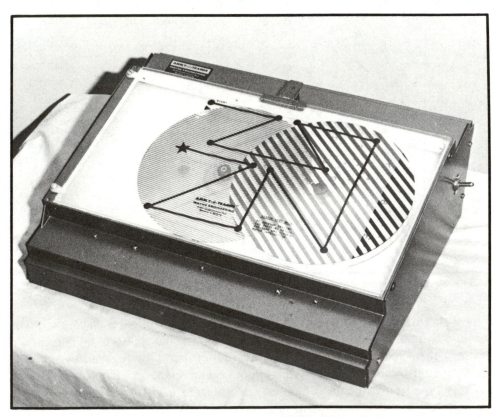

FIGURE 16-9 — Ambly-O-Trainer™. (Courtesy of Wayne Engineering.) Either a single square-wave-pattern disc or two discs can be used. When two discs are rotating, interesting Moiré fringe patterns are produced that may help hold the patient's attention doing monocular training activities, e.g., when combining Perceptuo-Motor Pen tracing on the overlay transparent sheet. A tic-tac-toe game can be played with the patient using either one or two discs of this instrument.

the various CAM-type devices can be used to hold the attention of young amblyopic patients during monocular activities, then positive results may justify using them.

Birnbaum et al.[33] made a literature search to analyze the success of amblyopia therapy for patients under the age of 7 years compared with the success rate for patients over the age of 7. They wrote: "It is commonly stated in the lay press and other media and from the professional lecture platform that amblyopia cannot be successfully treated in patients over the age of 6." They refuted this by showing that reported success was substantial for patients over the age of 6, with success rates of patients under age 6 not being significantly better when the criterion for success was achievement of 20/30 acuity or better. Amblyopia therapy should not necessarily be withheld just because the patient is an older child or adult.

AGE AND AMBLYOPIC THERAPY

A method for eliminating A R C effects in *some* patients when performing the Brock-Givner afterimage transfer test (see Chapter Two) was recommended by Wick.[34] Instead of using an occluder, the patient uses his own fingers to close the amblyopic eye when the nonamblyopic eye is receiving the flash of the afterimage generator. Likewise, the patient holds his nonamblyopic eye shut when viewing the transferred afterimage with his amblyopic eye. When A R C is "eliminated" under these conditions, the fovea of the amblyopic eye is "tagged" by the transferred afterimage. This allows the patient to know where his fovea is seeing, and it facilitates home training to eliminate eccentric fixation. Note that the "finger-closing" method does not always allow fovea-to-fovea afterimage transfer in patients with A R C; when it does, however, it can be very helpful in therapy for eccentric fixation and amblyopia.

HOME PLEOPTICS

Wick[35,36] described another method whereby the patient can view Haidinger's brushes with an eye and, at the same time, align the image of the brushes on a dark spot in the center of an annulus of an afterimage strobe. This superimposition can be accomplished either by using a special device for direct viewing or by using a half-silvered mirror that allows an eye to see two superimposable images. This allows the patient to have a circular afterimage, with foveal viewing being in the center, as well as having the fovea "protected" by the dark shadow and the eccentric point dazzled by the annulus afterimage. The patient can carry out his own home training with each new afterimage.

When patients are first trying to perceive Haidinger's brushes, it is good to let them see a demonstrator[d] (see Figure 16-10). This lets the patient know what he should be seeing and how Haidinger's brushes are to look to him.

Another effective use of Haidinger's brushes is to use a cheiroscope with a window[e] (see Figure 16-11). The patient can view a target with the

[d]Demonstration sheet for MITT is available from Bernell Corp.

[e]Cheiroscope available from Bernell Corp.

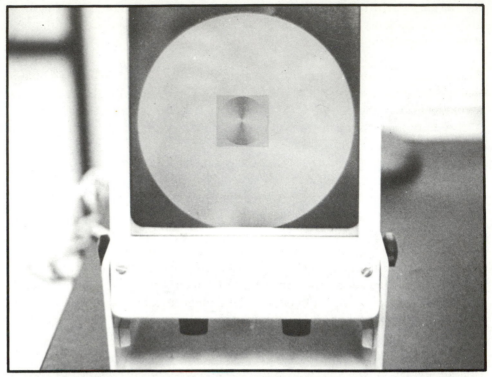

FIGURE 16-10 — Haidinger's brushes as seen in a demonstration sheet for the MITT.

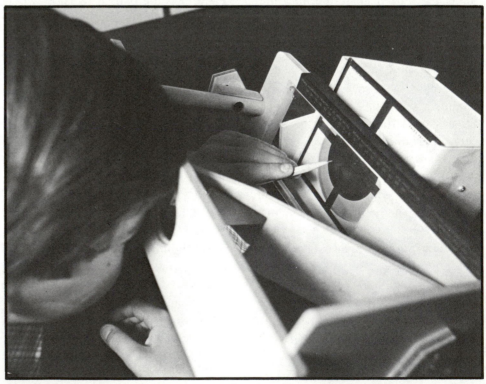

FIGURE 16-11 — Haidinger's brushes with the cheiroscope for use in the binocular phase of amblyopia therapy.

nonamblyopic eye in the mirror and see the brushes with the amblyopic eye. This is good in the binocular phase of amblyopia therapy in that bifoveal fixation can be encouraged. The patient can point to the brushes to superimpose the pencil tip onto the fixation target seen by the other eye. This is useful in A R C therapy and antisuppression training, as well as in working on amblyopia under binocular conditions.

According to Campbell and Maffei,[37] there is maximum contrast sensitivity for a simple sinusoidal grating pattern with a spatial frequency of about 3 cycles per degree (angular subtense representing 20/200), and the highest spatial frequency that can be seen (requiring maximum contrast and, therefore, minimum contrast sensitivity) is about 50 cycles per degree (angular subtense representing 20/12).

Bradley and Freeman[38] found that 10 anisometropic amblyopic subjects exhibited contrast sensitivity deficits over middle and high spatial frequencies when measured using sinusoidal gratings. The defect was correlated with the magnitude of anisometropia. Their results tended to agree with the contrast detection defect in other types of amblyopias (e.g., strabismic amblyopia), with the possible difference that in anisometropic amblyopia, there appears to be an absence of a low-frequency deficit. They thought evidence was that anisometropic amblyopia "is caused by blur-induced monocular contrast deprivation," and "these subjects have a neural deficit in mechanisms responsible for contrast detection." Nevertheless, Lennerstrand and Lundh[39] improved contrast sensitivity in the majority of 24 amblyopic children they treated. Therapy included CAM therapy, in addition to relatively extensive occlusion. Eight of the children had no improvement of visual acuity, but remarkably, four of these showed improved contrast sensitivity. The larger group with improved visual acuity also showed improvement in contrast sensitivity. The investigators concluded that the normalization of contrast sensitivity represents a valuable gain for the patient, even when visual acuity is not improved.

Kleinstein[40] stated that in amblyopia, contrast sensitivity is impaired, as it is in a host of ocular diseases, such as macular degeneration, retrobulbar neuritis, and multiple sclerosis. He cautioned, however, that "it remains to be determined if contrast sensitivity can uniquely diagnose or detect these and other conditions earlier than standard tests."

The visually evoked response (VER) is also known as the visually evoked cortical potential (VECP) or the visually evoked potential (VEP). The VER may provide information on the status of the visual pathways. Transient VER, which is a stroboscopically presented stimulus, will elicit a pattern (a graphical printout) that is evaluated in terms of (1) amplitude, (2) latency of occurrence of the major positive peak response, and (3) general waveform morphology. Amplitude reduction may indicate optic atrophy, but latency differences between each eye may indicate optic nerve demyelination (as in multiple sclerosis). Refer to Figures 16-12 and 16-13 for examples.

CONTRAST SENSITIVITY

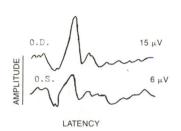

FIGURE 16-12 — Transient VER graph showing normal latency for each eye and normal amplitude for the right eye but reduced amplitude for the left eye, as in optic atrophy.

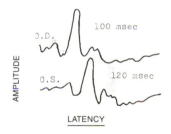

FIGURE 16-13 — Transient VER graph showing normal amplitude for each eye and normal latency for the right eye but increased latency for the left eye, a difference indicative of optic nerve demyelination.

VISUALLY EVOKED RESPONSE

Another type of VER is that of pattern stimuli of black and white checks that exchange places at a rapid rate. The black checks become white, and vice versa, as in Sherman's procedure.[41] The sustained response with this type of VER allows assessment of visual acuity. Refer to Figure 16-14, showing an amblyopic response of the right eye, from a clinical report by Lee et al.[42]

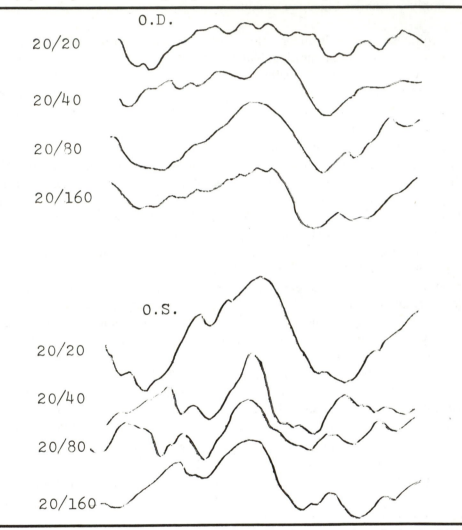

FIGURE 16-14 — Sustained VER graph for visual acuity assessment. Responses indicate visual acuity of 20/80 for the right eye and 20/20 for the left eye, judging from amplitude comparisons.[42]

BINOCULAR CELLS   Animal research has shown that binocular correspondency can be found in about 80 percent of the cells of the visual cortex.[43,44] As clinicians know, sensory obstacles (e.g., occlusion and anisometropia) and strabismus (motor obstacle) are amblyogenic. Such sensory and motor obstacles can act to place one eye at a "competitive disadvantage" over the other eye. Cool[45] summarized electrophysiological research and stated: "The end result is that one eye comes to dominate most, if not all, of the cells in visual cortex. The other eye (the amblyopic eye) winds up with little or no functional input to cortex at all."

Cool found that physiological research corroborated clinical impressions that "the amblyopia was a result of constant tonic, active inhibition of the amblyopic eye's inputs by the good eye." (Suppression is the cause of amblyopia after all.)

There has been some question recently whether the nonamblyopic eye can be called the "good" eye. Kandel et al.[46] prefer to use the term "dominant" rather than "normal" eye when referring to the nonamblyopic eye in the case of unilateral amblyopia. They found that the dominant eye (of amblyopic subjects) had reduced dark adaptation sensitivity, reduced acuity, and poorer fixation than normal eyes (of nonamblyopic subjects). These differences were slight, however, and they were found under laboratory testing conditions and were not clinically obvious. Reasons for the differences may be due either to the binocular nature of the amblyopic disorder or to adverse effects of treating amblyopia, e.g., long-term direct patching. (Refer to Chapter Seven for a discussion on the prevention of occlusion amblyopia.)

Visual acuity testing was discussed in Chapter Two, but some additional aspects of infants' vision are given in this section. Marg et al.[47] convincingly showed that visual acuity develops very early in life. They used VER results as an index to visual acuity in testing 16 infants on 19 different occasions, and they found that "adult acuity, which is defined as 20/20, is reached during the fourth to sixth month of life." Mohindra[48] pointed out that, although VER results show 20/20 by 4 to 6 months, this is a neurophysiological type of acuity, and that other *behavioral* tests indicate that visual acuity of 20/20 (6/6) can normally be expected by the age of 2 years. The acuity may be underestimated with the preferential looking method.[49,50] This type of testing is based on infants' preferring to gaze at a target with details (such as a disc with a grating of black and white stripes) to one without details (such as a plain gray disc).

VISUAL ACUITY OF INFANTS

Preferential looking methods for visual acuity assessment offer a means to study behavioral visual acuity development of the infant.[51] This may be more reliable when operant conditioning is applied.[52]

Although preferential looking may be useful for the investigation of visual acuity in the laboratory, it is my opinion that preferential looking methods will not be used widely and routinely in clinical practice because of the considerable time, space, and personnel required to perform this type of testing.

The important thing, however, is for the clinician to detect amblyogenic disorders early on in the infant's life. Preferential looking methods are not necessary; instead, traditional methods, such as the cover test to detect strabismus, and refraction to detect errors such as astigmatism and anisometropia, are recommended as routine tests for all infants.

Mohindra introduced a quick and reliable refractive method, termed "near retinoscopy." It can be used on young children without the necessity of cycloplegia.[53] It involves the patient's fixating the light of the retinoscope from a distance of 50 cm while the nonfixating eye is occluded in an otherwise dark room. Trial lenses are introduced to neutralize the retinoscopic reflex motion. The net refractive error is determined by simply adding $-1.25D$ to the gross lens power required for neutralization. For example, if it takes $+1.25D$ for neutralization, the eye is emmetropic. If no lens (plano) gives neutralization, the eye is myopic by 1.25D. Even though the test is at near, it is the *distance* refractive error that is determined. I have found that occlusion of an eye is not particularly necessary to obtain reliable refractive results, and this is supported by Mohindra.[54]

Early and careful refraction of infants can go a long way in the prevention of amblyopia as well as other binocular anomalies.

Special Uses of the Cover Test

The cover test was discussed in Chapter One, but because of its importance in evaluating binocular anomalies, a brief review of some of its uses is given in this section. There are two types of cover testing. The first is the *unilateral cover test*, also known as the *cover-uncover test*. The second type is the *alternating cover test*.

The main reason for performing the unilateral cover test is to detect strabismus and distinguish heterotropia from heterophoria. Take, for example, an esotropia of the right eye (as indicated in Figure 16-15). Assume the diplopic image of the right eye is suppressed. The patient is instructed to look at the straight-ahead target while the doctor occludes the left eye. The right eye would have to abduct so that its fovea could take up fixation on the target. The amount of movement of the right eye represents the horizontal objective angle of deviation (H). This strabismic angle can be either estimated or measured using the unilateral cover test. To measure it, the doctor must simultaneously occlude the left eye and place the correct magnitude of base-out prism before the right eye to neutralize any movement of that eye. Refer to Figures 16-16 and 16-17.

Another important use of the unilateral cover test is to determine if a strabismus is constant or intermittent. If, in our example, the right eye abducts with each trial on different occasions, constant esotropia is assumed. This would be confirmed if, on every occasion, the left eye never moved as the right eye was covered (unilateral, constant esotropia of the right eye).

When the strabismic angle is small (less that 10 p.d.) it may be helpful to verify the constancy of the esotropia of the right eye (in this example) by performing the *4-prism base-out test* (Figures 16-18 and 16-19). The prism is placed in a base-out orientation before the fixating left eye. The right eye will abduct if it is esotropic (just as when the left eye is covered with the occluder). Similarly, if the base-out prism is placed before the suppressing right eye, no movement of the left eye will occur (as when the right eye is occluded in the unilateral cover test). Note that exceptions may occur when the base-out prism is larger than the angle of deviation.

If the angle H is *esophoric* and not esotropic, the eye behind the prism would be expected to adduct (i.e., convergence would take place, since the binocular viewing conditions would allow fusional convergence to be feasible

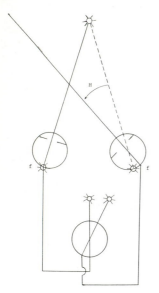

FIGURE 16-15 — Esotropia of the right eye with diplopia representing the subjective angle of directionalization.

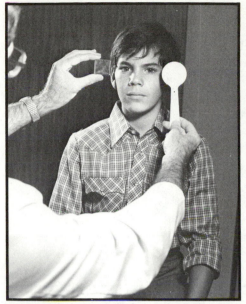

FIGURE 16-16 — Preparing for unilateral cover test neutralization of an esotropic right eye with base-out prism.

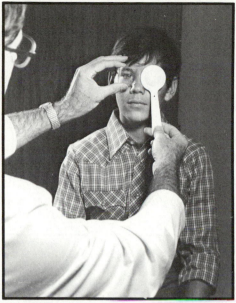

FIGURE 16-17 — Simultaneous cover of the left eye with an occluder and of the right eye with base-out prism. The prism power that equals the esotropic angle of the right eye neutralizes the angle of deviation so that no eye movement occurs on this procedure.

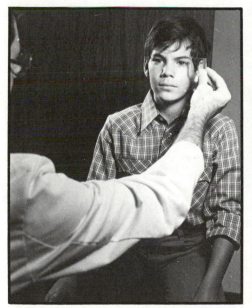

FIGURE 16-18 — Preparing for the 4-prism base-out test in the case of esotropia of the right eye.

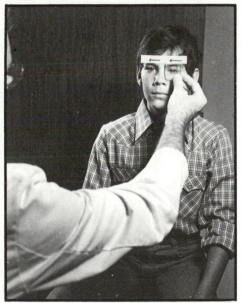

FIGURE 16-19 — The fixating left eye adducts toward the apex of the prism, and the esotropic right eye abducts. In other words, there is dextro*version* but no con*vergence* in this case of strabismus. If the patient had a heterophoria instead of heterotropia, a vergence would result rather than only a version movement.

in meeting the base-out prism demand). Likewise, the eye behind the occluder during the unilateral cover test would be expected to adduct (i.e., deviation would become manifest under monocular viewing conditions).

The supplementary use of the 4-prism base-out test with the unilateral cover test aids in differential diagnosis of strabismus versus phoria as well as the *objective* assessment of suppression of an eye.

A pitfall of the cover test is that its validity is vitiated if there is eccentric fixation. For example, suppose point "e" is located on point "zero" of the right eye; this would cause angle E to be equal to angle H, as can be visualized in Figure 16-15. In this case, the *measured* angle H would be ortho, although the *true* angle H would not. Eskridge[55] gave the following rules: Nasal eccentric fixation causes the measured angle H to be smaller than the true angle H in esotropia but larger than the true angle H in exotropia. Contrarily, temporal eccentric fixation causes the measured angle H to be larger in esotropia but smaller in exotropia. (Refer to Table 16A.)

TABLE 16A. *Effects of Eccentric Fixation on Measurement Results of the Cover Test*[55]		
Direction of Deviation	Nasal Eccentric Fixation	Temporal Eccentric Fixation
Eso	Smaller measurement	Larger measurement
Exo	Larger measurement	Smaller measurement

The alternate cover test is primarily used to measure angle H without differentiating between phoria and tropia. Angle H measurement is affected in the same way when there is eccentric fixation as it is with the unilateral cover test.

Alternate covering, at just the appropriate rate, allows the phi phenomenon to be perceived so that the subjective angle of directionalization (S) can be measured. The diplopic separation, shown in cyclopean projection (as in the "mind's eye") in Figure 16-15, represents angle S. In this case, the power of the base-out prism that neutralizes the phi movement is the magnitude of angle S. Anomalous correspondence can be evaluated quickly by comparing angle H with angle S in performing the alternate cover test objectively and subjectively, respectively. Remember that angle H is affected by eccentric fixation, but angle S is not (because eccentric fixation is not evident under binocular viewing conditions).

The judicious use of both types of the cover test provides the experienced clinician with enough information to make a fairly complete tentative diagnosis of strabismus and heterophoria.

Learning Theories Applied to Binocular Therapy

The attainment of clear, single, comfortable, efficient binocular vision is the goal of therapy when visual skills are found to be less than adequate. The means to achieving this end can be enhanced by applying educational psychology learning theories to vision therapy.

Suppose, for example, that a patient has convergence insufficiency. Assume that the patient's positive fusional vergence is poor and that convergence (base-out) training is to be emphasized. (Refer to Chapter Thirteen.) In such a case, pencil push-ups would be appropriate as one of the initial training procedures. This relatively simple task can be practiced successfully at home by very young children. Some children 2 years of age or younger can successfully perform push-up training.

Push-up training can continue until the patient has the ability to pursue the pencil tip from arm's length to a normal nearpoint of convergence. Monitoring bifixation during training is important; otherwise, subsequent practice by the patient will be to no avail. The therapist must watch the patient's eyes to ensure that proper vergences are made during push-ups.

Note that *practice* is defined as a recurrence of a set of responses in the presence of a certain stimulus. On the other hand, *training* is practice plus error correction. Mere practice without training may fail to accomplish anything positive, and adverse effects possibly can result if the patient practices improperly. Therefore, correct training (and learning) must be achieved.

It should also be pointed out that prior monocular training (e.g., pursuit and saccadic procedures) is usually advised. Only a few representative binocular procedures will be mentioned here for the purpose of relating learning theories to binocular therapy.

The introduction of a septum into nearpoint convergence training creates a more complex task for the patient. Additional learning on the part of the patient is required before this can be fully understood and practiced properly. The three-dot card available from Allbee has three red dots on one side and three blue dots on the other. The patient must learn to overcome the dissociative effect of the septum in order to fuse the red and blue images into a unified purple percept. Awareness of physiological diplopia is also part of the training involved in this procedure (see Figure 13-3 in Chapter Thirteen). Because learning requirements are more complex for this exercise than for pencil push-ups, the minimum age for training is higher for the three-dot card. Some toddlers over age 2 and most preschoolers can learn to perform this task.

Chiastopic fusion (Figure 12-14 in Chapter Twelve) involves a higher order of cognitive learning than do push-ups and three-dot card procedures. Because of this, the therapist generally has difficulty trying to teach chiastopic fusion to the preschooler. As a rule, it is more efficacious to begin this with patients who are at least 7 years old. Otherwise, failure and frustration on this procedure can cause the patient to reject the therapy in toto.

Learning theories may be included under two headings: stimulus-response and cognitive. Theorists of stimulus-response learning are generally thought of as behaviorists and include many advocates of behavior modification programs. Cognitive explanations of learning fall into two broad groups of theorists: the gestalt and cognitive field psychologists, and the cognitivists.[56]

(See Table 16B for an outline of basic learning theories in educational psychology.)

TABLE 16B. Basic Learning Theories in Educational Psychology

Learning theories			
Stimulus-response conditioning		Cognitive explanations	
Classical (e.g., Pavlov, Watson)	Reinforcement (e.g., Thorndike, Skinner)	Gestalt and cognitive field psychology (e.g., Wertheimer, Lewin)	Cognitivism (e.g., Bruner, Piaget)

STIMULUS-RESPONSE
CONDITIONING

Wilson et al.[57] described stimulus-response learning in terms of formation of cognitive associations. They subdivided this type of learning into two categories: *classical* and *reinforcement* (operant) conditioning. Both of these theories are based on bits of information linked together to produce effects on either the "pleasure" or "punishment" centers in the brain. The most familiar example of classical conditioning is Pavlov's experiment in which a dog would associate the ringing of a bell (conditioned stimulus) with food (unconditioned stimulus). In time, the mere ringing of the bell produced salivation (conditioned response). Thus, the salivation changed from being an unconditioned to a conditioned response.

Such notable learning theorists as Edwin Ray Guthrie and John B. Watson tried to explain human learning by the simultaneity of paired events, such as in the Pavlovian model. But for most practitioners using this approach, it has become apparent that there are serious shortcomings when more complex learning is involved. This is particularly so with human patients undergoing visual training.

To promote "shaping" of behavior more effectively than is likely by means of classical conditioning, many advocate reinforcement learning methods. Introduced by Thorndike, this theory is based on the "law of effect." It states that a satisfying stimulus is more likely to produce repeated responses than is an annoying stimulus. Presumably there are pleasure/punishment centers in the brain that are involved in such directing of behavior.

A more elaborate use of reinforcement in promoting learning—*operant conditioning*—was later developed and popularized by B. F. Skinner. Here, the emphasis is placed on the response rather than on the stimulus. Desired responses are reinforced by means of a reward (e.g., food or praise). In this type of learning, the original desirable response must be waited for ("emitted") and not elicited (as in classical conditioning). When this response occurs, a reward, often referred to as the *reinforcer*, is given. This is repeated with each "good" response so that the reward becomes a stimulus to promote repetition of the desired behavior. (Rewards will be discussed in more detail later in this chapter.)

Classical conditioning can be applied in vision therapy. Perhaps patients with convergence insufficiency can be able to achieve voluntary convergence by conditioning. For instance, the unconditioned stimulus could be a real target (e.g., a pencil) that is to be reflexly bifixated (the unconditioned response) at a near distance. The therapist could use the word "converge" as the conditioned stimulus. The ensuing convergence would promote the conditioned response. It is hoped that the patient would learn to associate this word (or any suitable word chosen) with the act of convergence so that voluntary convergence would result from the patient's mere saying of the word to himself.

The ability to voluntarily converge the eyes can be of great assistance to the patient when trying to learn three-dot card training. The dissociating effect of the septum can then be overcome by the patient, so fusion can be achieved in spite of the septum.

Another aspect of educational objectives must be considered in therapy. Bloom[58] listed three taxonomic parts of educational objectives, which are referred to as *domains*. The first is the *cognitive domain*, which "includes those objectives which deal with the recall or recognition of knowledge and the development of intellectual abilities and skills." The second part is the *affective domain*, which includes "changes in interest, attitudes, and values, and the development of appreciations and adequate adjustment." The third domain is the *manipulative* or *motor-skill* area. This part has been elaborated upon and called the *psychomotor domain* by Harrow.[59]

DOMAINS

All three domains are involved in binocular therapy to some extent, and all three must be considered for any particular training procedure. But the relative extent of each depends upon which training procedure is being used at the moment. For example, with pencil push-up training, there would probably be more reliance on the psychomotor domain than on the cognitive. On the other hand, chiastopic free-space fusion training requires considerable cognitive skill for the patient to grasp the procedure's essence. Therefore, emphasis would then be in the cognitive domain as opposed to the psychomotor skills chiefly needed for pencil push-ups.

It goes without saying that the affective domain must be considered in all procedures in visual training.

The psychomotor domain appears to be the major one involved in response conditioning as it relates to the teaching of push-up convergence. However, the affective domain must also be considered in stimulus-response (associative) conditioning. The development of proper affective associations by the patient may be the most important part of classical stimulus-response conditioning (and probably also of other learning theories). For example, say a father wanted his son to learn to appreciate classical music. To accomplish this goal, the appropriate classical music albums were played in the home each evening during dinner. In time, the son learned to like classical music, presumably because of the pleasant affective association of the music with the attendant olfactory-gustatory pleasures. This then would be a perfect example of "classical" conditioning.

The doctor can apply this same principle to vision training. If the patient forms unpleasant associations (e.g., unfriendliness or disinterest on the part of the doctor or therapist), the vision training program is doomed to be unsuccessful. But success is more likely if the patient can develop a good attitude toward training (and subsequent practice). The proper application of this concept can be one of the doctor's most important allies in therapy.

REWARDS   The Skinnerian approach to operant conditioning was summarized by Hershey and Lugo.[60] "Rewards are effective for learning only if the rewards are important to the person. Praise received from a loving parent or a respected teacher can be effective . . . only if given at the proper time . . . the greatest amount of learning occurs when the reward comes immediately after the correct response. . . ."

Rewards can be given to the young patient during pencil push-up training when he pursues the pencil in the appropriate manner. This is presumed to be a reflexive, and possibly a somewhat involuntary, response to the stimulus. Therefore, it is imperative to provide feedback to the patient. Again, it must be stressed that for operant behavior training to be effective to the learning process, the reward must be given *after* the desired behavior occurs, and this reward must be given *immediately* (within a second or two). It should be noted that a "token" reward program may be established in due course (e.g., poker chips as symbols for some meaningful prize to be obtained later).

To promote voluntary control of vergence via pencil push-ups, the doctor may recommend having the patient make the transition from the relatively reflexive following to the more voluntary near-far jump vergences. It is vitally important that the patient's responses be monitored carefully in this type of training. Otherwise, negative progress in therapy could result if the wrong responses are rewarded. However, with the proper application of operant conditioning to binocular training, the rewarding of correct responses (appropriate feedback) can lead to the voluntary effort becoming easier and more automatic.

Hershey and Lugo defined *learning* as "any permanent behavior change or modification as a result of experience." They summarized Skinner's sequence for long-range learning objectives in the following manner. First, there should be a *continuous reward*—that is, the reward should be given every time the patient makes the correct response (e.g., a reward for each time the patient makes the proper response when doing either following or jump vergences with the pencil target).

When this comes to be "habitlike" and automatic ("habit" meaning behavior without thinking), the therapist may begin giving *periodically intermittent rewards*. The praise (or other reward) is not given every time the correct response is made, but rather in a fixed and regular time sequence.

The next step in progress is *variably intermittent rewards* so the patient does not know when the reward is going to come. In the case of push-up training, the variable reward is more practical for the therapist (or the helper at home) to mete out. Continuous rewards create tedium, and they are only necessary at the onset of the particular training procedure in question. Furthermore, the quickly gained effectiveness is lost if the patient knows that the reward always follows each correct vergence response. The patient could become dependent on external stimuli from a "helper" and possibly discontinue the newly learned, correct binocular responses in everyday life.

It is hoped that the sequence of rewarding will progress to the point where primary rewards can be eliminated. The secondary reward—the patient's perception of good control of eye movements—can become foremost. In other words, it is hoped that training and practice will result in the proper vergence responses becoming automatic, with the reinforcement being the patient's awareness of having improved his binocularity. As a rule, patients who do not realize they have a binocular problem need stronger primary reinforcers; those who do realize the problem need reinforcers that are less strong.

Other feedback mechanisms are often necessary to ensure self-rewarding behavior for the patient so that external primary rewards are no longer required. Physiological diplopia training is one method. Training with the three-dot card also can provide effective feedback.

There are two main groups of theorists with cognitive explanations of learning: (1) the phenomenologists, composed of the gestaltists and the cognitive field psychologists, and (2) the cognitivists, such as Jerome S. Bruner and Jean Piaget.

COGNITIVE EXPLANATIONS

The gestalt type of phenomenological theory began in the 1920s. Psychologists such as Max Wertheimer, Wolfgang Köhler, and Kurt Koffka believed that insight is the key to learning (sometimes spoken of as the "ah-ha" phenomenon). Gestalt psychology refers to the structure of the "whole" rather than to smaller bits (parts), which distinguishes it from stimulus-response learning theories. Furthermore, gestaltists are concerned with perception, and many apply gestalt principles to thinking and problem solving. Wertheimer is considered to be the founder of gestalt psychology. It may have been his experiments with the phi phenomenon (the perception of motion) in the early 1900s that set the stage for his contributions to gestalt learning theory. Wertheimer formulated some basic laws of gestalt psychology, including those of *proximity, similarity, objective set, direction, closure* and *pragnanz*. Other gestaltists later contributed to gestalt learning theory. Köhler, for instance, expounded on learning by insight, and Koffka defined trace theory as related to memory and forgetting.

Hilgard and Bower[61] summed up the applicability of cognitive learning theory with the following principles. The first principle involves the importance of *perceptual features*, such as figure-ground relations. The second deals with the *organization of knowledge*. Learning should be from simple to complex, developing from "simplified wholes to more complex wholes." The third says that learning with *understanding* is more effective and lasting than is learning by rote. Fourth, *cognitive feedback* allows the learner to accept or reject what is tried. Fifth, *goal setting* is important for motivation. Sixth, *divergent* (inventive) and *convergent* (logical) thinking are important principles.

As an overview, consider the cognitive principles used in pencil push-up training. The gestalt of figure and ground relations can be developed by having the patient perceive the diplopic images of the background simultaneously with the pencil (which is the figure). The organization of knowledge is from simple reflexive vergences to the more complex task of converging while appreciating diplopia—either of background objects, with pencil bifixation, or of the pencil, when bifixation is lost momentarily. If the patient can understand why he is doing the training (and the subsequent practice at home), he will not think of the procedure as a rote exercise. Feedback allows the patient to correct faulty responses of bifixation while reaffirming his correct ones. Goal setting tells him what he has to do to attain success. Divergent and convergent thinking are important in that the patient can think of and apply new ways of performing the push-up procedure in similar but more interesting ways.

A variation on the pencil push-up exercise that may be interesting to a patient is the combination of framing with jump vergences as the pencil is advanced slowly. Framing is important in exo cases. The patient learns to perceive either a background object framing the pencil, or the pencil framing the background, depending on which is bifixated. (Refer to Chapter Thirteen.)

If the patient can achieve these complex embellishments of the pencil push-up procedure, he should then be able to advance to three-dot card and chiastopic fusion procedures. It is hoped that, with each new "ah-ha," the patient's face will brighten with pleasure.

Kurt Lewin has been the main spokesman for the cognitive field theory of learning. An excellent review of cognitive field psychology was presented by Sahakian.[62] Lewin spoke of a person's "life-space," his perception of two interdependent factors, the state of the person and his environment. According to Lewin, one's behavior is a function of one's life-space. This is an expansion of gestalt psychology in that it considers the whole person relating to the environment. It is as though the person perceives himself as the "figure" in a life-space "ground."

Lewin spoke of barriers in one's life-space. The boundary zone is affected by the person's social as well as physical world at the moment. For instance, objects in a room lead to different behavior for each person, e.g., toys to a child as compared with toys to an adult. In other words, the life-space is different for everyone.

It is difficult enough to understand Lewin's learning theories, without trying to apply them. One principle does shine through, however: considering the uniqueness of each individual patient. This must be taken into account even in such simple tasks as pencil push-up training, and it is even more important if more complex tasks, such as chiastopic fusion training, are prescribed.

Cognitivism is yet another basic learning theory. A brief overview of exemplary cognitive explanations of Bruner and Piaget are given along with suggestions as to how their theories may be applied to certain binocular therapeutic procedures, such as pencil push-ups, use of the three-dot convergence card, and chiastopic fusion in free space.

According to Bruner,[63] "Any subject could be taught in an intellectually honest manner to any age group if increments in the sequence were made small enough." Bruner stressed that basic *information* is the foundation for conceptualization. For example, with the three-dot convergence card, the patient would be taught, step-by-step, in small increments, toward mastery learning. The doctor (and/or therapist) may have to explain in detail how the right eye sees certain colored dots and the left eye sees other colored ones. Then the patient is told that if correspondingly sized dots are blended together (fused), the red and blue mixture will appear to be purple. If this can be achieved, the doctor points out that the other dots will be seen diplopically, heteronymously for the proximal and homonymously for the distal pairings if the middle dots are being fused. Finally, the patient develops voluntary control so that jump vergences are rapid and accurate.

Several additional teaching steps are often required, particularly with very young children, before the desired result is attained. One essential step in getting the patient to grasp the inherent relations involved in the three-dot card procedure may be the initial mastery of the pencil push-up procedure. Both the awareness of the act of convergence and the perception of physiological diplopia are necessary. When this is accomplished, the three-dot card can be introduced.

Initially it may be helpful to introduce the card with the top portion cut off, thereby removing the dissociative septum effect (Figure 16-20). A small pin can be stuck into one of the dots for bifixation. This makes the procedure similar to pencil push-ups in that the pin is bifixated in free space without a septum. The patient is instructed on how the dots should be perceived before going to the uncut card (a more complex demand because of the dissociative effect).

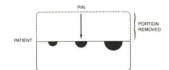

FIGURE 16-20 — The three-dot convergence card with the top portion cut off to facilitate bifixation. A pen is stuck into the card to promote fusion of the middle-sized pair of dots.

In going beyond the mere formation of cognitive associations by step-by-step teaching, Bruner emphasized the importance of building *intuitive thought*. For a patient being taught the three-dot card procedure, intuitive thought would enable him to *discover* what the procedure is "all about" in relation to his own *private world*. The patient then understands how and why to carry out this home training procedure on his own, as well as how to originate variations and embellishments of the procedure on his own initiative. When this level of "actualization" is reached for each and every procedure used in a patient's therapy program, success is imminent.

In summary, learning according to the Brunerian approach would best result from initial teaching in small increments so the learner can develop knowledge. From this knowledge base, the learner can then develop "intuitive thinking" and mastery through practice.

From the observations of the famous epistemologist, Jean Piaget, certain periods of cognitive development of children have been outlined. One such representative outline was listed by Wilson et al.[57] and is shown in Table 16C. (Piaget's theories are too complex and extensive to discuss in any detail here, but a brief exposition of how I see his periods relating to binocular therapy will be given.)

Age (Years)	Period
0–2	Sensorimotor intelligence
2–7	Preoperational representations
7–11	Concrete operations
>11	Formal operations

TABLE 16C. Cognitive Development According to Piaget[57]

Sensorimotor intelligence is built upon innate reflexes by means of motoric trial-and-error activity that may lead to the attainment of the desired results. Through this process, the infant begins to learn about cause and effect and the relationship of *real objects* in space. Thus, infants can usually learn to bifixate a pencil (real object) accurately enough to perform the pencil push-up procedure.

However, the sensorimotor child is "locked in" to interacting with real objects with respect to vision, so he lacks thought in terms of symbols. It follows that more complex tasks, such as the three-dot card procedure (diplopic images being somewhat "unreal"), cannot normally be achieved in the sensorimotor period of development. Therefore, the doctor should not normally expect to have an infant (ages 0 to 2 years) undergo procedures for convergence insufficiency that require more cognitive development than that required for bifixating a real object in free space.

A note of caution should be interjected at this point. Piaget found that the *age boundaries* are flexible, but the *sequence* is not. Each successive period is built in turn upon the previous developmental period. Getman[64] expressed this most aptly by saying that "the divisions, or categories, are never absolute because of individual differences, but the guide posts are always present, if observers are acute enough to see them, because there is general commonality, which is valid in all humans as they progress through time."

Whereas the child in the sensorimotor stage had to rely on the viewing of, and the physical interaction with, real objects, the *preoperational* child is not so restricted. He can begin to call on language to help in learning social organization as well as in understanding symbols requiring cognition. The dependence on, and the physical interaction with, "realia" become less than before.

There is, however, a considerable restriction for the preoperational patient when it comes to *conservation* (a term of Piaget implying being able to overcome through cognition an otherwise faulty judgment based on what is actually perceived). A famous experiment on the "conservation" of liquids illustrates how a preoperational child is duped by the "perceived image" of a tall, thin glass of water appearing to have greater volume than a short, fat glass (with water of equal volume in each vessel). That is, this child has incomplete thinking as opposed to an adult, who can use logical reasoning to determine the correct answer.

How can Piaget's theory be applied to binocular therapy? From the discussion, it seems reasonable to expect a preoperational child to be able to learn to perform well on the three-dot card. My clinical experience has borne this out in most cases, particularly with older patients in the later stages of this developmental period. (Piaget divided each period into a sequence of stages.)

When it comes to chiastopic fusion in free space, however, preoperational patients (normally under the age of 7) usually have trouble. It has been my experience and that of several colleagues that the patient must be in the period of *concrete operations* (normally from ages 7 to 11 years) before this procedure can be utilized effectively. The older, concrete operational patient probably is not "perception bound" like the younger, preoperational one. The patient can "conserve" (my usage of Piaget's term) the floating images in space while making the necessary vergences. This is too much to ask of the preoperational patient, who is perception bound by the two real targets—thus, vitiation of chiastopic fusion occurs.

The last developmental period of Piaget is that of *formal operations* (normally in ages greater than 11 years). The individual can now think in abstract terms and has become far less dependent on representations of reality than when he was in the concrete operational period. Most procedures for convergence insufficiency, including elaborate *embellishments* of chiastopic fusion, can be learned and practiced by patients who are in this advanced period of cognitive development. This may explain why older patients with convergence insufficiency are relatively easy to cure.

It should be pointed out that the learning theories of Bruner and Piaget only represent some of the many facets of cognitivism. Like most theories, these two conflict in certain respects. Bruner's theory would imply that poor teaching is why learning does not take place, whereas Piaget's theory would imply that, in spite of good teaching, learning is unlikely if the individual is not at the cognitive level of development commensurate with the level of what is being taught.

I follow Bruner's approach and optimistic philosophy whenever it is warranted. However, I have also found Piaget's classification of cognitive developmental periods to be very useful in practice.

Suchoff[65] has extended Piaget's concepts into visual spatial development in a way that promises to be very applicable to vision therapy. He states, "We can clinically determine the level of spatial maturity as the child cognitively grows."

Almost everyone would agree that as yet there is no one theory of learning that provides all the answers. It is hoped that visual training specialists will draw from the "best" of each of the many learning theories and appropriately apply them to each particular visual training patient.

Keep in mind that these principles can be applied to other types of vision therapy cases than the category of convergence insufficiency exemplified in this discussion.

Aniseikonia Summary

Testing for aniseikonia (unequal ocular images) in strabismic patients was discussed in Chapter Eight. However, when there is a significant amount of aniseikonia, it is more often the heterophoric than the strabismic patient who presents with symptoms.

The prevalence of aniseikonia is surprisingly high in the general population. However, the magnitude of aniseikonia that causes patient symptoms, including interference with binocular vision, occurs in a relatively small percentage of the population (i.e., 3 to 10 percent).[66,67] Many of the symptoms reported by patients with aniseikonia do not differ significantly from symptoms of ametropia, heterophoria, and heterotropia (e.g., headache, asthenopia, reading difficulties, and diplopia).[67] However, when ametropic and/or binocular anomalies are eliminated, the presence of such symptoms may assist in diagnosing aniseikonia. Other symptoms associated with aniseikonia are photophobia, nausea, nervousness, dizziness, vertigo, and general fatigue. However, these symptoms may also be associated with other systemic disorders. Symptoms of patients with aniseikonia are generally of long standing and are not relieved by conventional prescription lenses.

Clinically measurable aniseikonia may be manifested as a difference of the size of objects seen with each eye and/or spatial distortion of size and shape of the environment. The magnification differences between the eyes can occur in all meridians of the eye (overall aniseikonia), in a particular meridian (meridional aniseikonia), or a combination of the above (compound aniseikonia). The etiology of these size differences is primarily anisometropia. The nature and magnitude of aniseikonia will depend upon whether the ametropia is axial and/or refractive and the mode of correction (i.e., spectacle or contact lenses). Other etiologies of aniseikonia could conceivably be retinal and neural asymmetries independent of anisometropia.

Three methods are available to the practitioner for determining the nature and magnitude of aniseikonia: (1) standard, or *direct comparison, eikonometry;* (2) *space eikonometry;* and (3) an *estimation* method.

Standard eikonometry may utilize vectographic visual targets for comparison of image sizes in the horizontal, vertical, and (with some targets, e.g., American Optical Aniseikonia Nearpoint Card) oblique meridians. The percentage size difference between the two eyes can be measured by magnifying the *smaller* image with appropriate size lenses before that eye until equality of image size is achieved. Kleinstein[68] described a useful iseikonic trial lens set for such diagnostic purposes (see Table 16D). Ideally, this type of trial set should include meridional as well as overall size lenses. Direct comparison of image size can be accomplished, grossly, by alternate occlusion and by vertical prism dissociation. Size lenses can also be used with these techniques to help patients judge image size differences.

TABLE 16D. *Sample Iseikonic Trial Lenses Providing Overall Magnification for Aniseikonia Testing, Modified from Kleinstein[68] (Afocal Lenses of Glass with Index of Refraction of 1.53)*

Magnification (Percent)	Front Surface Power (F_1)	Back Surface Power (F_2)	Lens Thickness (in mm)
1	+6.75	−6.82	2.24
2	+11.25	−11.47	2.65
3	+12.00	−12.36	3.75
4	+12.00	−12.48	4.95
5	+12.00	−12.60	6.12

Space eikonometry utilizes an instrument once manufactured by the American Optical Company. The Space Eikonometer measures deviations from normal stereoscopic spatial perception induced by aniseikonia. The validity of measurements with this instrument depends upon at least 20/60 visual acuity, and normal fusion and stereopsis. Aniseikonia is measured in the horizontal, vertical, and oblique (declination error) meridians. Since the Space Eikonometer has not been manufactured for many years and therefore is difficult to obtain, the practitioner may have to use alternate methods of eikonometry.

A number of practitioners have attempted to *estimate*, rather than measure, the magnitude of aniseikonia from the differences of refractive correction due to anisometropia.[69-71] Ogle[69] suggested that 1.5 to 2.0 percent aniseikonia is induced per diopter of corrected anisometropia. As mentioned earlier, the percentage per diopter would depend upon the nature of the ametropia (myopia versus hyperopia, and axial versus refractive ametropia) and the mode of correction. Others disagreed with Ogle's estimate and proposed that 1.0 percent per diopter is a more realistic value.[70,71] I believe this is more likely, because axial anisometropia should produce little or no retinal size difference (Knapp's law) with spectacle lens correction. Polasky[70] described a viable noninstrumental clinical procedure using nomograms to determine the magnitude of aniseikonia based upon their estimation per diopter of anisometropia.

The correction of overall, meridional, or compound aniseikonia is accomplished by magnifying the smaller image in the appropriate meridian(s) until a reasonable image size match is achieved. (Overall magnification trial lenses can be used to measure separate meridians.) A certain percentage of undercorrection (e.g., 0.5 percent) is acceptable due to a presumed patient tolerance. Spectacle magnification can be accomplished by appropriate modification of the shape factor of an ophthalmic lens (which is dependent upon the front base curve and thickness of the lens) and/or the power factor (which is dependent upon the vertex power and vertex distance of the lens). Since the power factor can be modified only slightly without undercorrecting or overcorrecting the ametropia, the *shape factor* is the variable which is most often considered to create the desired magnification. Tables containing the different front base curve and thickness values for a given spectacle magnification effect are available in the literature.[68, 70] Iseikonic lenses are available through some local optical laboratories. When designing an aniseikonic correction, lens availability with the desired specifications and cosmesis should be serious considerations.

Kleinstein[68] gave the magnification formula for the shape factor as follows:

$$M = \left(\frac{1}{1 - ZF_v}\right)\left(\frac{1}{1 - CF_1}\right)$$

Where M = Magnification
Z = Vertex distance in meters, e.g. 0.013
F_v = Vertex power in diopters, e.g., +3.00
C = Thickness of lens (in meters) divided by the index of refraction, e.g., 0.002/1.53
F_1 = Front surface power in diopters, e.g., +9.00

Using this formula and calculating with the numbers in the examples, M = 1.05, or 5 percent magnification, say, for the lens of the right eye. However, say a lens for the left eye has the following specifications:

F_v = +5.00
C = 0.003/1.53 (i.e., it is a thicker lens compared with the lens of the right eye)
F_1 = +11.00

$$M = \left(\frac{1}{1 - 0.013(5)}\right)\left(\frac{1}{1 - 0.003/1.53(11)}\right)$$

= 1.09, or 9% spectacle magnification

Predicted aniseikonia = M left eye − M right eye
= 9% − 5%
= 4%

If the thickness of the lens of the right eye were 5 mm and the front surface power were increased to +11.00D, then M would be calculated as follows:

$$M = \left(\frac{1}{1 - 0.013(3)}\right)\left(\frac{1}{1 - 0.005/1.53(11)}\right)$$
$$= 1.08, \text{ or } 8\% \text{ spectacle magnification}$$

Predicted aniseikonia would then be

$$M \text{ left eye} - M \text{ right eye} = 9\% - 8\%$$
$$= 1\%$$

This 1 percent difference of ocular image size would probably be more tolerable to the patient (who has symptoms of aniseikonia) than the 4 percent difference if the front surface power and lens thickness had not been increased. (Note: This example applies to overall aniseikonia. Meridional aniseikonia would require direct comparison and calculations for various meridians for toric iseikonic prescription lenses.)

It should be noted that reduction of the retinal size difference from 4 to 1 percent was done by the shape factor. However, there is an anisometropia of 2.00D in this example; therefore, an estimated 2 percent size difference could also be induced by the anisometropic factor. The patient could have 1 percent plus the estimated 2 percent, for a total of 3 percent retinal size difference. This would still be more desirable than if 4 plus 2 percent, for a total of 6 percent difference, were the case (if the shape factor had not been modified). Fortunately, Knapp's law (*assuming* the patient has axial anisometropia) may account for the 2 percent anisometropic factor being almost 1 percent and may explain why many patients, as in this example, tolerate spectacle lenses very well. If, on the other hand, the patient has refractive anisometropia (different corneal curvature of each eye), the estimated 2 percent anisometropic factor may be considerably larger. In such a situation, the patient may develop foveal suppression and learn to live with the aniseikonia by being a monofixator. But if this adaptive binocular anomaly (i.e., suppression) does not exist, iseikonic lenses may be necessary.

Contact lenses may be recommended before prescribing iseikonic spectacle lenses. I have seen patients with refractive anisometropia who had suppression eliminated (and sometimes amblyopia cured) when contact lenses were tried; reduction (or elimination) of aniseikonia via the contact lenses may have been the reason.

A substantially high rate of cure for anomalous correspondence was reported by Greenwald,[72] who reemphasized the utilization of disruptive methods, such as overcorrecting lenses, occlusion, and fogging lenses. (Refer to discussions in Chapter Nine.)

Blakemore[73] reported a possible breakthrough in the prevention of irreparable loss of binocular function in cases of congenital strabismus. His studies have been with kittens, but there may be far-reaching implications for human infants. His concept is as follows: "These eye/brain binocular connections are

Some Things to
Consider and Remember

already established at birth and are geared for immediate operation." When strabismus prevents these conditions from being properly used, he advocates "exposing a young baby to a pattern of stripes several times a day, giving, in total, a daily exposure of about half an hour." Like strabismic kittens, human infants with strabismus could have coincident images in an environment of stripes.

Another study involved surgically induced strabismus in kittens followed by their being exposed a few hours daily to black and white stripe patterns so that equal imagery for both eyes would result, no matter which way the eyes were positioned. Binocular cell activity was normal after a few months of this kind of preventive therapy.[74]

It is reasonable to assume that human infants with strabismus should respond in a similar manner. If so, the advantage of this type of therapy is that it can begin as soon as the infant is able to open his eyes and look around. This could have a great positive impact on the prognosis of congenital strabismus.

Occasionally a patient has intractable diplopia that does not seem to be amenable to elimination through vision therapy of any kind. Kirschen and Flom[75] reported successful measurement of such a problem for one patient by degrading central vision of one eye using a disc of translucent tape on the spectacle lens. For another patient, the central portion of the spectacle lens was degraded with fingernail polish. This method of central attenuation allowed the patient to have full peripheral visual fields, yet without problems of diplopia when viewing centrally through the lenses.

The following are some very basic things to remember.
1. Give vision therapy as soon as possible; do not delay. This implies that infants and toddlers should be given professional eye/vision examinations for detection of problems so that treatment, if needed, can be given as soon as possible.
2. Be on guard against the possibility of creating occlusion strabismus or occlusion amblyopia when patching is prescribed.
3. Always make sure the patient's refractive status is known and accounted for. Watch for esotropia if there is hyperopia of 2.00D or more, and for suppression if there is anisometropia, which could lead to amblyopia.
4. Check for all pathologies, ocular and systemic, before beginning functional training procedures.
5. Make sure the patient can do a home training procedure correctly before you prescribe it.
6. *Ask* the patient to do his therapy rather than telling him to do it.
7. Give the patient goals, reinforcement, and reasons for his being in therapy.
8. Realize that a functional cure can be achieved in some cases and not in others.

9. Remember that the better the diagnosis and assessment of the total patient's attitudes and potentials, the more accurate is the prognosis.

Remember that the most important consideration is the patient's ability to achieve in school, play, work, and life in general. Try to help the patient achieve clear, single, comfortable, efficient, binocular vision. Keep in mind, however, that the binocular status is sometimes of minor importance in regard to an individual's success and achievement in life, but when binocular anomalies are handicapping the patient, recommend the appropriate procedures for vision therapy.

APPENDIX

Convergence — Components according to Maddox

1. Tonic convergence = $T_L + T_R$

   T_L is adduction of left eye from anatomic to physiologic position of rest. T_R is adduction of right eye.

   This illustration represents an example of an exo deviation, and thus, low tonicity. Assume the patient is 16 p.d. exo in this example. The absolute value of T_L or T_R is not known. Thus, tonic convergence is not measured, only the error from the ortho position is measured.

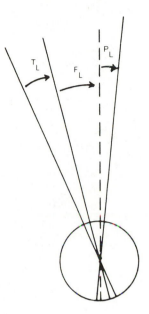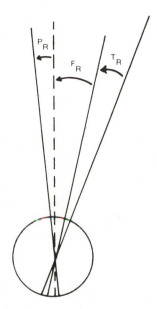

2. Fusional convergence = $F_L + F_R$

   F_L is the adduction of the left eye from the physiologic position of rest to the ortho demand position. The basic deviation, measured at the far point without accommodation in play, must be compensated by means of fusional convergence in order for the patient to properly fuse the target at optical infinity. The patient therefore converges a total of 16 p.d.

3. Proximal convergence = $P_L + P_R$

   Assume the patient is looking into a reduced environment; e.g., optical infinity. The average overconvergence is approximately 4 p.d.

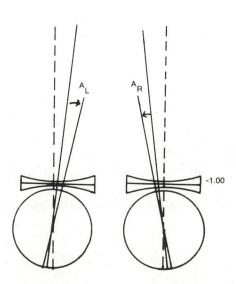

4. Accommodative convergence = $A_L + A_R$

   Assume minus one diopter lenses are placed before this patient and that the accommodative response is one diopter. If the patient has a 6/1 AC/A, the accommodative convergence would be 6 p.d. This combined with the 4 p.d. of proximal convergence would cause a posture of 10 eso.

Conversions of Prism Diopters and Degrees

Prism diopters	Degrees	Degrees	Prism diopters
1	0° 34'	1	1.75
2	1° 9'	2	3.49
3	1° 43'	3	5.24
4	2° 17'	4	6.99
5	2° 51'	5	8.75
6	3° 26'	6	10.51
7	4° 0'	7	12.29
8	4° 34'	8	14.05
9	5° 9'	9	15.84
10	5° 43'	10	17.63
15	8° 32'	15	26.80
20	11° 19'	20	36.40

Visual Acuity and Visual Efficiency

Snellen Acuity	Angle of Resolution	Visual Efficiency in Percent	Percentage Loss of Vision
20/20 (6/6)	1.0'	100.0	0
20/25 (6/7.5)	1.25'	95.6	4.4
20/30 (6/9)	1.50'	91.4	8.6
20/40 (6/12)	2'	83.6	16.4
20/50 (6/15)	2.5'	76.5	23.5
20/60 (6/18)	3'	69.9	30.1
20/70 (6/21)	3.5'	63.8	36.2
20/80 (6/24)	4'	58.5	41.5
20/100 (6/30)	5'	48.9	51.1
20/200 (6/60)	10'	20.0	80.0
20/300 (6/90)	15'	8.2	91.8
20/400 (6/120)	20'	3.3	96.7
20/800 (6/240)	40'	0.1	99.9

Stereoacuity calculations

To determine the stereoacuity when lateral displacement is known, first this must be expressed in terms of a theoretical value that represents the apparent linear displacement. This is the x value in the formula:

$$Eta = \frac{I.P.D. \quad (x)}{d^2} (206,000).$$

Assume, for instance, the eyes are bi-fixating a circle by means of polarization. Another target (such as the disparate circles in the Wirt Rings Test) is designed so that each can be seen by only one eye. Assume: The lateral displacement is 1 mm for this particular stereoscopic test, the I.P.D. is 60 mm, and the testing distance (d) is 40 cm (400 mm). Find x from the formula:

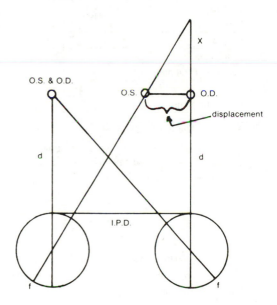

$$\frac{x}{displacement} = \frac{x + d}{I.P.D.}$$

$$\frac{x}{1} = \frac{x + 400}{60}$$

59x = 400

x = 6.78mm

Now substituting into the linear formula for stereoacuity,

$$Eta = \frac{60 \quad (6.78)}{(400)^2} (206,000)$$

Eta = 524 seconds of arc

Some Appropriate Tests in Strabismus/Amblyopia Diagnosis

VARIABLES and CONDITIONS	Hx	VA	DIR	KAP	HIR	UCT	ACT	4BO	3S	H-L	MR	VIS	HB	B-G	MA	H-B	BAG	GIES	BGHB	BIF	W4D	PM	CHS	PO	STE
Concomitancy	?		?		X	X	X		X	X	X														
Frequency	?		?		X	X		X																	
Eye Laterality	?		?		X	X		X							?										
Eye Dominancy	?		?		X	X		X							X						X	?	X		
Direction	?		?		X	X	X		X	?	?				X	?				?				?	
Magnitude	?		?	?	X	X			?	?	?				X		?							?	
AC/A Ratio					X	X					?				?										
Cosmesis	X		X	X																					
Variability	?		?		X	X	X			?	?				X										
Suppression	?					?		X		X	X				X	X			?	X	X	X	X	X	X
Amblyopia	?	X											?												?
Eccentric Fixation	?			X								X	X	X	?	?			X						
ARC												X	X	X	X	X	X	X	X					?	
Horror Fusionis										X	?				X									X	

X = excellent test for particular variable or condition

? = possible test, but not always appropriate or reliable (e.g., Hx may not be reliable as to magnitude or suppression, and MR may give the subjective angle of directionalization rather than the magnitude of the deviation)

Hx	= history	MR	= Maddox rod
VA	= visual acuity	VIS	= visuoscopy
DIR	= direct observation	HB	= Haidinger's brushes
KAP	= angle kappa	B-G	= Brock-Givner after-image transfer
HIR	= Hirschberg		
UCT	= unilateral cover	MA	= major amblyoscope
ACT	= alternate cover	H-B	= Hering-Bielschowsky afterimage
4BO	= 4Δ base-out		
3S	= 3-step method	BAG	= Bagolini lenses
H-L	= Hess-Lancaster		

GIES = Giessen
BGHB = Brock-Givner and Haidinger's brushes
BIF = bifoveal test (Cüppers)
W4D = Worth 4-Dot
PM = Pola-Mirror
CHS = cheiroscope
PO = Polachrome Orthopter
STE = stereoacuity testing

Strabismus/Amblyopia Testing Outline

STRABISMUS/AMBLYOPIA TESTING OUTLINE	Date_____ Patient_____ Age____

Reason for exam:_____

A. History:
   1. Is there an eye turn?_____ Which eye?_____ What direction?_____ Always the same eye?_____ Cosmetically noticeable to others?_____ Are you (or is the child) bothered by the cosmetic appearance?_____ Age of onset?_____ Gradual or sudden onset?_____ Is the eye turn getting worse?_____ Any symptoms?_____ Double vision?_____ When and where?_____ Any trauma, disease or health conditions associated with eye turn?_____ Family history of an eye turn?_____
   2. Record all previous vision therapy (e.g., occlusion, surgery, lenses) and other pertinent information.

B. Visual Acuity (State method of testing, e.g., Snellen line, Snellen letter, Flom Psychometric).

    $\overline{sc}$ V $\begin{array}{l} OD \\ OS \end{array}$ Present lenses   OD
                              and VA   OS

    Refraction (state if cycloplegic or manifest) and VA
       OD
       OS

C. Hirschberg test suggests:_____

D. Unilateral Cover Test (far and near):_____
_____

E. Alternate Cover Test (far and near):_____
_____ AC/A Calculated:_____

F. Concomitancy Testing (e.g., ductions, versions, Hess-Lancaster, Three-step method):_____
_____

G. Monocular Testing for eccentric and unsteady fixation (e.g., visuoscopy, Haidinger's brushes):_____
_____

H. Binocular testing for ARC (e.g., Bagolini, afterimages, amblyoscope):_____
_____

I. Sensory and motor fusion testing and suppression status (1st, 2nd, & 3rd degree fusion):_____
_____
_____

J. Additional Testing:_____

K. Diagnosis (including all variables of the deviation and any associated conditions):_____
_____
_____

L. Prognosis:_____

M. Recommendations, advice given and plan:_____
_____

Visual Skills Efficiency Evaluation (Testing Outline)

VISUAL SKILLS EFFICIENCY EVALUATION (TESTING OUTLINE)   Date:_____

Patient_____ Age_____ Reason for Exam_____

1. VISUAL ACUITY: @ Farpoint   @ Nearpoint

    Lenses worn   VA   s̄c V OD   s̄c V OD
                                  OS   OS
    OD   c̄c V OD
    OS   OS

                                        Comments

    Refractive data: OD
                      OS

2. SACCADIC EYE MOVEMENTS: e.g., Pierce Test, King-Devick, Eye-Trac,
                             penlight

    Results:

3. PURSUIT EYE MOVEMENTS: e.g., Keystone Rotator, Marsden Ball, penlight
    Results:

4. ACCOMMODATION EFFICIENCY: e.g., Insufficiency, excess, infacility,
                               ill-sustained
    Testing Results   (e.g., Dynamic retinoscopy, rock, amplitude):

5. VERGENCES:
    Ranges: Far BI   Far BO   Near BI   Near BO

    Facility:

    Stamina:

    Phoria/tropia data:

    Nearpoint of Convergence (in centimeters), blur, break, recovery
        Results: (one trial and after 5 trials):

    Fixation Disparity (ortho demand)
        Results:

6. SENSORY FUSION (ortho demand) @ Farpoint and @ Nearpoint
    Flat fusion s̄ suppression:
    Stereoacuity (specify tests used):

7. OTHER SENSORY-MOTOR FUSION RANGES: e.g., s̄ suppression, s̄ loss of
        stereoacuity, s̄ fixation disparity, s̄ discomfort
        Results:

8. DIAGNOSIS:

9. PROGNOSIS:

10. RECOMMENDATIONS AND ADVICE GIVEN:

Evaluation for Visually Related Learning Difficulties — John R. Griffin, O.D., M.S.Ed.

(Visual Skills and Developmental-Perceptual Profile)

Category	Tests	R.S.	A.E.	Comments	Very Weak 1	Weak 2	Average 3	Strong 4	Very Strong 5
VISUAL FUNCTIONS	Saccadic Eye Movements								
	Pursuit Eye Movements								
	Accommodation (sufficiency)								
	Accommodation (facility)								
	Accommodation (stamina)								
	Vergence (sufficiency)								
	Vergence (facility)								
	Vergence (stamina)								
	Stereopsis								
	Other								
GROSS MOTOR	Balance (eyes open)								
	Balance (eyes closed)								
	Angels (bilateral Integration)								
	Piaget (R-L)								
	Other								
VISUAL-MOTOR	Visual Motor Integration (VMI)								
	Visual Motor (speed)								
	Visual Motor (precision)								
	Wold (sentence copy)								
	Other								
VISUAL-PERCEPTUAL	Jordan Reversal Test								
	Motor Free Perceptual (MVPT)								
	So. Cal. Figure-Ground Test								
	Visual Attention Span (letters)								
	Other								
VISUAL-AUDITORY	Auditory Attention (digit span)								
	Birch-Belmont (A-V integration)								
	Wepman (auditory discrimination)								
	Dyslexia Determination (DDT)								
	Other								

Patient:
Date:
Comments:

Evaluation of Visually Related Learning Difficulties

Home Training Worksheet
recommended by Victoria M. Lupei, O.D., of Las Vegas, Nevada

RECORD THE TIME IN MINUTES THAT YOU WORKED ON EACH EXERCISE.

WEEK NUMBER_____

EXERCISE	SUNDAY	MONDAY	TUESDAY	WEDNESDAY	THURSDAY	FRIDAY	SATURDAY
1							
2							
3							
4							
5							
6							

COMMENTS:

Sample of Consultant's letter. (See case number one in Chapters 3 and 5)

SOUTHERN CALIFORNIA COLLEGE OF OPTOMETRY

2001 ASSOCIATED ROAD / FULLERTON, CALIFORNIA 92631 / (714) 870-7226

Richard R. Roe, O.D.
1234 Blank Street
Anywhere, CA 90001

Re: Ricky Doe, Age 7

Dear Doctor Roe:

Thank you for referring Ricky Doe to our Vision Therapy Clinic. As you
stated in your letter the patient has no complaints but was advised
by the school nurse to have an examination, and subsequently, by you to
have the binocular status also evaluated by us.

Case history indicates the patient's mother noticed the onset of esotropia
when Ricky was about three months of age. There was token treatment at
the age of four years. We have obtained this report which shows the refractive error then was: ≠ 0.75D. Sph. in each eye. Glasses were prescribed
(≠ 0.75 O.U.) at that time; but they were worn for only a few days.

Our testing at this time revealed refraction was OD plano 20/20, OS plano
20/20.

Binocular testing revealed that the deviation was a: concomitant, constant,
alternating (right eye dominant) esotropia of 15 prism diopters at far
and 13 at near. There was also a double hyper found upon dissociation. The
AC/A was normal and cosmesis good due to positive angle kappa. **There was lack**
of correspondence and no demonstrable motor fusion range.

Impressions: This case of congenital divergence insufficiency has no
chance for development of fusion. Cosmetic surgery is unnecessary at
this time because of good cosmesis.

Recommendations: No therapy required.

Advice given: Patient is to return to you for future care.

Thank you for giving us the opportunity to evaluate this case. We will be
glad to see Ricky in the future if you feel another binocular work-up
is needed then.

Sincerely,

John R. Dee, O.D.
Staff Optometrist

Joseph A. Jones
Student Clinician

JRD/rh

Sample Surgical Report

Operation: Bilateral medial rectus recessions with right lateral rectus resection and inferior oblique myectomy O.U.

FINDINGS AND PROCEDURE:

Charles Brown is a 2½-year-old male who has been followed in the eye clinic and found to have congenital esotropia of 45 prism diopters with overt inferior obliques. There is no A or V pattern. He was admitted for elective strabismus surgery. The patient was brought to the operating room. General anesthesia was instituted. The patient was prepped and draped in the usual manner. Attention was directed to the right eye. Lids were retracted with a lid retractor. Forced duction was performed and found to be normal. An inferior cul-de-sac incision was made on the medial aspect to the sclera, and a muscle hook was passed through the incision, engaging the tendon of the medial rectus muscle. The muscle was bluntly dissected and isolated. A double arm 5-0 Vycril suture was passed 1 mm from the insertion of the muscle in a locking fashion. The muscle was then severed from the globe. A distance of 4.5 mm was measured from the insertion of the medial rectus muscle with calipers, and the muscle was then sutured to this point by means of scleral suturing technique using a spatula needle. Attention was then directed to the inferior oblique muscle. This was approached through an inferior cul-de-sac incision on the lateral aspect of the eye. The inferior oblique muscle was isolated by grasping it with a muscle hook and was bluntly dissected to reveal approximately a 7 mm section of the inferior oblique muscle as far medial as the ligament of Lockwood and the inferior rectus muscle. Two hemostats were placed across the inferior oblique muscle, one at the ligament of Lockwood and another one approximately 7 mm lateral to this hemostat. The muscle in between the hemostats was then excised, and both cut ends of the muscle were cauterized to prevent bleeding. The hemostats were then released. Attention was then directed to the lateral rectus muscle. This muscle was isolated with the muscle hook and bluntly dissected, isolating the muscle. A muscle clamp was placed across the body of the lateral rectus muscle and positioned so that suturing could take place 8 mm from the insertion of the muscle. The muscle, after the muscle clamp had been placed, was cut free from the globe, and two 5-0 Vycril sutures with the spatula needle were placed through the insertion of the lateral rectus muscle and then placed through the body of the lateral rectus muscle 8 mm from its insertion. The lateral rectus was then pulled so that the areas of suturing were approximated, and these two sutures were tied in a mattress fashion. Excess lateral rectus muscle and lateral rectus muscle tendons were then cut free. The inferior cul-de-sac incision was then approximated by crushing the margins with forceps. Attention was then directed to the left eye. This eye was operated on in an identical manner as far as the medial rectus and inferior oblique muscles are concerned. No operation was done on the left eye on the lateral rectus muscle. The patient tolerated the procedure well, and there were no operative complications. The patient was brought out of general anesthesia and taken to the recovery room in stable condition.

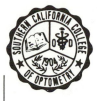

Southern California College of Optometry

2001 Associated Road · Fullerton · California 92631 · (714) 870-7226

September 10, 1981

TO WHOM IT MAY CONCERN:

Re: Charles Brown, Age 4

Charles has been under visual care at the Southern California College
of Optometry since July 22, 1981, when his mother brought him to see
us. He has a visual history of congenital esotropia. There is a
medical history of his having stopped breathing at about 6 months of
age. There was surgery for the esotropia at 2½ years of age. His
mother reported cosmetically straight eyes immediately after surgery.
Since them, however, she has noticed a gradually increasing exotropia.

A strabismic evaluation was performed and for the past four weeks
Charles has been in vision therapy at this facility. The tentative
diagnosis is as follows: nonconcomitant, constant, consecutive,
alternating exotropia of approximately 35 prism diopters when the
left eye is fixating and about 45 prism diopters when his right eye
is fixating. Adduction is severely restricted OD; also he is unable
to converge with OD. Mechanical restriction may be causing underaction
of the right medial rectus. There is also a right hypertropia of about
10 prism diopters. Cosmesis is poor. There is anomalous retinal
correspondence, probably of paradoxical type I. No sensory or motor
fusion is present. Visual acuities with Lighthouse cards are 10/15,
in each eye, at 10 feet and 20/25 with both eyes at 40cm; therefore,
there is no amblyopia. Refraction is +0.50 OD and +0.50 OS. Prognosis
for a functional cure with vision therapy is poor. Prognosis for a
cosmetic cure with further surgery is probably fair. At the present
time, we are seeing Charles at our clinic one day per week. We are
working on his monocular skills and trying to establish some second
degree fusion. Since the problem stems from a condition of congenital
esotropia, there is a very small chance of any central fusion being
achieved. A monofixation pattern, however, may be a more realistic goal.

The plan for future treatment of Charles will be as follows: surgical
evaluation by an ophthalmologist who specializes in strabismus surgery
is recommended. In the event of extraocular muscle surgery, it would
be desirable to have Charles return to our clinic to work on possible
development of sensory and motor fusion. His mother has been advised
of the above diagnosis and plan and is very willing to do what she can
to give Charles the best possible care.

Sincerely,

James C. Jones

James C. Jones
Clinician

John R. Dee

James R. Dee, O.D.
Faculty Consultant

JCJ/JRD/rch

Sample of Consultant's Letter to Parents
of Amblyopic Child

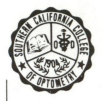

Southern California College of Optometry

2001 Associated Road · Fullerton · California 92631 · (714) 870-7226

January 30, 1981

Mr. and Mrs. Robert Roe
1234 Blank Street
Anywhere, California 90000

                              RE: Ted Roe
                              BD: 10-25-74, age 6-3

Dear Mr. and Mrs. Roe:

Ted was first seen in our Vision Therapy Clinic on August 20, 1980. He was diagnosed as having anisometropia (unequal refractive state between the two eyes) with moderate amblyopia (dull vision) in the right eye. Glasses were prescribed along with patching of the left eye to improve his vision of the right eye.

Eye movements (tracking) and accommodative facility (focusing) were poor as were vergence abilities. Therapy for these deficient skills should be considered in the future.

A vision therapy program was instituted, in September 1980, for the problems listed above. As of this date, Ted has shown an increase in vision in his right eye from approximately 20/70 to 20/30 (or about 60% to 90% visual acuity efficiency).

We feel at this time that the vision in the right eye has leveled off to the best we can obtain for now and that a break in the therapy would be appreciated by Ted. As we discussed, we would like to reevaluate his visual skills and consider more vision training in about six months for improvement of his visual problems.

In the meantime, we recommend that Ted continue to patch his left eye about 30 minutes to 1 hour a day while at home.

Please feel free to contact us if you have any further questions.

                              Sincerely,

Paul Doe   *John R. Dee*

Paul Doe   John R. Dee, O.D.
Clinician   Faculty Consultant

JRD/PD/bja

Case Report of Strabismus Therapy

A 9-year-old boy presented with a small-angle constant esotropia and, through training and with the help of lenses and prisms, became an intermittent esotrope, and later an esophore. Sensory fusion was improved from approximately 550 seconds of arc to 60 seconds of arc stereothreshold. Motor fusion amplitude was expanded from 3 to 42^Δ. Functional results were attained, which justified the relatively lengthy vision therapy process required for this patient.

Summary of Evaluation

I first saw the patient on October 3, 1969. Prior to this he had been given pleoptics for amblyopia of the left eye under Dr. Cüppers' supervision in West Germany. The patient's father was in the U.S. Army and was stationed near Dr. Cüppers' renowned clinic.

Complete records of the patient's treatment in Europe were never attained, but supposedly some degree of amblyopia had been present at one time. Apparently this was treated effectively, but there was no indication that anything had been done to try to achieve a functional cure of the existing constant esotropia.

My diagnosis of the case on October 3 was the following: concomitant, constant, alternating, O.D. preferred eye to fixate, esotropia of 10^Δ at far and 12^Δ at near. Associated conditions included central suppression, no significant amount of amblyopia, fixation central and steady, correspondence normal, some peripheral sensory fusion, and poor motor fusion ranges.

Best correctable vision was O.D.: $20/25^{+2}$, O.S.: $20/25^{-1}$. The subjective manifest refraction was O.D.: $+3.25 -0.25$ x 95, O.S.: $+3.75 -0.25$ x 90. The patient was wearing the following lenses:

O.D.: $+3.25 -0.25$ x 95, 3^Δ base-out
O.S.: $+3.75 -0.25$ x 90, 3^Δ base-out
$+2.25$ add (25 mm straight top bifocal)

This had been prescribed 6 months previously. The patient was cooperative about wearing the glasses for general wear, and he wore them most of the time. The lenses worn prior to the above were:

O.D.: $+4.00 -0.25$ x 105 20/50
O.S.: $+4.25 -0.25$ x 90 20/50

They were single vision lenses without prisms.

The patient had complained of blur at distance. The prognosis for a functional cure of the strabismus by means of vision therapy appeared to be fair to good from the diagnosis and quantification of several test results. These test results included 550 seconds of arc stereoacuity, and motor fusion range being from 1^Δ base-out to 4^Δ base-out with 3^Δ base-out recovery. At least some small motor fusion range was present. (This was measured through the patient's spectacles so that the range in absolute terms would really be 7^Δ to 10^Δ base-out.)

Procedures for Therapy

A series of 12 vision therapy visits was recommended for the patient to determine what results could be achieved. These visits were from October 10, 1969, to January 9, 1970.

Procedures for training included:

1. Cheiroscopic drawing (in-office and out-of-office).
2. Loose (base-in) prism training (in-office).
3. Stereopsis perception training with vectograms (in-office).

4. Brock Posture Board antisuppression training (in-office; see Figure 12-18 in Chapter Twelve).

5. Motor fusion range training on the Vectotrainer (in-office and out-of-office).

6. Bausch & Lomb Orthofusor (out-of-office).

7. Mirror Stereoscope (in-office; see Figure 2-15 in Chapter Two).

8. Red glass technique: fuse red and white at centration point (in-office).

9. Brief periods of patching of O.D., dominant eye (in-office).

10. Major amblyoscope (Synoptophore in-office).

11. Accommodation facility training, monocular and binocular (in-office and out-of-office).

12. Root Rings for peripheral stereopsis, with walkaway technique (in-office; see Figure 2-10 in Chapter Two).

An evaluation of results as of January 9, 1970, showed these changes: improved stereopsis, from 550 seconds of arc originally to 300 seconds of arc; and increased motor fusion amplitude, being from 6^Δ base-out to 1^Δ base-in (total of 7^Δ, which was an increase from the previous total of 3^Δ). Most of the central suppression appeared to be eliminated when testing was done on macular-sized targets in the major amblyoscope. However, central suppression was revealed when more sensitive tests were done, such as when very small foveal targets were used. Also, the 4^Δ base-out prism test indicated central suppression (alternating type, but mainly confined to the left eye).

Additional Training Advised

Additional recommended procedures were very similar to those used in the first series. As is so frequently found in vision therapy patients, progress appeared to wax and wane from one visit to the next. For example, stereoacuity was 400 seconds of arc on January 14, 800 seconds of arc on February 25, 100 seconds of arc on April 10, and 140 seconds of arc on May 22.

Although no consistent findings regarding the status of fusion could be reported, I felt that the patient's binocularity was being improved gradually with training.

An additional training device included was the Pola-Mirror and Vis-A-Vis (Figure 2-4 in Chapter Two) for in-office and out-of-office training for antisuppression. Testing via this method revealed that fusion was a function of the patient's concentration. Without concentration, the patient would alternately suppress, usually suppressing his left eye. With this type of testing/training, the patient can monitor his own suppression. This proved to be an interesting and effective home training method.

Third Series

Recommendations were made for another series of 12 visits, from June 8, 1970, to November 17, 1970. Motor fusion training was heavily emphasized in this series. Originally, the patient had a relatively remote nearpoint of convergence (N P C), notwithstanding this being a case of esotropia. The N P C was 28 cm when I first saw the patient. Now it was improved to 5 cm.

In addition to the above-mentioned training devices and procedures, several other out-of-office training procedures were instituted, such as Allbee 3-dot Card, Brock String, Acetate Eccentric Circles (Keystone), and increased use of vectograms for motor fusion. The motor fusion ranges seemed to have improved as a result of training.

On the major amblyoscope:

Base-in: 12^Δ break with 10^Δ recovery

Base-out: $12^\triangle$ break with $9^\triangle$ recovery

On the Polachrome Orthopter using Topper Slide:

Base-in: $11^\triangle$ break with $9^\triangle$ recovery

Base-out: $31^\triangle$ break with $24^\triangle$ recovery

With loose prisms:

Base-in: $7^\triangle$ to break (fixation on penlight)

On the last visit of the series (November 17), a Fresnel Press-on Membrane Prism was prescribed ($4^\triangle$ base-out for the right eye). This was regionally placed only on the major portion of the lens (not over the bifocal segment). Since the right eye was the preferred eye, the prism was placed over it and thereby acted as a very mild occluder. This made the patient favor the left eye, which usually was the one with suppression.

A final series of 12 visits was recommended, from November 24, 1970, to April 29, 1971. During this period a cycloplegic (with Cyclogel) refraction was done and showed the following:

Last Series

$$O.D.: +5.00 -1.25 \times 90$$
$$O.S.: +4.50 -1.25 \times 85$$

Manifest refraction (postcycloplegic, 1 week later) gave the following results.

Retinoscopy:

$$O.D.: +4.50 -2.00 \times 90$$
$$O.S.: +4.25 -1.00 \times 90$$

Subjective:

$$O.D.: +3.75 -1.00 \times 90 \ 20/20$$
$$O.S.: +3.75 -1.00 \times 90 \ 20/20$$

(This was the best visual acuity with the most plus acceptance.)

The following is a summary of the results of therapy during this last period of visits. The Fresnel prism was worn for about 3½ months until the patient was able to be weaned from it. This was accomplished successfully. The status of sensory fusion had become much more favorable, as evidenced by the fact there was now 60 seconds of arc, stereothreshold. Also, the patient got 1 through 10 correct (passing) on the Keystone Skills Stereopsis Card (Test 7, DB-6D).

Results of Therapy

The cover test with spectacles worn showed the following: at far, $2^\triangle$ esophoria (the patient had a total of $6^\triangle$ base-out in the lenses; therefore, the angle of deviation was actually $8^\triangle$ eso); at near, the patient was ortho (through the bifocal addition). The cover test revealed that, using loose trial lenses and prisms, the patient could maintain fusion for several minutes without the help of base-out prisms, but he could do so only briefly when not wearing his lenses for the hyperopic condition. This being the case, he would lapse into esotropia. At near, the deviation would become an intermittent esotropia through the distance correction, but there was orthophoria most of the time through the bifocal addition.

Because of the above findings, I felt it wise to continue full-time wearing of spectacles with base-out prisms, full acceptable plus correction for far, and bifocal additions for near vision. With this help, the patient showed no appreciable central suppression. He passed the Keystone Visual Skills test—all 15 cards. His motor fusion on the major amblyoscope (checking for suppression) was from $8^\triangle$ base-in to $34^\triangle$ base-out, or a total of $42^\triangle$. The cover test showed the patient to be heterophoric, and not heterotropic, provided his spectacles were worn.

In-Office Procedures End

After these results had been obtained, the patient was dismissed from therapy and reminded to return as necessary for a complete evaluation and possible short-term training. He was told to continue home training in the meantime.

He wanted a new pair of glasses (since the old frame had cracked), and the following prescription was given on February 8, 1973:

$$\text{O.D.: } +3.75 \, -1.00 \text{ x } 90 \, 3^\Delta \text{ base-out}$$
$$\text{O.S.: } +3.75 \, -1.00 \text{ x } 80 \, 3^\Delta \text{ base-out}$$
$$+2.00 \text{ add (Executive bifocal)}$$

Vision with correction was O.D.: 20/20, O.S.: 20/20.

Some of the findings at that time included positive relative convergence, 31^Δ; negative relative convergence, 17^Δ; negative relative accommodation and positive relative accommodation findings were normal.

The patient subsequently moved from the area, but throughout this lengthy case, the father and the patient became very aware of proper training procedures. Therefore, I felt I could depend on them to carry out limited vision training at home until the patient could be seen by another practitioner in a different locale.

Comments

While this case is not spectacular in that cosmesis was never a great problem as long as spectacles were worn, I did find it rewarding to achieve an *almost* complete functional cure.[a] Admittedly, it was a long process, but I believe the results attained made it all worthwhile. I also might add that the judicious use of optical aids helped play an important role in this case.

The history as to time of onset of strabismus was not definite, but it is my impression that the patient originally had a unilateral esotropia of the left eye. This seemed to have been an accommodative esotropia acquired early (about the age of 2 years). With early institution of lenses to correct the hyperopia, the angle of deviation became progressively smaller, but a residual manifest deviation was present at all times. Thus, the amblyopia of the deviating left eye continued. Although pleoptic therapy was undoubtedly efficacious, this case points out the need for additional therapy to treat the remaining binocular problems.

---

[a] According to the criteria of Flom (Chapter Five), up to 5^Δ may be worn in glasses in "functional cure." Therefore, the patient's wearing of 6^Δ would qualify him only as being "almost cured."

Case Report of Therapy for Visual Skills Inefficiency[a]

An 18-year-old female, Mary, presented with complaints of sharp pain in her left eye which was usually accompanied by headaches. She had noticed these symptoms for many months. They were consistent in that they would begin after approximately 15 minutes of reading. The symptoms subsided, however, in about 30 minutes after cessation of reading. She also reported skipping lines and losing her place while reading. Mary was a freshman in college with a history of being an excellent reader in the past, but not recently because of her symptoms. She mentioned that she was able to read on a college level when she was in junior high school.

At the first visit further history indicated that Mary had an eye examination 1 year before. Accommodative rock training was recommended at that time, but this was not carried out. She reported that her mother has intermittent exotropia. There is no other remarkable eye health history in her family. Medical health history for her and her family was negative, with the exception that there is hypertension on her father's side of the family. Mary's blood pressure was normal.

First Visit

Subjective refraction was O.D. plano -0.25 x 180 20/15-1/6; O.S. plano 20/15-1/6.

Mary has $\frac{1}{2}^\Delta$ exophoria at farpoint and 5^Δ exophoria at nearpoint. Base-in to break at far was 5^Δ, and recovery was 3^Δ. Base-in to blur at near was 10^Δ, to break 16^Δ, and to recover 4^Δ. Base-out to blur at far was 4^Δ, to break 9^Δ, and to recover 8^Δ. Base-out to blur at near was 12^Δ, to break 18^Δ, and to recover 6^Δ. Vergence ranges were considered to be slightly below normal.

Accommodative amplitude of the right eye was 11.00D, but was only 8.50D for the left eye. Negative relative accommodation was $+1.75$D, and the positive relative accommodation was -5.25D. Accommodative facility with ±2.00D was 15 cycles per minute O.D., O.S., and binocularly. Accommodative skills were considered fairly normal with the exception of insufficient amplitude of the left eye. The cause of less accommodative amplitude of the left eye could not be explained on any organic basis.

Mary appeared to have problems with saccadic eye movements. She scored an equivalent age of about 10 years on the Pierce Saccade Test. (Refer to Chapter Fifteen.) A problem with position maintenance and saccadic eye movements could also be seen on the results of Eye-Trac® testing. Her nearpoint of convergence was normal, being 2 cm from the bridge of the nose.

To summarize, on the first visit Mary seemed to have a significant problem with saccadic eye movements, possible accommodative insufficiency of the left eye, and possible vergence insufficiency and poor facility. Prescribed home vision therapy consisted of monocular pencil push-ups (to work on accommodative amplitude) for 5 minutes per day.

The second visit was approximately 2 months later. Accommodative facility was tested and found to be 21 cycles per minute for the right eye, 19 for the left eye, and 17 under binocular viewing conditions, using ±2.50D. These values are within normal limits. Base-out to blur on the Vodnoy Aperture Rule Trainer was 20^Δ.

Second Visit

---

[a]Camuccio, D., and J.R. Griffin: Visual Skills Therapy: A Case Report. *Optom. Monthly*, 73(2), pp. 94-96, Feb. 1982.

Home training was prescribed as follows:

1. Monocular pencil push-ups, right eye 5 minutes/day, and left eye 5 minutes/day.
2. Binocular pencil push-ups 5 minutes/day.
3. Accommodative rock using +2.50D: monocularly right eye 5 minutes/day and left eye 5 minutes/day, binocularly 5 minutes/day.
4. Landolt C charts and star-like charts for saccadic eye movement training (identification of the direction of open portion of C's) for 5 minutes/day. (Refer to Figure 2-21 in Chapter Two and Figure 7-5 in Chapter Seven.)

Third Visit   The third visit was 1 week later, and Mary reported doing her home therapy faithfully, with no problems doing the tasks except for occasionally having trouble seeing clearly with the plus lenses during accommodative rock.

Mary was able to converge greater than 33^Δ with clear, single vision on the Aperture Rule Trainer, and she could diverge 16^Δ with clear, single vision using the Polachrome Orthopter. Saccadic eye movements were judged normal on the Pierce Saccade Test.

Prescribed home therapy consisted of the following:

1. Eccentric Circles (Keystone) combined with Hart Chart (Figure 15-24 in Chapter Fifteen) 5 minutes/day. She was instructed on how to do chiastopic fusion at near with the circles and to shift fixation to the farpoint Hart Chart to read successive Snellen letters, thus working on fusional convergence, accommodative facility, and saccadic eye movements in this procedure.
2. Michigan Tracking pages (Figure 15-20 in Chapter Fifteen) for saccadic training, 5 minutes/day.
3. Circling vowels in newspaper print along with "dive bombing" them with the pencil from above, i.e., quick pointing (fast pointing).

Fourth Visit   Mary reported at the fourth visit that she noticed improvement during the previous week from home training. Office therapy included work with the La Barge Electro Therapist (Figure 15-10 in Chapter Fifteen) for saccadic eye movement training. She was able to fuse with clearness and singleness on the Vodnoy Aperture Rule Trainer over 30^Δ base-out and 22^Δ base-in.

Our impression is that Mary showed excellent compliance with home and office training and is a highly motivated VT patient.

Home therapy prescribed was the following:

1. Orthopic and chiastopic fusion (vergence rock) in free space, 5 minutes/day. This was at nearpoint and for the purpose of improving both vergence sufficiency (ranges) and facility.
2. Procedure 1 combined with shifts of fixation to a farpoint Hart Chart, 5 minutes/day.
3. Combination of procedure 1 with Landolt C chart, 5 minutes/day.
4. Michigan Tracking activities continued 5 minutes/day.

Fifth Visit   The fifth visit was 3 weeks later. Using the "SOAP" format (i.e., subjective, objective, analysis, plan), we found the following results:

S: There were no subjective complaints. Mary is doing a great deal of reading in college and has experienced no headaches or pain in the eye for the past few weeks. She reported "noticing a greatly increased reading speed."

O: Phorometry: Orthophoria at farpoint, 5^Δ exo at nearpoint. Base-in at farpoint was x/5/4; base-in at nearpoint was 20/24/18. Base-out at farpoint was 14/24/12; base-out at nearpoint was 18/24/18. Accommodative amplitude was 11.00D O.D. and 11.00D O.S. Nearpoint of convergence was 2 cm. Keystone Eccentric Circles, 55^Δ base-out with chiastopic fusion, and 37^Δ base-in with orthopic fusion in free space at nearpoint. Eye-Trac® revealed an apparent great improvement in eye movements with fewer regressions during saccades, better return sweeps, and improved position maintenance.

A: All subjective and objective problems seem to have abated.

P: Mary was dismissed for 6 months. However, she was put on a "maintenance" program with the following home vision therapy being prescribed:

1. Pencil push-ups, monocular and binocular, 5 minutes/week.
2. Binocular pencil saccades (two pencils), 5 minutes/week.
3. Keystone Eccentric Circles for orthopic-chiastopic vergence rock with fixation shifts to a farpoint Hart Chart, 5 minutes/week.

List of Equipment Suppliers

Alfred P. Poll, Inc., 40 W. 55th St., New York, NY 10019

Allbee and Son Co., 515 Washington St., Box 177, Waterloo, IA 50704

Allied Ophthalmic Products Co., c/o Fred Marvin, P.O. Box 71, 1923 Elmore Rd., Downers Grove, IL 60515

American Optical Corp., 14 Mechanic St., Southbridge, MA 01550; or American Optical Corp., Scientific Instrument Division, Buffalo, NY 14215

Ann Arbor Publishers, Inc., P.O. Box 7249, Naples, FL 33940

Archer-Elliott Ltd., 8–9 Spring Place, Kentish Town, London NW5, England

Dr. George Ariyasu, 8783 Parthenia Pl., Sepulveda, CA 91343

AV Scientific Aids, 12601 Industry St., Garden Grove, CA 92641

Bernell Corp., 422 East Monroe St., South Bend, IN 46601

Clement Clarke, Instrument Division, 15 Wigmore St., London, W1H 9LA, England

Cook Inc., P.O. Box 498, Bloomington, IN 47401; Pierce Saccade Test, V.P.R., Route 2, Box 174-W, McCalla, AL 35111

Creative Associates, *see* Efficient Seeing Publications

Efficient Seeing Publications (formerly Creative Associates), 7510 Soquel Dr., Aptos, CA 95003

G&W Applied Science Laboratories, 335 Bear Hill Rd., Waltham, MA 02154

Highlights for Children, 2300 W. Fifth Ave., Columbus, OH 43216

IMED, 1520 Cotner Ave., Los Angeles, CA 90025

Keeler Optical Products, Inc., 456 Parkway, Broomall, PA 19008

Keystone View Division of Mast/Keystone, 2212 E. 12th St., Davenport, IA 52803

Lafayette Instrument Co., Box 5729, North 9th St. and Sagamore Pkwy., Lafayette, IN 47903

Manico, P.O. Box 395, Clute, TX 77531

Mentor, Division of Codman and Shurtleff, Inc., Randolph, MA 02368

Minnesota Manufacturing and Mining Co., 3M Center, St. Paul, MN 55101

Multimedia Center, University of California, School of Optometry, Berkeley, CA 94720

Neitz Instruments Co. Ltd., 20–10 San-Eicho, Shinjuku-Ku, Tokyo 160, Japan

New York Association of the Blind (Lighthouse), Low Vision Services, 111 E. 59th St., New York, NY 10022

Oculus Products, Dutenhofen, Kr. Wetzlar, West Germany

The Ohio State University College of Optometry, Columbus, OH 43210

Omega Instrument Co. Inc., 215 E. 37th St., New York, NY 10016

Ophthalmix, La Grange, IL 60525

Optical Science Group, 24 Tiburon St., San Rafael, CA 94901

Rader Child Development Products, Dr. Kenneth Rader, 5623 S. Lewis, Tulsa, OK 74105

Stereo Optical Company, Inc., 3539 N. Kenton Ave., Chicago, IL 60641

Stewart Film Screen Corp., 1161 W. Sepulveda Blvd., Torrance, CA 90502

Titmus Optical Co., Inc., P.O. Box 191, Petersburg, VA 23803

Transilwrap Co., 2740 N. 4th St., Philadelphia, PA 19133

Vision Analysis, P.O. Box 14390, Columbus, OH 43214

Visual Data Corp., 11917 Borman Dr., St. Louis, MO 63141

Wayne Engineering, Orthoptic Division, 4120 Greenwood, Skokie, IL 60076

Western Optical, 1200 Mercer St., Seattle, WA 98109

Self-Assessment Test in Vision Therapy of Binocular Anomalies

Questions 1–20 pertain to the diagnosis of a deviation of the visual axes, 21–30 to the diagnosis of anomalous retinal correspondence, 31–40 to the diagnosis of amblyopia and eccentric fixation, 41–50 to the testing of stereopsis and evaluation of suppression, 51–60 to prognosis in strabismus, 61–70 to vision therapy for conditions commonly associated with strabismus, 71–80 to motoric aspects of vision therapy for eso and exo deviations, 81–90 to efficiency of visual skills, and 91–100 to miscellaneous new considerations and methods in the evaluation of therapy of binocular anomalies.

Questions

1. The diagnostic variables of strabismus associated with frequency are constant and _____; with eye laterality they are _____ and _____.
   a. alternating; unilateral, intermittent
   b. unilateral; intermittent, alternating
   c. alternating; intermittent, unilateral
   d. unilateral; alternating, intermittent
   e. intermittent; unilateral, alternating

2. An esotropic patient has 12^Δ strabismus at far and near. Cosmesis would be favored if the patient had _____.
   a. a positive angle kappa and a narrow bridge of the nose
   b. a wide face and a negative angle kappa
   c. a positive angle kappa and a wide bridge of the nose
   d. a negative angle kappa and a wide bridge of the nose
   e. a negative angle kappa and a narrow bridge of the nose

3. The most important diagnositc variable of the deviation to be evaluated in strabismus is _____, and the second is _____.
   a. frequency, magnitude
   b. concomitancy, magnitude
   c. eye laterality, frequency
   d. concomitancy, frequency
   e. direction of deviation, magnitude

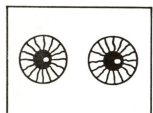

FIGURE 1

4. You do the Hirschberg test on a patient with constant strabismus whose right eye is dominant. (See sketch of the results in Figure 1.) Assume the pupillary width is 4 mm in diameter. The strabismus is estimated as _____.
   a. 22^Δ of esotropia
   b. 22^Δ of exotropia
   c. 44^Δ of exotropia
   d. 44^Δ of esotropia
   e. orthotropia (patient has proper alignment of the visual axes but is suppressing one eye)

5. Strabismus is defined as having a magnitude as small as _____.
   a. 1 minute of arc
   b. 1 degree of arc
   c. 1^Δ
   d. 2^Δ
   e. 2 degrees of arc

6. The comparison of the primary and secondary angles found on the alternate cover test is a test for _____.

   a. eye laterality
   b. nonconcomitancy
   c. eccentric fixation
   d. both a and b
   e. both b and c

7. A disjunctive movement resulting from the four-prism test indicates _____.

   a. first-degree fusion
   b. heterophoria
   c. heterotropia
   d. nonconcomitancy
   e. all of the above

8. Which of the following is true?

   a. nonconcomitancy means there is paresis
   b. paresis probably means there is concomitancy
   c. nonconcomitancy means there is either palsy, paresis, or paralysis
   d. all of the above
   e. none of the above

9. A patient has a paresis of the right superior rectus. The head posture would be _____.

   a. face down and to the left, with head tilt to the left
   b. face up and to the right, with head tilt to the left
   c. face down and to the right, with head tilt to the right
   d. face up and to the right, with head tilt to the right
   e. face down and to the left, with head tilt to the right

10. In the three-step method, the patient has a left hypertropia (LHT) that increases on dextroversion and further increases on right head tilt (Bielschowsky's head tilt test). The suspected isolated paretic extraocular muscle is the _____.

    a. left superior rectus (LSR)
    b. right superior rectus (RSR)
    c. left superior oblique (LSO)
    d. left inferior rectus (LIR)
    e. right inferior oblique (RIO)

11. A "monofixation pattern" would probably be related to the following condition: _____.

    a. $5^\triangle$ of esotropia without foveal fusion and without peripheral fusion
    b. $5^\triangle$ of esotropia without foveal fusion but with peripheral fusion
    c. $15^\triangle$ of esotropia without foveal fusion
    d. $20^\triangle$ of esotropia without foveal fusion
    e. $15^\triangle$ of esophoria with a fixation disparity manifest deviation that is greater than zero but less than $1^\triangle$ magnitude

12. A good sequence of procedures for the detection of strabismus is _____.

    a. direct observation, listening to the history, the Hirschberg test, 4 base-out prism test, unilateral cover test
    b. listening to the history, direct observation, the Hirschberg test, 4 base-out prism test

c. listening to the history, direct observation, unilateral cover test, the Hirschberg test, 4 base-out prism test

d. listening to the history, the Hirschberg test, direct observation, unilateral cover test, 4 base-out prism test

e. listening to the history, direct observation, the Hirschberg test, unilateral cover test, 4 base-out prism test

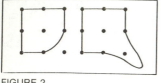

FIGURE 2

13. The Hess-Lancaster results from a complaining patient are shown in Figure 2. You would expect past pointing on _____.

a. dextroinfraduction
b. levoinfraduction
c. dextroinfraversion
d. levoinfraversion
e. dextroversion

14. The patient in Question 13 is 8 years old. Your case history would immediately center around questions of _____.

a. vascular disease
b. viral disease
c. obstetrics trauma causing nonconcomitancy
d. faulty muscle insertion
e. accommodation infacility

15. The affected extraocular muscle (Question 13) was probably the _____ and the condition was a _____.

a. right inferior rectus (RIR), faulty muscle insertion
b. left superior oblique (LSO), faulty muscle insertion
c. RIR, paresis
d. LSO, paresis
e. left inferior rectus (LIR), paresis

16. A patient has an amblyopic left eye with a +0.5 mm angle kappa and a right eye with a +1 mm angle kappa. The type of deviation is _____.

a. esotropia of the left eye
b. eccentric fixation of both eyes, but more central in the left eye
c. nasal eccentric fixation of the left eye
d. nasal eccentric fixation of the right eye
e. esotropia of the right eye

17. The patient in Question 16 has a true angle H of 22^Δ of esotropia. On alternate cover testing you would expect to measure _____.

a. ortho
b. 11^Δ eso
c. 22^Δ eso
d. 33^Δ eso
e. 44^Δ eso

18. The patient in Question 16 has normal correspondence and is tested with the Maddox rod. His subjective angle (angle S) would be _____.

a. ortho
b. 11^Δ eso
c. 22^Δ eso
d. 33^Δ eso
e. 44^Δ eso

19. The patient in Question 16 is given the phi phenomenon test via rapid alternate cover testing. You would expect to measure _____.

    a. ortho
    b. 11^Δ eso
    c. 22^Δ eso
    d. 33^Δ eso
    e. 44^Δ eso

20. An esotropic patient has 20^Δ eso on supraversion and 10^Δ eso on infraversion. This is an example of _____.

    a. "A" pattern esotropia
    b. "V" pattern esotropia
    c. periodic esotropia
    d. esotropia with anomalous retinal correspondence
    e. concomitant esotropia

21. Patient #21 views a penlight from a distance of 1 meter and reports perception of homonymous (uncrossed) diplopia of the light. The two images are separated by a distance of 18 cm. Upon alternate cover testing, the eye movement is neutralized with an 18^Δ base-out loose prism. Assume the patient has 20/20 acuity in each eye. The type of retinal correspondence indicated is _____.

    a. harmonious
    b. unharmonious, typical type
    c. unharmonious, atypical paradoxical, type 1
    d. unharmonious, atypical paradoxical, type 2
    e. normal

22. Patient #22 sees the same diplopia as Patient #21. On alternate cover testing, however, the eye movement is neutralized with 38^Δ base-out. The type of correspondence indicated for Patient #22 is _____.

    a. harmonious
    b. unharmonious, typical type
    c. unharmonious, atypical paradoxical, type 1
    d. unharmonious, atypical paradoxical, type 2
    e. normal

23. Patient #23 gives the same diplopic response as Patients #21 and #22. However, on cover testing you discover the patient has 23^Δ of exotropia. The type of correspondence suggested here is _____.

    a. harmonious
    b. unharmonious, typical type
    c. unharmonious, atypical paradoxical, type 1
    d. unharmonious, atypical paradoxical, type 2
    e. normal

24. Patient #24 has an esotropia of 8^Δ as found via the cover test. On subjective testing, however, this patient has the same diplopic response as Patients #21, #22, and #23. The type of retinal correspondence indicated here is _____.

    a. harmonious
    b. unharmonious, typical type
    c. unharmonious, atypical paradoxical, type 1
    d. unharmonious, atypical paradoxical, type 2
    e. normal

25. Patient #25 has a subjective angle of directionalization (angle S) of zero, although his esotropic angle (H) is 8^Δ. Correspondence in this case is _____.

    a. harmonious
    b. unharmonious, typical type
    c. unharmonious, atypical paradoxical, type 1
    d. unharmonious, atypical paradoxical, type 2
    e. normal

26. Suppose you see Patient #25 and perform the Hering-Bielschowsky afterimage test. The right eye is the esotropic eye. The fixating left eye gets the horizontal afterimage, and the deviating right eye gets the vertical afterimage. The patient's response to this afterimage would be the following configuration: _____.

    a. perfect cross
    b. vertical line displaced 8^Δ to the right of the center
    c. vertical line displaced 8^Δ to the left of the center
    d. vertical line displaced 16^Δ to the right of the center
    e. vertical line displaced 16^Δ to the left of the center

27. Patient #27 has 8^Δ nasal eccentric fixation of the right eye. He also has an esotropia of the right eye of 8^Δ and harmonious anomalous retinal correspondence (HARC). His response to the Hering-Bielschowsky afterimage test would be _____.

    a. perfect cross
    b. vertical line displaced 8^Δ to the right of the center
    c. vertical line displaced 8^Δ to the left of the center
    d. vertical line displaced 16^Δ to the right of the center
    e. vertical line displaced 16^Δ to the left of the center

28. You perform the alternate cover test with neutralizing prisms on Patient #27. The response would be _____.

    a. ortho (no movement)
    b. 8^Δ of esotropia
    c. 8^Δ of exotropia
    d. 16^Δ of esotropia
    e. 16^Δ of exotropia

29. Suppose you place Patient #27 in a Synoptophore® (major amblyoscope). What subjective angle of directionalization would you expect to find?

    a. ortho
    b. 8^Δ base-out
    c. 8^Δ base-in
    d. 16^Δ base-out
    e. 16^Δ base-in

30. You perform the Bagolini striated lens test on Patient #27. The expected report of the patient would be _____.

    a. intersection of lines on the fixation light (ortho response)
    b. intersection of lines above the fixation light by 8^Δ
    c. intersection of lines below the fixation light by 8^Δ
    d. intersection of lines above the fixation light by 16^Δ
    e. intersection of lines below the fixation light by 16^Δ

31. In performing the Hirschberg test, you observe the eyes of your patient, a young

child, as shown in Figure 1. The right eye is the fixating eye. What is the angle kappa of each eye?

a. O.D. +1 mm, O.S. +1 mm
b. O.D. +1 mm, O.S. +2 mm
c. O.D. +1 mm, O.S. −1 mm
d. O.D. −1 mm, O.S. unknown
e. O.D. +1 mm, O.S. unknown

32. Suppose for the patient in Question #31, the light reflection for the left eye under monocular conditions is in the same place as is shown in Figure 1. The condition would therefore be _____.

a. temporal eccentric fixation of the right eye
b. nasal eccentric fixation of the right eye
c. temporal eccentric fixation of the left eye
d. nasal eccentric fixation of the left eye
e. central fixation of the left eye

33. The test designed for detecting eccentric fixation by means of comparison of angles kappa is known as the _____.

a. Bangerter test
b. Cüppers test
c. Worth test
d. Hirschberg test
e. Krimsky test

34. A patient has nasal eccentric fixation of the right eye of 3 degrees. Haidinger's brushes testing is done at a distance of 40 cm, at which a small black spot is fixated. The patient would be expected to report seeing the brushes approximately _____.

a. 20 mm to the right of the spot
b. 20 mm to the left of the spot
c. superimposed on the spot
d. 5 mm to the right of the spot
e. 5 mm to the left of the spot

35. An estimated visual acuity can be calculated (according to the formula of Flom[2]) for an amblyopic eye with eccentric fixation. What would this be for a patient with 1 degree of eccentric fixation?

a. 20/35
b. 20/45
c. 20/55
d. 20/65
e. 20/75

36. The distance from the center of the fovea to the center of the optic disc is 15.5 degrees. The doctor sees the Visuscope star approximately halfway between the center of the disc and the center of the fovea, while the patient reports superimposition of the star with a fixation target. This indicates _____.

a. a nasal angle of eccentric fixation of approximately 8 degrees
b. a temporal angle of eccentric fixation of approximately 8 degrees
c. an angle of anomaly of zero

d. an angle of anomaly of approximately 15.5 degrees

e. none of the above

37. For a patient with an angle of eccentric fixation (angle E) of 1 degree, you must predict that this patient will have visual acuity of that eye that is _____.

a. 20/30

b. 20/55

c. either fair or poor

d. between 20/30 and 20/55

e. between 20/20 and 20/30

38. According to this text, if the eccentric fixation point (point "e") is on the nasal retina 2 degrees from the center of the fovea, the magnitude of the angle of eccentric fixation (angle E) is considered to be _____.

a. foveal

b. foveal off-center

c. parafoveal

d. paramacular

e. peripheral

39. Cüppers modified the ophthalmoscope for testing purposes by adding a graticule to project and to focus a star pattern onto the fundus. This instrument is known as the _____, and monocular testing is _____.

a. Euthyscope, visuoscopy for anomalous correspondence

b. Visuscope, visuoscopy for eccentric fixation

c. Projectoscope, visuoscopy for anomalous correspondence

d. Euthyscope, visuoscopy for eccentric fixation

e. Visuscope, visuoscopy for anomalous correspondence

40. Which type of amblyopia is not classified as being functional?

a. nutritional amblyopia

b. isoametropic amblyopia

c. anisometropic amblyopia

d. strabismic amblyopia

e. hysterical amblyopia

41. You perform the 4 base-out prism test on a patient and find no eye movement when the prism is placed before the patient's left eye, but a conjugate (version) movement when the prism is placed before the right eye. You would suspect your patient has _____.

a. heterophoria with suppression of the right eye

b. heterotropia with suppression of the right eye

c. heterotropia with suppression of the left eye

d. heterotropia with suppression of both eyes

e. heterophoria without suppression

42. Suppose a patient shows an eye movement on the alternate cover test and also shows a vergence when a 4 base-out prism is placed before either eye. You would suspect the patient has _____.

a. heterophoria with suppression of either eye

b. heterotropia with suppression of the right eye

c. heterotropia with suppression of the left eye

d. heterotropia with suppression of both eyes

   e. heterophoria without suppression of either eye

43. A patient has been sent to you from a colleague for a strabismus evaluation. The patient is reported to have "suppression." Based on the naturalness of testing conditions, the test most likely to detect any evidence of suppression would be _____.

   a. Pola-Mirror
   b. Brewster stereoscope and stereograms
   c. Wheatstone stereoscope and stereograms
   d. penlight with red-green filters
   e. Maddox rod test

44. Your patient states that "one eye appears blackened" on the Pola-Mirror test. According to Griffin and Lee,[3] you would suspect the patient's stereoacuity to be worse than _____.

   a. 20 seconds of arc
   b. 30 seconds of arc
   c. 40 seconds of arc
   d. 50 seconds of arc
   e. 60 seconds of arc

45. Suppression may be evaluated in either the Brewster stereoscope or the Wheatstone stereoscope using sensory targets classified as _____.

   a. simultaneous perception
   b. superimposition
   c. flat fusion
   d. stereopsis
   e. all of the above

46. Your patient has 40 seconds of arc stereoacuity. You are requested to state this in terms of percentage of stereopsis. This would be _____.

   a. 72 percent
   b. 78 percent
   c. 95 percent
   d. 100 percent
   e. 106 percent

47. Bar reading and Turville balance testing can be used at near and far, respectively, for testing of suppression. This involves _____.

   a. simultaneous perception
   b. superimposition
   c. flat fusion
   d. stereopsis
   e. all of the above

48. A child with a newly acquired strabismus may have diplopia and/or confusion in his visual space. To eliminate such annoyances, he may first develop _____.

   a. amblyopia
   b. anomalous retinal correspondence
   c. eccentric fixation
   d. horror fusionis
   e. suppression

49. Your patient has an esotropic right eye and suppression. According to Jampolsky,[5]

an ophthalmoscopic view of the zone of suppression would resemble a _____.

a. football, horizontal dimension larger than vertical
b. football, vertical dimension larger than horizontal
c. basketball
d. letter "D"
e. reversed letter "D"

50. Assume the suppression zone extends 8 degrees from the fovea to point zero. The suppression would be classified according to size as _____.

a. peripheral
b. paramacular
c. parafoveal
d. foveal
e. center of the fovea

CASE HISTORY A

The deviation is a concomitant, constant, unilateral exotropia of the right eye of 25^Δ at far and 15^Δ at near with a high AC/A ratio (10/1). Cosmesis is poor due to the magnitude of the deviation and to a large positive angle kappa ($+1\frac{1}{2}$ mm). The associated conditions include deep peripheral suppression; deep amblyopia; unsteady, temporal, parafoveal, eccentric fixation; typical, unharmonious, anomalous correspondence; and no motor fusion. The 10-year-old patient has a history of exotropia of the right eye. Onset was intermittent from 7 months through 1 year of age. The strabismus has been constant since then. Direct patching was attempted for a few weeks at age 3, but only token occlusion was accomplished. No other treatment has been given since. Refraction is

O.D. $-1.00 -1.00 \times 180$ 20/100
O.S. Plano 20/20

There is no history of strabismus in the family.

51. Certain favorable factors in the prognosis for a functional cure can be found in the diagnosis of Case History A. Examples of these favorable factors are _____.

a. no family history of strabismus, concomitant deviation, and exo direction of the deviation
b. no family history of strabismus, constant deviation, and exo direction of the deviation
c. no family history of strabismus, concomitant deviation, and constant deviation
d. constant deviation, concomitant deviation, and patient's age (10 years old)
e. exo direction of the deviation, concomitant deviation, and patient's age (10 years old)

52. Unfavorable factors in the prognosis for a functional cure of strabismus in Case History A would be _____.

a. anomalous correspondence (A R C)
b. constant strabismus
c. concomitant deviation
d. both a and b
e. both a and c

53. Flom[6] presented a schema for the prognosis of esotropia and exotropia relating each type of strabismus to the factors of constancy of the deviation and the type of retinal correspondence. According to this model, you would predict the chance for a functional cure for Case History A by all means of vision therapy to be about _____.

    a. 5 percent, constant esotropia with A R C
    b. 20 percent, constant exotropia with A R C
    c. 35 percent, constant exotropia with N R C
    d. 50 percent, intermittent exotropia with A R C
    e. 60 percent, intermittent exotropia with N R C

54. A five-point qualitative prognosis range (Table 5C) was advocated and a case similar to Case History A was discussed in the "Case Studies" section of Chapter Five. Looking at the case as a whole, the qualitative judgment as to prognosis for a functional cure would be _____.

    a. poor (equivalent to approximately 10 percent)
    b. poor to fair (approximately 30 percent)
    c. fair (approximately 50 percent)
    d. fair to good (approximately 70 percent)
    e. good (approximately 90 percent)

55. Age at strabismus onset is another important factor to consider in the prognosis for functional cure. Considering Case History A, the prognosis would be affected _____.

    a. unfavorably because of congenital strabismus
    b. favorably because of congenital strabismus
    c. unfavorably because of late-acquired strabismus
    d. favorably because of late-acquired strabismus
    e. possibly favorably, early-acquired strabismus notwithstanding

CASE HISTORY B

The deviation is concomitant (except for a slight V pattern), intermittent (10 percent at far and 80 percent at near), alternating (O.D. dominant) esotropia of 5^Δ at far and 10^Δ at near. There is a high AC/A ratio (8/1) and good cosmesis. Variability of the basic deviation was undetermined at this one visit, but the magnitude appeared to remain stable during the visit. Associated conditions include intermittent, alternating, parafoveal suppression (mostly O.S.); eso fixation disparity (associated heterophoria of 2^Δ eso); and probably normal correspondence. (N R C response was elicited with afterimages and on the major amblyoscope, but an A R C response was found occasionally on the Bagolini test.) The motor fusion range was poor, 2 base-in to break to 10 base-out to break. The base-in recovery was "negative." Stereoacuity with or without trial plus adds was 125 seconds of arc. The patient is 8 years old and loves to read, but complains of headaches. Refraction is

O.D. +0.50 20/25
O.S. +0.50 20/25

As to history of strabismus in the family, the patient's father and paternal grandmother have esotropia.

56. Favorable factors in the prognosis for a functional cure can be found in the diagnosis of Case History B. An example of such factors is _____.

    a. concomitant deviation
    b. intermittent strabismus
    c. family history of strabismus
    d. status of motivation
    e. all of the above

57. Unfavorable factors relating to the prognosis for a functional cure of strabismus in Case History B would be _____.

    a. concomitant deviation
    b. intermittent strabismus
    c. family history of strabismus
    d. both a and b
    e. none of the above

58. The prognostic schema of Flom[6] would predict the chance for functional cure for Case History B by all means of vision therapy to be about _____.

    a.   0 percent
    b.   5 percent
    c. 20 percent
    d. 35 percent
    e. 50 percent

59. A range of values as to prognosis can be made by looking at Case History B as a whole. An appropriate judgment on the prognosis for a functional cure would be _____.

    a. 0 percent
    b. poor to fair (approximately 30 percent)
    c. fair (approximately 50 percent)
    d. fair to good (approximately 70 percent)
    e. 100 percent

60. Age of strabismus onset is another important factor to consider in the prognosis for functional cure. Considering Case History B, the prognosis would be affected _____.

    a. unfavorably because of congenital strabismus
    b. favorably because of congenital strabismus
    c. unfavorably because of early-acquired strabismus
    d. favorably because of late-acquired strabismus
    e. possibly favorably, early-acquired strabismus notwithstanding.

61. More than 100 years ago, Javal advocated certain procedures for treatment of cases of strabismus. The first step was the correction of refractive errors. Next was to eliminate amblyopia by means of occlusion. However, even when the amblyopic condition was cured, occlusion was continued for the prevention of _____.

    a. esotropia
    b. exotropia
    c. fixation disparity
    d. accommodation infacility
    e. suppression

62. You examine an infant who has constant, unilateral esotropia and is suspected of

having functional amblyopia of the left eye. *Initially,* the recommended occlusion therapy would be _____.

   a. direct, for the first day
   b. inverse (indirect)
   c. a patch to be worn over the right (not left) eye, for the first day
   d. both a and c
   e. both b and c

63. You consider prescribing occlusion for the infant patient in Question 62. The preferable scheduling of patching for the first few weeks of therapy would be a _____.

   a. constant, unilateral, and opaque occluder
   b. periodic, unilateral, and opaque occluder
   c. constant, alternating, and opaque occluder
   d. periodic, unilateral, and attenuating occluder
   e. constant, alternating, and attenuating occluder

64. The therapeutic regimen originated by Bangerter for curing amblyopia would include _____.

   a. dazzling the eccentric fixation point
   b. stimulating the fovea (previously protected by a shadow) with flashes of light
   c. creating a negative afterimage with the fovea having been protected by a shadow
   d. both a and b
   e. both a and c

65. You examine a patient who has intermittent exotropia of 28^Δ at far and near. Anomalous retinal correspondence (A R C) is elicited, but only when the exo deviation is manifested. Occlusion therapy would most likely be _____.

   a. advised to eliminate suppression
   b. advised to eliminate A R C
   c. advised to prevent the exo deviation from becoming manifest, rather than latent
   d. both a and b
   e. not advisable

66. Therapy for an individual who has constant esotropia with A R C may include _____.

   a. occlusion
   b. prism overcorrection (e.g., with Fresnel prisms)
   c. major amblyoscopic procedures
   d. use of luster
   e. all of the above

67. You find that a patient has suppression of the left eye. A procedure to avoid at the start of antisuppression therapy would be the use of _____.

   a. a small target before the left eye
   b. a dim target before the left eye
   c. a nonmoving target before the left eye
   d. low-contrast and colorless targets
   e. all of the above

68. Bi-ocular antisuppression procedures should be considered somewhere during the course of strabismus therapy and may include _____.

   a. monocular occlusion

b. physiological diplopia awareness
c. pathological diplopia awareness
d. both a and b
e. both b and c

69. You see a patient who has deep suppression. Several approaches may be used in antisuppression therapy:

1. colored filters (e.g., red-green)
2. diplopia of natural objects in free space
3. septums with optical systems (e.g., Brewster's stereoscope)
4. vectographic targets

Theoretically, the best sequencing for therapy would be _____.

a. 1, 2, 3, 4
b. 2, 3, 4, 1
c. 2, 4, 3, 1
d. 1, 3, 4, 2
e. 4, 3, 2, 1

70. Whenever there is strabismus—either constant or intermittent—therapy should be considered for any associated conditions such as _____.

a. suppression, A R C, and horror fusionis
b. amblyopia and abnormal fixation
c. accommodation infacility
d. poor fusional vergences and fixation disparity
e. all of the above

71. A patient has esotropia on right lateral gaze that is the result of an automobile accident with apparent VI cranial nerve damage causing paresis of the right lateral rectus. Therapy you should consider is _____.

a. alternate occlusion
b. unilateral occlusion
c. ocular calisthenics
d. both a and c
e. both b and c

72. A patient has 18^Δ of constant esotropia at far. Initially, functional training procedures may be done with the major amblyoscope. The most appropriate targets should be for _____, and the setting of the tubes of the major amblyoscope should be at _____.

a. flat fusion, the objective angle of strabismus
b. superimposition, the objective angle of strabismus
c. flat fusion, 18^Δ base-out demand
d. superimposition, ortho
e. both a and c

73. An ideal goal to achieve in the training of motor fusion is the Sheard criterion. For example, your patient has an intermittent esotropia of 8^Δ and has poor motor fusion ranges. You would attempt to expand the _____ range with your patient's having single, _____ binocular vision to _____ prism diopters.

a. base-in, clear, 16
b. base-out, clear, 16
c. base-in, blurred, 8

d. base-out, blurred, 8

e. base-in, clear, 8

74. For another patient, you use the Rémy separator with a fixation distance of 40 cm and a target separation (laterally displaced) of 6 cm. To fuse these targets, the patient would have to meet a _____ demand of _____ prism diopters. This would be a good procedure to use in _____ deviations, either heterotropia or heterophoria.

a. base-in, 0, eso

b. base-out, 0, eso

c. base-in, 0, exo

d. base-out, 15, exo

e. base-in, 15, eso

75. Assume you have a patient who has a 6 cm interpupillary distance and a constant esotropia of 15^Δ at 6 meters. You wish to do some testing and training at the patient's centration point to determine what sensory fusion abilities are present. For this procedure, the patient would wear a _____ diopter addition over each eye and view a test target from a distance of _____ cm.

a.   0, 15

b. +1.50, 40

c. −2.50, 40

d. +2.50, 40

e. +2.50, 15

76. Suppose a patient with divergence insufficiency has an esophoria of 2^Δ at 40 cm and 10^Δ intermittent esotropia at 6 meters. You use split vectograms at a fixation distance of 40 cm that are separated by 8^Δ base-in demand. The patient is to do fusion walk-aways from near to far fixation distances while maintaining fusion of the vectograms. This would help promote fusional _____, with the fusional demand being _____ when the patient moves from a near fixation distance to a far distance from the targets.

a. divergence, harder

b. divergence, the same

c. divergence, easier

d. convergence, easier

e. convergence, harder

77. There are various ways to promote increased fusional ranges of convergence and divergence. One is a stereoscopic training procedure using motion pictures in which the patient wears an appropriate vertical prism before one eye so that three images are seen—the top image by one eye, the middle image by both eyes, and the bottom image by the other eye. Specifically, this would be _____ fusion training.

a. chiastopic

b. orthopic

c. chiastopic-orthopic

d. Cine-Ortho™

e. vectographic

78. Your patient is orthophoric at 6 meters but 10^Δ esophoric at 40 cm. Difficulty in fusing would be expected with _____.

a. hand-held vectograms having a 15^Δ base-in demand

    b. hand-held vectograms having a 15^Δ base-out demand

    c. accommodation facility training (accommodative rock) with $\pm 2.00D$ lenses when the minus lenses are introduced

    d. both a and b

    e. both a and c

79. Patients who have high exotropic deviations at far distance as compared with relatively low exo deviations at near distance are classified as having _____, and optical treatment initially may be the use of _____ because of the effect of the _____ AC/A ratio in such cases.

    a. divergence excess, minus overcorrection at farpoint, high

    b. divergence insufficiency, plus overcorrection at nearpoint, low

    c. convergence insufficiency, minus overcorrection at farpoint, high

    d. convergence insufficiency, minus overcorrection at farpoint, high

    e. convergence insufficiency, plus overcorrection at nearpoint, high

80. An exophoric patient with convergence insufficiency would probably need fusional convergence training. A logical sequence of training procedures would be _____.

    a. chiastopic fusion, pencil push-ups, three-dot card

    b. three-dot card, chiastopic fusion, pencil push-ups

    c. pencil push-ups, three-dot card, chiastopic fusion

    d. pencil push-ups, chiastopic fusion, three-dot card

    e. three-dot card, pencil push-ups, chiastopic fusion

81. The goal in vision therapy is the patient's achievement of _____.

    a. clear binocular vision

    b. single binocular vision

    c. comfortable binocular vision

    d. efficient binocular vision

    e. all of the above

82. The sequence of emphasis in the practice of optometric vision therapy, from a historical perspective, is _____.

    a. clear, single, comfortable, efficient, binocular vision.

    b. efficient, clear, single, comfortable, binocular vision

    c. binocular, efficient, clear, single, comfortable vision

    d. comfortable, efficient, clear, single, binocular vision

    e. single, comfortable, efficient, clear, binocular vision

83. A normed test for saccadic eye movements in which a time score is obtained and in which the patient is asked to name single-digit numbers (two numbers for each line) is the _____.

    a. Eye-Trac® test

    b. Sequence Fixator test

    c. LaBarge Electro Therapist test

    d. Pierce Saccade test (indirectly assessing saccadic eye movements)

    e. Two-object gross saccade test (objects held in front of the patient at a distance of 40 cm and separated approximately 20 cm)

84. As a therapy goal for pursuit eye movements, the patient should be able to _____.

    a. have the right and left eye approximately equal in skill

b. achieve smooth (not jerky) pursuits

c. sustain good pursuit eye movements for a reasonable period (e.g., 1 minute of rotations) without breaking down into saccades

d. simultaneously perform cognitive tasks (e.g., number counting) without interfering with pursuit eye movements

e. all of the above

85. The Nott method[9] and the monocular estimate method (MEM) are both ways, _____, to estimate _____ lag, and one that is _____ may be of concern.

a. subjectively, vergence, 1^{Δ}

b. objectively, accommodative, $+1.00D$ or greater

c. subjectively, accommodative, $+1.00D$ or greater

d. objectively, vergence, 1^{Δ}

e. objectively, either accommodative or vergence, either $+1.00D$ or 1^{Δ}

86. Suppose a teenage patient has 20 cycles/minute on $\pm2.00D$ accommodative rock when tested monocularly. However, he has only 5 cycles/minute with lenses of the same power when tested binocularly. You suspect problems with _____.

a. fusional convergence

b. accommodative amplitude

c. accommodative lag

d. accommodative sustaining ability

e. tonic convergence

87. A logical set of criteria for vergence facility for either exophoria or esophoria can be advocated as a goal in therapy. This would be, in prism diopters, a range of _____.

a. 8 base-in to 8 base-out, 10 cycles/minute

b. 8 base-in to 12 base-out, 10 cycles/minute

c. 5 base-in to 15 base-out, 20 cycles/minute

d. 4 base-in to 8 base-out, 10 cycles/minute

e. 4 base-in to 8 base-out, 20 cycles/minute

88. On the vis-à-vis test, having the patient point to and name (right or left) your "black" eye is a test for _____.

a. directionality

b. monofixation pattern

c. suppression

d. foveal fusion

e. all of the above

89. A patient has fixation disparity. When possible, the goals in therapy are to _____.

a. increase the value on the ordinate (y-intercept) and flatten the fixation disparity curve

b. decrease the value on the ordinate (y-intercept) and steepen the fixation disparity curve

c. increase the value on the ordinate (y-intercept) and steepen the fixation disparity curve

d. decrease the value on the ordinate (y-intercept) and flatten the fixation disparity curve

e. decrease the value on the abscissa (x-intercept) and steepen the fixation disparity curve

90. Your patient has 50 seconds of arc stereoacuity. What is the percentage of stereopsis according to Shepard, using the formula of Fry?

    a. 50
    b. 72
    c. 78
    d. 95
    e. 100

91. A random dot type of test for stereopsis that has the "figure" on one side of a transparent Plexiglas plate and the "ground" on the other side and that does not require the patient to wear either polarizing or colored filters is the _____.

    a. Bernell Reindeer Stereotest
    b. Frisby Stereo Test
    c. Random Dot E Test
    d. Titmus Stereo Test (Fly)
    e. TNO Test

92. The stereopsis test(s) most likely to be certain to differentiate between heterophoria and heterotropia in young children would be the _____.

    a. Bernell Reindeer Stereotest
    b. Frisby Stereo Test
    c. Titmus Stereo Test (Fly)
    d. TNO Test
    e. Both a and c

93. The stereopsis test completely dependent upon changing of testing distance for various stereoacuity levels would be the _____.

    a. A.O. Vectographic Near Point Card No. 3
    b. Bernell Reindeer Stereotest
    c. Random Dot E Test
    d. Titmus Stereo Test (Fly)
    e. TNO Test

94. According to the concepts of Piaget, you could normally expect your 4-year-old patient in vision therapy to learn to perform _____.

    a. pencil push-ups, three-dot card, and free-space chiastopic fusion
    b. pencil push-ups, use of prisms and/or lenses to stimulate vergence, and three-dot card
    c. pencil push-ups and three-dot card only
    d. pencil push-ups only
    e. use of prisms and/or lenses to stimulate vergence only

95. A patient with intermittent exotropia might be expected to have a _____ identical-visual-direction horopter that is _____ toward the patient's eyes and _____ the Vieth-Mueller circle.

    a. flat, concave, inside
    b. steep, concave, inside
    c. flat, convex, outside
    d. steep, concave, outside
    e. steep, convex, inside

96. A patient has 15^Δ of constant esotropia of the right eye and harmonious anomalous (retinal) correspondence (A R C). The patient fixates a target 2 meters away while wearing colored filters, red over the right eye and green over the left eye. The three-light test (three lights positioned horizontally in a frontal plane) is performed at a distance of 1.5 meters from the patient and such that the central light is placed in in the "notch" of the identical-visual-direction horopter with the outer lights being to the left and right of the "notch." Your patient would be expected to be able to see a total of _____ lights.

a. two
b. three
c. four
d. five
e. six

97. Consider the identical-visual-direction horopter in five types of retinal correspondence in the case of a patient who has constant, unilateral esotropia. Assume the patient is fixating a target approximately 2 meters away. Five types of correspondence are listed as follows:

1. normal correspondence
2. harmonious correspondence
3. unharmonious anomalous correspondence (typical type)
4. paradoxical anomalous correspondence, type 1 (atypical unharmonious)
5. paradoxical anomalous correspondence, type 2 (atypical unharmonious)

Rank the horopters as to distance from the patient for the five types of correspondence above. Proceeding from the most distant to the nearest horopter, the rank order is

a. 5, 4, 2, 3, 1
b. 4, 2, 3, 1, 5
c. 2, 3, 1, 5, 4
d. 3, 1, 5, 4, 2
e. 1, 5, 4, 2, 3

98. The concept of checking the base-in and base-out ranges in which there is no _____ was recommended by Dr. Byron Newman.[22]

a. blur
b. diplopia
c. fixation disparity
d. suppression
e. discomfort

99. In vision training, _____ should be adequate to prevent consecutive strabismus in case there is a possibility of the patient undergoing subsequent extraocular muscle surgery.

a. fixation disparity range with angle F being zero
b. base-in to blur, break, and recovery
c. base-out to blur, break, and recovery
d. base-in and base-out to blur, break, and recovery
e. range of accommodative convergence without suppression

100. The goal in vision therapy is the patient's achievement of clear, single, comfortable, efficient, binocular vision in such activities as _____.

a. work

b. play
c. school
d. hobbies
e. all of the above

Answers

1. e. Frequency of strabismus is either constant (i.e., 100 percent of the time) or intermittent (i.e., from 1 to 99 percent of the time). Some authorities use the word *occasional* synonymously with *intermittent*.

2. a. A positive angle kappa (actually angle lambda) in a case like this gives the individual a less eso or more exo appearance, as an eye with a positive angle kappa is anatomically positioned outward (temporally) even though the eye may be centrally fixating in the primary position of gaze. Likewise, a narrow bridge of the nose gives a less eso appearance than would a wide bridge.

3. d. Acute diseases may cause the deviation to be nonconcomitant (e.g., hemorrhage, viral disease, or brain tumor). Since these may be life threatening, the evaluation of concomitancy is most important. Frequency is next in importance, because the prognosis for a functional cure is related (to a great extent) to the percentage of time the deviation is manifest.

4. d. Assume the light reflection is nasal by 1 mm ($+1$ mm). Assume the deviating (nonfixating) left eye has a reflection displaced 1 mm temporally (-1 mm). The 2 mm total equals 44^Δ (assuming 1 mm equals 22^Δ).

5. c. One prism diopter is about the smallest deviation that can practically be measured via the cover test. It is unlikely that a fixation disparity (at least in the central fovea) could exceed this value. Therefore, strabismus would exist, as true bifoveal fixation would not be in play. Such a patient would probably show evidence of a small central suppression.

6. b. Hering's law of equal innervation would cause the angles to be different in the right eye fixating versus the left eye. For example, if the right lateral rectus were paretic, more innervation would go to its yoke muscle, the left medial, causing an existing eso deviation to be larger with the right eye fixating than with the left.

7. b. Suppose your patient has heterophoria, say 6 exophoria, and is bifixating a target. Now, if a 4^Δ base-out prism is placed over an eye, a convergence (disjunctive movement) response will be expected. Actually the magnitude or direction of the heterophoria does not matter so long as there is foveal fusion (bifixation) during the test.

8. e. An individual may have a nonconcomitant deviation due to other conditions (e.g., a faulty muscle insertion or a mechanical restriction of eye movement).

9. b. A convenient rule to remember is that the abnormal head posture will be such that the face is directed toward the diagnostic action field of the affected extraocular muscle. In this case, the face would be up and to the right. Since the superior rectus muscle intorts, the face would be tilted toward the patient's left.

10. b. Paresis of the right superior rectus muscle would cause the right eye to be hypotropic (relative left hypertropic). On right gaze the hypotropia of the right eye would be worse, as the superior rectus becomes a "pure" elevator on abduction. A right head tilt would cause the other intorting muscle of the right eye, which

is the superior oblique, to come into play and further worsen the hypotropia deviation. Also, the yoke muscle of the right superior rectus is the left inferior oblique. The tilt would cause an overaction of the left inferior oblique (more left hypertropia) due to Hering's law.

11. b. The concept of a monofixation pattern was reported by Parks[1] and was previously called a "monofixational phoria." For example, a patient with a small-angle constant esotropia of 5^Δ will not have bifixation (foveal fusion). However, he may have peripheral fusion, as Panum's areas may be large enough in the extreme peripheral field to allow some sort of gross fusion. In many such individuals, the angle of eso deviation increases upon prolonged occlusion. The "latent" deviation was incorrectly called a "phoria." The patient was *esotropic,* not esophoric, although in clinical terms the additional eso deviation can be thought of as though there were an "esophoric" component.

Assume that the manifest deviation (esotropia) was measured via the prism and unilateral cover test to be 5^Δ eso. Now, on the alternate cover test with prism neutralization, the patient's eso deviation is found to be 15^Δ eso. The difference of 10^Δ represents the so-called phoria (latent deviation). As stated earlier, the use of "phoria" is not appropriate for this patient with the diagnosis of strabismus (as determined via the unilateral cover test). Therefore, such a condition was called a "monofixation syndrome" rather than a "phoria." However, the word *syndrome* did not seem appropriate either. Rather, the word *pattern* seems to be a more acceptable term. A manifest esotropia greater than 8 or 9^Δ would probably not allow for peripheral fusion, as the size of Panum's areas would be exceeded. An eso deviation less than 1^Δ would not be called an esotropia. Although it is possible that there could be central suppression to prevent bifixation (i.e., monofixation resulting), the answer to Question 11 could not with certainty be said to be "e." There could be a fixation disparity present without significant suppression, and, therefore, bifixation (inexactness notwithstanding) could also be present. Fixation disparity is a *manifest* deviation of the visual axes that is too small to be considered strabismic.

12. e. Always listen to the patient's history first. For example, he may say his right eye turns outward some of the time. Before dissociating the visual field of his right eye from his left, directly observe your patient to see if a deviation is manifest or not. Next, perform the Hirschberg test if the angle is small and you are unable to detect any strabismus by direct observation alone. If the strabismus is quite small, say 5^Δ or less, go to the unilateral cover test. A "flick" as small as 1^Δ can be seen with very careful observation. As to whether there is bifixation or monofixation, a strabismus means that there is monofixation only. To be sure, however, place a 4^Δ base-out prism over an eye. If there is an absence of convergence, assume monofixation (e.g., suppression). If the prism is placed over the other eye and a version (conjugate movement) occurs, monofixation is confirmed. (*Caveat:* If the strabismus is smaller than the testing prism, a combination of version and vergence may occur. This requires careful interpretation.)

13. a. The patient would have past pointing when looking monocularly with the left eye at an object down and to his right. Disruption of normal retinomotor values in the particular action field of the extraocular muscle would cause this.

14. b. Viral diseases or history of recent illness should be suspected. Vascular causes for such a condition are more common in the elderly than in the young. An acute

condition would more likely cause symptoms than a chronic condition, therefore ruling out birth trauma or muscle insertion anomalies. Accommodation problems would not likely cause a nonconcomitant pattern like this.

15. d. The probable recent onset would indicate a paresis, and the underaction shown on the Hess-Lancaster chart in Figure 2 is the left superior oblique. Note also the overaction of its yoke, the right inferior rectus.

16. c. Angle kappa testing is done monocularly. Therefore, no statement can be made regarding heterotropia (strabismus). An eccentric fixation is indicated for the amblyopic left eye, since angles kappa are different. The left eye should normally have a +1 mm value, but the +0.5 mm would mean that the left eye turned inward (more nasal) upon fixating monocularly to reduce the angle kappa from +1 mm to +0.5 mm. Therefore, there is nasal eccentric fixation of the left eye. Such a testing procedure is known as the Worth test for eccentric fixation. Although not very sensitive (compared with visuoscopy), it is credited as being one of the first methods originated to test for eccentric fixation.

17. b. The angle of eccentric fixation (E) is approximately 11^Δ ($0.5 \times 22 = 11$). Use this formula:

$$Ht = Hm + E$$
$$\text{or}$$
$$Hm = Ht - E$$

In this case, the true angle of deviation was given as 22^Δ of esotropia. Label this Ht. Now, angle E is $+11^\Delta$ (nasal eccentric fixation having a positive value, as opposed to temporal having a negative value). Therefore,

$$Hm = 22 - 11$$
$$= +11, \text{ or } 11^\Delta \text{ eso}$$

18. c. Normal (retinal) correspondence means that the objective angle (Ht) is equal to the subjective angle (the angle of subjective directionalization), which is angle S. Therefore, angle S would be 22^Δ of eso (the same magnitude as the objective angle). This *binocular* measurement is not affected by the *monocular* finding of eccentric fixation.

19. c. The phi phenomenon test, if done properly, shows the magnitude of angle S. Therefore, prism neutralization of the apparent movement of a fixation target would be achieved with 22^Δ base-out.

20. a. The "A" pattern means the eso deviation increases on upward gaze and is less eso on downward gaze. Another way of thinking of this is that there is more exo on downward gaze, as symbolized by the letter "A."

21. e. Normal retinal correspondence (N R C) is indicated. The patient's subjective angle of directionalization (angle S) is 18^Δ, as is his objective angle of deviation (angle H). Using the formula A = H − S, A = 18 − 18, or 0. When the angle of anomaly (angle A) is zero, there is normal correspondence. In other words, if H and S are equal, there is N R C. If A happens to be other than zero, there is anomalous retinal correspondence (A R C). See Table 2K in Chapter Two for a system of correspondence for esotropia.

22. b. This situation exemplifies a condition of typical unharmonious retinal correspondence. From the formula A = H − S, A = 38 − 18, or 20. In this type of anomalous correspondence, the angle of anomaly (A) is less than H. Also, S is less than H.

23. c. Patient #23 is an exotrope but perceives diplopically as if he were an esotrope. This occurs in paradoxical, type 1 unharmonious A R C. A = $-23 - 18$, or -41. The angle of anomaly is greater in magnitude than the strabismic deviation. This indicates paradoxical, type 1 A R C (PARC 1). Another way to know if there is PARC 1 is to compare the direction of deviation of H and S. PARC 1 is indicated if the directional values are different, e.g., exotropic angle H and eso angle S in Patient #23.

24. d. Paradoxical type 2 (PARC 2) is indicated when S is greater than H. In this case Patient #24 has an esotropia of only 8^Δ, but subjectively he directionalizes as though the eso deviation were 18^Δ.

25. a. Harmonious A R C (HARC) is indicated when the subjective angle (S) is zero. From the formula A = H $-$ S, A = $8 - 0$, or 8^Δ. The type of A R C is HARC when A is equal to H.

26. c. The vertical afterimage would be projected by the fovea of the right eye toward the left of the center of the horizontal line. The 8^Δ represents the magnitude of the angle of anomaly, in this case of HARC.

27. a. The patient would report seeing a perfect cross, because the right eye would monocularly fixate with a nasal eccentric point 8^Δ from the fovea. In HARC, the anomalous associated point is located the same distance away from the fovea as point zero (the magnitude of the strabismus). For Patient #27, the eccentrically fixating point coincides with this anomalous associated point. Therefore, the angle of eccentric fixation's being of the same magnitude as the angle of anomaly gives the false impression of N R C.

28. a. Even though the patient has an esotropia of 8^Δ, he will not abduct his right eye when the left eye is occluded. This is because he will fixate eccentrically and nasally by 8^Δ, the same amount as his angle H. Therefore, no movement of his eyes should occur on the cover test.

29. a. For patients with HARC, the subjective angle of directionalization (S) is zero. There is no effect of the angle of eccentric fixation, since the viewing conditions are binocular. Eccentric fixation is found during testing under *monocular* viewing conditions.

30. a. The patient has HARC. Therefore, the subjective angle of directionalization is zero. Note that angle S would also be zero for an individual with N R C who is bifixating the target. Therefore, an ortho response would be reported in either case.

31. e. The right eye is fixating, and angle kappa can be estimated in an eye that is fixating. However, the strabismic left eye is not fixating, leaving angle kappa unknown. The Hirschberg test is done with the patient in *binocular* viewing conditions. The right eye would have to be occluded, with the left eye being tested under *monocular* viewing conditions, in order for angle kappa to be determined for the left eye.

32. d. Under monocular conditions for the left eye, a point nasal to the fovea is used for fixation. A nasalward movement of the left eye causes the light reflection to be shifted temporally.

33. c. The Worth test was one of the original procedures that helped explain the relationship between amblyopia and eccentric fixation.

34. b. The brushes would be seen to the left of the spot by the nasally fixating right eye.

With a viewing distance of 40 cm, a 20 mm separation between the brushes and the spot would represent an angle of approximately 3 degrees.

35. c. According to Flom,[2] the minimal angle of resolution (in minutes of arc) is equal to the angle of eccentric fixation (in prism diopters) plus 1. One degree equals 1.75^Δ. $1.75^\Delta + 1 = 2.75$ minutes of arc, which represents 20/55 visual acuity:

$$\frac{1}{20} = \frac{2.75}{x}, x = 55$$

36. e. Superimposition of the Visuscope star and another target of fixation implies binocular viewing, as in the bifoveal test of Cüppers. An angle of anomaly could be estimated under these circumstances, but an angle of eccentric fixation could not. (Eccentric fixation is evaluated under monocular conditions.)

If the anomalous associated point of one eye (that which corresponds to the fovea of the other eye) is located halfway between the fovea and the center of the optic disc, the angle of anomaly would be positive (nasal) of approximately 8°.

37. c. The visual acuity cannot be predicted with certainty. It is possible, for example, to have poor vision (e.g., 20/200 with central-fixation amblyopia) with eccentric fixation of 1 degree or greater. However, it is almost impossible to have very good visual acuity (e.g., 20/20).

38. c. Parafoveal eccentric fixation is considered to 3 degrees or less from the center of the fovea, but greater than 1 degree away from the center.

39. b. The Visuscope (Visuskop®) is the instrument designed by Cüppers. Monocular testing is for eccentric fixation. Binocular testing would be for anomalous retinal correspondence.

40. a. Nutritional amblyopia is considered by most authorities to be an organic amblyopia. Poor diet in alcoholism is an example.

41. c. Heterotropia (strabismus) is suspected, because the right eye was fixating, whereas the left eye was not. When the prism was placed before the patient's fixating right eye, an adduction was made, which in turn caused the suppressing left eye to passively abduct. The conjugate movement occurred without any vergence. Furthermore, when the prism was placed before the left eye, no eye movement at all was elicited, thus indicating suppression of the left eye. A vergence would likely occur if a heterophoria were present (assuming no suppression).

42. e. The alternate cover test revealed some type of deviation of the visual axes, whether it was a heterotropia or a heterophoria. On the 4 base-out prism test, however, a vergence (presumably convergence) was noted. This indicates the absence of suppression and the presence of sensory and motor fusion. This would mean the patient probably has a heterophoria rather than a heterotropia.

43. a. The Pola-Mirror procedure[3] is vectographic and is considered natural relative to the more laboratorylike tests employing septums or colored filters. Suppression is not apt to be detected when testing conditions are unnatural, such as in a dark room with a bright fixation light and with the patient looking through red and green filters.

44. e. The Pola-Mirror test was studied with 17 patients.[3] All who had worse than 60 seconds of arc failed the Pola-Mirror test; those who had better than 60 seconds of arc passed. The patient's report of a "black eye" indicates suppression of that eye, presumably resulting in poor stereoacuity.

45. e. Suppression would be evaluated indirectly via stereoacuity testing in that the larger and deeper the suppression, the poorer the expected stereoacuity. The other targets would have direct suppression clues incorporated into them.

46. b. This value can be calculated using the formula of Fry:[4]

$$\text{percentage of stereopsis} = \frac{10100}{\text{eta} + 81} - 5 \, ,$$

with eta representing seconds of arc stereoacuity.

47. c. The reading of a page of print or the Snellen chart is a flat fusion demand. The septum merely provides a suppression clue.

48. e. Suppression probably occurs first. Confusion is probably eliminated first via foveal suppression, and diplopia is eliminated afterward by means of extrafoveal suppression.

49. d. Jampolsky[5] would contend that the suppression zone extends from the fovea of the right eye to a point-zero located nasal to the fovea. A vertical hemianopticlike demarcation would run through the fovea, with the zone becoming smaller in the vertical dimension toward point zero. A letter "D" would be the resulting shape of the zone.

50. a. A system of classifying size of suppression was given in Table 2B in Chapter Two. Central suppression is considered to exist when the distance from the fovea to point zero is 5 degrees or less, where that zone is the area being suppressed. This could be measured clinically, for example, by knowing the separation distance for stereograms between the center of the fused homologous points and the suppression clue.

51. e. Factors in the prognosis for a functional cure were reported by Flom[6,7] and discussed in Chapter Five. Exotropia is considered favorable relative to esotropia. Concomitancy is more favorable than nonconcomitancy. Between ages 7 and 11 years were reported as being the most favorable for vision therapy.

   The question of family history of strabismus is not very relevant for exotropia. But surprisingly, a positive relationship between esotropia and a family history of strabismus was found to be favorable by Flom.[6] Reasons why are not known.

   Constant strabismus (i.e., existing 100 percent of the time) is less favorable than intermittent strabismus, whether esotropia or exotropia.

52. b. According to Flom,[6] the prognosis for functional cure is not greatly influenced by the type of retinal correspondence in *exotropia*. However, A R C in *esotropia* is considered to be unfavorable.

53. b. Constant exotropia with A R C was found by Flom[6] to have a probability of functional cure of 20 percent. He also listed as unfavorable factors marked suppression, amblyopia, and eccentric fixation, which tends to lower the expectation for cure for the patient in Case History A. (These associated conditions would be even more unfavorable, however, in esotropia.)

54. a. A poor prognosis would be in agreement with the prediction of Flom.[6] Some possible reasons for pessimism follow. There is constant strabismus. The long duration and many associated conditions make the prognosis unfavorable, particularly since there was only token therapy in the past. Future motivation and cooperation are questionable.

   Note that any value judgments made in such an instructive exercise as this are speculative. Professional judgments involving actual clinical patients vary according to circumstances.

55. e. In Case History A, the age of strabismus onset was 7 months. This is after the 4 to 6 month cutoff period that most authorities say differentiates between congenital and acquired problems. Similarly, most authorities would hold that the age of onset in this case would be classified as early-acquired (if age 2 years is the cutoff), and not late-acquired. The best option is Answer e. Regarding the "possibly favorably" prognosis, one cannot be too optimistic in this case, considering all the facts. Although "e" is the best answer for the test, many things are unknown about a patient's diagnosis described on paper. The doctor-patient relationship fills in much of the information, aided by the supplemental testing the doctor uses in the prognostic process.

56. e. It is likely that this patient will be cooperative in therapy; he seems to have the motivation. (This is based on circumstantial evidence of his desire to read and eliminate headaches.) The history of esotropia in the family may also tend to motivate the parents to do something about their child's strabismic problem (now that it has been identified and diagnosed). Answers a and b also apply (see discussion of Case History A above).

57. e. All the options listed are considered favorable.

58. e. The schema of Flom[6] would give a 50 percent chance for a functional cure in this case of occasional (intermittent) esotropia if there is normal retinal correspondence. Since there appears to be probable normal retinal correspondence, this prediction probably would apply in this case. However, there is no amblyopia, the suppression is not marked, the deviation is concomitant, and there is some degree of sensory and motor fusion. Therefore, the prediction would likely be somewhat higher than 50 percent, considering these favorable factors.

59. d. Although some clinicians would predict a 100 percent chance for cure in this case, a prediction for a functional cure somewhere between this and the 50 percent in Question 58 may be better. It is wise to be conservative when estimating and stating prognoses to patients. For example, a cure rate of 100 percent is not always possible, even in the "easy" cases. Likewise, stating a 0 percent chance is not wise, because unanticipated functional cures may result in "difficult" cases. (How many times have you heard patients say that their other doctor gave them no hope at all?) In short, it is better to avoid stating either 0 or 100 percent when telling a prognosis to a patient.

60. d. It is probable that this was late-acquired esotropia. Since the cosmesis is good, the age of onset is difficult to pinpoint. However, the fact that the associated conditions are few and not too deeply embedded seems to indicate a relatively short duration of strabismus. The high AC/A ratio also tends to support the contention that the strabismus is accommodative, rather than congenital, esotropia. Furthermore, the deviation is manifested only a small portion of the time at far. This can be interpreted possibly to mean the strabismus has not "deteriorated," and the onset may be late (i.e., after the age of 2 years).

61. e. Javal is generally credited as being the originator of modern functional training procedures in strabismus, and he is particularly known for studying the nature of suppression. Occlusion is thought to be a passive form of antisuppression therapy. Presumably, the inhibitory mechanism of suppression does not function during occlusion of an eye.

62. d. Direct occlusion is usually recommended as the first choice of therapy for the infant amblyopic patient. In this case, the nonamblyopic right eye would be patched initially before alternate occlusion is begun.

63. c. Alternate occlusion should be recommended to prevent occlusion amblyopia, which might occur with unilateral occlusion that is prolonged in the case of an infant. Constant occlusion would prevent the inhibitory effects of suppression, whereas intermittent occlusion would allow suppression (thus exacerbating the amblyopia) to occur when the patch was not worn. Therefore, any gains made during patching could be lost when the patient was not patching an eye. An opaque occluder would definitely be dissociative (to prevent suppression), but an attenuating lens (e.g., neutral density filter) might be questionable in this regard. However, the technique of penalization using attentuation might be effective in later stages of amblyopic therapy.

64. d. The negative afterimage technique is that of Cüppers, not Bangerter.

65. e. Although A R C may occur when exotropia is present, the phenomenon of co-variation is often present in such intermittent exotropia cases where normal retinal correspondence is present when there is bifixation (i.e., foveal fusion). Although occlusion is often useful for eliminating suppression and A R C, it is not useful in this case, because normal retinal correspondence may be occurring whenever the patient has bifixation. The objective of therapy would be to keep the patient bifixating as much as possible. Occlusion would work against this objective by the dissociative effects of patching. In fact, constant strabismus possibly could result from prolonged occlusion.

66. e. The number of possible approaches to A R C therapy is great.

67. e. Antisuppression procedures are enhanced by the use of large, bright, moving, high-contrast, colored targets. As the patient gradually improves, these qualities gradually may be modified; e.g., smaller and dimmer targets can be used.

68. e. Bi-ocular training means there is stimulation of noncorresponding points when diplopia is perceived. Appreciation of diplopia is frequently useful in breaking down suppression and promoting proper fusional responses in patients with strabismus.

69. d. A patient with deep suppression is more likely to suppress under natural conditions than under unnatural conditions. Therefore, it is logical to begin with unnatural testing and training procedures so the patient will tend to appreciate diplopia rather than suppress it. In this example, the use of colored filters is considered to be the most unnatural, then the Brewster stereoscope, the vectographic targets, and objects in free space.

70. e. Therapy being addressed to all associated conditions should be considered in cases of strabismus.

71. d. There is a chance of remission, particularly if appropriate procedures are carried out to prevent secondary contractures. Alternate occlusion is preferable to unilateral occlusion for preventing contracture of either the homolateral antagonist (right medial rectus) or the contralateral synergist (left medial rectus). A modified form of alternate occlusion is the use of bi-nasal occluders, which may be useful in a case like this. Ocular calisthenics designed to force the paretic eye to move in the action field of the affected muscle (right lateral rectus) may help. Also, relaxation of the homolateral antagonist may be aided by calisthenics.

72. e. Flat fusion targets (testing second-degree fusion) are similar in design and allow the patient to hold the fusible images, whereas superimposition targets are dissimilar, causing the patient to let go of the images, and they are not truly fusible. Since the esotropia is constant in this example and the deviation is moderately large, there is little to be gained by starting the patient with an ortho demand. It is unlikely that fusional divergence (if any were present) would be great enough to allow true fusion of the targets in the major amblyoscope set

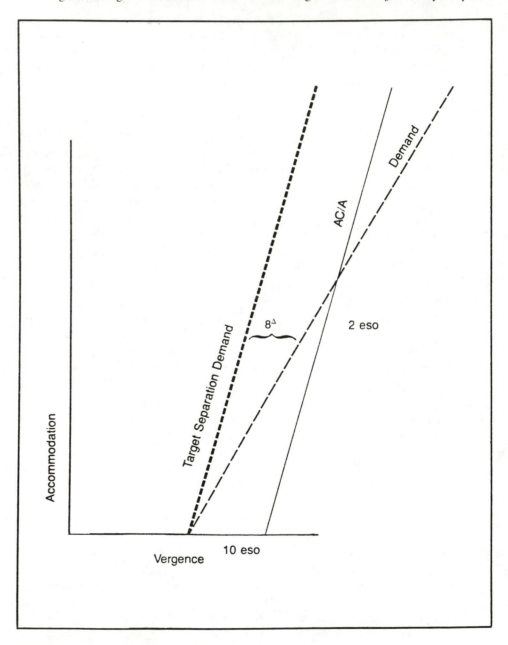

FIGURE 3 — Vergence demands for fusion for a patient with eso deviation viewing split vectograms that are separated by 8^Δ and viewed at various distances ranging from near to far.

at the ortho setting. (*Caveat:* The ortho setting could be a stimulation for the development of a harmonious anomalous retinal correspondence response in a case like this.) Regarding the objective angle of strabismus, the 18^Δ base-out demand is identical to the objective angle in this case.

73. a. The Sheard criterion is satisfied if the opposing vergence (with clear, single, binocular vision) is twice the magnitude of the deviation of the visual axes.

74. e. The Rémy separator is a T-shaped device having no lenses or prisms, but merely a septum to dissociate the visual field of one eye from the other eye. If the targets are 6 cm apart and viewed from a fixation distance of 40 cm, the relative divergence (base-in) demand is 15^Δ. This is useful in the training of patients with eso deviations.

75. d. The visual axes of a 15^Δ esotrope would intersect at the 40 cm distance if no accommodative convergence were provided. Optical infinity at 40 cm would be simulated by the patient's wearing $+2.50D$ addition lenses. A convenient way to calculate the lenses needed for centration point testing is to divide the objective angle (H) by the interpupillary distance (PD). $D = H/IPD$, or, in this example, $15/6 = +2.50D$.

76. b. Mathematically, the demand lessens with increased fixation distance with split vectograms when only the targets (but not the patient's AC/A ratio and deviations) are considered. For example, if the vectograms are separated by 32 mm, then at 40 cm this is equivalent to 8^Δ. But at a fixation distance of 80 cm, the demand would be half, i.e., 4^Δ. Theoretically, there would be no demand at infinity. Thus, the mathematical fusional demand for the targets decreases as the fixation distance increases. The concept works well if the patient's AC/A ratio parallels the demand line (e.g., 6/1). However, the patient in this example has an AC/A of 3/1 (see Figure 3). If the targets are separated by 8^Δ at the near fixation distance, the vergence demand created by the target separation can be represented by a dotted line, and this becomes parallel to the AC/A line. It can be seen that the patient in this example must diverge a total of 10^Δ at the near fixation distance as well as 10^Δ at far to fuse the split vectographic targets. (*Note:* If the separation of the split vectograms were greater than 8^Δ, the divergence demand would be easier with fusion walk-aways. Conversely, if the separation were less than 8^Δ, the divergence demand would be more difficult with increasing fixation distances.)

77. d. Cine-Ortho™ fusion training was developed by optometrist and ophthalmologist Kenneth Oakley, and these films are available from Keystone View Co.

78. e. This esophoric patient would probably have difficulty with hand-held targets (i.e., nearpoint) that have a base-in demand of 15^Δ. The patient's total fusional divergence would have to be 25^Δ, which may pose some difficulty in fusing. Accommodative stimulus achieved by using minus lenses would tend to exacerbate the existing eso condition caused by an added accommodative convergence resulting from an accommodative response.

79. a. Because of the high AC/A ratio in the case of divergence excess, minus overcorrections may be advisable for far distance but probably not for near. Suppose a patient is almost orthophoric at nearpoint. The minus addition, along with the high AC/A ratio, could result in an eso deviation when the patient accommodated for a nearpoint target. Fusional divergence would be necessary, and this is contrary to the purpose of initial therapy in these cases, i.e., fusional convergence

improvement. Plus additions in the form of bifocals for nearpoint viewing may be recommended.

80. c. This ranking from easy to difficult is in accord with the vision therapy philosophy. The three-dot card procedure is more difficult than pencil push-ups because a septum is dissociative. Chiastopic fusion requires fusional convergence responses without the help of accommodative convergence, and thus is more difficult than the three-dot card.

81. e. The ultimate goal in therapy for binocular anomalies, whether in cases of heterotropia or heterophoria, is for the patient to have clear, single, comfortable, and efficient binocular vision.

82. a. Early practitioners primarily addressed the patient's problem of poor eyesight, and thus the concern was which lenses could be used to reduce or eliminate blurred vision. Later in the 19th century, effective orthoptic regimens for strabismus therapy were introduced. These helped emphasize the importance of the development of clear, single (not diplopic), binocular vision. Optometrists in the first half of the 20th century originated "models of vision" to explain the relationship of the patient's discomfort to accommodation and vergence (e.g., the analytical approach of case typing and graphical analysis). From these models arose the modern concepts of "learning lenses" and functional training procedures to promote efficient binocular vision, which imply as prerequisites the qualities of clearness, singleness, and comfort. This attention to providing therapy for inefficient vision has led many optometrists to work with visually related scholastic learning abilities, occupational vision, sports vision, and so on.

83. d. The Pierce Saccade test is composed of three plates on which digits are placed (independent variables) for gross saccadic eye movement testing. The dependent variables, time and errors, can be calculated into corrected scores to be compared with expected norms for various age groups.

84. e. This is conventional wisdom, and many practitioners who prescribe functional training procedures in their practice advocate similar approaches to therapy for pursuit eye movements. Arthur C. Heinsen, O.D., and Ralph E. Schrock, O.D.,[8] of San Jose and San Diego, California, respectively, originated an evaluation rating system (called the Visual Performance Scale) for pursuit eye movements, as well as for other visual efficiency skills. Important factors in pursuits are smoothness, freedom of head movement, automation of movements, and adequate stamina.

85. b. The Nott method[9] and the monocular estimate method (MEM)[10-12] are variations of dynamic retinoscopy (objective testing). In the Nott method, the linear difference between the fixation distance (usually 40 cm) and the distance of the retinoscope from the patient is converted into diopters to determine the accommodative lag. The patient fixates reading material at 40 cm (2.50D) while retinoscopy, performed through a hole in the card, shows a neutral reflex at, say, 67 cm (1.50D). The accommodative lag, according to the Nott method, would be 1.00D in this example.

The MEM is similar theoretically. However, the retinoscopic distance is kept constant. This is often at the Harmon distance (the distance from the patient's elbow to his first knuckle), but varying distances may be chosen, e.g., the patient's customary working distance. The patient is told to read appropriate reading material mounted on the retinoscope. A trial lens is interposed in the spectacle plane of the patient to neutralize the reflex. The lens is removed from the eye within a split second, because the latency for the accommodation response is short. The lens power (addition of plus) necessary to achieve retinoscopic neutralization is the estimated accommodative lag of the eye being tested at the moment. (Minus power required for neutralization is a cause for concern.) The MEM is called "monocular," although the patient has both eyes open, with testing being under binocular viewing conditions. Using the Nott or MEM procedures, a lag of 1.00D (or greater) of accommodation (behind the point of convergence) is cause for further investigation.[13] A high lag time suggests the possibility of accommodation anomalies, e.g., infacility and insufficiency of accommodation, ill-sustained accommodation, and possibly performance inefficiencies in school, work, and play. Margach[14] discussed several different types of nearpoint retinoscopies, and each more thoroughly than the two presented herein.

86. a. Monocular accommodative facility of 20 cycles/minute on ±2.00D before therapy would be good.[15] An ideal after-therapy goal would be 20 cycles/minute with clear vision of ±2.50D (see Chapter Two, "Accommodation Infacility"). The ideal goal of Pierce and Greenspan,[16] however, is 20 cycles/minute on +2.50 and −4.00D. All the above values apply to monocular and binocular accommodative rock.

Because monocular rock was fairly adequate, the amplitude of accommodation would probably be adequate, as was evident for accommodative sustaining ability in this case. The great discrepancy between monocular and binocular findings in this case strongly suggests poor fusional vergence ability. For example, the patient may be esophoric with minus lenses and exophoric with plus lenses, demanding negative and positive fusional vergence, respectively, to fuse with single, clear, binocular vision. (Comfort should be a goal in accommodation facility procedures.)

Tonic convergence sometimes indirectly affects binocular accommodation facility. For example, a patient has 20^Δ of esophoria at 6 cm (high tonic convergence). You would expect at least some esophoria at 40 cm (even with low AC/A ratio). This would necessarily make it more difficult for such a patient to fuse (with clear, comfortable, binocular vision) when viewing through the minus lenses than through the plus lenses.

Whether accommodative lag would be found in the teenage patient with poor binocular accommodative rock cannot be predicted with certainty. Although a lag is suggested by poor facility, there are many exceptions to such a rule. I have seen many cases of high accommodative lag—either by the Nott method or MEM—that are esophoric and many that are exophoric at near, with varying fusional vergence abilities.

87. c. A training goal for vergence facility that I advocate is 20 cycles/minute for 5^Δ base-in to 15^Δ base-out. This is a "dynamic" evaluation and probably relates to real-life demands of patients more than do our more "static" measurements of vergence. (The factor of time, unfortunately, is not adequately considered in such classic approaches to case analysis as the analytic and graphic approaches.)

I believe it is logical to require only 5^Δ base-in. For example, it would be unreasonable to expect a highly esophoric patient to diverge much past the ortho demand, especially after coming from a posture of 15^Δ convergence. The important consideration is the vergence facility, not the vergence amplitude.

Similarly, a 15^Δ base-out demand is reasonable for an exophoric patient. Again, for the patient's welfare, it is more the facility than mere amplitude that is important. I call this procedure the "20/20 vergence rock" (range of 20^Δ for 20 cycles/minute). This applies to both testing and training. There are numerous ways to perform this procedure, e.g., loose prisms, prism flippers, B.I.-B.O. dual vectographic sets, and so on.

88. e. The Vis-A-Vis (vis-à-vis) test, when done at relatively long distances greater than 50 cm, is sensitive in detecting foveal suppression. This also tests for a monofixation pattern. Directionality can be tested in a cursory manner by having the patient tell you which of your eyes is blacked out (representing either the patient's suppressed eye or one that he purposely closes).

89. d. If the y-intercept is reduced to zero, there is no fixation disparity as to the particular point of regard at which the patient is fixating. Saladin and Sheedy[17] concur with the concept that one therapy goal is for the patient to have a curve with a flat slope.

90. b. A Shepard percentage of 72 percent stereopsis corresponds to 50 seconds of arc stereoacuity. This can be calculated using the formula of Fry (Table 2G in Chapter Two).

91. b. In the Frisby Stereo Test (Clement Clarke), various stereothresholds are produced using plates of different thicknesses and by increasing or decreasing the viewing distance. The Reindeer Stereotest (Bernell Corp.), the Random Dot E Test (Stereo Optical Co.), and the Fly Test (Titmus Optical Co.) require the patient to view the target through polarizing filters. The TNO Test (distributed in the United States by Alfred Poll, Inc.) requires red-green filters.

92. d. Clinical experience has shown that random dot stereograms indicate strabismus (by an absence of stereopsis on the test) more reliably than those tests having contours. The contours may act as monocular clues that give rise to a response of "This one is the different one." Both the Reindeer and Fly tests have contours; not surprisingly, one-eyed individuals often come up with appropriate answers on these tests, simulating stereopsis (usually gross, but not fine, stereopsis). This rarely happens when random dot stereograms are used; they are almost foolproof in this respect. Random dot designs contain no monocular clues that tend to promote "correct" guessing. Horizontal disparities, necessary for binocular depth perception, are not as obvious as they are in most contoured vectographic or anaglyphic stereograms. In addition to monocular clues, it is quite possible that another type of perception is involved when stereopsis is being tested via random dot patterns, but this is not yet fully understood. The Frisby Stereo Test uses the random dot principle, but Cooper and Feldman[18] point out a possible drawback of this test for young children. They believe that young children are not as cooperative as older patients, and that head movements can give motion parallax clues. Thus, "false" correct answers may be reported in such instances.

93. c. The Random Dot E Test (Stereo Optical Co.) is designed to be used at varying distances, giving a range of 42 to 1,261 seconds of arc.

94. b. Although the convergence reflex may not be seen at birth, it is well developed by the age of 6 months.[19] Therefore, reflex vergence enhancement would be appropriate for a 4-year-old patient. Likewise, the sensorimotor task (ages 0 to 2 years, according to Piaget) of pencil push-ups could normally be learned by a 4-year-old patient.

The stage of preoperational representations, according to Piaget, is from ages 2 to 7 years. It is reasonable to expect a preoperational patient to be able to learn to perform well on a three-dot convergence card. However, patients usually must be at least in the stage of concrete operations (ages 7 to 11) before free-space chiastopic fusion can be achieved.[20]

95. b. Flom[21] states that it is possible that unusual distributions of corresponding retinal points, as found on the horopter, may drive the eyes via fusional vergence. The resulting eso or exo deviation may then become tonic. In exo deviations, for example, it is typical (according to Flom) that peripheral objects (to the side of the fixated one) will be off the horopter. They will thus be seen in diplopia. It may be reasoned that a divergence (e.g., fusional) movement would move the horopter backward so as to eliminate peripheral diplopia. However, central suppression would consequently be necessary to eliminate any resulting central diplopia (assuming an exotropia is manifested in relation to the fixation target). Conversely, convergence from the exotropic position of the eyes would eliminate the central diplopia. But again, peripheral diplopia would be resumed. Such actions may occur in cases of intermittent exotropia and may often be a cause of the instability of fusion in them.

96. e. The three-light test as used in this example would be such that the central light (in the "notch") would be behind the horopter. Therefore, homonymous (red light seen to the right) diplopia would be perceived. The outer two lights, placed in a frontal plane, would be in front of the horopter (in this case of esotropia with harmonious anomalous correspondence). This would give rise to heteronymous diplopia (red light seen to the left). The same would be perceived for each of the laterally displaced test lights, which causes a total of six lights to be perceived under these circumstances. (*Note:* On page 693 of Flom's work,[21] there was an apparent typographical error as to right and left directions in an example given for the purpose of explaining this phenomenon.)

97. b. The esotropic patient with paradoxical type 1 A R C would directionalize as though he were exotropic. Therefore, his horopter would be farther away than the fixation point. If the patient had harmonious A R C, the horopter would be approximately the same distance as the fixation point (i.e., in "harmony" with true space). The typical type of unharmonious A R C for an esotrope would place the horopter somewhere between the fixation point and the point where the visual axes cross. If the esotropic patient had normal correspondence, the horopter would be at the approximate distance of the point of crossing of his visual axes. If the esotropic patient had paradoxical type 2 unharmonious A R C, the horopter would be nearer than the point of crossing of the visual axes. This type of patient would directionalize more eso than he really was.

98. e. Newman[22] recommended recording the patient's remarks when doing vergence testing. Use the exact words of the patient, e.g., "pain" or "strain." Of course, blur, diplopia, fixation disparity, and suppression should be recorded. However, if the goal is to have your patient achieve clear, single, efficient, and *comfortable* binocular vision, it may be important to note the remarks of discomfort during testing procedures.

99. d. Consecutive strabismus refers to surgical overcorrection, e.g., an intermittent exotropic patient becoming a constant esotrope following extraocular muscle surgery. It is always recommended that the patient achieve good base-in and

base-out ranges. The occurrence of consecutive esotropia may possibly be prevented in such instances if the base-in ranges for blur, break, and recovery are adequate. Both magnitude and facility are important.

100. e. This goal is important in all facets of life.

References to Self-Assessment Test

1. *Parks, M.M.: The Monofixation Syndrome, in Symposium on Strabismus, Transactions of New Orleans Academy of Ophthalmology. St. Louis: C.V. Mosby Co., 1971, pp. 122-153.*

2. *Flom, M.C.: Cited by M. Schapero, Amblyopia. Philadelphia: Chilton Book Co., 1971, p. 92.*

3. *Griffin, J.R., and J.M. Lee: The Polaroid Mirror Method. Optom. Weekly, 61(40), p. 29, 1970.*

4. *Fry, G.: Measurement of the Threshold of Stereopsis. Optom. Weekly, 33(37), pp. 1029-1032, 1942.*

5. *Jampolsky, A.: The First International Congress of Orthoptists. St. Louis: C.V. Mosby Co., 1968, p. 23.*

6. *Flom, M.C.: Treatment of Binocular Anomalies of Vision, in M.J. Hirsch and R.E. Wick, editors, Vision of Children. Philadelphia: Chilton Book Co., 1963.*

7. *Flom, M.C.: The Prognosis in Strabismus. Am. J. Optom., 35(10), pp. 509-514, Oct. 1958.*

8. *Heinsen, A.C., and R.E. Schrock: Personal communication, January 1980.*

9. *Nott, I.S.: Dynamic Skiametry, Accommodation and Convergence. Am. J. Physiol. Optics, 6, pp. 490-503, 1925.*

10. *Haynes, H.M.: Clinical Observations with Dynamic Retinoscopy. Optom. Weekly, 51, pp. 2306-2309, 1960.*

11. *Greenspan, S.B.: MEM Retinoscopy, in The Refraction Letter. Rochester, N.Y.: Bausch and Lomb, Dec. 1974.*

12. *Greenspan, S.B.: The Use of MEM Retinoscopy to Determine Nearpoint Prescriptions, in The Refraction Letter. Rochester, N.Y.: Bausch and Lomb, May 1975.*

13. *Bieber, J.C.: Why Nearpoint Retinoscopy with Children? Optom. Weekly, 65, pp. 54-57, 78-82, 1974.*

14. *Margach, C.B.: Nearpoint Retinoscopies. Optometric Extension Program, Inc., Curriculum 2, Series 3, No. 12, Sept. 1978.*

15. *Hoffman, L.G., and M. Rouse: Referral Recommendations for Binocular Function and/or Developmental Perceptual Deficiencies. J. Am. Optom. Assoc., 51, pp. 119-125, 1980.*

16. *Pierce, J.R., and S.B. Greenspan: Accommodation Rock Procedure in VT, A Clinical Guide: Part Two. Optom. Weekly, 62(34), pp. 25-29, Aug. 26, 1971.*

17. *Saladin, J.J., and J.E. Sheedy: Paper presented at the Garland W. Clay Award Lecture at the American Academy of Optometry, Anaheim, Calif., Dec. 9, 1979.*

18. *Cooper, J. and J. Feldman: Assessing the Frisby Stereo Test under Monocular Viewing Conditions. J. Am. Optom. Assoc., 50(7), pp. 807-809, July 1979.*

19. *Solomons, H.: Binocular Vision: A Programmed Text. London: William Heinemann Medical Books, 1978, p. 334.*

20. *Griffin, J.R.: Learning Theories Applied to Binocular Therapy: Part 4. Optom. Weekly, 68(8), pp. 224-227, Feb. 24, 1977.*

21. *Flom, M.C.: Corresponding and Disparate Retinal Points in Normal and Anomalous Correspondence. Am. J. Optom., 57(9), pp. 656-665, 693, Sept. 1980.*

22. *Newman, B.Y.: Add a Measurement, in The Refraction Letter. Rochester, N.Y.: Bausch and Lomb, Jan. 1974.*

REFERENCES

CHAPTER 1

1. Hugonnier, R., Hugonnier, S. and S. Troutman: Strabismus, Heterophoria, Ocular Motor Paralysis. St. Louis: C.V. Mosby, Co., 1969, p. 263.
2. Parks, M. M.: Isolated Cyclovertical Muscle Palsy. Arch. Oph., 60 (6), pp. 1027-1035, Dec. 1958.
3. Borish, I.: Clinical Refraction, Third Edition. Chicago: Professional Press, 1970, p. 1216.
4. Jones, R. and J. B. Eskridge: The Hirschberg Test—A Re-evaluation. Am. J. Optom., 47 (2), pp. 105-114, 1970.
5. Griffin, J. R. and F. Boyer: Strabismus: Measurement with the Hirschberg Test. Optom. Weekly, 65 (31), pp. 863-866, Sept. 12, 1974.
6. Hugonnier, R., Hugonnier, S. and S. Troutman: Strabismus, Heterophoria, Ocular Motor Paralysis. St. Louis: C.V. Mosby Co., 1969, p. 598.
7. Von Noorden, G. and A.E. Maumenee: Atlas of Strabismus. St. Louis: C.V. Mosby Co., 1967, p. 20.
8. Hugonnier, R., Hugonnier, S. and S. Troutman: Strabismus, Heterophoria, Ocular Motor Paralysis. St. Louis: C.V. Mosby Co., 1969, p. 417.
9. Krimsky, E.: The Corneal Light Reflex. Springfield, Ill.: Charles Thomas, 1972, pp. 22-24.
10. Flom, M.: in Vision of Children, "Treatment of Binocular Anomalies of Vision," by Hirsch, M. and R. Wick. Philadelphia: Chilton, 1963, p. 216.
11. Hebbard, F.: Measuring Tonic Convergence. Am. J. Optom, 29 (5), pp. 221-230, May, 1952.

CHAPTER 2

1. Jampolsky, A.: Arch. Oph., Vol. 54, pp. 683-696, 1955.
2. Jampolsky, A.: in The First International Congress of Orthoptists. St. Louis: C.V. Mosby, Co., 1968, p. 23.
3. Worth, C., cited by Revell, M. J.: Strabismus. London: Barrie and Jenkins, 1971, p. 32.
4. Griffin, J.R. and J.M. Lee: The Polaroid Mirror Method. Opt. Weekly, 61 (40), p. 29, Oct. 1, 1970.
5. Griffin, J.R.: Screening for Anomalies of Binocular Vision by Means of the Polaroid Mirror Method. Am. J. Optom., 48 (8), pp. 689-692, Aug. 1971.
6. Blum, H., Peters, H.B., and J. Bettman: Vision Screening For Elementary Schools; the Orinda Study. Berkeley: University of California Press, 1959.
7. Heikkla, R. and A. Dennis: Southern California College of Optometry, Senior Student Research, unpublished study, 1971.
8. Vodnoy, B.E.: The Practice of Orthoptics and Related Topics, Fourth Ed. South Bend, Ind.: Bernell Corp., 1970, Topic No. 32.
9. Apell, R., cited by M.J. Revell: Strabismus—A History of Orthoptic Techniques. London: Barrie and Jenkins, 1971, p. 73.
10. Borish, I.: Clinical Refraction, Third Ed. Chicago: Professional Press, 1970, p. 1216.
11. Gibson, H.: Textbook of Orthoptics. London: Hatton, 1955, p. 134.
12. Turville, A.: Outline of Infinity Balance, Raphael's Limited. London: Hatton Garden, 1946. Cited by Borish, op. cit., p. 757.
13. Hugonnier, R., Hugonnier, S., and S. Troutman: Strabismus, Heterophoria, Ocular Motor Paralysis. St. Louis: C.V. Mosby, Co., 1969, p. 356.
14. Winter, J.: Striated Lenses and Filters in Strabismus. Opt. Weekly, pp. 531-534, June 10, 1971.
15. Jampolsky, A.: Arch. Ophthal., 54, pp. 683-696, 1955.
16. Cline, D., Hofstetter, H., and J. Griffin: Dictionary of Visual Science, 3rd edition. Radnor, Pa.: Chilton Book Co., 1980.
17. Schapero, M.: Amblyopia. Philadelphia: Chilton Book Co., 1971.
18. Schapero, M.: Ibid., p. 42.
19. Humphriss, D., and E. Woodruff: Refraction by Immediate Contrast. B.J. Physiol. Opt., 19, 1962.

20. *Schapero, M.: op. cit., p. 62.*

21. *Von Noorden, G.: in The First International Congress of Orthoptists. St. Louis: C.V. Mosby, Co., 1968, p. 116.*

22. *Chavasse, F.: Worth's Squint, 7th Ed. Philadelphia: Blakiston's Son and Co., Inc., 1939.*

23. *Flom, M., Weymouth, F., and D. Kahneman: Visual Resolution and Contour Interaction. J. Opt. Soc. Am., 53(9), pp. 1026-1032, 1963.*

24. *Flom, M.: New Concepts on Visual Acuity. Opt. Weekly, 57(28), pp. 63-68, July 14, 1966.*

25. *Fry, G.: Measurement of the Threshold of Stereopsis. Opt. Weekly, 33, p. 1032, Oct. 22, 1942.*

26. *Allen, H.F.: A New Picture Series for Preschool Vision Testing. Am. J. Ophth., 44(1), pp. 38-41, 1957.*

27. *Schapero, M.: op. cit., p. 88.*

28. *Dayton, G., Jones, M., Aiv, P., Rawson, R., Steele, B., and M. Rose: Developmental Study of Coordinated Eye Movements in the Human Infant, I. Visual Acuity in the Newborn: A Study Based on Induced Optokinetic Nystagmus Recorded by Electro-oculography. Arch. Ophth., 71(6), pp. 865-870, 1964.*

29. *White, C.T. and R.G. Eason: Evoked Cortical Potentials in Relation to Certain Aspects of Visual Perception, Psychology Monogram. 80(24), 1966.*

30. *Harding, G.F.A.: The Visual Evoked Response. Adv. Ophthal., 28 (Karger, Basal 1974), pp. 2-28.*

31. *Harter, M.R. and C.T. White: Evoked Cortical Responses to Checkerboard Patterns, Effect of Check-size as a Function of Visual Acuity. Electro-enceph. Clinic. Neurophysiol., 28: 48-54, 1970.*

32. *Von Noorden, G.K., and H. Burian: Visual Acuity in Normal and Amblyopic Patients Under Reduced Illumination. Arch. Ophth., 61(4), pp. 533-535, 1959.*

33. *Burian, H.: in The First Congress of the International Strabismological Association, edited by Peter Fells. St. Louis: C.V. Mosby, Co., 1971, p. 181.*

34. *Verin, P.: in The First Congress of the International Strabismological Association, edited by Peter Fells. St. Louis: C.V. Mosby, Co., 1971, p. 175.*

35. *Caloroso, E., and M. Flom: Influences of Luminance on Visual Acuity in Amblyopia. Am. J. Optom., 46(3), pp. 189-195, 1969.*

36. *Ball, G.: Anomalies of Vision in Low Illumination. Am. J. Optom. 50(3), p. 200, March 3, 1973.*

37. *Harrington, D.: The Visual Fields, 3rd Ed. St. Louis: C.V. Mosby, Co., 1971, p. 65.*

38. *Schapero, M.: Amblyopia, op. cit., p. 162.*

39. *Irvine, S.R.: Amblyopia ex anopsia. Observations on Retinal Inhibition, Scotoma, Projection, Sight Difference, Discrimination, and Visual Acuity. Trans. Am. Ophth. Soc., 46, p. 531, 1948.*

40. *Tsujimoto, E., and E. Caloroso: Visual Field Screening with an Ophthalmoscope. Am. J. Optom., 47(6) pp. 496-498, 1970.*

41. *Krueger, G., Wolleat, W., and J. Griffin: Visual Fields Testing by Means of Ophthalmoscopy. Optom. Weekly, 64, pp. 176-179, Feb. 8, 1973.*

42. *Awaya, S., Takeaki, O. and A. Toshiki: Spot Scotometry—A New Method to Examine Scotomas Under Direct Ophthalmoscopy by Using Visuscope (Euthyscope). Japanese J. Ophth., 16(3), pp. 145-157.*

43. *Winter, J.: Clinical Management of Amblyopia. Houston, Tex.: Univ. of Houston, College of Optom., 1973, p. 37.*

44. *Schapero, M.: Amblyopia, op. cit., p. 64.*

45. *Schapero, M.: Amblyopia, op. cit., pp. 41-42.*

46. *Winter, J.: Clinical Management of Amblyopia, op. cit., p. 38.*

47. *Schapero, M.: Amblyopia, op. cit., p. 57.*

48. *Davson, H.: The Physiology of the Eye, Third Ed. New York: Academic Press, 1972, pp. 126-127.*

49. *Wolff, E.: The Anatomy of the Eye and Orbit, Fourth Ed. New York: McGraw-Hill, 1955, pp. 114 and 134.*

50. *Cogan, D.: Neurology of the Visual System. Springfield, Ill.: Charles Thomas, 1966, p. 17.*

51. Harrington, D.: The Visual Fields, Second Ed. St. Louis: C.V. Mosby, Co., 1964, p. 115.
52. Schapero, M.: Amblyopia, op. cit., p. 145.
53. Brock, F.: Visual Training. Optom. Weekly, 41, pp. 1715-1719, Nov. 16, 1950.
54. Brock, F., and I. Givner: Fixation Anomalies in Amblyopia. Arch. Oph., 47(6), pp. 1465-1466, 1952.
55. Flom, M., and F. Weymouth: Centricity of Maxwell's Spot in Strabismus and Amblyopia. Arch. Ophth., 66(2), pp. 266-268, 1961.
56. Flom, M.: cited by Schapero, M.: Amblyopia, op. cit., p. 93.
57. Schapero, M.: Amblyopia, op. cit., p. 23
58. Alpern, M., Petrauskas, R., Sandall, G. and R. Vorenkamp: Recent Experiments on the Physiology of Strabismus Amblyopia. Am. Orth. J., 17, pp. 62-72, 1967.
59. Hugonnier, R., et al.: Strabismus, Heterophoria, Ocular Motor Paralysis, op. cit., p. 183.
60. Parks, M.: The Monofixation Syndrome, in Symposium on Strabismus. Trans. of New Orleans Acad. of Ophth., St. Louis: C. V. Mosby Co., 1971, pp. 121-153.
61. Ludlam, W.: Speaker at San Jose Vision Training Seminar, 1970, San Jose, Cal.
62. Bagolini, B., and N. Capobianco: Subjective Space in Comitant Squint. Am. J. Ophth., 59, 1965.
63. Von Noorden, G. and A. Maumenee: Atlas of Strabismus. St. Louis: C.V. Mosby, Co., 1967.
64. Borish, I.: Clinical Refraction, op. cit., p. 1233.
65. Hugonnier, R., et al.: Strabismus, Heterophoria, Ocular Motor Paralysis, op. cit., pp. 396-399.
66. Halldén, V.: Fusional Phenomena in Anomalous Correspondence. Copenhagen, Ejnar Munksgaard, Acta Ophthalmological Suppl., 37, 1952.
67. Cüppers, C.: cited by Hugonnier, R. et al., Strabismus, Heterophoria, Ocular Motor Paralysis, op. cit., pp. 404-406.
68. Burian, H.M.: Anomalous Retinal Correspondence, Its Essence and Its Significance in Prognosis and Treatment. Am. J. Ophth., 34, 1951, pp. 237-253.
69. Flom, M.C. and K.E. Kerr: Determination of Retinal Correspondence, Multiple-testing Results and the Depth of Anomaly Concept. Arch. Ophthal., Vol. 77, pp. 200-213, February 1967.
70. Flom, M.C. and K.E. Kerr: Ibid., p. 211.

71. Burian, H.M.: Anomalous Retinal Correspondence, Its Essence and Its Significance in Prognosis and Treatment, op. cit., pp. 242-243.
72. Morgan, M.W.: Anomalous Correspondence Interpreted as a Motor Phenomenon. Am. J. Optom., 38(3), pp. 131-148, 1961.
73. Fitton, M.: in The First International Congress of Orthoptists. St. Louis: C.V. Mosby, Co., 1968, p. 32.
74. Griffin, J. and C. Scheffel: Unpublished case report on vertical anomalous correspondence. Southern California College of Optometry, 1974.
75. Enos, M.V.: Anomalous Correspondence. Am. J. Ophth., 33, pp. 1907-1916.
76. Hugonnier, R., et al.: Strabismus, Heterophoria, Ocular Motor Paralysis, op. cit., p. 199.
77. Parks, M.: Audio Digest Ophthalmology, 7(9), Side A, May 8, 1969.
78. Schapero, M., et al.: Dictionary of Visual Science, op. cit.
79. Lyle, T.K. and K. Wybar: Practical Orthoptics in the Treatment of Squint, 5th Ed. Springfield, Ill.: Charles C. Thomas, 1967, p. 617.
80. Kramer, M.: Clinical Orthoptics, 2nd Ed. St. Louis: C.V. Mosby, Co., 1953, p. 337.
81. Burian, H.M.: Anomalous Retinal Correspondence, op. cit., p. 242.
82. Krimsky, E.: The Management of Binocular Imbalance. Philadelphia, Penn.: Lea and Febiger, 1948, p. 204.
83. Borish, I.: Clinical Refraction, op. cit., p. 1179.
84. Bielschowsky, A.: Congenital and Acquired Deficiencies of Fusion. Am. J. Ophth., 18(10), pp. 925-937, 1935.
85. Vodnoy, B.E.: Bernell Corporation Bulletin, 422 E. Monroe St., South Bend, Ind., 46601, April 1974, p. 13.

86. *Crane, H.D.: Automatic Focus by the Human Eye. Optom. Weekly, 57(33), pp. 36-41, 1966.*

87. *Pierce, J.R., and S.B. Greenspan: Accommodative Rock Procedure in V.T. ----A Clinical Guide, Part One. Optom. Weekly, 62(33), pp. 19-23, Aug. 19, 1971.*

88. *Pierce, J.R., and S.B. Greenspan: Accommodative Rock Procedures in V.T. ----A Clinical Guide, Part Two. Optom. Weekly, 62(34), pp. 25-29, Aug. 26, 1971.*

89. *Ogle, K.N., Mussey, F. and A. deH Prangen: Fixation Disparity and the Fusional Processes in Binocular Single Vision. Am. J. Ophth., 32, pp. 1069-1087, 1949.*

90. *Jampolsky, A.J.: in Symposium on Strabismus. Trans. of New Orleans Acad. of Ophth., op. cit., p. 35.*

91. *Morgan, M.W.: Anomalies of Binocular Vision, in Vision of Children, ed. by M.J. Hirsch, and R.E. Wick. Philadelphia: Chilton Book Co., 1969, p. 176.*

92. *Flom, M.C.: Some Interesting Eye Movements Obtained During the Cover Test. Am. J. Optom., 35(2), pp. 69-71, 1958.*

93. *Parks, M.: The Monofixation Syndrome, in Symposium on Strabismus. Trans. of New Orleans Acad. of Ophth., op. cit.*

94. *Ogle, K.N., Martens, T.G., and J.A. Dyer: Oculomotor Imbalance in Binocular Vision and Fixation Disparity. Philadelphia: Lea and Febiger, 1967, p. 366.*

95. *Cole, R.G., and R.P. Boisvert: Effect of Fixation Disparity on Stereo-Acuity. Am. J. Optom., 51(3), pp. 206-213, 1974.*

96. *Levin, M. and B. Sultan: Unpublished study at Southern California College of Optometry, Senior student research study, 1972.*

97. *Ogle, K.N., Mussey, F., and A. deH Prangen: Fixation Disparity and the Fusional Processes in Binocular Single Vision, op. cit., pp. 1069-1087.*

CHAPTER 3

1. *Costenbader, F.D.: Symposium: Infantile Esotropia, Clinical Characteristics and Diagnosis, presented at the joint meeting of the American Association of Certified Orthoptic Council and the American Association of Certified Orthoptists, Chicago, Oct. 29, 1967.*

2. *Jampolsky, A.J.: in Section in the First Congress of the International Strabismological Association. edited by Peter Fells, St. Louis: C.V. Mosby, Co., 1971, p. 24.*

3. *Parks, M.M.: in Section in the First Congress of the International Strabismological Association, op. cit., p. 31.*

4. *Forrest, E.B. and R. Fitzgerald: Analyzing Infant's Vision: the Evaluation of Basic Data. J. Am. Optometric Assoc., 45(11), pp. 1318-1319, Nov. 1974.*

5. *Costenbader, F.D., cited in Hugonnier, R., Hugonnier, S., and S. Troutman: Strabismus, Heterophoria, Ocular Motor Paralysis. St. Louis: C.V. Mosby Co., p. 6 of foreword, 1969.*

6. *Parks, M.M.: Audio Digest Ophthalmology, 10(18), Side A, Sept. 14, 1972.*

7. *Fisher, N.F.: General Principles of Esotropia. Audio Digest Ophthalmology, 10(18), Side B, Sept. 14, 1972.*

8. *Illingworth, R.S.: The Development of the Infant and Young Child, Normal and Abnormal, Fourth Edition. Edinburgh and London: E. and S. Livingstone, 1971.*

9. *Jampolsky, A.J.: in Symposium on Strabismus. Trans. of New Orleans Acad. of Ophth., op. cit., 1971, pp. 66-75.*

10. *Aust, W. and L. Welge-Lussen: in the First Congress of the International Strabismological Association, op. cit., pp. 211 and 218.*

11. *Alpern, M.B. and H.W. Hofstetter: The Effect of Prism on Esotropia—A Case Report. Am. J. Optom., 25(2), pp. 80-91, Feb. 1948.*

12. *Postar, S.H.: Ophthalmic prism and extraocular muscle deviations—the effect of wearing compensatory prisms on the angle of deviation in cases of esotropia (Senior Research Paper, 1972). Los Angeles College of Optometry (now in library of Southern California College of Optometry, 2001 Associated Rd., Fullerton, Cal. 92631).*

13. *Carter, D.B.: Effects of Prolonged Wearing of Prism. Am. J. Optom., 40(5), pp. 265-272, May 1963.*

14. *Griffin, J.R.: The Kinetic Cover Test. Unpublished work at Southern California*

College of Optometry, 2001 Associated Rd., Fullerton, Cal. 92631, 1971.

15. Brignull, R., and G. Mueller: *The Kinetic Cover Test in Relation to the Alternate Cover Test.* Senior Research Paper at the Southern California College of Optometry, March 15, 1973 (paper is in the SCCO library, 2001 Associated Rd., Fullerton, Cal. 92631).

16. Romano, P.E.: *Optical Aid for Performing Hirschberg and Krimsky Tests at Distance.* J. Ped. Ophth., 10(3), pp. 208-209, Aug. 1973.

17. Marlow, F.W.: *The Relative Position of Rest of the Eyes and the Prolonged Occlusion Test.* Philadelphia: F.A. Davis Co., 1924, p. 11.

18. Bergin, D.A., Griffin, J.R. and M.I. Levin: *Hyperphoria of Large Magnitude—A Case Report.* Am. J. Optom., 49(11), pp. 947-950, Nov. 1972.

19. Marlow, F.W.: *The Relative Position of Rest of the Eyes and the Prolonged Occlusion Test,* op. cit., p. 71.

20. Flom, M.C.: *Treatment of Binocular Anomalies of Vision, in Vision of Children,* ed. M.J. Hirsch and R.E. Wick. Philadelphia: Chilton Book Co., 1963, pp. 209-210.

21. Flax, N.: *Address to C.O.V.D. Meeting,* Chicago, Ill., 1974, quoted in the Am. Optom. News, 13(20), p. 2, Dec. 15, 1974.

22. Hirsch, M.J.: *The Refraction of Children, in Vision of Children,* ed. by M.J. Hirsch and R.E. Wick. Philadelphia: Chilton, 1969, pp. 149-150.

23. Ludlam, W.M.: *statement in lecture,* presented at the American Academy of Optometry, Continuing Education Courses, Miami, Florida, Dec. 1974.

CHAPTER 4

1. Allen, M.J.: *Occlusion Syllabus.* J. Am. Optom. Association, 44(6), pp. 636-639, June, 1973.

2. Diorio, P.C. and R.D. Friedman: *A New Occlusion Aid in the Treatment of Amblyopia.* J. Pediatric Ophth., 11(1), p. 41, Feb. 1974.

3. Enoch, J.M.: *The Fitting of Hydrophilic (Soft) Contact Lenses to Infants and Young Children.* Contact Lens Medical Bulletin, 5, pp. 41-46, 1973.

4. Gillie, W.: *in The First Congress of the International Strabismological Association,* edited by Peter Fells. St. Louis: C.V. Mosby, Co., 1971, p. 88.

5. Donders, F.C., cited by Revell, M.J.: *Strabismus, A History of Orthoptic Techniques.* London: Barrie and Jenkins Limited, 1971, pp. 10-14.

6. Dowaliby, M. and J.R. Griffin: *Pediatric Ophthalmic Dispensing.* Am. J. Optom., 50(4), p. 322, April, 1973.

7. Eakin, R.: *in Vision of Children—An Optometric Symposium,* edited by M. Hirsch and R. Wick. Philadelphia: Chilton Book Co., 1969, p. 283.

8. Jampolsky, A.J., Flom, M.C. and J. Thorsen: *in The First Congress of the International Strabismological Association,* edited by Peter Fells. St. Louis: C.V. Mosby Co., 1971, p. 188.

9. Fleming, A., Pigassou, R. and J. Garipuy: *Adaptation of a Method of Prismatic Overcorrection, for Treating Strabismus in Children One and Two Years Old.* J. Ped. Ophth., 10(2), pp. 154-159, May 1973.

10. Dobson, M., cited by Revell, M.J.: *Strabismus—A History of Orthoptic Techniques.* London: Barrie and Jenkins, 1971, p. 228.

11. Mallett, R.F.: *The Investigation of Heterophoria at Near and a New Fixation Disparity Technique,* from instruction manual, The Mallett Fixation Disparity Test, Mark 2. London: Archer-Elliott, Ltd. (8-9 Spring Place, Kentish Town, London, N.W. 5), p. 4, circa 1970.

12. Bangerter, A., cited by Shapero, M.: *Amblyopia.* Philadelphia: Chilton Book Co., 1971, p. 207.

13. Landolt, E.: *Refraction and Accommodation of the Eye,* 1886, cited by Gibson, H.W., *Textbook of Orthoptics.* London: Hatton Press Ltd., 1955, p. 11 of introduction.

14. Dyer, J.A.: *in Symposium on Strabismus.* Trans. New Orleans Acad. of Ophth. St. Louis: C.V. Mosby Co., 1971, pp. 160-193.

15. Hugonnier, R., Hugonnier, S. and S. Troutman: *Strabismus, Heterophoria, Ocular Motor Paralysis.* St. Louis: C.V. Mosby Co., 1969, pp. 595-664.

16. *Hurtt, J., Rasicovici, A. and C.E. Windsor: Comprehensive Review of Orthoptics and Ocular Motility. St. Louis: C.V. Mosby Co., 1972, pp. 202-238.*

17. *Abraham, Samuel V.: The Use of Miotics in the Treatment of Convergent Strabismus and Anisometropia. Am. J. Ophth., 32(2), p. 233, February 1949.*

18. *Gellman, M.: The Use of Miotics for the Correction of Hypermetropia and Accommodative Esotropia. Am. J. Optom., 40(2), pp. 93-101, February 1963.*

19. *Smith, M.B.: Handbook of Ocular Pharmacology. Acton, Mass.: Publishing Sciences Group Inc., 1974, p. 52.*

20. *Manley, D.R.: Symposium on Horizontal Ocular Deviations. St. Louis: C.V. Mosby Co., 1971, p. 68.*

CHAPTER 5

1. *Flom, M.C.: The Prognosis in Strabismus. Am. J. Optom., 35(10), pp. 509-514, Oct. 1958.*

2. *Manley, D.R.: Symposium on Horizontal Ocular Deviations. St. Louis: C.V. Mosby Co., 1971, p. 28.*

3. *Ludlam, W.M.: Orthoptic Treatment of Strabismus. Am. J. Optom., 38(7), pp. 369-388, July 1961.*

4. *Etting, G.: Visual Training for Strabismus—Success Ratio in Private Practice. Optom. Weekly, 64(48), pp. 23-26, Nov. 29, 1973.*

5. *Taylor, D.M.: Congenital Esotropia—Management and Prognosis. New York: Intercontinental Medical Book Corp., 1973, pp. 75-79.*

6. *Wybar, K.: in Section in the First Congress of the International Strabismological Association, edited by Peter Fells. St. Louis: C.V. Mosby Co., 1971, p. 243.*

7. *Parks, M.M.: in Symposium on Strabismus, Trans. of New Orleans Acad. of Ophth., Section on Monofixation. St. Louis: C.V. Mosby Co., 1971, p. 122.*

8. *Winter, J.: Clinical Management of Amblyopia, Houston: Univ. of Houston, College of Optometry, 1973, p. 39.*

9. *Aust, W.: in the First Congress of the International Strabismological Association, edited by Peter Fells. St. Louis: C.V. Mosby Co., 1971, p. 163.*

10. *Goodier, H.M.: Some Results of Occlusion in Cases of Noncentral Fixation, from section in Orthoptics, edited by J. Mein. Amsterdam: Excerptal Medica, 1972, p. 369.*

11. *Kavner, R.S. and I.B. Suchoff: Pleoptics Handbook. New York: Optometric Center of New York, 1969, p. 18.*

12. *Chavasse, F.B.: Worth's Squint, 7th edition. Philadelphia: Blakiston's Son and Co., Inc., 1939.*

13. *Flom, M.C.: Treatment of Binocular Anomalies of Vision, chapter in Vision of Children, edited by M.J. Hirsch M.J. and R.E. Wick. Philadelphia: Chilton Book Co., 1969, p. 201.*

14. *Manas, L.: The Effect of Vision Training upon the ACA Ratio. Am. J. Optom., 35(8), pp. 428-437, Aug. 1958.*

15. *Flom, M.C.: On the Relationship Between Accommodation and Accommodative Convergence. Am. J. Optom., 37(12), pp. 630-631 Dec. 1960.*

16. *Costenbader, F.D.: Diagnosis and Clinical Significance of the Fusional Vergences. Am. Orth. J., 15, pp. 14-20, 1965.*

17. *Jones, B.A.: Orthoptic Handling of Fusional Vergences. Am. Orth. J., 15, pp. 21-29, 1965.*

18. *Griffin, J.R. and R.J. Baldwin: Absence of Stereopsis During Fusion. J. Calif. Optom. Association, 42(3), pp. 138-139, July/August 1974.*

CHAPTER 6

1. *Revell, M.J.: Strabismus—A History of Orthoptic Techniques. London: Barrie and Jenkins, 1971, pp. 21-22.*

2. *Cantonnet, A. and J. Filliozat: Strabismus—Its Re-education: The Physiology and Pathology of Binocular Vision. London: M. Wiseman and Co., 1934.*

3. *Gibson, H.W.: Textbook of Orthoptics. London: Hatton Press Ltd., 1955, pp. 289-290.*

4. *Worth, C.: Squint—Its Causes, Pathology, and Treatment. Philadelphia: P. Blakiston's Son and Co., 1921.*

5. *Chavasse, F.B.: Worth's Squint, the Binocular Reflexes and the Treatment of Strabismus, 7th ed. Philadelphia: P. Blakiston's Sons and Co., 1939.*

6. *Lyle, T.K., and G.J. Bridgeman: Worth and Chavasse's Squint—The Binocular Reflexes and the Treatment of Strabismus, 9th ed. London: Bailliere, Tindall and Cox, 1959.*

7. *Optometric Extension Program Papers, Duncan, Okla. Refer to monthly publications from 1928 to present.*

8. *Getz, D.J.: Optometric Extension Program, Continuing Education Courses, Vol. 46, p. 69, Sept. 1974.*

9. *Brock, F.W.: A Simple and Direct Clinical Method of Controlling the Squinter to Normal Visual Habits. J. Am. Opt. Assoc., 13(4): 132-145, Nov. 1941.*

10. *Brock, F.W.: Vision Training Part II—The Problems Pertaining to the Loss of Binocular Vision. Optom. Weekly, p. 1157, June 28, 1956.*

11. *Brock, F.W.: Vision Training Part III—The Problems Pertaining to the Loss of Binocular Vision. Optom. Weekly, pp. 1521-1523, Aug. 30, 1956.*

12. *Smith, W.S.: Clinical Orthoptic Procedures, 2nd edition. St. Louis: C.V. Mosby Co., 1954.*

1. *Winter, J.: Clinical Management of Amblyopia. Houston, Tex.: Univ. of Houston, College of Opt., 1973, p. 42.*

2. *Curry, G.I.: Winter Haven's Perceptual Testing and Training Handbook for First Grade Teachers. Winter Haven, Florida: Winter Haven Lions Research Foundation, Inc., P.O. Box 111, 1969, pp. 40-41.*

3. *Sedan, J.: Re-educative Treatment of Suppression Amblyopia, English Translation by Lyle, T.K., Douthwaite, C. and J. Wilkinson. Edinburgh: E. and S. Livingston, Ltd., 1960, p. 7 of preface.*

4. *Brinker, W.R. and S.L. Katz: A New and Practical Treatment of Eccentric Fixation. Am. J. Ophth., 55(5), pp. 1033-1035, 1963.*

5. *Cüppers, C.: cited by Amigo, G., Present Trends in Orthoptics and Pleoptics in Giessen. Am. J. Optom., 47(9), pp. 709-714, Sept. 1970.*

6. *Pigassou, R., and J. G. Toulouse: Treatment of Eccentric Fixation. J. Ped. Ophth., 4(2), pp. 35-43, May 1967.*

7. *Sedan, J.: Re-educative Treatment of Suppression Amblyopia, op. cit., pp. 128-129.*

8. *Bangerter, A.: Amblyopiebehandlung. Basel, Switzerland: S. Karger, 1953.*

9. *Bangerter, A.: Notre Devoir Envers Les Enfants Amblyopes. Bulletin des Societes d'Ophtalmologie de France, 62(5), 332-340, 1962.*

10. *Priestley, B.S., Byron, H.M. and A.C. Weseley: Pleoptic Methods. Am. J. Ophth., 48(3), pp. 490-502 (part I), 1959.*

11. *Allen, M.J.: Shock Treatment for Visual Rehabilitation. Opt. J. and Rev. Optom., 106(24), pp. 27-29, Dec. 15, 1969.*

12. *Otwell, H.C.: Therapeutic Orthoptics. Optom. World, 53(9), pp. 28-32, 1966.*

13. *Priestley, B.S., Hermann, J.S. and A.H. Nutter: Home Pleoptics. Arch. Ophth., 70(5), pp. 616-624, 1963.*

14. *Backman, H.A.: Pleoptics. Am. J. Optom., 43(1), p. 49, Jan. 1966.*

15. *Vodnoy, B.E.: Personal Communications, 1974.*

16. *Kavner, R.S.: Speaker at American Academy of Optometry, Miami, Fla., Dec. 18, 1974.*

17. *Irvine, S.R.: Amblyopia Ex Anopsia—Observations on Retinal Inhibition, Scotoma, Projection, Light Difference Discrimination and Visual Acuity. Transactions of the American Ophthalmological Society, Vol. 46, pp. 527-575, 1948.*

18. *Pigassou-Albouy, R.: Is the Treatment of Amblyopia Worthwhile. Annals of Ophth., 2(5), pp. 494-497, Aug. 1970.*

CHAPTER 7

CHAPTER 8

1. Folk, E.R.: Treatment of Strabismus. Springfield, Ill.: Charles Thomas, 1965, p. 72.
2. Smith, C.J.: Unusual Case of "Horror Fusionalis." Optom. Weekly, 64(4), pp. 88-89, Jan. 25, 1973.
3. Fisher, H.M. and W.M. Ludlam: An Approach to Measuring Aniseikonia in Non-Fusing Strabismus—A Preliminary Report. Am. J. Optom., 40 (11), pp. 653-665, Nov. 1963.
4. Walton, H.N.: Associate Professor at Southern California College of Optometry, Personal Communications.
5. Borish, I.M.: Clinical Refraction, 3rd Ed. Chicago, Ill. The Professional Press, 1970, p. 1197.
6. Bielschowsky, A.: Congenital and Acquired Defect of Fusion. Am. J. Ophth., 18(10), pp. 925-937, Oct. 1935.
7. Jaques, L.: Half-Black is Beautiful. The Oregon Optometrist, pp. 8-10, Jan,-Feb. 1972.
8. Revell, M.J.: Strabismus—A History of Orthoptic Techniques. London: Barrie and Jenkins, 1971, p. 124.
9. Flom, M.C.: Corresponding and Disparate Retinal Points in Normal and Anomalous Correspondence. Am. J. Optom., 57(9), pp. 656-665, Sept. 1980.

CHAPTER 9

1. Folk, E.R.: Treatment of Strabismus. Springfield, Ill.: Charles Thomas, 1965, p. 69.
2. Greenwald, I.: Re-evaluation of Binasal Occlusion. Optom. Weekly, 65(4) pp. 21-22, Jan. 24, 1974.
3. Fleming, A., Pigassou, R. and J. Garipuy: Adaption of a Method of Prismatic Overcorrection for Testing Strabismus in Children One·and Two Years Old. J. Ped. Ophth., 10(2), pp. 154-159, May 1973.
4. Amigo, G.: Present Trends in Orthoptics and Pleoptics in Giessen. Am. J. Optom., 47(9), p. 713, Sept. 1970.
5. Arruga, A.: in The First International Congress of Orthoptists. St. Louis: C.V. Mosby Co., 1968, p. 69.
6. Ludlam, W.M.: Lecture at San Jose Vision Training Seminar, San Jose, California, 1970.
7. Gibson, H.W.: Textbook of Orthoptics. London: Hatton Press Ltd., 1955, p. 219.
8. Walraven, F.: cited by M.E. Kramer: Clinical Orthoptics—Diagnosis and Treatment. St. Louis: C.V. Mosby Co., 1953, pp. 384-386.
9. Revell, M.J.: Strabismus—A History of Orthoptic Techniques. London: Barrie and Jenkins, 1971, pp. 160-163.
10. Vodnoy, B.E.: Orthoptics with the PSC Variable Prismatic Mirror Stereoscope—Cheiroscope Kit with Correlary Techniques. Am. J. Optom., 40(2), p. 84, Feb. 1963.
11. Allen, M.J.: The Bartley Phenomenon and Visual Rehabilitation—A Home Training Technique. Optom. Weekly, 57(30), pp. 21-22, July 28, 1966.
12. Ronne, G. and E. Rindziunski: The Diagnosis and Clinical Classification of Anomalous Correspondence, Acta Ophthalmologica, 31, cited by Borish, I., Clinical Refraction, 3rd edition. Chicago: Professional Press, 1970, p. 1235.
13. Hugonnier, R., Hugonnier, S. and S. Troutman: Strabismus, Heterophoria, Ocular Motor Paralysis. St. Louis: C.V. Mosby Co., 1969, pp. 573-580.
14. Hugonnier, S. and C. Bernard: in Orthoptics, edited by J. Mein et al. Amsterdam: Excerpta Medica, 1972, pp. 115-116.
15. Parks, M.M.: in Symposium on Horizontal Ocular Deviations, edited by D.R. Manley. St. Louis: C.V. Mosby Co., 1971, p. 85.
16. Wick, B.: Visual Therapy for Small Angle Esotropia. Am. J. Optom., 51(7), pp. 490-496, July 1974.

CHAPTER 10

1. Flynn, J.T., Grundmann, S., and M. Mashikian: Binocular Suppression Scotoma: Its Role in Phorias and Intermittent Tropias. Am. Orthoptic J., 20, pp. 54-67, 1970.
2. Getz, D.J.: Strabismus and Amblyopia, Optometric Extension Program, Duncan, Oklahoma, Vol. 46, Series 1, No. 12, 1974.

3. Vodnoy, B.E.: Single Oblique Mirror Stereoscope-Cheiroscope Orthoptics. Optom. Weekly, 66(5), pp. 31-34, Feb. 6, 1975.
4. Cantonnet, A. and J. Filliozat: Strabismus-Its Re-education: The Physiology and Pathology of Binocular Vision. London: M. Wiseman and Co., 1934.

1. Hugonnier, R., Hugonnier, S. and S. Troutman: Strabismus, Heterophoria and Ocular Motor Paralysis. St. Louis: C.V. Mosby Co., 1969, p. 277.
2. Hurtt, J., Rasicovi, A., and C.E. Windsor: Comprehensive Review of Orthoptics and Ocular Motility. St. Louis: C.V. Mosby Co., 1972, p. 228.
3. Burian, H.M., and G.K. Von Noorden: Binocular Vision and Ocular Motility. St. Louis: C.V. Mosby Co., 1974, p. 363.

CHAPTER 11

1. Wick, B.: A Fresnel Prism Bar for Home Visual Therapy. Am. J. Optom., 51(8), pp. 576-578, August 1974.
2. Vodnoy, B.E.: The Basis and Practice of Orthophtics. Optom. Weekly, 63(25), p. 16, June 22, 1972.
3. Wick, B.: Visual Therapy for Small Angle Esotropia. Am. J. Optom., 51(7), p. 491, July 1974.
4. Smith, W.: The Right View of Vision Training. Optometric Management, 10, pp. 45-51, Oct. 1974.
5. Oakley, K.H.: Personal Communication, 164 Hawthorne St., Bend, Oregon 97701.
6. Gillie, J.C.: Orthoptics—A Discussion of Binocular Anomalies. London: Hatton Press, 1969.
7. Burian, H.M. and G.K. Von Noorden: Binocular Vision and Ocular Motility—Theory and Management of Strabismus. St. Louis: C.V. Mosby Co., 1974, pp. 381-382.
8. Greene, E.: Cyclic Esotropia. J. Am. Optom. Assoc., 45(6), pp. 737-740, June 1974.
9. Crone, R.A.: Diplopia. New York: American Elsevier Publishing Co., Inc., 1973, p. 80.
10. Brock, F.W. and W.C. Folsom: A Clinical Measure of Fixation Disparities. J.A.O.A., 33(7), pp. 497-502, Feb. 1962.
11. Christian, P.: The Management of Small-Angle Esotropia with Abnormal Retinal Correspondence. Am. Orthoptic J., 21, pp. 92-95, 1971.

CHAPTER 12

1. Flax, N.: Address at C.O.V.D. Meeting, Chicago, Nov., 1974, cited in Am. Optom. Assoc. News, 13(20), p. 2, Dec. 15, 1974.
2. Long, W.S.: Manual of Strabismus and Orthoptics. Waterloo, Ontario: School of Optometry, 1975, p. 50.
3. Ryan, V.I. and E.D. Pronchick: Manual of Orthoptics. Philadelphia: College of Optometry, 1967, p. i68.
4. Vodnoy, B.E.: Aperture Orthoptics for the Non-Strabismic. Am. J. Optom., 33(10), p. 540, Oct. 1956.
5. Tsukamoto, K.: Personal Communications, Hoya Glass Works, Ltd., Shinkyobashi Bldg., 4, 3-Chrome, Takara-Cho, Chuo-Ku, Tokyo 104, Japan.
6. Crone, R.A.: Diplopia. New York: American Elsevier Publishing Co., Inc., 1973, p. 184.
7. Ellin, R.I.: Treatment of Exotropia Due to Anisometropia. Optom. Weekly, 65(41), pp. 27-28, Dec. 5, 1974.
8. Wick, B.: Visual Therapy for Constant Exotropia with Anomalous Retinal Correspondence—A Case Report. Am. J. Optom., 51(12), pp. 1005-1008, Dec. 1974.
9. Flom, M.C.: Corresponding and Disparate Retinal Points in Normal and Anomalous Correspondence. Am. J. Optom., 57(9), pp. 656-665, Sept. 1980.

CHAPTER 13

CHAPTER 14

1.   Payne, C.R., Grisham, J.D., and K.L. Thomas: *A Clinical Evaluation of Fixation Disparity. Am. J. Optom.*, 51(2), p. 90, Feb. 1974.
2.   Borish, I.M.: *Clinical Refraction, Third Edition. Chicago: The Professional Press*, 1970, pp. 875-894.
3.   Hofstetter, H.W.: *The Zone of Clear Single Binocular Vision, Part One. Am. J. Optom.*, 22(7), pp. 301-333, July 1945.
4.   Hofstetter, H.W.: *The Zone of Clear Single Binocular Vision, Part Two. Am. J. Optom.*, 22(8), pp. 361-384, Aug. 1945.
5.   Ogle, K.M. and A. de H. Prangen: *Further Considerations of Fixation Disparity and the Binocular Fusional Processes. Am. J. Ophth.*, 34(5), Part Two, p. 70, May 1951.
6.   Carter, D.B.: *Fixation Disparity with and without Foveal Contour. Am. J. Optom.* 41(12), p. 732, Dec. 1964.
7.   Sheedy, J.E.: *Fixation Disparity Analysis of Oculomotor Imbalance. Am. J. Optom.*, 57(9), pp. 632-639, 1980.
8.   Sheedy, J.E., and J.J. Saladin: *Phoria, Vergence, and Fixation Disparity in Oculomotor Problems. Am. J. Optom.*, 54(7), pp. 474-478, 1977.
9.   Sheedy, J.E., and J.J. Saladin: *Association of Symptoms with Measures of Oculomotor Deficiencies. Am. J. Optom.*, 55(10), pp. 670-676, 1978.
10. Saladin, J.J., and J.E. Sheedy: *A Population Study of Relationships between Fixation Disparity, Heterophorias, and Vergences. Am. J. Optom.*, 55(11), pp. 744-750, 1978.

CHAPTER 15

1.   Moses, R.A.: *Adler's Physiology of the Eye, 7th edition. St. Louis: C.V. Mosby Co.*, 1981, p. 137.
2.   Gay, A.J., Newman, N.M., Keltner, J.L., and M.H. Stroud: *Eye Movement Disorders. St. Louis: C.V. Mosby Co.*, 1974, pp. 2-8.
3.   Solomons, H.: *Binocular Vision: A Programmed Text. London: William Heinemann Medical Books*, 1978, p. 151.
4.   Hoffman, L.G., and M. Rouse: *Referral Recommendations for Binocular Function and/or Developmental Perceptual Deficiencies. J. Am. Optom. Assoc.*, 51(2), pp. 119-125, Feb. 1980.
5.   Marcus, S.E.: *A Syndrome of Visual Constrictions in the Learning Disabled Child. J. Am. Optom. Assoc.*, 45(6), pp. 746-749, June 1974.
6.   Heinson, A., and R. Schrock: *Personal communication*, 1981.
7.   Griffin, D.C., Walton, H.N., and V. Ives: *Saccades as Related to Reading Disorders. J. Learning Disabilities*, 7(5), pp. 52-58, May 1974.
8.   King, A.J., and S. Devick: *The Proposed King-Devick Saccade Test and Its Relation to the Pierce Saccade Test and Reading Levels. Chicago: Illinois College of Optometry, Senior Research Study*, 1976.
9.   Cohen, A., and S. Lieberman: *Personal communication, Lake Ronkonkoma, New York, in press.*
10. Rosner, J.: *Perceptual Skills Curriculum, Program One: Visual-Motor Skills. New York: Walker Educational Book Corp.*, 1973.
11. Cline, D., Hofstetter, H., and J. Griffin: *Dictionary of Visual Science, 3rd edition. Radnor, Pa., Chilton Book Co.*, 1980, p. 409.
12. Michaels, D.D.: *Visual Optics and Refraction: A Clinical Approach. St. Louis: C.V. Mosby Co.*, 1980, p. 417.
13. Bajandas, F.J.: *Neuro-Ophthalmology Board Review Manual. Thorofare, N.J.: Charles B. Slack*, 1980, pp. 48-54.
14. Gay, A.J., Newman, N.M., Keltner, J.L., and M.H. Stroud: *op. cit.*, pp. 50-54.
15. Hoffman, L.G., and M. Rouse: *op cit.*, p. 122.
16. Heinsen, A., and R. Schrock: *op. cit.*
17. Marcus, S.E.: *op. cit.*
18. Schapero, M.: *Amblyopia. Philadelphia: Chilton Book Co.*, 1971, pp. 88-89.
19. Griffin, J.R.: *Pursuit Fixations: An Overview of Training Procedures. Optom. Weekly*, 67(20), pp. 534-537, May 13, 1976.
20. Gay, A.J., Newman, N.M., Keltner, J.L., and M.H. Stroud: *op. cit.*, pp. 15-17, 27.
21. Gay, A.J., Newman, N.M., Keltner, J.L., and M.H. Stroud: *op. cit.*, p. 10.
22. Gay, A.J., Newman, N.M., Keltner, J.L., and M.H. Stroud: *op. cit.*, p. 13.

23. Cline, D., Hofstetter, H., and J. Griffin: op. cit., p. 5.
24. Day, R., Miller, S., and R. Wilson, editors: *Current Optometric Information and Terminology*, 3rd edition. St. Louis: Am. Optom. Assoc., 1980, pp. 1-2.
25. Nott, I.S.: Dynamic Skiametry: Accommodation and Convergence. *Am. J. Physiol. Optics*, 6, pp. 490-503, 1925.
26. Haynes, H.M.: Clinical Observations with Dynamic Retinoscopy. *Optom. Weekly*, 51, pp. 2306-2309, 1960.
27. Tucker, J., and W.N. Charman: Reaction and Response Times for Accommodation. *Am. J. Optom.*, 56(8), pp. 490-503, 1979.
28. Bieber, J.C.: Why Nearpoint Retinoscopy with Children? *Optom. Weekly*, 65, pp. 54-57, 78-82, 1974.
29. Keller, J.T., and J.F. Amos: Low Plus Lenses and Visual Performance: A Critical Review. *J. Am. Optom. Assoc.*, 50(9), pp. 1005-1011, Sept. 1979.
30. Greenspan, S.B.: Behavioral Effects of Children's Nearpoint Lenses. *J. Am. Optom. Assoc.*, 46(10), pp. 1031-1036, Oct. 1975.
31. Pierce, J.R.: A Response to Low Plus Lenses and Visual Performance: A Critical Review. *J. Am. Optom. Assoc.*, 51(5), pp. 453-459, May 1980.
32. Day, R., Miller, S., and R. Wilson: op. cit., p. 3.
33. Cline, D., Hofstetter, H., and J. Griffin: op. cit., p. 5.
34. Borish, I.M.: *Clinical Refraction*, 3rd edition. Chicago: Professional Press, 1975, p. 1232.
35. Liu, J.S., Lee, M., Jang, J., Ciuffreda, K.J., Wong, J.H., Grisham, D., and L. Stark: Objective Assessment of Accommodation Orthoptics, 1: Dynamic Insufficiency. *Am. J. Optom.*, 56(5), pp. 285-294, 1979.
36. Griffin, J.R., Britz, D., and M. Zundell: A Study of Variables Influencing the Facility of Accommodation. On file in the library of the Southern California College of Optometry, 1972.
37. Griffin, J.R., Clausen, D., and G. Graham: A New Apparatus for Accommodative Rock. On file in the library of the Southern California College of Optometry, 1977.
38. Burge, S.: Suppression during Binocular Accommodative Rock. *Optom. Monthly*, 79(12), pp. 867-872, Dec. 1979.
39. Alpert, T., and J. Zellers: A Normative Study of Accommodative Facility. On file in the library of the Southern California College of Optometry, 1980.
40. Schlange, D., Kostelnik, K., and D. Paterson: Accommodative Facility: A Normative Study. On file in the library of the Illinois College of Optometry, 1979.
41. Hoffman, L., Espe, R., and J. Roberts: Accommodative Facility Evaluation of Successfully Achieving Grade School Children. On file in the library of the Southern California College of Optometry, 1978.
42. Hoffman, L.G., and M. Rouse: op. cit.
43. Borish, I.M.: op. cit., p. 169.
44. Cline, D., Hofstetter, H., and J. Griffin: op. cit., p. 251.
45. Borish, I.M.: op. cit., p. 186.
46. Cline, D., Hofstetter, H., and J. Griffin: op. cit., p. 399.
47. Streff, J.W.: Preliminary Observations on a Non-Malingering Syndrome. *Optom. Weekly*, 53(12), pp. 536-537, Mar. 22, 1962.
48. Gilman, G.D.: A Case in Point: Optometric or Psychological Problem? *J. Am. Optom. Assoc.*, 52(7), pp. 609-610, Aug. 1981.
49. Hoffman, L.G.: The Effect of Accommodative Deficiencies on the Developmental Level of Perceptual Skills. Fullerton, Calif.: Southern California College of Optometry, Research Study, 1981.
50. Manas, L.: The Effect of Visual Training upon the AC/A Ratio. *Am. J. Optom.*, 35(8), pp. 428-437, 1958.
51. Flom, M.C.: On the Relationship between Accommodation and Accommodative Convergence, 3: Effects of Orthoptics. *Am. J. Optom.*, 37(12), pp. 619-632, 1960.
52. Grosvenor, T.: Can the AC/A Ratio Change? *Optom. Weekly*, 67(27), pp. 744-746, 1976.
53. Bergin, D.A., Griffin, J.R., and M.I. Levin: Hyperphoria of Large Magnitudes: A Case Report. *Am. J. Optom.*, 49(11), pp. 947-950, Nov. 1972.
54. Morgan, M.W., in I.M. Borish, *Clinical Refraction*, 3rd edition. Chicago: Professional Press, 1970, p. 910.
55. Grisham, J.D.: The Dynamics of Fusional Vergence Eye Movements in Binocular Dysfunction. *Am. J. Optom.*, 57(9), pp. 645-655, Sept. 1980.

56. *Sheedy, J.E., and J.J. Saladin: Phoria, Vergence and Fixation Disparity in Oculomotor Problems. Am. J. Optom., 54(7), pp. 474-478, 1977.*

57. *Sheedy, J.E., and J.J. Saladin: Association of Symptoms with Measures of Oculomotor Deficiencies, Am. J. Optom., 55(10), pp. 670-676, 1978.*

58. *Newman, B.Y.: Add a Measurement. The Refraction Letter, Bausch and Lomb, Jan. 1974.*

59. *Grisham, J.D.: op. cit.*

60. *Kenyon, R.V., Ciuffreda, K.J., and L. Stark: Dynamic Vergence Eye Movements in Strabismus and Amblyopia: Symmetric Vergence. Investigative Ophthal. and Vis. Science, 19(1), pp. 60-74, Jan. 1980.*

61. *Pierce, J.R.: Lecture at Northern Central States Optometric Conference, Minneapolis, Minn., 1973.*

62. *Stuckle, L.G., and M. Rouse: Norms for Dynamic Vergences. On file in the library of the Southern California College of Optometry, 1979.*

63. *Mitchell, R., Stanich, R., and M. Rouse: Norms for Dynamic Vergences. On file in the library of the Southern California College of Optometry, 1980.*

64. *Moser, J.E., and W.F. Atkinson: Vergence Facility in a Young Adult Population. On file in the library of the Southern California College of Optometry, 1980.*

65. *Rosner, J.: Lecture notes of Course #551, New England College of Optometry, Fall 1976.*

66. *Rosner, J.: Lecture notes of Course #548, University of Houston, College of Optometry, Spring 1979.*

67. *Jacobson, M., Goldstein, A., and J.R. Griffin: The Relationship between Vergence Range and Vergence Facility. On file in the library of the Southern California College of Optometry, 1979.*

68. *Griffin, J.R.: Lecture notes of Course #453, Southern California College of Optometry, Spring 1981.*

69. *Hoffman, L.G., and M. Rouse: op. cit.*

70. *Schapero, M.: The Characteristics of Ten Basic Visual Training Problems. Am. J. Optom., 32(7), pp. 333-342, July 1955.*

71. *Michaels, D.D.: Visual Optics and Refraction, op. cit., p. 194.*

72. *Simons, K.: Stereoacuity Norms in Young Children. Arch. Ophthal., 99(3), pp. 439-445, 1981.*

73. *Cooper, J., Feldman, J., and D. Medlin: Comparing Stereoscopic Performance of Children Using the Titmus, TNO, and Randot Stereo Tests. J. Am. Optom. Assoc., 50(7), pp. 821-825, July 1979.*

74. *Hofstetter, H., and J.D. Bertsch: Does Stereopsis Change with Age? Am. J. Optom., 53(10), pp. 664-667, Oct. 1976.*

75. *Cooper, J., and J. Feldman: Operant Conditioning and Assessment of Stereopsis in Young Children. Am. J. Optom., 55(8), pp. 532-542, Aug. 1978.*

76. *Fagin, R.R., and J.R. Griffin: Stereoacuity Tests: Comparison of Mathematical Equivalents. Am. J. Optom., 59(5), pp. 427-435, May 1982.*

77. *Shipley, T.: The First Random-Dot Texture Stereogram. Vision Research, 11, pp. 1491-1492, 1971.*

78. *Julesz, B.: Binocular Depth Perception of Computer-Generated Patterns. Bell System Technical Journal, 39, pp. 1125-1162, 1960.*

79. *Cooper, J., and J. Feldman: Assessing the Frisby Stereo Test under Monocular Viewing Conditions. J. Am. Optom. Assoc., 50(7), pp. 807-809, July 1979.*

80. *Vodnoy, B.E.: Personal communication.*

81. *Hine, N.A.: Random-Dot Stereogram: Survey of the Clinical Uses and Reliability. Aust. J. Optom., 63(3), pp. 123-129, May 1980.*

82. *Richards, W.: Stereopsis and Stereoblindness. Exp. Brain Res., 10, pp. 380-388, 1970.*

83. *Cooper, J., and J. Warshowsky: Lateral Displacement as a Response Cue in the Titmus Stereo Test. Am. J. Optom., 54(8), pp. 537-541, Aug. 1977.*

84. *Walraven, J.: Amblyopia Screening with Random-Dot Stereograms. Am. J. Ophthal., 80(5), pp. 893-899, Nov. 1975.*

85. *Rosner, J.: The Effectiveness of the Random Dot E Stereotest as a Preschool Vision Screening Instrument. J. Am. Optom. Assoc., 49(10), pp. 1121-1124, Oct. 1978.*

86. *Cooper, J., and J. Feldman: Random-Dot Stereogram Performance by Strabismic, Amblyopic, and Ocular-Pathology Patients in an Operant-Discrimination Task. Am. J. Optom., 55(9), pp. 599-609, Sept. 1978.*

87. *Birnbaum, M.H.: Observations of Peripheral Stereopsis in Strabismus. J. Am. Optom. Assoc., 46(2), pp. 151-155, Feb. 1975.*

88. *Cline, D., H. Hofstetter, and J. Griffin: op. cit., p. 587.*

89. *Hamsher, K. de S.: Stereopsis and Unilateral Brain Disease. Investigative Ophthal. and Vis. Science, 17(4), pp. 336-343, April 1978.*

90. *Wittenberg, S.: Brock's Research in Stereopsis. Am. J. Optom., 58(8), pp. 663-666, Aug. 1981.*

CHAPTER 16

1. *Scobee, R.G.: Rehabilitation of a Child's Eyes, 3rd edition. St. Louis: C.V. Mosby Co., 1969. Cited by E. Greene: Cyclic Esotropia. J. Am. Optom. Assoc., 45(6), p. 738, 1974.*

2. *Hugonnier, R., Hugonnier, S., and S. Troutman: Strabismus, Heterophoria, Ocular Motor Paralysis. St. Louis: C.V. Mosby Co., 1969, p. 131.*

3. *Michaels, D.D.: Visual Optics and Refraction. St. Louis: C.V. Mosby Co., 1980, p. 677.*

4. *Vodnoy, B.E.: The Basis for and Practice of Orthoptics. Optom. Weekly, 63(25), p. 15, June 22, 1972.*

5. *Vodnoy, B.E.: Orthoptics for the Advanced Presbyope. Optom. Weekly, 66(8), pp. 34-36, March 6, 1975.*

6. *Wick, B.: Vision Training for Presbyopic Nonstrabismus Patients. Am. J. Optom., 54(4), pp. 244-247, 1977.*

7. *Swanson, W.J.: Visually Related Learning Disorders. J. Calif. Optom. Assoc., 34(7), p. 343, Dec. 1971.*

8. *Hoffman, L.G.: Incidence of Vision Difficulties in Children with Learning Disabilities. J. Am. Optom. Assoc., 51(5), pp. 447-451, May 1980.*

9. *Weber, G.Y.: Visual Disabilities: Their Identification with Academic Achievement. J. Learning Disabilities, 13(6), pp. 13-19, 1980.*

10. *Sherman, A.: Relating Vision Disorders to Learning Disability. J. Am. Optom. Assoc., 44(2), pp. 140-141, Feb. 1973.*

11. *Burg, A.: Vision Test Scores and Driving Record: Additional Findings. Los Angeles: University of California, Department of Engineering, Report No. 68-27, 1968.*

12. *Brod, N., and D. Hamilton: Binocularity and Reading. Optom. Weekly, 64(46), p. 35, Nov. 15, 1973.*

13. *Flax, N.: The Contribution of Visual Problems to Learning Disability. J. Am. Optom. Assoc., 41(10), p. 844, Oct. 1970.*

14. *Griffin, D.C., Walton, H.N., and V. Ives: Saccades as Related to Reading Disorders. J. Learning Disabilities, 7(5), pp. 52-58, May 1974.*

15. *Griffin, J.R., and H.N. Walton: Dyslexia Determination Test (DDT): Examiner's Instruction Manual. Los Angeles: I-MED, 1981.*

16. *Norn, M.S., Rindziunski, E., and H. Skydsgaard: Ophthalmologic and Orthoptic Examinations of Dyslectics. Acta Ophthalmologica, 47, pp. 147-160, 1969.*

17. *Adler-Grinberg, D., and L. Stark: Eye Movements, Scanpaths, and Dyslexia. Am. J. Optom., 55(8), pp. 557-570, Aug. 1978.*

18. *Hoffman, L.G.: An Optometric Learning Disability Evaluation: Part 1. Optom. Monthly, 70(2), pp. 118-121, Feb. 1979.*

19. *Hoffman, L.G.: An Optometric Learning Disability Evaluation: Part 2. Optom. Monthly, 70(3), pp. 201-205, March 1979.*

20. *Hoffman, L.G.: An Optometric Learning Disability Evaluation: Part 3. Optom. Monthly, 70(4), pp. 279-283, April 1979.*

21. *Getz, D.J.: Learning Enhancement through Visual Training. Academic Therapy, 15(4), pp. 457-466, March 1980.*

22. *Burian, H.M., and G.K. von Noorden: Binocular Vision and Ocular Motility. St. Louis: C.V. Mosby Co., 1974, p. 406.*

23. *Cline, D., Hofstetter, H., and J. Griffin: Dictionary of Visual Science, 3rd edition. Radnor, Pa.: Chilton Book Co., 1980, p. 613.*

24. *Ciuffreda, K.J., Goldrich, S., and C. Neary: Auditory Biofeedback as a Potentially Important New Tool in the Treatment of Nystagmus. J. Am. Optom. Assoc., 51(6), pp. 615-617, June 1980.*

25. *Van Brocklin, M.D., Vasché, T.R., Hirons, R.R., and R.L. Yolton: Biofeedback Enhanced Strabismus Therapy. J. Am. Optom. Assoc., 52(9), pp. 731-736, Sept. 1981.*

26. *Flom, M.C., New Concepts on Visual Acuity. Optom. Weekly, 57(28), pp. 63-68, 1966.*

27. *Kirschen, D.G.: Clinical case study at the Southern California College of Optometry, 1982.*

28. *Davidson, D.W., and J.B. Eskridge: Reliability of Visual Acuity Measures of Amblyopic Eyes. Am. J. Optom., 54(11), pp. 756-766, Nov. 1977.*

29. *Banks, R.V., Campbell, F.W., Hess, R., and P.G. Watson: A New Treatment for Amblyopia. Brit. Orthoptic J., 35, pp. 1-12, 1978.*

30. *Schor, C., Gibson, J., Hsu, M., and M. Mah: The Use of Rotating Gratings for the Treatment of Amblyopia: A Clinical Trial. Am. J. Optom., 58(11) pp. 930-938, Nov. 1981.*

31. *Griffin, J.R., Sherban, R.J., and P. Seibert: Amblyopia Therapy: A Case Report. Optom. Monthly, 69(9), pp. 619-620, June 1978.*

32. *Dalziel, C.C.: Strabismic Amblyopia: Case Report. Am. J. Optom., 58(9), pp. 777-779, Sept. 1981.*

33. *Birnbaum, M.H., Koslowe, K., and R. Sanet: Succes in Amblyopia Therapy as a Function of Age: A Literature Survey. Am. J. Optom., 54(5), pp. 269-275, May 1977.*

34. *Wick, B.: Anomalous After-image Transfer: An Analysis and Suggested Method of Elimination. Am. J. Optom., 51(11), pp. 862-871, 1974.*

35. *Wick, B.: A Home Pleoptic Method. Am. J. Optom., 53(2), pp. 81-84, Feb. 1976.*

36. *Wick, B.: Modified Strobe Flash for Home Pleoptics. Am. J. Optom., 54(3), pp. 187-188, March 1977.*

37. *Campbell, F.W., and L. Maffei: Contrast and Spatial Frequency. Scientific American, 231(5), pp. 106-114, Nov. 1974.*

38. *Bradley, A., and R.D. Freeman: Contrast Sensitivity in Anisometropic Amblyopia. Investigative Ophthal. and Vis. Science, 21(3), pp. 467-476, Sept. 1981.*

39. *Lennerstrand, G., and B.L. Lundh: Improvement of Contrast Sensitivity from Treatment for Amblyopia. Acta Ophthalmologica, 58, pp. 292-294, 1980.*

40. *Kleinstein, R.N.: Contrast Sensitivity. Optom. Monthly, 72(4), pp. 38-40, April 1981.*

41. *Sherman, J.: Visual Evoked Potential (VEP): Basic Concepts and Clinical Applications. J. Am. Optom. Assoc., 50(1), pp. 19-30, Jan. 1979.*

42. *Lee, R.A., Wolfe, P.J., and J.R. Griffin: Visually Evoked Cortical Potential. Optom. Monthly, in press.*

43. *Hubel, D.H., and T.N. Wiesel: Receptive Fields of Single Neurones in the Cat's Striate Cortex. J. Physiol., 148(3), pp. 574-591, Oct. 1959.*

44. *Hubel, D.H., and T.N. Wiesel: Receptive Fields: Binocular Interaction and Functional Architecture in the Cat's Visual Cortex. J. Physiol., 160(1), pp. 106-154, Jan. 1962.*

45. *Cool, S.J.: The Amblyopic Eye: Is It Downtrodden or Just Lazy? J. Am. Optom. Assoc., 50(6), pp. 694-698, June 1979.*

46. *Kandel, G.L., Grattan, P.E., and H.E. Bedell: Are the Dominant Eyes of Amblyopes Normal? Am. J. Optom., 57(1), pp. 1-6, Jan. 1980.*

47. *Marg, E., Freeman, D.N., Peltzman, P., and P.J. Goldstein: Visual Acuity Development in Human Infants: Evoked Potential Measurements. Invest. Ophthal., 15(2), pp. 150-153, Feb. 1976.*

48. *Mohindra, I.: Lecture notes of Course #85, American Academy of Optometry, Orlando, Fla., Dec. 12, 1981.*

49. *Held, R., Gwiazda, J., Brill, S., Mohindra, I., and J. Wolfe: Infant Visual Acuity Is Underestimated because Near Threshold Gratings Are Not Preferentially Fixated. Vis. Res., 19(12), pp. 1377-1379, 1979.*

50. *Dobson, V., and D.Y. Teller: Visual Acuity in Human Infants: A Review and Comparison of Behavioral and Electrophysiological Studies. Vis. Res., 18, p. 1469, 1978.*

51. *Gwiazda, J., Wolfe, J.M., Brill, S., Mohindra, I., and R. Held: Preferential Looking Acuity in Infants from Two to Fifty-eight Weeks of Age. Am. J. Optom. and Physiol. Optics, 57, pp. 428-432, 1980.*

52. *Mayer, D.L., and V. Dobson: Assessment of Vision in Young Children: A New Operant Approach Yields Estimates of Acuity. Invest. Ophthal., 19, pp. 566-570, 1980.*

53. *Mohindra, I., and J.F. Molinari: Near Retinoscopy and Cycloplegic Retinoscopy in Early Primary Grade School Children. Am. J. Optom., 56(1), pp. 34-38, Jan. 1979.*

54. *Mohindra, I.: Personal communication, 1981.*

55. *Eskridge, J.B.: The Complete Cover Test. J. Am. Optom. Assoc., 44(6), pp. 601-609, 1973.*

56. *Lefrancois, G.R.: Psychological Theories and Human Learning: Kongor's Report. Monterey, Calif.: Brooks/Cole Publishing Co., 1972, pp. 185-262.*

57. *Wilson, J.A.R., Robeck, M.C., and W.B. Michael: Psychological Foundations of Learning and Teaching. New York: McGraw-Hill Book Co., 1974.*

58. *Bloom, B.S., editor: Taxonomy of Educational Objectives: The Classification of Educational Goals, Handbook 1: Cognitive Domain. New York: David McKay Co., 1972, p. 7.*

59. *Harrow, A.J.: A Taxonomy of the Psychomotor Domain: A Guide for Developing Behavioral Objectives. New York: David McKay Co., 1972.*

60. *Hershey, G.L., and J.O. Lugo: Living Psychology: An Experimental Approach. London: Macmillan Company, 1970.*

61. *Hilgard, E.R., and G.H. Bower: Theories of Learning. New York: Appleton-Century-Crofts, 1966.*

62. *Sahakian, W.S.: Psychology of Learning: Systems, Models, and Theories. Chicago: Markham Publishing Co., 1971.*

63. *Bruner, J.S., cited by Wilson, J.A.R., Robeck, M.C., and W.B. Michael: op. cit., p. 90.*

64. *Getman, G.N.: Techniques and Diagnostic Criteria for the Optometric Care of Children's Vision. Duncan, Okla.: Optometric Extension Program Foundation, 1960.*

65. *Suchoff, I.B.: Visual-Spatial Development in the Child. New York: State University of New York, 1975, p. 18.*

66. *Duke-Elder, S., and D. Abrams: Systems of Ophthalmology, vol. 5: Ophthalmic Optics and Refraction. St. Louis: C.V. Mosby Co., 1970.*

67. *Bannon, R.E.: Clinical Manual on Aniseikonia. Buffalo, N.Y.: American Optical Company, 1976.*

68. *Kleinstein, R.N.: Iseikonic Trial Lenses: An Aid in Diagnosing Aniseikonia. Optom. Monthly, 69, pp. 132-137, March 1978.*

69. *Ogle, K.N.: Researches in Binocular Vision. Philadelphia: W.B. Saunders Co., p. 264, 1950.*

70. *Polasky, M.: Aniseikonia Cookbook. Columbus, Ohio: Ohio State University, School of Optometry, 1974.*

71. *Ryan, V.I.: Predicting Aniseikonia in Anisometropia. Am. J. Optom., 52, pp. 96-105, 1975.*

72. *Greenwald, I.: Effective Strabismus Therapy, Duncan, Okla. Optometric Extension Program Foundation, 1979.*

73. *Blakemore, C.: Infants' Squint Cured in the Cat. New Scientist, Oct. 10, 1974. Also cited from Modern Problems in Pediatrics, Proceedings of International Symposium on Nutrition, Growth and Development, May 1973.*

74. *Blakemore, C., and R.C. Van Sluyters: Experimental Analysis of Amblyopia and Strabismus. Brit. J. Ophthal., 58(3), pp. 176-182, March 1974.*

75. *Kirschen, D., and M.C. Flom: Monocular Central-Field Occlusion for Intractable Dioplopia. Am. J. Optom., 54(5), pp. 325-331, May 1977.*

GLOSSARY

This glossary is intended to serve as a reference for brief definitions pertaining to some of the more frequently used terms, and to those terms having a particular meaning, as well as for clarification of certain abbreviations used throughout this text.

Abduction Outward horizontal movement of the eye

Abnormal fixation Fixation in which the fovea is not used and/or the fixation is unsteady

AC/A ratio The accommodative-convergence to accommodation ratio

Adduction Inward horizontal movement of the eye

A.I. Abbreviation for afterimage

Alpha rhythm Intermittent photic stimulation of 7 to 10 cycles per second

Angle A (angle of anomaly) In the deviating eye this is represented by the distance from point "a" to the center of the fovea

Angle E (angle of eccentric fixation) Magnitude of the angle of eccentric fixation which is represented by the distance on the retina from point "e" to the center of the fovea

Angle eta Designation for stereoacuity

Angle F Angle of fixation disparity

Angle H Horizontal angle of deviation of the visual axes measured by objective testing methods

Angle K (angle kappa) Angle subtended by the visual axis and the pupillary axis at the nodal point; *see* angle lambda

Angle lambda Angle subtended at the center of the entrance pupil of the eye by the intersection of the pupillary axis and the visual axis; this angle is inappropriately referred to as "angle kappa" in clinical testing; angle kappa testing actually determines angle lambda, not angle kappa

Angle S Subjective angle of directionalization; it should be the same as angle H if there is NRC but different if there is ARC

ARC (anomalous retinal correspondence) Condition in which the two foveas do not correspond (this is more correctly referred to as "anomalous correspondence," since correspondence is cortical rather than retinal)

Associated phoria This is determined by the amount of compensatory prism needed to reduce angle F to zero

Attenuation A form of occlusion in which the transmission of light is altered by means of certain filters and/or lenses (this is sometimes referred to as "graded occlusion")

Bifixation Implication of central fusion in which the center of the fovea of each eye participates in viewing a fixated object

Bifoveal test of Cüppers (maculo-macular test) Estimation of angle A by means of visuoscopy when the patient is seeing under binocular conditions

Concomitancy Condition in which the angle of deviation is measured to be approximately the same magnitude in all positions of gaze

Contracture Inability of an extraocular muscle to relax may

result in permanent structural changes with the inelasticity becoming irreversible

Co-variation Intermittency of ARC and NRC in the case of intermittent strabismus, particularly in exotropia

DAF (diagnostic action field) Six positions of gaze used to evaluate the action of the six extraocular muscles of each eye

Eccentric fixation Fixation (designated by point "e") not employing the center of the fovea; it may vary in magnitude and/or direction from moment to moment or day to day and may be relatively steady or unsteady

ET Abbreviation for esotropia at far

ET' Abbreviation for esotropia at near

First-degree fusion Term used interchangeably with "superimposition"

Fixation disparity A slight error of vergence in cases of heterophoria; the limit of the magnitude of the angle of fixation disparity (angle F) is considered to be less than 30 minutes of arc.

Free space Patient is directly viewing a fixation object that is not housed inside an instrument such as a stereoscope, or that is not viewed through any optical system, the apparent position of the object not being altered; *see* true space

Functional amblyopia Central visual acuity reduction not attributable to pathological causes, but due to functional causes (e.g., refractive, strabismic, and hysterical)

Functional cure Criteria used in this text are clear, comfortable, single, binocular vision at all distances from the farpoint to a normal NPC with a stereoacuity of 67 seconds of arc or better and with no central suppression; a deviation may be manifest up to 1 percent of the time providing diplopia is experienced whenever this happens

Giessen Test ARC is tested by means of a white light, a deep red filter, an afterimage, and a tangent scale; angles H, S, and A can be measured

H.B. (Haidinger's brushes) Entoptic phenomenon used to tag the projected location of the center of the macula

Heterophoria A latent deviation of the visual axes from the ortho position which requires vergence for bifixation to be maintained; (the direction may be horizontal, vertical, or torsional)

Heterotropia (strabismus) Manifest deviation of 1^Δ or more (the direction of the deviation may be horizontal, vertical, or torsional)

IPD Abbreviation for interpupillary distance; this is often inappropriately referred to as the pupillary distance (P.D.)

KCT (kinetic cover test) A test for estimating angle H by

means of a moving fixation target and occlusion

Maddox cross A graduated vertical and horizontal ruler in the form of a cross with a light source placed at the intersection for the purpose of subjectively measuring vertical and horizontal angles of directionalization, synonym, "Maddox scale"

Mental effort A concept of the patient attempting to make vergence movements by imagining fixation is above or below the horizon or using other willful means to produce voluntary vergence

MITT Abbreviation for the Macula Integrity Tester-Trainer of Bernell (instrument used to produce the entoptic phenomena of Haidinger's brushes)

M.S. (Maxwell's spot) Entoptic phenomena used to tag the projected location of the center of the macula

Negative fusional vergence The ability to diverge the visual axes behind the object of regard without blurring (this is stimulated by base-in prism)

Nonvariable eccentric fixation A condition in which point "e" has a fixed site, although fixation may be unsteady as to the point used for fixation

NPC (nearpoint of convergence) Single vision with bifixation, but not necessarily clear vision, normally expected to be about 3 cm from the bridge of the nose as an ideal

NRC (normal correspondence) The condition in which the two foveas correspond

Organic amblyopia Central visual acuity loss attributable to pathological causes that are not obvious by means of ophthalmoscopy

Partial occlusion Less than the full visual field of an eye is occluded (some texts refer to it as the same as attenuation)

Past pointing The demonstration of faulty eye-hand localization ability by inaccurately pointing to one side or the other of a fixated object (this is common in cases of amblyopia with eccentric fixation and in cases of extraocular muscle paresis of recent onset)

PAT (prism adaptation test) A prognostic test in cases of esotropia to determine if base-out prism causes angle H to increase

Pathological diplopia Perception of a doubled image of a fixated target

Physiological diplopia Perception of a doubled image of a nonfixated target

Point "a" The place on the retina of the deviating eye corresponding to the fovea of the nondeviating eye

Point "e" The time-averaged point used for fixation under monocular conditions

Point "f" The center of the fovea of an eye

Positive fusional vergence The ability to converge the visual axes in front of the object of regard without blurring (this is stimulated by base-out prism)

Secondary angle of deviation The measured angle of deviation found with the paretic eye fixating

Second-degree fusion Term used interchangeably with "flat fusion"

Steady fixation The condition determined on visuoscopy in which the point on the retina used for fixation (either "f" or "e") is seen to be relatively stationary as the patient fixates the nonmoving target of an instrument (e.g., Linksz star)

T.B.I. Abbreviation for Translid Binocular Interaction Trainer

Third-degree fusion Term used interchangeably with "stereopsis" and in reference to stereoacuity

True space Viewing conditions in which the patient is directly looking at a fixation object without intervening optics causing reflection or refraction; in clinical usage, filters may be used (e.g., polarizing) with this definition being satisfied; *see* free space

Unsteady fixation In central fixation, point "f" is seen on visuoscopy to be moving rapidly in a nystagmoid manner about the center of the star; in eccentric fixation, this rapid movement would be seen for point "e" during visuoscopy

Variable eccentric fixation The condition in which the time-averaged point "e" changes site from one measurement to the next on visuoscopy, although fixation may be relatively steady at any particular moment; synonym, "wandering eccentric fixation"

VER (visual evoked response or visually evoked response) This is the same as VECP (visually evoked cortical potential) or VEP (visually evoked potential)

Vergence Disjunctive movement of the eyes

Version Conjugate movement of the eyes

Visual axis This line of sight extending from the fixated target through the nodal point to the center of the fovea

XT Abbreviation for exotropia at far

XT' Abbreviation for exotropia at near

Zero point The point on the retina of the deviating eye representing no vergence demand (if there is bifixation, point "zero" is at point "f," the center of the fovea)

INDEX